OXFORD MEDICAL PUBLICATIONS

Oxford Handbook of Respiratory Medicine

Published and forthcoming Oxford Handbooks

Oxford Handbook of Clinical Medicine 6/e (also available for PDAs and in a Mini Edition)
Oxford Handbook of Clinical Specialties 7/e
Oxford Handbook of Acute Medicine 2/e
Oxford Handbook of Anaesthesia 2/e
Oxford Handbook of Applied Dental Sciences
Oxford Handbook of Cardiology
Oxford Handbook of Clinical Dentistry 4/e
Oxford Handbook of Clinical and Laboratory Investigation 2/e
Oxford Handbook of Clinical Diagnosis
Oxford Handbook of Clinical Haematology 2/e
Oxford Handbook of Clinical Immunology and Allergy 2/e
Oxford Handbook of Clinical Pharmacy
Oxford Handbook of Clinical Surgery 2/e
Oxford Handbook of Critical Care 2/e
Oxford Handbook of Dental Patient Care 2/e
Oxford Handbook of Dialysis 2/e
Oxford Handbook of Emergency Medicine 3/e
Oxford Handbook of Endocrinology and Diabetes
Oxford Handbook of ENT and Head and Neck Surgery
Oxford Handbook for the Foundation Programme
Oxford Handbook of Gastroenterology and Hepatology
Oxford Handbook of General Practice 2/e
Oxford Handbook of Genitourinary Medicine, HIV and AIDS
Oxford Handbook of Geriatric Medicine
Oxford Handbook of Medical Sciences
Oxford Handbook of Nephrology and Hypertension
Oxford Handbook of Neurology
Oxford Handbook of Obstetrics and Gynaecology
Oxford Handbook of Oncology 2/e
Oxford Handbook of Ophthalmology
Oxford Handbook of Palliative Care
Oxford Handbook of Practical Drug Therapy
Oxford Handbook of Psychiatry
Oxford Handbook of Public Health Practice 2/e
Oxford Handbook of Rehabilitation Medicine
Oxford Handbook of Respiratory Medicine
Oxford Handbook of Rheumatology 2/e
Oxford Handbook of Tropical Medicine 2/e
Oxford Handbook of Urology

Oxford Handbook of Respiratory Medicine

SECOND EDITION

Stephen Chapman

Clinical Lecturer in Respiratory Medicine,
University of Oxford

Grace Robinson

Consultant in Respiratory Medicine,
Royal Berkshire Hospital, Reading

John Stradling

Professor of Respiratory Medicine,
University of Oxford

Sophie West

Consultant in Respiratory Medicine,
Oxford

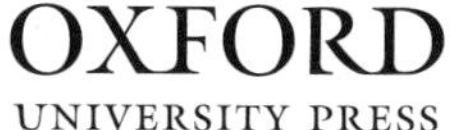

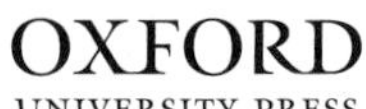

Great Clarendon Street, Oxford OX2 6DP

Oxford University Press is a department of the University of Oxford. It furthers the University's objective of excellence in research, scholarship, and education by publishing worldwide in

Oxford New York

Athens Auckland Bangkok Bogotá Buenos Aires Cape-Town Chennai Dar-es-Salaam Delhi Florence Hong-Kong Istanbul Karachi Kolkata Kuala-Lumpur Madrid Melbourne Mexico-City Mumbai Nairobi Paris São-Paulo Shanghai Singapore Taipei Tokyo Toronto Warsaw

with associated companies in Berlin Ibadan

Oxford is a registered trade mark of Oxford University Press in the UK and in certain other countries

Published in the United States by Oxford University Press Inc., New York

First edition published 2005
Second edition published 2009
Reprinted 2009

Typeset by Cepha Imaging Private Ltd., Bangalore, India
Printed in China
on acid-free paper through
Asia Pacific Offset

ISBN 978-0-19-954516-2

10 9 8 7 6 5 4 3 2

Oxford University Press makes no representation, express or implied, that the drug dosages in this book are correct. Readers must therefore always check the product information and clinical procedures with the most up to date published product information and data sheets provided by the manufacturers and the most recent codes of conduct and safety regulations. The authors and the publishers do not accept responsibility or legal liability for any errors in the text or for the misuse or misapplication of material in this work.

► Except where otherwise stated, drug doses and recommendations are for the non-pregnant adult who is not breast-feeding.

Preface

This *Handbook of Respiratory Medicine* has been written largely by specialist registrars, for specialist registrars. Three of the four authors, Stephen Chapman, Grace Robinson, and Sophie West, are specialist registrars on the Oxford rotation and John Stradling is Professor of Respiratory Medicine in Oxford. It is in a format that the authors would like to have had when they started their specialist registrar training. However, we hope that any health worker or student with an interest in respiratory medicine will find this text a rapid and useful reference source.

The layout of the book tries to fulfil the requirement to be able to look up a topic quickly when the clinical need arises, but also to provide a bit more insight into the more difficult areas. Therefore the chapters are of necessity different in style and reflect the authors' own views on how to best approach and understand an area.

The handbook is divided into five sections: clinical presentations and approaches to symptoms and problems; the clinical conditions themselves; supportive information; procedures; and useful appendices (also on the inside covers), containing more technical and reference information.

We hope you find it helpful. Feedback on errors and omissions would be much appreciated. Please post your comments via the OUP website: *www.oup.com/uk/medicine/handbooks*.

Stephen Chapman
Grace Robinson
John Stradling
Sophie West
June 2005

The second edition of this book has allowed us to make several improvements in response to readers' suggestions. We have changed the order of chapters within each section to alphabetical, and improved the index, to make the contents more rapidly accessible. We have added new content such as more detailed radiology, pandemic influenza, and pulmonary complications of sickle cell disease. In addition, we have updated and enhanced topics where there have been new guidelines and relevant publications. The overall aim of the book, to provide a rapid and comprehensive resource for all those involved in respiratory medicine, has remained paramount.

October 2008

Acknowledgements

We would like to offer our grateful thanks to the following friends and colleagues for their reviewing and advice on various sections of this book.

First edition

Dr Nicholas Bates, Dr Lesley Bennett, Dr Rachel Bennett, Dr Malcolm Benson, Dr Penny Bradbury, Mrs Debbie Buttar, Dr James Calvert, Dr Jane Collier, Dr Graham Collins, Dr Chris Conlon, Dr Chris Davies, Dr Helen Davies, Dr Rob Davies, Dr Thearina de Beer, Mrs Joan Douglass, Dr Rachael Evans, Dr Fergus Gleeson, Dr Maxine Hardinge, Dr Ling Pei Ho, Dr Andrew Jeffreys, Dr Nick Maskell, Dr Phil Mason, Dr Kim McAnaulty, Dr Fiona McCann, Dr Sarah Menzies, Dr Annabel Nickol, Dr Jayne Norcliffe, Dr Jeremy Parr, Mrs Lisa Priestley, Dr Naj Rahman, Dr Catherine Richardson, Mrs Jo Riley, Dr Peter Sebire, Mrs Gerry Slade, Dr Mark Slade, Dr S Rolf Smith, Dr Catherine Swales, Dr Denis Talbot, Dr David Taylor, Dr Catherine Thomas, Dr Estée Török, Dr David Waine, Dr Chris Wathen, Dr John Wiggins, and Dr Eleanor Wood.

Second edition: additional acknowledgements

Dr Luke Howard, Dr Clare Jeffries, Dr Stuart Mucklow, Dr Andrew Stanton, and Mrs Jan Turner-Wilson. Dr Fergus Gleeson and Dr Rachel Benamore provided considerable help with the radiology section.

Contents

Appendices

Abbreviations

A–a	alveolar to arterial gradient
ABG	arterial blood gas
ABPA	allergic bronchopulmonary aspergillosis
ACE	angiotensin-converting enzyme
ADH	antidiuretic hormone
AFB	acid-fast bacillus
AFP	alpha-fetoprotein
AIA	aspirin-induced asthma
AIDS	acquired immune deficiency syndrome
AIP	acute interstitial pneumonia
ANA	antinuclear antibody
ANCA	antinuclear cytoplasmic antibody
ANP	atrial natriuretic peptide
APTT	activated partial thromboplastin time
ARDS	acute respiratory distress syndrome
ATRA	all-trans retinoic acid
ATS	American Thoracic Society
AVM	arteriovenous malformation
A&E	accident and emergency
BAL	bronchoalveolar lavage
BCG	bacille Calmette–Guérin
bd	twice a day
BHR	bronchial hyperreactivity or hyperresponsiveness
BIPAP	bi-level positive airways pressure
BMI	body mass index (kg/m^2)
BNP	B-type natriuretic peptide
BOOP	bronchiolitis obliterans organizing pneumonia
BP	blood pressure
BPD	bronchopulmonary dysplasia
BSAC	British Subaqua Club
BTS	British Thoracic Society
CABG	coronary artery bypass graft
CAP	community-acquired pneumonia
CCB	calcium-channel blocker
CCF	congestive cardiac failure
CF	cystic fibrosis

CFA	cryptogenic fibrosing alveolitis
CFT	complement fixation test
CFTR	cystic fibrosis transmembrane conductance regulator
CHART	continuous hyperfractionated accelerated radiotherapy
CI	contraindication
CLL	chronic lymphocytic leukaemia
CMV	cytomegalovirus
CNS	central nervous system
CO	carbon monoxide
CO_2	carbon dioxide
COHb	carboxyhaemoglobin
COP	cryptogenic organizing pneumonia
COPD	chronic obstructive pulmonary disease
CPAP	continuous positive airway pressure
CRP	C-reactive protein
CSA	central sleep apnoea
CSF	cerebrospinal fluid
CT	computed tomography
CTPA	computed tomographic pulmonary angiogram
CVA	cardiovascular accident
CVD	cardiovascular disease
CVP	central venous pressure
CXR	chest radiograph
DIC	disseminated intravascular coagulation
DIP	desquamative interstitial pneumonitis
dsDNA	double-stranded DNA
DVLA	Department of Vehicle Licensing Authority
DVT	deep vein thrombosis
EBUS	endoscopic bronchial ultrasound
ECG	electrocardiogram
Echo	echocardiogram
ECOG	Eastern Cooperative Oncology Group
EEG	electroencephalogram
EGFR	epidermal growth factor receptor
EIA	enzyme immunoassay
ELCAP	Early Lung Cancer Action Project
ELISA	enzyme-linked immunosorbent assay
EMG	electromyogram
ENT	ear, nose, and throat
EOG	electro-oculogram

EPAP	expiratory positive airways pressure
ERS	European Respiratory Society
ESR	erythrocyte sedimentation rate
ESS	Epworth sleepiness scale/score
EUS-FNA	endoscopic ultrasound fine-needle aspiration
FBC	full blood count
FEV_1	forced expiratory volume in 1 s
FiO_2	fractional inspired oxygen
FNA	fine-needle aspirate
FOB	fibre optic bronchoscopy
FPAH	familial pulmonary arterial hypertension
FRC	functional residual capacity
FVC	forced vital capacity
g	gram
GBM	glomerular basement membrane
GCS	Glasgow coma scale
GI	gastrointestinal
GORD	gastro-oesophageal reflux disease
GP	general practitioner
GU	genitourinary
GVHD	graft-versus-host disease
h	hour
H2	histamine receptors, type 2
HAART	highly active antiretroviral therapy
HACE	high altitude cerebral oedema
HAPE	high altitude pulmonary oedema
Hb	haemoglobin
HCG	human chorionic gonadotrophin
HCO^-_3	bicarbonate
HHT	hereditary haemorrhagic telangiectasia
HIV	human immunodeficiency virus
HLA	human leucocyte antigen
HOOF	home oxygen order form
HP	hypersensitivity pneumonitis
HRCT	high resolution computed tomography
HSCT	haematopoietic stem cell transplant
HSV	herpes simplex virus
ICU	intensive care unit
IDDM	insulin-dependent diabetes mellitus
IFA	indirect immunofluorescence assay

IgE	immunoglobulin E
IgG	immunoglobulin G
IgM	immunoglobulin M
IIP	idiopathic interstitial pneumonia
ILD	interstitial lung disease
IM	intramuscular
INR	international normalized ratio
IPAH	idiopathic pulmonary arterial hypertension
IPAP	inspiratory positive airways pressure
IPF	idiopathic pulmonary fibrosis
IRIS	immune reconstitution inflammatory syndrome
ITU	intensive therapy unit
IV	intravenous
IVC	inferior vena cava
JVP	jugular venous pressure
kCO	carbon monoxide transfer factor
l	litre
LAM	lymphangioleiomyomatosis
LCH	Langerhans cell histiocytosis
LDH	lactate dehydrogenase
LFT	liver function test
LIP	lymphoid interstitial pneumonia
LMWH	low molecular weight heparin
LOS	lower oesophageal sphincter
LTOT	long-term oxygen therapy
LVRS	lung volume reduction surgery
M, C & S	microscopy, culture, and sensitivity
MDI	metered dose inhaler
MDR-TB	multidrug-resistant TB
MDT	multidisciplinary team
mg	milligram
MGUS	monoclonal gammopathy of uncertain significance
MI	myocardial infarction
min	minute
MND	motor neuron disease
MRI	magnetic resonance imaging
MRSA	methicillin (or multiply) resistant *Staphylococcus aureus*
MTB	mycobacterium tuberculosis
ng	nanogram
NIPPV	non-invasive positive pressure ventilation

NIV	non-invasive ventilation
NNRTI	non-nucleoside reverse transcription inhibitor
NO	nitric oxide
NO_2	nitrogen dioxide
non-REM	non-rapid eye movement sleep
NSAID	non-steroidal anti-inflammatory drug
NSCLC	non-small cell lung cancer
NSIP	non-specific interstitial pneumonia
NTM	non-tuberculous mycobacteria
NYHA	New York Heart Association
OCP	oral contraceptive pill
od	once a day
OSA	obstructive sleep apnoea
OSAHS	obstructive sleep apnoea/hypopnoea syndrome
OSAS	obstructive sleep apnoea syndrome
$PaCO_2$	arterial carbon dioxide tension
PAF	platelet-activating factor
PaO_2	arterial oxygen tension
PAP	pulmonary artery pressure
PAS	para-aminosalicylic acid
PAVM	pulmonary arteriovenous malformations
PC_{20}	provocative concentration (of histamine or methacholine) causing a 20% fall in FEV_1
PCD	primary ciliary dyskenesia
PCO_2	carbon dioxide tension
PCP	*Pneumocystis carinii* (now *jiroveci*) pneumonia
PCR	polymerase chain reaction
PCT	primary care trust
PE	pulmonary embolus
PEEP	positive end expiratory pressure
PEFR	peak expiratory flow rate
PEG	percutaneous endoscopic gastrostomy
PET	position emission tomography
PFT	pulmonary function test
PHLS	Public Health Laboratory Service
PHT	pulmonary hypertension
PO	orally/by mouth
PO_2	oxygen tension
PPH	primary pulmonary hypertension
prn	as required
PSA	prostate-specific antigen

PSB	protected specimen brush
PSG	polysomnography
PT	prothrombin time
PTH	parathyroid hormone
qds	four times a day
RADS	reactive airways dysfunction syndrome
RAST	radioallergosorbent test
RBBB	right bundle branch block
RB-ILD	respiratory bronchiolitis-associated interstitial lung disease
RCP	Royal College of Physicians
RCT	randomized controlled trial
REM	rapid eye movement
RFA	radiofrequency ablation
RNP	ribonuclear protein
RSV	respiratory syncytial virus
RT-PCR	reverse transcriptase polymerase chain reaction
RV	residual volume
RVH	right ventricular hypertrophy
SaO_2	arterial oxygen saturation
SARS	severe acquired respiratory syndrome
SBE	subacute bacterial endocarditis
SC	subcutaneous
SCL-70	scleroderma antibody (to topoisomerase 1)
SCLC	small cell lung cancer
SCUBA	self-contained underwater breathing apparatus
SBOT	short burst oxygen therapy
SE	side-effect
SLE	systemic lupus erythematosus
SO_2	sulphur dioxide
SOB	shortness of breath
SVC	superior vena cava
SVCO	superior vena caval obstruction
TB	tuberculosis
TBB	transbronchial biopsy
tds	three times a day
Th2	T-helper 2 cell
TIA	transient ischaemic attack
TLC	total lung capacity
TLCO	total lung carbon monoxide transfer factor
TNF	tumour necrosis factor

TPMT	thiopurine methyltransferase
TRALI	transfusion-related acute lung injury
TSH	thyroid-stimulating hormone
U&E	urea and electrolytes
UIP	usual interstitial pneumonia
UK	United Kingdom
URT	upper respiratory tract
URTI	upper respiratory tract infection
USS	ultrasound scan
V/Q	ventilation/perfusion ratio
VAP	ventilator-acquired pneumonia
VATS	video-assisted thoracoscopic surgery
VC	vital capacity
VTE	venous thromboembolism
WBC	white blood cell count
WCC	white cell count
WHO	World Health Organization
ZN	Ziehl–Neelsen
α_1-AT	α_1-antitrypsin
β_2	beta-2 adrenergic receptor
βHCG	beta human chorionic gonadotrophin
μg	micrograms

Part 1

Clinical presentations—approaches to problems

Chapter 1

Breathlessness

Clinical assessment and causes

Physiological mechanisms of breathlessness

Dyspnoea refers to the abnormal and uncomfortable awareness of breathing. Its physiological mechanisms are poorly understood; possible afferent sources for the sensation include receptors in respiratory muscles, juxtacapillary (J) receptors (sense interstitial fluid), and chemoreceptors (sensing ↑CO_2 and ↓O_2).

Clinical assessment

All patients need a full history and examination. Key points in the assessment are:

- Duration and onset of breathlessness. The box opposite groups the causes of breathlessness by speed of onset, although in practice some variability and overlap exists. Patients often underestimate the duration of symptoms—enquiring about exercise tolerance over a period of time is a useful way of assessing duration and progression
- Severity of breathlessness. Assess the level of handicap and disability by asking about effects on lifestyle, work, and daily activities
- Exacerbating factors. Ask about rest and exertion, nocturnal symptoms, and body position. The timing of nocturnal breathlessness may provide clues to the likely cause: left ventricular failure causes breathlessness after a few hours of sleep, and resolves after about 45 min; asthma tends to occur later in the night; laryngeal inspiratory stridor causes noisy breathlessness of very short duration (<1 min); and Cheyne–Stokes apnoeas result in breathlessness that is recurrent and clears each time in less than 30 s. Orthopnoea is suggestive of left ventricular failure or diaphragm paralysis, although it is also common in many chronic lung diseases. Breathlessness during swimming is characteristic of bilateral diaphragm paralysis. Trepopnoea refers to breathlessness when lying on one side as a result of ipsilateral pulmonary disease
- Associated symptoms, such as cough, haemoptysis, chest pain, wheeze, stridor, fever, loss of appetite and weight, ankle swelling, and voice change. Wheeze may occur with pulmonary oedema, pulmonary embolism, bronchiolitis, and anaphylaxis, in addition to asthma and COPD
- Personal and family history of chest disease
- Lifetime employment, hobbies, pets, travel, smoking, illicit drug use, medications
- Examination of the cardiovascular and respiratory systems. Observe the pattern and rate of breathing. Assess for signs of respiratory distress. Look for paradoxical abdominal movement if the history suggests diaphragmatic paralysis. A useful bedside test is to exercise the patient (e.g. by stepping on and off a 15–20-cm block) until their breathlessness occurs, and then measure oximetry immediately on stopping when the finger is still; a fall in oxygen saturation is expected with organic causes of dyspnoea.

Investigations

Initial investigations typically include resting oximetry, peak flow and spirometry, CXR, and ECG. Further tests depend on clinical suspicion; options include full PFTs with measurement of lung volumes lying and standing, gas transfer and flow-volume loop, bronchial hyperresponsiveness or reversibility testing, maximal mouth or inspiratory sniff pressures, ABGs (with measurement of A–a gradient, see p 793), exercise oximetry, ventilation perfusion scanning and CTPA, HRCT, blood tests (full blood count and TSH), echo, exercise ECG, and cardiac catheterization.

Causes of breathlessness grouped by speed of onset

Instantaneous

- Pneumothorax
- Pulmonary embolism.

Acute (minutes–hours)

- Airways disease (asthma, exacerbation of COPD, upper airways obstruction)
- Parenchymal disease (pneumonia, pulmonary oedema, pulmonary haemorrhage, acute hypersensitivity pneumonitis)
- Pulmonary vascular disease (pulmonary embolism)
- Cardiac disease (e.g. acute myocardial infarction, arrhythmia, valvular disease, tamponade, aortic dissection)
- Metabolic acidosis
- Hyperventilation syndrome.

Subacute (days)

- Many of the above, plus:
  - Pleural effusion
  - Lobar collapse
  - Acute interstitial pneumonia
  - Superior vena cava obstruction
  - Pulmonary vasculitis.

Chronic (months–years)

- Some of the above, plus:
  - Obstructive airways disease (COPD, asthma)
  - Diffuse parenchymal disease (including idiopathic pulmonary fibrosis, sarcoidosis, bronchiectasis, lymphangitis carcinomatosis)
  - Pulmonary vascular disease (chronic thromboembolic disease, idiopathic pulmonary hypertension, veno-occlusive disease)
  - Hypoventilation (chest wall deformity, neuromuscular weakness, obesity)
  - Anaemia
  - Thyrotoxicosis.

Specific situations

Causes of breathlessness with a normal CXR

- Airways disease (asthma, upper airways obstruction, bronchiolitis)
- Pulmonary vascular disease (pulmonary embolism, idiopathic pulmonary hypertension, intrapulmonary shunt)
- Early parenchymal disease (e.g. sarcoid, interstitial pneumonias, infection—viral, PCP)
- Cardiac disease (e.g. angina, arrhythmia, valvular disease, intracardiac shunt)
- Neuromuscular weakness
- Metabolic acidosis
- Anaemia
- Thyrotoxicosis
- Hyperventilation syndrome (p 255).

Causes of episodic/intermittent breathlessness

- Asthma
- Pulmonary oedema
- Angina
- Pulmonary embolism
- Hypersensitivity pneumonitis
- Vasculitis
- Hyperventilation syndrome.

Distinguishing cardiac and respiratory causes of breathlessness

This can be difficult. Many of the clinical features of left heart failure are non-specific and easily confused with respiratory disease (e.g. orthopnoea, wheeze). In chronic cardiac failure, crackles on auscultation and radiological features of pulmonary oedema may be absent even when the pulmonary capillary wedge pressure is significantly raised (due to adaptive changes from vascular remodelling). The presence of emphysema may also render crackles inaudible and lead to atypical CXR appearances of pulmonary oedema. Chronic left heart failure commonly leads to a restrictive ventilatory defect and reduced gas transfer on PFTs, and may also result in pulmonary hypertension. HRCT features of left heart failure include septal and peribronchovascular interstitial thickening, ground-glass shadowing, pleural effusions, and cardiomegaly. Resting ECG is useful—in practice, a cardiac cause of breathlessness is unlikely in the setting of a completely normal ECG. Exercise ECG, echo, and cardiac catheterization may be required. Measurement of B-type natriuretic peptide (BNP) is a recent development that may be of value in the diagnosis of cardiac failure; in patients presenting as an emergency with breathlessness, a serum BNP level <50 ng/L makes cardiac failure very unlikely. Cardiac and respiratory diseases can, of course, coexist.

Further information

Maisel AS, Krishnaswamy P *et al.* Rapid measurement of B-type natriuretic peptide in the emergency diagnosis of heart failure. *N Engl J Med* 2002; **347**: 161–7

Chapter 2

Chest pain

The majority of patients with chest pain referred to the respiratory team have either acute pleuritic pain or persistent, well-localized pain. Cardiac pain rarely presents in this manner, although it should be considered in exertional pain or in the presence of risk factors for ischaemic heart disease. Within the respiratory system, pain may arise from the parietal pleura, major airways, chest wall, diaphragm, and mediastinum; the lung parenchyma and visceral pleura are insensitive to pain. Processes involving the upper parietal pleura cause a pain localized to that part of the chest. The lower parietal pleura and outer region of diaphragmatic pleura are innervated by the lower six intercostal nerves, and pain here may be referred to the abdomen. The central region of the diaphragm is supplied by the phrenic nerve (C3, 4, and 5), and pain may be referred to the ipsilateral shoulder tip. Tracheobronchitis tends to be associated with retrosternal pain.

Acute pleuritic chest pain

- Pleuritic pain is sharp, well-localized, worse on coughing and inspiration, and the subsequent limitation of inspiration often leads to a degree of breathlessness
- Causes of acute pleuritic chest pain include:
  - Pulmonary infarction (following embolism)
  - Pneumonia
  - Pneumothorax
  - Pericarditis
  - Pleural infection (empyema, tuberculous)
  - Autoimmune disease (e.g. systemic lupus erythematosus, rheumatoid arthritis)
  - Musculoskeletal
  - Fractured rib
- In addition, consider atypical presentations of serious conditions such as myocardial infarction, aortic dissection, oesophageal rupture, and pancreatitis. Consider angioinvasive fungi, such as aspergillus, as a cause of chest pain in the immunocompromised
- Diagnosis is typically based on 'pattern recognition' of clinical features followed by selected investigations. Initial investigations typically include CXR, ECG, ABGs, serum inflammatory markers, and D-dimers. Further investigations may include V/Q scanning or CT pulmonary angiography, pleural aspiration, and measurement of serum autoantibodies
- Pulmonary embolism (p 401) commonly presents with pleuritic pain and exclusion of this diagnosis is the usual reason for referral. Assess risk factors for thromboembolic disease. Normal oxygen saturations and PaO_2 in the 'normal' range do not exclude the diagnosis; calculate the A–a gradient (p 793). The presence of a pleural rub is a non-specific sign that occurs with pleural inflammation of any cause
- In young adults, pneumococcal pneumonia may present with acute onset pleuritic chest pain, although systemic symptoms such as fever usually predate the pain by hours

- The pain from pericarditis is pleuritic, but central, and relieved on leaning forward; there may also be a pericardial rub, characteristic ECG features, and a small pericardial effusion on echo
- Musculoskeletal pain may occur as a result of cervical disc disease, arthritis of the shoulder or spine, a fractured rib, or costochondritis (Tietze's syndrome), which often follows a viral infection
- The presence of chest wall tenderness does not invariably indicate a benign, musculoskeletal cause; tenderness may be seen in malignant chest wall infiltration and sometimes following pulmonary infarction
- Other features besides pleurisy that may suggest a diagnosis of systemic lupus erythematosus include rash, photosensitivity, oral ulcers, arthritis, pericarditis, renal or neurological disease, cytopenia, positive ANA, and dsDNA.

Chronic chest pain

- Persistent chest pain that is well localized is typically caused by chest wall or pleural disease. Causes include:
  - Malignant pleural disease or chest wall infiltration
  - Benign musculoskeletal pain
  - Pleural infection (empyema, tuberculous)
  - Benign asbestos pleural disease
  - Autoimmune disease (e.g. systemic lupus erythematosus, rheumatoid arthritis)
  - Recurrent pulmonary infarction (emboli, vasculitis)
- Pain from malignant chest wall infiltration is often 'boring' in character, and may disturb sleep; it is frequently not related to respiration. Causes include primary lung cancer, secondary pleural malignancy, mesothelioma, and rib or sternal involvement from malignancy (including myeloma and leukaemia)
- Chronic thromboembolic disease tends to present with breathlessness; when chest pain occurs, it is usually episodic, rather than persistent
- As with acute pleuritic pain, investigations are directed by initial clinical suspicion. Consider CT chest, bone scan, serum autoantibodies, full blood count and film, serum electrophoresis. CXR may appear normal in malignant chest wall disease.

Chapter 3

Chronic cough and normal CXR

Aetiology and clinical assessment

Cough is a frequent symptom of many respiratory diseases and is often associated with underlying lung pathology and an abnormal CXR. Cough can occur in otherwise healthy people and is often a self-limiting symptom. Persistent coughing can be a socially disabling and distressing symptom, for which help is often sought. **Cough syncope** is loss of consciousness following violent coughing, a Valsalva type manoeuvre, which impairs venous return to the heart and provokes bradycardia and vasodilatation (similar to an ordinary faint). Important as car drivers must cease driving until liability to cough syncope has ceased, confirmed by medical opinion; commercial drivers must cease driving and have no cough syncope or pre-syncope for 5 years if they have a chronic respiratory condition, including smoking. If they have asystole due to cough, driving can be considered after pacemaker insertion.

- **Acute cough** = cough lasting less than 3 weeks, usually due to viral upper respiratory tract infection. May linger for 3–8 weeks as a 'post-viral cough'
- **Chronic cough = cough lasting more than 8 weeks**
- Patients with a normal CXR and persistent cough are often grouped under the heading **'chronic cough'**
- It can sometimes be difficult to determine the underlying cause
- Susceptible individuals have a heightened cough reflex
- Investigation is warranted, but successful response to therapeutic trials may aid determination of the underlying cause. Centres vary in their approach to this
- Specialist cough clinics suggest they achieve diagnosis and effective treatment in over 80% of patients referred with chronic cough.

Aetiology In practice, over 90% of cases of chronic cough with a normal CXR are caused by one or more of:

- Cough variant asthma or eosinophilic bronchitis
- Gastro-oesophageal reflux disease
- Post-nasal drip, due to perennial or allergic rhinitis, vasomotor rhinitis, or chronic sinusitis.

In clinic: full history can be unhelpful. Although cough is most commonly due to asthma, reflux, or post-nasal drip, there may be no specific symptoms to suggest these diagnoses.

- Duration of cough
- When it tends to occur—night or early morning, after exertion, on exposure to dust, pollen, or cold air (asthma), after meals or on sitting or bending over (GORD), nocturnal (post-nasal drip and asthma)
- Non-productive or productive and, if so, how much sputum and colour. Significant amounts of sputum usually indicate a primary lung pathology
- Haemoptysis
- Fever

- Associated symptoms:
  - Shortness of breath or wheeze
  - Throat clearing or sensation of post-nasal drip
  - Chest pain
  - Ankle swelling/orthopnoea/paroxysmal nocturnal dyspnoea
  - Dyspepsia
- Previous respiratory disease, such as childhood asthma, eczema, or hay fever
- History of sinus disease or perennial rhinitis
- History of previous severe respiratory infections, such as whooping cough, that may have caused bronchiectasis
- Known cardiac disease or valvular heart disease
- Drug history ?ACE inhibitor
- Occupation ?Workplace irritants
- Pets/birds
- Smoker
- Use of recreational drugs.

Examination can also be unhelpful, as it is usually normal. Look for signs of underlying lung disease or other medical conditions, such as heart failure, neurological disease (particularly bulbar involvement).

Investigations

Initially

- **Ensure CXR is normal**
- **Spirometry** may indicate restrictive or obstructive defect. Performance of spirometry may provoke cough and bronchospasm
- **Methacholine provocation test** (p 769) provides the best positive predictive value for cough due to asthma. A lack of response suggests cough variant asthma is extremely unlikely. PC_{20} is normal in eosinophilic bronchitis
- **Serial peak flow recordings** twice daily for 2 weeks. Greater than 20% diurnal variation suggests asthma. Can be normal in cough variant asthma
- **Induced sputum examination,** if available, for eosinophil count, to suggest either asthma or eosinophilic bronchitis. Usually a research tool.

Later

- **Consider chest HRCT** if any features suggestive of lung cancer or interstitial lung disease, as a small proportion may present with a normal CXR (central tumour)
- **Consider ENT examination** if predominantly upper respiratory tract disease, resistant to treatment. Consider sinus CT
- **Consider bronchoscopy** if foreign body possible, or history suggestive of malignancy, small carcinoid, endobronchial disease. Perform after CT to help guide bronchoscopist
- **Consider oesophageal pH monitoring.**

Treatment

The initial treatment of patients with a chronic cough is determined by what the most likely underlying cause is, based on the history and investigations. The key is to give any drug treatment at a high enough dose, and for a long enough time (such as 3 months), to be effective.

Symptomatic treatment for cough

Over the counter medicines may provide relief, although there is little evidence of a specific pharmacological effect. Below is a list of possible treatments:

- **Honey and lemon**—home remedies
- **Dextromethorphan**—a non-sedating opiate. Component of many over the counter cough remedies. Dose response, with maximum cough reflex suppression at 60 mg. (Benylin® preparations, Actifed® preparations, Vicks Vaposyrup® preparations, Sudafed Linctus®, Night Nurse®)
- **Menthol**—short lived cough suppressant (Benylin® preparations, Vicks Vaposyrup® preparations)
- **Sedative antihistamines**—suppress cough, but cause drowsiness. Good for nocturnal cough
- **Codeine or pholcodine**—opiate antitussives—codeine requires prescription. No greater efficacy than dextromethorphan and greater side-effect profile
- **Opiates**—prescription. Low dose morphine sulphate 5–10 mg showed significant improvement in patients with intractable cough in RCT (Morice AH *et al Am J Crit Care Med* 2007). Side-effect profile of opiates, so should be used with caution.

Causes of cough (with or without CXR abnormality)

Respiratory
- Infection: viral upper and lower respiratory tract infection, bacterial pneumonia, TB, pertussis
- Chronic bronchitis
- Obstructive airways disease: COPD, asthma
- Cough variant asthma
- Eosinophilic bronchitis
- Obstructive sleep apnoea (nocturnal only)
- Lung cancer
- Bronchiectasis, cystic fibrosis
- Interstitial lung disease
- Airway irritants: smoking, dusts and fumes, acute smoke inhalation
- Airway foreign body.

Mediastinal
- External compression of trachea by enlarged lymph nodes (e.g. lymphoma, TB)
- Mediastinal tumours/cysts/masses.

Cardiac
- Left ventricular failure
- Left atrial enlargement (e.g. severe mitral stenosis).

ENT
- Acute or chronic sinusitis
- Post-nasal drip due to perennial, allergic, or vasomotor rhinitis.

GI
- GORD
- Oesophageal dysmotility, stricture, or pharyngeal pouch causing repeated aspiration
- Oesophago-bronchial fistula.

CNS

Neurological disease affecting swallowing causing repeated aspiration, such as stroke, multiple sclerosis, motor neurone disease, or Parkinson's disease.

Drugs
- ACE inhibitors
- Some inhaled preparations can cause cough—particularly ipratropium.

Other
- Idiopathic
- Ear wax (vagal nerve stimulation)
- Psychogenic/habitual.

Causes of chronic cough: asthma, GORD

Asthma or 'cough variant asthma', 'cough predominant asthma'. This represents one end of the asthma spectrum, with airway inflammation, but may have minimal bronchoconstriction. There is not always a typical asthma history, but ask about wheeze, atopy, hay fever, or childhood asthma or eczema. Cough may be the only symptom. Cough is typically worse after exercise, in cold air, or in the mornings.

- ***Spirometry*** may be normal, without evidence of airflow obstruction. There may be typical asthmatic diurnal peak flow variability of >20%, or peak flows may be stable.
- ***Methacholine challenge*** should be positive. If negative, other causes of cough should be sought.
- ***Treatment*** should be for at least 2 months, with high-dose inhaled steroids. Response may take days or weeks. Bronchodilators may make little difference. If inhaled steroid therapy has been tried unsuccessfully, ensure inhaler technique is optimal and a high dose has been used. Alternatively prescribe a 2-week course of oral prednisolone 30mg/day and assess response. If the cough improves, high-dose inhaled steroids should be continued and slowly reduced after about 2 months.
- ***Eosinophilic bronchitis*** Airway eosinophilia, rarely with peripheral blood eosinophilia, causing heightened cough reflex, but no bronchial hyperresponsiveness/wheeze or peak flow variation. Diagnosis based on negative asthma investigations and induced sputum eosinophilia. Improves with inhaled corticosteroids, usually after 2–3 weeks, or trial of oral prednisolone. Sputum eosinophil count also reduces with treatment. If there is no response, the cough is unlikely to be due to eosinophilic airway inflammation.

Gastro-oesophageal reflux disease (GORD)

Cough may be related to distal reflux at the lower oesophageal sphincter (LOS) or due to micro-aspiration of acid into the trachea. There may be associated oesophageal dysmotility. LOS reflux is often longstanding and is associated with a productive or non-productive daytime cough, and minimal nocturnal symptoms. It is worse after meals and when sitting down, due to increased intra-abdominal pressure being transmitted to the LOS. Micro-aspiration is associated with more prominent symptoms of reflux or dyspepsia, although these are not always present. Patients may have an intermittent hoarse voice, dysphonia, and sore throat. Cough may be the only symptom.

Laryngoscopy may reveal posterior vocal cord inflammation, but this is not a reliable sign.

A trial of treatment for both is recommended. This is with a high-dose proton pump inhibitor for at least 2 months, although longer treatment may be required to control cough. H_2 receptor blockers are also effective and pro-kinetics like metoclopramide may help. Other reflux avoidance measures should be carried out: avoiding caffeine, wearing loose fitting clothes, sleeping with an empty stomach (avoid eating <4 h before bed), sleeping propped up.

Investigation, if required, due to either treatment failure or because of diagnostic uncertainty, is with 24 h ambulatory pH monitoring, which determines the presence of reflux events. These may not necessarily be responsible for the cough, so it is not a very specific or sensitive test. Oesophageal manometry can be used to measure the LOS pressure and oesophageal contractions after swallowing to determine the presence of oesophageal dysmotility.

Causes of chronic cough: rhinitis, post-infectious, ACE inhibitors, idiopathic

Rhinitis and post-nasal drip

Rhinitis is defined as sneezing, nasal discharge, or blockage for more than an hour on most days for either a limited part of the year (seasonal) or all year (perennial). Rhinitis may be allergic (e.g. hay fever), non-allergic, or infective. The associated nasal inflammation may irritate cough receptors directly or produce a post-nasal drip. These secretions may pool at the back of the throat, requiring frequent throat clearing, or drip directly into the trachea, initiating cough. A history of facial pain and purulent nasal discharge suggests sinusitis, which can also predispose to post-nasal drip. Symptoms of cough can occur on lying, but can be constant, regardless of position.

ENT examination may reveal swollen turbinates, nasal discharge, or nasal polyps.

Treatment Nasal preparations should be taken by kneeling with the top of the head on the floor ('Mecca' position) or lying supine with the head tipped over the end of the bed.

- **Non-allergic rhinitis** Trials suggest the best results are with an initial 3 weeks of nasal decongestants with first-generation antihistamines (which have helpful anticholinergic properties) and pseudoephedrine. Alternatives are nasal ipratropium bromide or xylometazoline. This is then followed by 3 months of high-dose nasal steroids, which are ineffective when used as first-line treatment. Second-generation antihistamines (i.e. non-sedating) are of no use in non-allergic rhinitis
- **Allergic rhinitis** Second-generation antihistamine and high-dose nasal steroids for 3 months at least
- **Vasomotor rhinitis** Nasal ipratropium bromide for 3 months.

Sinusitis is an infection of the paranasal sinuses, which may complicate an URTI and is frequently caused by *Haemophilus influenzae* or *Streptococcus pneumoniae*. It causes frontal headache and facial pain. Chronic sinusitis may require further investigation with CXR or CT, which shows mucosal thickening and air-fluid levels. Surgery may be indicated.

- **Chronic sinusitis** Treat as for non-allergic rhinitis, but include 2 weeks of antibiotics active against *H. influenzae*, such as doxycycline or co-amoxiclav.

Post-infectious Respiratory tract infections, especially if viral in nature, can cause cough. This may take weeks or months to resolve spontaneously, although most settle within 8 weeks. The cough is related to a heightened cough reflex. Associated laryngospasm can occur, which is a sudden hoarseness, with associated stridulous inspiratory efforts and a sensation of being unable to breathe.

Treatment with antitussives, such as codeine linctus, may ease the symptoms. Inhaled steroids have been tried, but there is no trial evidence that these work.

ACE inhibitor cough occurs with any ACE inhibitor and is related to bradykinin not being broken down by angiotensin-converting enzyme, and accumulating in the lung. Occurs in 10% of people on ACE inhibitors; more frequent in women. Can occur 3–6 months after starting the drug; the cough may be initiated by a respiratory tract infection, but persists thereafter. Cough usually settles within a week of stopping the drug, but may take months. Avoid all ACE inhibitors thereafter and may need to change to an angiotensin receptor antagonist. Stop ACE inhibitor in any patient with a troublesome cough.

Idiopathic cough accounts for 20% of referrals to a specialist cough clinic. It is diagnosed after a thorough assessment. Typically, there is lymphocytic airway inflammation, but there may also be a history of reflux cough.

Further information

BTS guidelines: Recommendations for the management of cough in adults. *Thorax* 2006; **61** (suppl 1) www.thoraxjnl.com

Review Series on Cough. Morice A, Kastelik J. *Thorax* 2003; **58**: 901–5; Fontana GA, Pistolesi M, *Thorax* 2003; **58**: 1092–5; Dicpinigaitis PV 2004; **59**: 71–2; McGarvey LP 2004; **59**: 342–6.

Birring SS *et al.* Eosinophilic bronchitis: clinical features, management and pathogenesis. *Am J Resp Med* 2003; **2**: 169–73.

Irwin RS, Madison JM. The diagnosis and treatment of cough. *NEJM* 2000; **343**: 1715–21.

Chapter 4

Critically ill patient with respiratory disease

Patients often present critically ill to the Emergency or the Acute Medical Department with respiratory disease. This may be due to a deterioration or exacerbation of an existing condition, a first presentation of a previously undiagnosed disease, or respiratory involvement of an acute systemic disease. As with any critically ill patient, standard management is required initially to stabilize, with the focus moving to diagnosis and treatment. Often these need to take place in parallel. Depending on the presence of any pre-existing respiratory disease and the nature and severity of this, it may be important to determine disease-specific treatment and/or treatment limitations, and senior physician input should be sought for this.

1. Initial assessment

Airway—is the patient maintaining their airway? Is there snoring or gurgling? Tilt head, lift chin, use suction if good views. Is an airway adjunct necessary? Consider inserting Guedel airway or nasopharyngeal airway if GCS reduced <8 (p 741). Consider calling ITU if intubation and ITU care likely to be necessary, or if the patient is rapidly deteriorating/peri-arrest and full assessment has not yet been possible (p 689).

Breathing—cyanosis? What is the SaO_2 and associated FiO_2?

- Exclude tension pneumothorax clinically (p 382).
- What is the respiratory rate?
- Has a blood gas been taken and what does it show? (p 791)
- Oxygenation adequate? If not, likely to need increased FiO_2 (p 704), or if this is already maximal, need ventilatory support—involve ITU
- Is the CO_2 low? If hyperventilation, already working hard breathing to maintain O_2 at current level. May need to increase FiO_2, or if already maximal, need ventilatory assistance—involve ITU
- Is the CO_2 high (p 791)? Hypoventilating, tiring, or CO_2 narcosis in COPD—consider ventilatory support
- Request an urgent portable CXR.

Circulation—what is pulse rate, BP, rhythm on cardiac monitor/ECG? What is fluid balance status? Aim to optimize. Ensure IV access secured and blood tests sent. Look at BP, JVP, urine output, peripheral perfusion (capillary refill time). If they are hypotensive, are they underfilled? Consider fluids (crystalloid). If they are euvolaemic/over filled but hypotensive with poor urine output, they may need inotropic support. Likely to need central venous access to enable CVP monitoring, and this will aid drug administration.

Disability—Conscious level: GCS or AVPU (alert, responsive to verbal commands, responsive to pain, unresponsive). Are they confused? Check blood glucose, temperature, pupils, signs of acute neurological disease—neck stiffness, plantar reflexes, tone.

Examination—temperature, sputum, asterixis, chest signs (pneumothorax, wheeze, silent chest, effusion, consolidation, pulmonary oedema), cardiac murmurs, palpable abdominal organomegaly, skin/nail signs, rash

Investigations—immediate tests include FBC, clotting screen, CRP, U&E, blood cultures before antibiotics.

2. Consider underlying cause

If known respiratory disease, this will enable more targeted therapy. Try and obtain recent hospital notes. Ask patient or their relatives about disease severity, current treatment, plans of clinicians for long-term care (immunosuppression, transplant list, home NIV, advanced directive, lasting power of attorney, etc.). What is their usual current health status—exercise tolerance, activities of daily living? What has caused this deterioration—a potentially reversible process (e.g. infection, drugs, pneumothorax, PE) or gradual progression of underlying disease? Review CXR and compare with old films if possible.

- For more details regarding exacerbations of chronic lung diseases, see p 128 (asthma), p 714 (COPD), p 565 (CF), p 176 (bronchiectasis), p 216 (IPF), p 154 (lung cancer), p 264 (sickle cell).

If no known respiratory disease, full history required to obtain diagnosis. The patient's cardiovascular status and illness severity will determine how brief/full this is. Ask about recent symptoms, travel, contact illness, risk factors for immunocompromise, usual health status, drugs.

For presentation-based differential diagnoses and initial investigation plans see p 3 (breathlessness), p 8 (chest pain), p 40 (haemoptysis), p 67 and p 79 (immunocompromise), p 91 (unexplained respiratory failure), p 29 (diffuse lung disease), p 25 (diffuse alveolar haemorrhage), p 45 (pleural effusion), p 61 (pregnancy), p 57 (post-operative), p 419 (pneumonia), p 401 (pulmonary embolism), p 373 (pneumothorax), p 593 (toxic agents), p 639 and p 642 (upper airway disease and anaphylaxis), and p 300 (SVCO).

3. Determine treatment aims

In patients with known severe respiratory disease, with poor pre-morbid state (e.g. very limited exercise tolerance, comorbidities, severe dementia), intubation and invasive ventilation may not be appropriate. The patient may have their own views on this or have made a living will/advanced directive. Old notes should be reviewed if possible, and this decision should be discussed with their respiratory consultant or the consultant on call. Non-invasive ventilation (p 693) may be appropriate.

In patients with known respiratory disease, with an acute exacerbation (infective or non-infective), respiratory and organ support may be indicated to enable them to survive this episode. This should be discussed with their respiratory consultant or the consultant on call and ITU.

In patients with no known respiratory disease, respiratory and organ support may well be indicated to enable them to survive this episode. This should be discussed with the consultant on call and ITU. If they have significant pre-existing comorbidity from a non-respiratory disease (severe cardiac failure, severe dementia), the details of this should be ascertained and discussed with their usual consultant if possible.

If there is any doubt about a patient's usual health status, or no previous history or notes available, or they are deteriorating before full assessment can be made, they should be considered for full ventilatory and organ support.

Chapter 5

Diffuse alveolar haemorrhage

Diffuse alveolar haemorrhage

A triad of:

- diffuse alveolar infiltrates
- haemoptysis (although not always present)
- a fall in haemoglobin or haematocrit.

Bleeding into the alveoli is often a feature of a small vessel vasculitis of the lungs. This blood tends to remain in the lungs and is not expectorated. Patients with diffuse alveolar haemorrhage may have a background history of vasculitis over the preceding weeks to months. They can present with slowly progressive dyspnoea with haemoptysis, or be acutely unwell with hypoxia. They may require ventilatory support.

Presentation Abrupt onset haemoptysis is the most common symptom, although this is not present in one-third of cases. Also cough, dyspnoea, low-grade fever, weight loss, arthralgia, myalgia. There may be a history of chronic sinusitis (Wegener's).

Examination May be non-specific, or may have signs of underlying vasculitis with skin rashes, nail fold infarcts, digital gangrene. Episcleritis, corneal ulceration, epistaxis, nasal crusting, or deafness may be present. Neurological signs including mononeuritis multiplex should raise the possibility of vasculitis. Patients may be breathless. Haematuria and proteinuria on urine dip.

Investigations

- May be hypoxic—check $SaO_2 \pm$ ABG
- FBC—?falling haemoglobin
- CXR showing bilateral alveolar infiltrates—difficult to distinguish from pulmonary oedema or infection
- Consider chest HRCT
- Raised kCO as increased intra-alveolar haemoglobin is available to combine with carbon monoxide. Abnormal if raised by more than 30%. If breathless at rest, they will not be able to perform this test as it requires breath-holding of an air, carbon monoxide, and helium mixture for 10 s. This test can be used to monitor disease progress
- BAL shows bloodstained lavage, which becomes sequentially more so with each washing. Cytology shows haemosiderin-laden macrophages
- Renal involvement: blood and/or protein in the urine, red cell casts, raised urea and creatinine
- Send blood for urgent ANA, ANCA (PR3 and MPO), anti-GBM, dsDNA, and rheumatoid factor
- Consider biopsy of lung, kidney (if acute glomerulonephritis present), or other affected site if well enough to make a tissue diagnosis. Transbronchial biopsy specimens are usually insufficient to make a diagnosis of vasculitis and a surgical lung biopsy is required. Capillaritis (a neutrophilic vasculitis of capillaries and venules), haemorrhage, or diffuse alveolar damage with haemorrhage seen on lung biopsy.

►► Management of alveolar haemorrhage

- Admit to hospital
- Supportive treatment, with intravenous fluids, blood transfusion, and oxygen if necessary
- Monitor, paying particular attention to oxygen saturations and keeping them above 92% with oxygen therapy. May need respiratory support with intubation and ventilation or CPAP. Monitor haemoglobin and transfuse if necessary. Monitor urine output and renal function
- Aim to establish the underlying diagnosis, usually with tissue biopsy
- Treatment with plasma exchange, high dose steroids and cyclophosphamide, and dialysis if required.

Key questions

- Is this isolated lung disease?
- Is there accompanying renal disease?
- Are there other features of an underlying disease?—ENT, joints, etc.

Causes of alveolar haemorrhage

First three are most common

Goodpasture's disease*	p 658
Wegener's granulomatosis*	p 652
SLE*	p 190
Rheumatoid arthritis	p 188
Microscopic polyangiitis*	p 656
Progressive systemic sclerosis	p 194
Mixed connective tissue disease	
Polyarteritis nodosa	p 662
Behçet's disease	p 198
Essential mixed cryglobulinaemia	
Vasculitis: endocarditis- or tumour-related	
Idiopathic rapidly progressive glomerulonephritis	
Idiopathic pulmonary haemosiderosis	p 620
Drugs: D-penicillamine, cocaine	
Chemicals: trimellitic anhydride, lymphangiography	
Leptospirosis	p 462
Isolated pauci-immune pulmonary capillaritis	
Coagulopathy, such as disseminated intravascular coagulation	

* Indicates conditions commonly considered in the differential diagnosis of **pulmonary-renal syndrome** (diffuse alveolar haemorrhage with glomerulonephritis). Note: conditions causing diffuse CXR infiltrate and renal failure may mimic these, e.g. severe cardiac failure, severe pneumonia, leptospirosis.

Chapter 6

Diffuse lung disease

Causes

Diffuse lung disease is common and its diagnosis is frequently challenging. This chapter describes a diagnostic approach based on clinical features, imaging, and other investigations; more detailed descriptions of the diseases themselves are presented later in the book. The term 'diffuse lung disease' is used here to describe any widespread pulmonary disease process. Patients typically present with breathlessness and bilateral CXR shadowing. The rate of onset and severity of breathlessness are extremely variable, however, and presentations range from an asymptomatic patient with longstanding radiological changes to an acute onset of breathlessness over a period of days, leading rapidly to respiratory failure and death.

Anatomy of diffuse lung disease

An understanding of lung anatomy is helpful when considering the causes of diffuse lung disease and their appearance on HRCT. Many diffuse lung diseases primarily affect the interstitium ('interstitial lung disease', also described as 'diffuse parenchymal lung disease'), a poorly defined term that refers to the connective tissue fibrous framework of the lung. Centrally, connective tissue surrounds bronchovascular bundles (each consisting of a bronchus and its accompanying pulmonary artery) that originate at the hila. Peripherally, these connective tissue sheaths are in continuity with fibrous interlobular septa, which organize the lung into units called 'secondary pulmonary lobules', polyhedral structures with approximately 2-cm sides (see diagram p 817). Interlobular septa, which define and separate secondary pulmonary lobules, contain lymphatics and venules. A secondary pulmonary lobule contains around 5–12 acini, and is supplied at its centre by a bronchiole and pulmonary arteriole.

The term 'interstitial lung disease' is confusing because many primarily interstitial processes also involve the airways, vasculature, and alveolar airspaces. Disease processes that primarily affect the airways (e.g. bronchiectasis), vessels (e.g. vasculitis), or airspaces (e.g. pneumonia) may also present with diffuse CXR shadowing and so are included in this chapter.

Causes

There are several hundred causes of diffuse lung disease, and it is useful to divide these into groups based on their rate of onset and aetiology/disease mechanism (see Table 6.1).

Further information

Picture of secondary pulmonary lobule, available on-line at: *www.vh.org/adult/provider/radiology/DiffuseLung/AnatImages/2LobuleRadiograph Schema.html*

British Thoracic Society. BTS guidelines on the diagnosis, assessment and treatment of diffuse parenchymal lung disease in adults. *Thorax* 1999; **54** (suppl. 1): S1–30

Table 6.1. Causes of diffuse lung disease

Disease onset	Cause/ mechanism	Examples (common conditions in bold)
Acute (days–weeks)	Infection	**Bacterial** (pneumococcal, staphylococcal, Gram-negative, anaerobic, TB, anaerobic, TB, atypical), viral (influenza, para-influenza, adenoma, RSV, measles, varicella, hanta), fungal (aspergillosis, histoplasmosis, PCP)
	Miscellaneous	**Adult respiratory distress syndrome**, acute interstitial pneumonia (AIP), acute hypersensitivity pneumonitis
Acute or chronic	Drugs	Immunosuppressants (methotrexate, azathioprine, cyclophosphamide); treatment of connective tissue disease (gold, penicillamine, sulfasalazine); cytotoxics (chlorambucil, melphalan, busulfan, lomustine, carmustine, bleomycin, mitomycin); antibiotics (nitrofurantoin, cephalosporins); anti-arrhythmics (amiodarone); illicit (cocaine inhalation, heroin, methadone, IV talc)
	Toxins	Radiotherapy, high concentration oxygen, paraquat
	Vasculitis/ alveolar haemorrhage	Wegener's granulomatosis, Churg–Strauss syndrome, Goodpasture's syndrome, SLE, microscopic polyangiitis, idiopathic haemosiderosis
	Pulmonary venous hypertension	**Cardiogenic pulmonary oedema**, pulmonary veno-occlusive disease
	Miscellaneous	**Sarcoidosis**, cryptogenic organizing pneumonia (COP), eosinophilic pneumonia, lipoid pneumonia
Chronic (months–years)	Idiopathic interstitial pneumonias	**Idiopathic pulmonary fibrosis (IPF)**, non-specific interstitial pneumonia (NSIP), desquamative interstitial pneumonia (DIP), lymphocytic interstitial pneumonia (LIP), respiratory bronchiolitis-associated interstitial lung disease (RB-ILD)
	Inhalational Inorganic	Asbestosis, coal worker's pneumoconiosis, silicosis, metals, e.g. cobalt, aluminium
	Organic	Hypersensitivity pneumonitis, e.g. bird fancier's lung, farmer's lung
	Connective tissue disease	**Rheumatoid arthritis**, SLE, scleroderma, poly- and dermatomyositis, enclosing spondylitis, Sjögren's syndrome, Behçet's disease
	Malignancy	Lymphangitis carcinomatosa, bronchoalveolar cell carcinoma, pulmonary lymphoma
	Miscellaneous	**Bronchiectasis**, Langerhans cell histiocytosis, amyloidosis, lymphangioleiomyomatosis, alveolar proteinosis, microlithiasis

Clinical assessment and imaging

History Clinical features may provide useful clues to the underlying diagnosis. Key points in the history are:

Presenting symptoms

- Breathlessness is the most common symptom, and its rate of onset may be useful diagnostically (see Table 6.1)
- Causes of truly *episodic* breathlessness/diffuse CXR shadowing include eosinophilic pneumonia, vasculitis, Churg–Strauss syndrome, hypersensitivity pneumonitis, cryptogenic organizing pneumonia, allergic bronchopulmonary aspergillosis, and pulmonary oedema
- Cough may occur, although its diagnostic value is uncertain; it may be a prominent symptom in lymphangitis carcinomatosis, hypersensitivity pneumonitis, cryptogenic organizing pneumonia, sarcoid, and eosinophilic pneumonia. Chronic production of purulent sputum suggests bronchiectasis. Bronchorrhoea (production of large volumes of sputum) may occur with bronchoalveolar cell carcinoma. Haemoptysis suggests alveolar haemorrhage, malignancy, or pulmonary venous hypertension
- Wheeze may occur in asthma associated with eosinophilic pneumonia or Churg–Strauss syndrome
- Weight loss and fever are non-specific symptoms associated with many diffuse lung diseases.

Other medical conditions e.g. malignancy, connective tissue disease, HIV infection, other immunosuppression. Ask about old CXRs, which may be helpful in assessing disease duration.

Drugs

- See Table 6.1 for common drug causes of diffuse lung disease
- Delays of months or even years may occur between starting the drug and developing lung involvement
- Illicit drug abuse (crack cocaine or heroin—pulmonary oedema, eosinophilic pneumonitis, diffuse alveolar haemorrhage, interstitial pneumonia; intravenous drug use—IV talcosis, septic emboli)
- Oily nose drops (lipoid pneumonia).

Occupation, lifestyle, hobbies, and pets

- May involve inhalation of inorganic or organic dusts. Document lifelong employment history, including probable exposure levels, use of protective equipment, and names of employers
- Inorganic dusts associated with development of diffuse lung disease include asbestos, silica, cobalt, beryllium, aluminium, isocyanates, copper sulphate, iron, tin, barium, and antimony
- Hypersensitivity pneumonitis may result from inhalation of organic dusts such as *Thermoactinomycetes* in mouldy hay (farmer's lung), avian proteins or feathers (bird fancier's lung), mushroom compost, mouldy cheese, cork or sugar cane, and isocyanates
- Risk factors for immunocompromise (opportunistic infection, LIP, lymphoma)

- Smoking history (Langerhans cell histiocytosis, respiratory bronchiolitis-associated interstitial lung disease, desquamative interstitial pneumonia, and Goodpasture's syndrome are more common in smokers).

Evidence of extrapulmonary disease Manifestations of connective tissue disease, vasculitis, sarcoidosis, e.g. arthralgia, skin rash, ocular symptoms, muscular pain and weakness, Raynaud's, nasal/sinus disease, haematuria. Infertility in males (immotile cilia syndrome, cystic fibrosis).

Travel Tuberculosis, pulmonary eosinophilia from parasites (tropics), histoplasmosis (north and central United States, parts of South America and Africa), hydatid disease (Middle East, Australasia, Mediterranean).

Family history α_1-antitrypsin deficiency, rare familial forms of UIP and sarcoidosis.

Examination

- Cyanosis and signs of cor pulmonale in severe disease
- Clubbing (usual interstitial pneumonitis, asbestosis, bronchiectasis)
- Basal crackles (usual interstitial pneumonitis, asbestosis, connective tissue disease, pulmonary oedema, lymphangitis, drugs); crackles in bronchiectasis are characteristically coarse
- Absence of crackles despite a significant CXR abnormality may be suggestive of sarcoidosis, pneumoconiosis, hypersensitivity pneumonitis, or Langerhans cell histiocytosis
- Squeaks suggest the presence of bronchiolitis
- Skin, joint, and eye disease (connective tissue disease, sarcoidosis, vasculitis).

Imaging

CXR is an essential test and is diagnostic in at least 50% of cases. Up to 10% of patients with biopsy-proven diffuse lung disease have a normal CXR, however. Previous CXRs are helpful in assessing disease duration and progression.

High-resolution CT (HRCT) chest is more sensitive and specific than CXR for diagnosing diffuse lung disease (see following page and Appendix 4). HRCT is often in itself diagnostic and should always precede biopsy in the investigation of diffuse lung disease. HRCT also enables assessment of disease extent, and optimal biopsy site if required. HRCT appearance correlates to some extent with disease activity in the interstitial pneumonias: a predominantly 'ground-glass' appearance may signify a steroid-responsive inflammatory state, whereas reticulation and honeycombing are often associated with fibrosis, poor response to treatment, and a worse prognosis.

HRCT diagnosis

HRCT (and to a limited extent CXR) appearances can be classified according to the pattern and distribution of disease, and the presence of additional features (see also Appendix 4).

1. Imaging pattern

Reticular (or linear) pattern Causes include:

- Interstitial pulmonary oedema
- Usual interstitial pneumonitis (UIP; reticular shadowing is typically patchy, subpleural, and basal; other features include loss of architecture of secondary pulmonary lobules, honeycombing, ground-glass change, traction bronchiectasis)
- Asbestosis (similar features to UIP, often with pleural plaques)
- Connective tissue disease associated fibrosis (similar features to UIP)
- Chronic hypersensitivity pneumonitis (often associated with regions of ground-glass change, air-trapping on expiration, and centrilobular micronodules)
- Drug-induced fibrosis
- Sarcoidosis.

Nodular pattern consists of numerous discrete, round opacities 0.1–1 cm in diameter.

- Interstitial processes result in nodularity within interlobular septa, around bronchovascular bundles, and subpleurally (e.g. sarcoidosis, which may demonstrate associated perihilar reticular shadowing and lymphadenopathy)
- Airspace diseases may lead to affected acini becoming visible as nodules (e.g. hypersensitivity pneumonitis, miliary TB, COP, malignancy).

Ground-glass change is an increase in lung density through which pulmonary vasculature is still visible (compare the lung density with that of air within the bronchi). May occur as a result of airspace or interstitial disease, and may be patchy or diffuse. Causes include:

- Pulmonary oedema or haemorrhage, ARDS
- Hypersensitivity pneumonitis
- Drugs
- Certain idiopathic interstitial pneumonias (NSIP, RB-ILD, DIP, AIP)
- PCP
- Sarcoidosis
- Bronchoalveolar cell carcinoma
- Alveolar proteinosis.

Ground-glass appearance may be artefactual, the increased density resulting from breath-holding during expiration. It may also be confused with 'mosaic perfusion', where densities vary in different regions of the lung as a result of variable perfusion, e.g. in chronic thromboembolic disease, small airways disease.

Consolidation (or airspace shadowing) is an increase in attenuation characterized by air bronchograms (air-filled bronchi superimposed against opacified alveoli) and the loss of visibility of adjacent vessels. It occurs as disease processes infiltrate and fill alveolar airspaces, for example, with water, blood, pus, malignant cells, or fibrous tissue. Causes include:

- Pneumonia
- Pulmonary oedema or haemorrhage, ARDS
- Drugs
- Cryptogenic organizing pneumonia (COP)
- Bronchoalveolar cell carcinoma, lymphoma
- Other rare conditions (e.g. eosinophilic pneumonia, alveolar proteinosis).

Cystic change refers to well-defined air spaces with a thin wall. Causes include:

- Langerhans cell histiocytosis (bizarrely shaped cysts and nodules, apical predominance)
- Usual interstitial pneumonitis (subpleural honeycombing)
- PCP
- Lymphocytic interstitial pneumonia
- Septic emboli
- Lymphangioleiomyomatosis (thin-walled cysts, otherwise normal lung)
- Centrilobular emphysema may simulate cystic disease, but there is absence of a well-defined wall.

Interlobular septal thickening occurs as a result of processes affecting the lymphatics or venules within interlobular septa, such as:

- Pulmonary oedema (smooth thickening)
- Lymphangitis carcinomatosis (irregular, nodular thickening of interlobular septa and bronchovascular bundles, no architectural distortion)
- Sarcoidosis
- Usual interstitial pneumonitis.

2. Imaging distribution

- Upper zone: silicosis, pneumoconiosis, chronic sarcoidosis, hypersensitivity pneumonitis, ankylosing spondylitis, tuberculosis, Langerhans cell histiocytosis
- Lower zone: UIP, connective tissue diseases, asbestosis
- Mid-zone: sarcoidosis, pulmonary oedema, *Pneumocystis carinii* pneumonia
- Peripheral: UIP, eosinophilic pneumonia, drugs (amiodarone), COP
- Sharp borders: radiation pneumonitis.

Additional imaging features

- Lymphadenopathy: sarcoidosis, lymphoma, malignancy, infection, silicosis, berylliosis, LIP
- Pleural effusion/involvement: pulmonary oedema, connective tissue diseases, infection, malignancy, asbestosis, drugs, LAM.

Further information

Ryu JH *et al.* Diagnostic approach to the patient with diffuse lung disease. *Mayo Clin Proc* 2002; **77**: 1221–7

Further investigations

Urine and blood tests

Consider the following investigations:

- Urine dipstick and microscopy for detection of renal disease associated with vasculitis/connective tissue disease
- ESR, CRP, FBC (look specifically at the eosinophil count), renal and liver function, calcium (increased in >10% of patients with sarcoidosis)
- Autoantibodies (including anti-Jo-1, occurs with myositis-associated interstitial pneumonia; positive rheumatoid factor or ANA may occur in infection, malignancy, and UIP as well as in connective tissue disease)
- ANCA (vasculitis), anti-GBM (Goodpasture's syndrome)
- Serum precipitins (to antigens in hypersensitivity pneumonitis; poor specificity)
- Serum ACE levels may be increased in sarcoidosis, but this is a non-specific and relatively insensitive test and is unhelpful diagnostically.

Sputum

- Cytology may be diagnostic in bronchoalveolar cell carcinoma
- Induced sputum may be useful in the diagnosis of PCP and TB.

Pulmonary function tests

- Useful in assessing severity of disease and response to treatment, but often unhelpful diagnostically
- Typically show restrictive pattern with reduced vital capacity and transfer factor. Normal values do not exclude mild, early lung disease
- Obstructive pattern rare, but may be seen in sarcoidosis, Langerhans cell histiocytosis, and lymphangioleiomyomatosis; may see mixed picture if coexisting COPD
- Transfer factor may be increased transiently (days) in alveolar haemorrhage. Reduced transfer factor with preserved lung volumes in scleroderma is suggestive of pulmonary vascular disease (such as pulmonary arterial hypertension or vasculitis)
- Disease progression and response to treatment are best assessed by serial measurements of vital capacity and transfer factor
- Check oxygen saturation and consider ABGs. A fall in oxygen saturation on simple exercise may be performed in the clinic setting, and is a useful clue to underlying lung disease in patients with normal saturation and lung function at rest and an unremarkable CXR.

Cardiac investigations

- **ECG** Conduction abnormality in sarcoidosis; cardiogenic pulmonary oedema is unusual in the presence of a completely normal ECG
- **Echocardiography** Assess left ventricular and valvular function if cardiac pulmonary oedema suspected, and measure pulmonary arterial pressure in scleroderma and suspected pulmonary veno-occlusive disease.

Bronchoalveolar lavage

- Most useful in diagnosis of opportunistic infection (bacterial or fungal pneumonia, tuberculosis, PCP), malignancy, alveolar proteinosis, eosinophilic pneumonia, and alveolar haemorrhage
- BAL differential cell counts usually unhelpful diagnostically.

Lung biopsy

Which patients need a lung biopsy?

In cases of uncertain aetiology, despite clinical assessment and HRCT, lung biopsies often provide a definitive diagnosis. Ideally, they should be taken before treatment is started. The decision to biopsy varies amongst clinicians, and should take into account the individual patient's clinical condition and wishes, and the likely benefit of a definitive diagnosis in terms of predicting treatment response and prognosis. Some take a pragmatic approach when a diagnosis (or group of diagnoses with the same treatment) is likely, but not biopsy-proven, and treat empirically. In some cases, the patient may be too unwell for biopsy and require empirical treatment. Biopsy of end-stage fibrosis is unhelpful in eliciting an underlying aetiology.

Biopsy techniques

Transbronchial biopsy provides small samples, but relatively high diagnostic yield in diseases with a 'centrilobular' distribution, e.g. sarcoidosis, hypersensitivity pneumonitis, malignancy, infection (fungi, tuberculosis), and cryptogenic organizing pneumonia. Take 4–6 samples. Additional blind endobronchial biopsies may be diagnostic in sarcoidosis.

Open lung biopsy via thoracotomy or video-assisted thoracoscopic (VATS) biopsy provide larger samples than TBB and have diagnostic yields of at least 90%. Both require general anaesthesia. VATS probably has a lower morbidity and is generally preferred in stable patients; open biopsy is required in ventilator-dependent patients.

Open or VATS biopsy (rather than TBB) is required for diagnosis of idiopathic interstitial pneumonias, vasculitis, lymphoma, lymphangioleiomyomatosis, and Langerhans cell histiocytosis.

Percutaneous image-guided biopsy may be useful in the diagnosis *of* well-localized and dense peripheral infiltrates. A cutting needle biopsy technique is best and, if the lesion(s) abuts the pleural surface, pneumothorax is uncommon.

Chapter 7

Haemoptysis

Clinical assessment and causes

Haemoptysis is a common and non-specific feature, and can be a sign of significant underlying lung disease. In up to one-third of cases, no cause is found. An early assessment of the likely underlying cause needs to be made and investigated accordingly.

Diagnostic approach to haemoptysis Small volume haemoptysis is a commonly encountered problem in the out-patient department. It can be safely and efficiently investigated as an out-patient. Massive haemoptysis is usually encountered in the accident and emergency department or in a patient already on the ward with known underlying lung disease. The approaches to small volume and massive haemoptysis are different.

History

- Past history of lung disease?
- Document volume of blood and whether old (altered) or fresh
- Time course (intermittent, constant)
- Definitely from the airway, and not from the nose or mouth, or haematemesis? (haemoptysis may be swallowed and then vomited)
- Presence of systemic features—associated infection, symptoms consistent with underlying malignancy or vasculitis?

Examination May be normal or show signs of underlying lung disease, e.g. bronchiectasis, bronchial carcinoma, or symptoms of circulatory collapse.

In practice the usual differential diagnosis lies between:

- Malignancy
- Bronchiectasis
- Tuberculosis/infection
- PE.

Causes of haemoptysis

Common

- Bronchial tumour (benign, e.g. carcinoid or malignant). Haemoptysis is a common presenting feature of bronchogenic malignancy, indicating endobronchial disease, which may be visible endoscopically
- Bronchiectasis. Small volume haemoptysis is a common feature of bronchiectasis, particularly during exacerbations. It can be a cause of massive haemoptysis from dilated and abnormal bronchial artery branches that form around bronchiectatic cavities
- Active tuberculosis. Haemoptysis occurs in cavitating and non-cavitating disease, active disease and inactive disease (e.g. from an old bronchiectatic cavity, which might contain a mycetoma)
- Pneumonia (especially pneumococcal disease)
- Pulmonary thromboembolic disease
- Vasculitides/alveolar haemorrhage syndromes, e.g. Wegener's granulomatosis, SLE, Goodpasture's syndrome
- Warfarin with any of the above.

Rare

- Lung abscess
- Mycetoma
- Fungal/viral/parasitic infections
- Fat embolism
- Arteriovenous malformation, e.g. in hereditary haemorrhagic telangiectasia (HHT) (see p 618)
- Severe pulmonary hypertension (see p 385)
- Mitral stenosis (rare)
- Congenital heart disease
- Aortic aneurysm
- Aspergillus—invasive fungal disease (intracavity mycetoma) can be a cause of massive haemoptysis
- Coagulopathy, including disseminated intravascular coagulation
- Endometriosis
- Pulmonary haemosiderosis
- Iatrogenic, e.g. lung biopsy, bronchoscopy.

Investigations

The investigation of haemoptysis can often be carried out as an out-patient, but patients with significant bleeding or a likely serious underlying cause should be admitted if there are concerns.

NB. Beware of the apparently small bleed, which is a sentinel/herald bleed for massive bleeding. This is fortunately rare.

Out-patient investigations and management

First-line investigations

- ***Blood tests*** FBC, clotting, group and save. If systemic vasculitis is suspected, renal function and a urine dip and microscopy for casts are necessary, as well as autoantibodies—ANCA, anti-GBM, and ANA
- ***Sputum cytology*** and M, C, & S and AFB if infection suspected
- ***CXR*** may show mass lesion, bronchiectasis, consolidation, or an AVM
- ***CT chest*** should be done prior to bronchoscopy, as prior knowledge of the site of abnormality leads to increased pick-up rates at bronchoscopy. Similarly, a definitive diagnosis, e.g. AVM, may be made from the CT, obviating the need for further investigations. This depends on local resources CT may miss an upper airway abnormality, but bronchoscopy should not
- ***Bronchoscopy*** to visualize the airways and localize the site of bleeding. May also be therapeutic, for example if a bleeding tumour can be injected with a vasoconstricting agent (adrenaline) or a catheter inserted for tamponade (see massive haemoptysis)
- ***Transbronchial biopsies***—if vasculitis suspected.

Second-line investigations

Usually done if first-line investigations fail to demonstrate a cause.

- ***CTPA*** to exclude PE
- ***Bronchial angiogram*** Diagnostic and therapeutic. Rare for the actual bleeding site to be identified; more often the bleeding site is assumed from visualizing a mesh of dilated and tortuous vessels, e.g. around a bronchiectatic cavity. Usually done during an episode of bleeding to maximize the chance of identifying the site of bleeding
- ***Bronchial artery embolization*** Therapeutic approach to embolize the bleeding artery, usually with coils or glue (specialist centre only). There is a small risk of paraplegia (<1%) if the anterior spinal artery originates from the bronchial arterial circulation
- ***ENT review*** The source of the bleeding may be the upper airway
- ***Echocardiogram*** Moderate/severe PHT can cause haemoptysis, especially in a patient on anticoagulants.

Cryptogenic haemoptysis In around one-third of cases, despite appropriate investigations as above, no cause for the haemoptysis can be found. This has a good prognosis. Often the haemoptysis will settle without treatment and will become less worrying to the patient over time, especially as investigations have failed to determine the cause. Massive haemoptysis (100–600 mL blood in 24 h) is a life-threatening emergency, with a mortality of up to 80%.

▶▶ Management of massive haemoptysis

Massive haemoptysis (100–600 mL blood in 24 h) is a life-threatening emergency, with a mortality of up to 80%. It is extremely distressing for the patient, relatives, and medical staff, but is fortunately rare. Investigations will follow treatment, which may be difficult, and is often unsuccessful. In some cases, active treatment may be inappropriate, and palliative treatment with oxygen and diamorphine may be warranted.

- Airway protection and ventilation

Protection of the non-bleeding lung is vital to maintain adequate gas exchange. This may involve lying on the bleeding side (to prevent blood flowing into the unaffected lung), or intubation with a double lumen tube. If intubation is not needed, or not appropriate, give high flow oxygen.

- Cardiovascular support:
  - large bore/central intravenous access
  - clotting factors, group and save
  - fluid resuscitation ± transfusion
  - reverse anticoagulants
  - inotropes
- Nebulized adrenaline (5–10 mL of 1 in 10,000)
- Oral tranexamic acid (500 mg tds, not if in severe renal failure)
- CXR ± chest CT (depending on stability of patient)
- Early bronchoscopy—diagnostic and therapeutic
- Rigid bronchoscopy (with general anaesthesia) is preferable. May allow localization of the site of bleeding; balloon tamponade with a Fogarty catheter
- Bronchial artery embolization—therapeutic approach to embolize bleeding artery, usually with coils or glue (specialist centre only)
- Surgery—resection of bleeding lobe (if all other measures have failed).

Chapter 8

Pleural effusion

Clinical assessment

Pleural effusion is a common presentation of a wide range of different diseases.

Commonest causes in UK and USA (in order): cardiac failure, pneumonia, malignancy, pulmonary embolism.

Priority is to make a diagnosis and relieve symptoms with minimum number of invasive procedures. The majority of patients do not require a chest drain and can be managed as out-patients. Procedures such as therapeutic thoracentesis may be performed readily on a day unit. Consider admission and chest drain insertion for:

- Patients with malignant effusions who are candidates for pleurodesis
- Empyema or parapneumonic effusion with purulent fluid or a pleural fluid pH <7.2 (the majority of these effusions are unlikely to resolve without drainage and antibiotics)
- Patients who are unwell with an acute massive effusion.

Key steps in the management of the patient with a pleural effusion (see also abbreviated algorithm in following section).

1. History, examination, CXR (PA and lateral).

2. Does the patient have heart failure? If so, this should be treated, with no need for pleural tap unless atypical features (such as very asymmetrical bilateral effusions, unilateral effusion, chest pain, or fever) or fails to respond within 3 days (75% of cardiac failure effusions resolve following 48 h of diuresis).

3. Thoracentesis (= 'pleural tap' or pleural fluid aspiration) may be diagnostic and/or therapeutic, depending on the volume of fluid removed. See p 782 for procedure details, and pp 52-55 for pleural fluid analysis. Following diagnostic tap:

- Note pleural fluid ***appearance***
- Send sample in sterile pot to biochemistry for measurement of ***protein*** and ***LDH***
- Send a fresh 20-mL sample in sterile pot to **cytology** for examination for malignant cells and differential cell count
- Send samples in sterile pot and blood culture bottles to ***microbiology*** for Gram stain and microscopy, culture, and AFB stain and culture
- Process non-purulent heparinized samples in arterial blood gas analyser for ***pH***
- Consider measurement of cholesterol and triglycerides, haematocrit, glucose, and amylase, depending on the clinical circumstances.

If the patient is breathless they may benefit from removal of a larger volume of fluid (therapeutic tap, p 783).

4. Is the pleural effusion a transudate or exudate? Helpful in narrowing the differential diagnosis. In patients with a normal serum protein, pleural fluid protein <30 g/L = transudate and protein >30 g/L = exudate. In borderline cases (protein 25–35 g/L), or in patients with abnormal serum protein, apply Light's criteria—effusion is exudative if it meets one of following criteria.

- Pleural fluid protein/serum protein ratio >0.5
- Pleural fluid LDH/serum LDH ratio >0.6
- Pleural fluid LDH >two-thirds the upper limit of normal serum LDH.

These criteria are very sensitive in the diagnosis of exudative effusions, although may occasionally falsely identify transudates as being exudates, e.g. patients with partially treated heart failure on diuretics may be misidentified as exudates.

5. Further investigations if the diagnosis remains unclear:

- CT chest with pleural contrast (ideally scan prior to complete fluid drainage, to improve images of pleural surfaces; useful in distinguishing benign and malignant pleural disease, p 346).
- Repeat pleural fluid cytology
- Further pleural fluid analysis (p 54), e.g. cholesterol, triglyceride, haematocrit, glucose, amylase, fungal stains
- Pleural tissue biopsy for histology and TB culture (ultrasound- or CT-guided, closed Abrams', or thoracoscopic biopsy; image-guided biopsies are superior to Abrams' for malignant disease; use Abrams' biopsy only in cases when tuberculosis is suspected; thoracoscopy is 'gold-standard'; biopsies have sensitivity of 90% for malignancy and allow therapeutic talc pleurodesis at the same time)
- Reconsider pulmonary embolism and tuberculosis
- Consider thoracoscopy if persistent undiagnosed pleural effusion.

Bronchoscopy has no role in investigating undiagnosed effusions unless the patient has haemoptysis or a CXR/CT pulmonary abnormality. Pleural fluid may compress the airways and limit bronchoscopic views, and so if bronchoscopy is indicated it is best performed following drainage of the effusion.

Further information

Holm KA, Antony VB. Pleural effusions: the workup and treatment. *J Respir Dis* 2001; **22**: 211–19

Light RW. Pleural effusion. *N Engl J Med* 2002; **346**: 1971–7

Maskell NA, Butland RJA. BTS Guidelines for the investigation of a unilateral pleural effusion in adults. *Thorax* 2003; **58** (suppl. II) ii8–17

Diagnostic algorithm for the patient with a pleural effusion

1. History, examination, CXR

2. Does the patient have heart failure with no atypical features (such as asymmetrical bilateral effusions, unilateral effusion, normal heart size on CXR, chest pain, fever)?

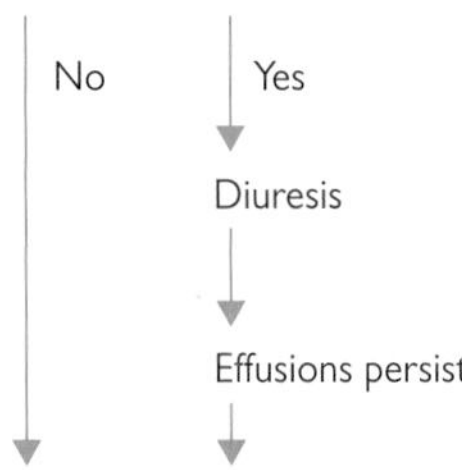

3. Thoracentesis (diagnostic ± therapeutic). Pleural fluid analysis: appearance, protein, LDH, cytology, microbiology, pH (± cholesterol, triglyceride, haematocrit, glucose, amylase).

4. Is the pleural effusion a transudate or exudate?

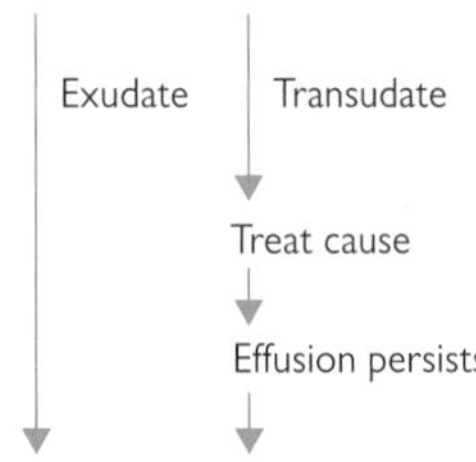

5. Further investigations if diagnosis remains unclear:

- CT chest with contrast to enhance pleura
- Repeat pleural fluid cytology
- Further pleural fluid analysis, e.g. cholesterol, triglyceride, haematocrit, glucose, amylase, fungal stains
- Pleural tissue biopsy for histology and TB culture (ultrasound- or CT-guided, closed Abrams', or thoracoscopic biopsy)
- Reconsider pulmonary embolism and tuberculosis
- Consider thoracoscopy if persistent undiagnosed pleural effusion.

Transudative pleural effusions

Mechanisms involve either increased hydrostatic pressure or reduced osmotic pressure (due to hypo-albuminaemia) in the microvascular circulation.

Differential diagnosis

Table 8.1 Causes of transudative pleural effusions

Cause	Notes
Common	
Left ventricular failure	Investigate further if atypical features (very asymmetrical bilateral effusions, unilateral effusion, chest pain, fever); frequently complicated by pulmonary embolism (up to one-fifth of cases at autopsy)
Cirrhotic liver disease ('hepatic hydrothorax')	Ascites often but not invariably present; majority right-sided; remove ascites and treat hypo-albuminaemia (p 244)
Pulmonary embolism	10–20% are transudates (p 401)
Peritoneal dialysis	Pleural fluid analysis resembles dialysis fluid, with protein <1 g/dl and glucose >300 mg/dl
Nephrotic syndrome	Usually bilateral; consider secondary pulmonary embolism if atypical features
Atelectasis	Common on ITU or post-operatively; usually small effusion, may be bilateral; rarely needs investigation
Less common	
Constrictive percarditis	May be unilateral or bilateral
Hypothyroidism	May be transudate or exudate; pleural effusions occur most commonly in association with ascites, pericardial effusion, and cardiac failure, although may be an isolated finding
Meigs' syndrome	Unilateral (often right-sided) or bilateral pleural effusions and ascites; occurs in women with ovarian or other pelvic tumours; resolves following removal of tumour
Urinothorax	Effusion ipsilateral to obstructed kidney with retro-peritoneal urine leak, resolves after treatment of obstruction; pleural fluid smells of urine, pH usually low; pleural fluid creatinine >serum creatinine is diagnostic
Malignancy	Up to 5% are transudates

Treatment of transudative effusions is directed at the underlying cause; consider further investigation if fails to respond.

Exudative pleural effusions

Mechanisms involve an increase in capillary permeability and impaired pleural fluid resorption.

Differential diagnosis

Table 8.2 Causes of exudative pleural effusions.

Cause	Notes
Common	
Parapneumonic effusion	Occurs in 40% of bacterial pneumonias; commonest exudative effusion in young patients (p 420)
Malignancy	Commonest exudative effusion in patients >60 years (p 279)
Pulmonary embolism	80–90% are exudates (p 401)
Rheumatoid arthritis	Typically low pleural fluid glucose, often <1.6 mmol/L (p 188)
Mesothelioma	Pleural fluid cytological analysis has low sensitivity (p 114)
Less common	
Empyema	Pleural fluid pH <7.2; clinical features of infection, e.g. fever, sweats (p 352)
Tuberculosis	Typically lymphocytic effusion; pleural fluid AFB smear positive in 10% of cases, culture positive in 25%, Abrams' biopsy histology sensitivity 90% (p 490)
Other infections	Very rare; include viral, parasitic, rickettsial, and fungal (e.g. aspergillus, histoplasma, coccidioidomycosis)
Hepatic, splenic, or subphrenic abscess	
Oesophageal rupture	Initially sterile exudate, followed by empyema; pH <7.2, raised salivary amylase, often history of vomiting
Pancreatitis	Pleural fluid pancreatic amylase may be raised
SLE	Lupus erythematosus cells in fluid are diagnostic; may respond quickly to prednisolone
Other autoimmune diseases	Churg–Strauss syndrome (intensely eosinophilic fluid), Sjögren's syndrome, scleroderma, dermatomyositis, Wegener's granulomatosis
Sarcoidosis	Effusions are uncommon
Post-cardiac injury syndrome (Dressler's syndrome)	Pleural effusions common; may be blood-stained
Post-coronary artery bypass surgery	(p 361)

Table 8.2 Causes of exdative pleural effusions (*cont.*)

Cause	Notes
Less common	
Radiotherapy	May cause small, unilateral effusions up to 6 months after treatment
Uraemia	Effusions frequently resolve after starting dialysis
Chylothorax	Presence of chylomicrons or pleural fluid triglyceride level >110 mg/dl (p 54)
Benign asbestos-related pleural effusion	(p 110)
Drug-induced	Drugs include amiodarone, bromocriptine, methotrexate, phenytoin, and nitrofurantoin; see www.pneumotox.com for full list; effusions usually resolve following discontinuation of drug
Other, rare causes	Include yellow nail syndrome, cryptogenic organizing pneumonia, amyloidosis, familial Mediterranean fever

Treatment of exudates involves treatment of the underlying cause, as well as measures to improve breathlessness and remove pleural fluid, e.g. therapeutic thoracentesis (p 783), intercostal drainage (p 760), and pleurodesis (p 776).

Pleural fluid analysis 1

'Routine' pleural fluid analysis comprises assessment of:

- Pleural fluid appearance
- Biochemistry (protein and LDH)
- Cytology (for malignant cells and differential cell count; ideally fresh 20-mL sample)
- Microbiology (Gram stain and microscopy, culture, and AFB stain and culture; inoculation of blood culture bottles with pleural fluid may increase yield)
- pH

Although considered routine, some of these investigations may be unnecessary and even misleading, depending on the clinical picture (e.g. microbiological analysis on patients suspected as having transudates).

Additional pleural fluid investigations such as measurement of cholesterol and triglycerides, haematocrit, glucose, and amylase may be helpful in certain clinical circumstances.

Appearance

Appearance	Possible causes
Bloody	Trauma, malignancy, pulmonary infarction, pneumonia, post-cardiac injury syndrome, pneumothorax, benign asbestos-related pleural effusion, aortic dissection/rupture; defined as haemothorax if pleural fluid haematocrit >50% of peripheral blood haematocrit (p 360)
Turbid or milky	Empyema, chylothorax, pseudochylothorax (clear supernatant after centrifuging favours empyema; cloudy after centrifuging suggests chylothorax or pseudochylothorax, p 54)
Putrid odour	Anaerobic empyema
Viscous	Mesothelioma
Food particles	Oesophageal rupture
Urine odour	Urinothorax
Black	Aspergillus infection
Brown, 'anchovy sauce'	Amoebic liver abscess draining into pleural space

Differential cell count

Predominant cell type	Possible causes
Neutrophils	Any acute effusion, e.g. parapneumonic, pulmonary embolus
Mononuclear cells	Any chronic effusion, e.g. malignancy, tuberculosis
Lymphocytes	Tuberculosis, especially if over 80%; other causes include malignancy, sarcoidosis, lymphoma, rheumatoid pleurisy, post-CABG
Eosinophils	Often unhelpful; associations include air or blood in pleural space (haemothorax, pulmonary infarct, pneumothorax, previous tap), malignancy, infection (parapneumonic, tuberculous, fungal, parasitic), drug- and asbestos-induced effusions, Churg–Strauss syndrome or idiopathic
Mesothelial cells	Predominate in transudates; variable numbers in exudates, typically suppressed in inflammatory conditions, e.g. tuberculosis
Lupus erythematosus cells	Diagnostic of systemic lupus erythematosus

Pleural fluid analysis 2

Pleural fluid pH and glucose Pleural fluid pH may be measured using an arterial blood pH analyser. The sample should be appropriately heparinized, e.g. aspirate a few mL of pleural fluid into a pre-heparinized blood gas syringe. Frankly purulent samples should not be analysed—it is unnecessary, and might damage the machine.

Normal pleural fluid pH is about 7.6. An abnormally low pH (<7.3) suggests pleural inflammation and is often associated with a low pleural fluid glucose (<3.3 mmol/L or pleural fluid/serum glucose ratio <0.5). The mechanism probably involves increased neutrophil phagocytosis, and bacterial or tumour cell breakdown, resulting in the accumulation of lactate and carbon dioxide.

Causes of low pH and low glucose effusions

- Parapneumonic effusion and empyema (pH <7.2 indication for drainage of pleural space, as unlikely to resolve spontaneously)
- Rheumatoid pleuritis (glucose <1.7 mmol/L in 66% and <2.8 mmol/L in 80% of cases)
- Malignant pleural effusion (associated with advanced disease and poor survival, higher sensitivity of pleural fluid cytological analysis, and failure of pleurodesis)
- Tuberculous pleural effusion
- Oesophageal rupture
- Lupus pleuritis.

Urinothorax is the only transudative effusion that can cause a pH <7.3. An abnormally high (alkaline) pH may rarely occur in the setting of *Proteus* pleural infection.

Pleural fluid triglyceride and cholesterol Measure in turbid or milky effusions or where chylothorax is suspected.

Chylothorax occurs following disruption of the thoracic duct, and pleural fluid may appear turbid, milky, serous, or blood-stained. The presence of pleural fluid chylomicrons or a pleural fluid triglyceride level >110 mg/dl confirms the diagnosis. Causes of chylothorax:

- Malignancy (particularly lymphoma)
- Trauma
- Following thoracotomy
- Pulmonary lymphangioleiomyomatosis.

Pseudochylothorax occurs due to cholesterol crystal deposition in chronic effusions, most commonly due to rheumatoid pleurisy or tuberculosis, and may cause a milky effusion; raised pleural fluid cholesterol (>200 mg/dl) and cholesterol crystals at microscopy distinguish it from chylothorax.

Pleural fluid amylase Abnormal if pleural fluid amylase > upper normal limit for serum amylase, or if amylase pleural fluid/serum ratio >1.0. Causes include:

- Pleural malignancy and oesophageal rupture (both associated with raised ***salivary*** amylase)
- Pancreatic disease (acute and chronic pancreatitis, pancreatic pseudocyst; associated with raised ***pancreatic*** amylase).

NB. May be normal early in the course of acute pancreatitis or oesophageal rupture.

Chapter 9

Post-operative breathlessness

The respiratory physician is often asked to see patients post-operatively who have become dyspnoeic following an operative procedure. The risk of pulmonary complications is greatest with thoracic or upper abdominal surgery, when a degree of pulmonary dysfunction and consequent breathlessness due to atelectasis is inevitable. Always rule out upper airway obstruction.

The four most likely common causes are:

- Infection/atelectasis
- Pulmonary emboli
- Left ventricular failure (fluid overload)
- Exacerbation of underlying lung disease, such as COPD or UIP.

Points to consider when assessing these patients

- Is the patient acutely unwell, needing immediate resuscitation and ventilatory support?
- Comorbid disease and past medical history, especially pulmonary, cardiac, or thromboembolic disease
- Type of surgery
  - ***Thoracic surgery:*** consider lobar gangrene (torsion of the remaining lobe causing vascular occlusion) leading to pulmonary infarction with fever and haemoptysis, bronchopleural fistula, often associated with an infected pleural space, leading to sepsis and failure of the underlying lung to re-expand
- Time since surgery:
  - ***Early complications (hours)*** related to residual anaesthetic effect not adequately reversed, atelectasis, respiratory failure, hypovolaemic shock, infection, PE, fat embolism, air embolism, left ventricular failure and fluid overload, myocardial ischaemia
  - ***Later complications (hours–days)*** related to PE, ARDS, infection, myocardial ischaemia.

Initial tests to consider performing in these patients

- Oxygen saturations and arterial blood gas breathing room air and on oxygen
- ECG
- CXR—compare with pre-operative CXR, if available
- Full blood count and clotting screen
- U&E and bicarbonate
- See if they had pre-operative oximetry and spirometry performed. There should be a record of the oxygen saturation in the anaesthetic room.

A D-dimer level is unhelpful as it will be raised by many different intra- and post-operative mechanisms.

CRP and WCC are also largely unhelpful as these are frequently raised post-operatively.

Table 9.1 Assessment of dyspnoea

Possible cause of dyspnoea	Management options
Basal atelectasis (commoner in smokers and following abdominal or trans-thoracic procedures. Mucus in bronchial tree causes small airway obstruction, subsequent alveolar air reabsorption, and collapse of lung segments); collapsed lobe—mucus plugging	Adequate analgesia to encourage expectoration, nebulized saline, chest physiotherapy, deep breathing. If lung does not reinflate, consider bronchoscopy to suction out secretions
Pneumonia—follows atelectasis and collapse. Possible aspiration also	If fever and chest signs, give antibiotics for hospital-acquired pneumonia (see p 436), adequate analgesia to encourage expectoration, chest physiotherapy
Thromboembolic disease	Oxygen as required. Measure A–a gradient on blood gas. Start treatment dose of unfractionated heparin (if not contraindicated by the operation), arrange VQ scan or CTPA, check D-dimers (although unhelpful unless negative). If in extremis consider urgent CT or echocardiogram and thrombolysis (see p 401)
Respiratory failure	Opiate overdose or anaesthetic agents causing neuromuscular block not reversed. Undiagnosed respiratory muscle weakness
Metabolic acidosis	Check U&E, look for underlying problem, such as renal failure or sepsis
Myocardial ischaemia	Oxygen, check cardiac enzymes and 12-h troponin. Sublingual or IV glyceryl trinitrate if required for pain. Start prophylactic heparin (if not contraindicated by the operation)
Myocardial infarction or acute coronary syndrome	Thrombolysis likely to be contraindicated by recent surgery, so consider referral for primary angioplasty. Consider aspirin, clopidogrel, low molecular weight heparin
Cardiac failure/fluid overload	Oxygen, IV furosemide, central line, and ionotropes if required. Echocardiogram to assess left ventricle
ARDS	Supportive, likely to need mechanical ventilatory assistance (see p 101)
Phrenic nerve damage causing diaphragmatic paralysis. May occur with thoracic operations such as CABG	Diagnose on lung function tests, CXR, and clinically decreased diaphragm movement. Advise to tilt whole bed (head up) when sleeping. Phrenics may recover, but can take 2+ years
Fat embolism following long bone fracture, especially with reaming and manipulation	Oxygen, IV fluids, supportive care
Laryngeal spasm	Reassurance, oxygen if required
Anaemia	Cross-match and transfuse. Identify if ongoing bleeding source
Myasthenia gravis crisis precipitated by anaesthetic agents	May need intubation and ventilation. Stop all anti-cholinesterases. Consider plasma exchange and IV immunoglobulin. Urgent neurology input

Chapter 10

Pregnancy and breathlessness

Causes

Normal physiological changes of pregnancy

- Elevated serum progesterone levels stimulate respiratory drive and lead to an increased tidal volume and raised minute ventilation, with only a modest increase in oxygen consumption. The subsequent fall in maternal pCO_2 facilitates fetal CO_2 transfer across the placenta; any cause of maternal hypercapnia leads quickly to fetal respiratory acidosis. Respiratory rate is unaffected by pregnancy. Elevation of the diaphragm occurs due to the enlarging uterus, leading to a reduced functional residual capacity, although diaphragm function is normal and vital capacity is unaffected. Peak flow and FEV_1 are unaffected by pregnancy
- Increased cardiac output occurs due to an increase in heart rate (by about 15 beats/min) and stroke volume; peripheral resistance falls. Blood pressure is reduced in the first and second trimesters by 10–20 mmHg, but is normal at term. Peripheral pulses tend to be increased in volume. Dependent oedema is common. Third heart sound and ejection systolic murmurs are commonly heard. May hear venous hums in the neck
- Raised levels of coagulation factors and impaired fibrinolysis, combined with venous stasis, result in a 5-fold increased risk of venous thromboembolism
- Upper airway oedema, particularly in the setting of pre-eclampsia, may predispose to upper airways obstruction during sleep, but rarely frank obstructive sleep apnoea. OSA tends to occur in obese women, and may be associated with impaired fetal growth and pre-eclampsia. Snoring in pregnancy is a poor predictor of OSA.

Causes of breathlessness in pregnancy

Causes are listed in the box opposite. In general, breathlessness may be due to:

- Normal physiological changes of pregnancy. Up to 75% of pregnant women experience a degree of breathlessness, perhaps as a result of the increase in ventilation. Tachypnoea is a useful sign, as it is abnormal in pregnancy and suggests an underlying disease process
- New disease process. Pulmonary embolism is the commonest and is a major cause of maternal death. Other rare, but serious, causes include amniotic fluid embolism and ARDS
- Exacerbation of chronic respiratory or cardiac disease. Asthma is the commonest. Unsuspected underlying disease may present for the first time in pregnancy, e.g. structural heart disease such as mitral stenosis, lymphangioleiomyomatosis. Pulmonary hypertension is associated with a particularly poor prognosis during pregnancy. Patients with interstitial lung disease and vital capacity <1 L should also consider avoiding pregnancy. In patients with cystic fibrosis, the presence of pulmonary hypertension or FEV_1 <50% predicted are associated with a poor outcome.

Causes of breathlessness in pregnancy

Pulmonary

- Exacerbation of pre-existing lung disease, e.g. asthma (p 140), cystic fibrosis, lymphangioleiomyomatosis
- Pneumonia (p 419)
  - Bacterial: usual organisms, including tuberculosis (p 502) and aspiration (p 442)
  - Viral: particularly varicella, influenza (p 538, 532)
  - Fungal: particularly coccidioidomycosis (p 483)
- Aspiration pneumonitis
- Pulmonary metastases from choriocarcinoma (very rare).

Pleural

- Pneumothorax (p 373), particularly during labour
- Small asymptomatic effusions post-partum
- Ovarian hyperstimulation syndrome (very rare).

Vascular

- Pulmonary embolism (p 401)
- Amniotic fluid embolism (p 416)
- Air embolism (p 416)
- Pulmonary hypertension (p 385).

Cardiogenic pulmonary oedema

- Exacerbation of pre-existing cardiac disease, e.g. mitral stenosis
- Peripartum cardiomyopathy.

Non-cardiogenic pulmonary oedema

- Iatrogenic fluid overload
- Tocolytic therapy (ß-agonists used to inhibit uterine contractions in preterm labour)
- ARDS due to pre-eclampsia, sepsis, massive haemorrhage, amniotic fluid embolism.

Other

- Anaemia
- Oesophageal rupture
- Hemidiaphragm rupture.

Investigations

Liaise with your obstetrics team, as well as with paediatricians and anaesthetists, if delivery is approaching. Management of specific conditions is discussed in the individual disease chapters in Part 2.

The following investigations may be affected by the pregnancy itself:

- ***ABGs.*** Normal maternal pO_2 >13.3 kPa and pCO_2 3.7–4.3 kPa. A compensatory fall in serum bicarbonate (to 18–22 mmol/L) occurs, resulting in an average pH of 7.44. During the third trimester, perform ABGs in an upright position, as pO_2 may be 2.0 kPa lower when supine. A–agradient is unaffected during pregnancy, except when supine near term
- ***Blood tests.*** In normal pregnancy, WCC, platelets, ESR, D-dimers, and fibrinogen are usually raised, and serum creatinine levels reduced. CRP is not significantly affected. D-dimer is increased from about 6 weeks gestation to 3 months post-partum
- ***CXR*** may show increased pulmonary vasculature due to normal increase in cardiac output. Required for diagnosis of pneumonia and pneumothorax. With abdominal shielding, the radiation doses to mother and baby are very small and CXR should be performed if clinically necessary. Lateral CXR carries a greater radiation exposure and should be avoided
- ***Ventilation–perfusion scans*** are considered relatively safe in pregnancy, and are the investigation of choice if pulmonary embolism is suspected (although some experts suggest performing leg vein ultrasound first; if an asymptomatic DVT is confirmed in the setting of clinical features suggestive of pulmonary embolism, then treatment may be started without the need for radiation exposure from further imaging). If V/Q is non-diagnostic, consider pulmonary angiography; the radiation exposure from the combination of CXR, V/Q, and angiography is not thought to be associated with fetal injury. CT pulmonary angiography carries a greater radiation dose and, in the setting of the hormonal changes within the breast during pregnancy, leads to an increased risk of breast cancer in the mother.

Chapter 11

Pre-operative assessment

The respiratory physician may be asked to assess a patient prior to elective or emergency surgery. These patients are usually those with pre-existing respiratory disease, such as COPD.

- The usual functional status of the patient should be determined
- Their respiratory function should be optimized if possible, with medication changes where appropriate.

These patients may require ventilatory support post-operatively. Ultimately the decisions regarding fitness for surgery rest with the surgeon and the anaesthetist.

Assessing the pre-operative patient

- Usual functional state and exercise tolerance (those with an exercise tolerance of <5 m will not come off a ventilator)
- Oxygen saturations on air and after exertion, such as walking or climbing up and down a step for 2 min
- Arterial blood gas on air, if saturations <94%. **Risk of surgery increases as the CO_2 increases**
- Spirometry, with bronchodilator reversibility testing. **Risk of surgery increased if FEV_1 <0.8 L**
- CXR—if 65+ and no CXR in last year, or if acute respiratory symptoms
- History of snoring or OSA
- ECG
- Echocardiogram, if cardiac function compromised.

Options for management of the pre-operative patient

- Regular inhaled or nebulized bronchodilators, if air flow obstruction
- Regular inhaled steroid, if evidence of steroid reversibility
- Pre-operative course of oral steroids, if evidence of steroid reversibility
- Pre-operative course of antibiotics, if evidence of infection
- Consider pulmonary rehabilitation
- Consider chest physiotherapy with deep breathing exercises
- Referral for CPAP if OSA present
- Optimize nutrition
- Lose weight
- Advise to stop smoking—ideally 8 weeks prior to surgery; reduces post-operative complication rate.

Risk factors for peri-operative complications

- Thoracic or upper abdominal surgery
- Anaesthetic length >3.5 h
- Smoker
- Chronic lung disease
- Raised $PaCO_2$
- Current respiratory symptoms
- Poor performance status
- Concurrent cardiac disease
- Obesity
- Older age.

Chapter 12

Pulmonary disease in the immunocompromised (non-HIV)

Clinical assessment

Respiratory disease is a significant cause of morbidity and mortality in the immunocompromised, and its diagnosis and management are challenging. In the UK this is encountered most commonly in the setting of immunocompromise secondary to cytotoxic chemotherapy, haematological malignancy, immunosuppression post-transplant (particularly renal and haematopoietic stem cell transplant [HSCT, including bone marrow, fetal cord blood, and growth-factor-stimulated peripheral blood transplantation]), prolonged corticosteroid use, and AIDS (p 79).

Most pulmonary diseases present in a similar manner in the setting of immunocompromise, with fever, dyspnoea, dry cough, chest pain, and often hypoxia. This non-specific clinical presentation, combined with the large number of possible causes, makes reaching a precise diagnosis difficult; the diagnosis remains unclear in up to 10% of cases even at autopsy. There is limited evidence to demonstrate that obtaining a definitive diagnosis leads to an overall improvement in mortality, although, in subgroups such as patients with respiratory infection, early identification and treatment of pathogens has been shown to improve outcome.

Causes of pulmonary infiltrates in the non-HIV-infected immunocompromised are presented on p 72, and treatment on p 76. Specific conditions are described separately (e.g. invasive aspergillosis, p 470; PCP, p 476).

Key steps in the management of these patients are as follows.

Clinical assessment In the ***history***, the underlying cause of immunocompromise and the timing and location of respiratory disease onset may provide clues to the diagnosis. The rate of disease onset may also suggest possible causes:

- ***Acute onset*** (<24 h) Bacterial pneumonia, viral pneumonitis (e.g. CMV), pulmonary oedema or haemorrhage, pulmonary emboli, ARDS
- ***Subacute onset*** (days) Fungi (e.g. *Pneumocystis, Aspergillus*), bacteria (e.g. *Nocardia, Legionella*), viral (e.g. CMV), drug-induced pneumonitis
- ***Chronic onset*** (weeks) Malignancy, mycobacteria, fungi.

Chest ***examination*** may suggest the extent of pulmonary involvement, although this can be misleading and there are often no abnormal signs (e.g. PCP, or bacterial pneumonia in the setting of neutropenia). Assess fluid status; pulmonary oedema is common following transplantation. Extrapulmonary involvement may be helpful in suggesting a pathogen, e.g. cutaneous lesions (herpes simplex and varicella-zoster; necrotic lesions from *Pseudomonas* and other Gram-negative bacteria, mycobacteria, and fungi; subcutaneous abscesses in *Staphylococcus aureus* and *Nocardia*), central nervous system involvement (*Pseudomonas, Aspergillus, Cryptococcus, Nocardia,* mycobacteria, *Streptococcus pneumoniae, Haemophilus influenzae*, varicella-zoster).

Initial investigations

- ***CXR*** appearance is very variable; may be normal or show consolidation, nodular infiltrate, or diffuse shadowing. CXR is of limited diagnostic value, as appearances are non-specific and atypical presentations are common; the 'first-choice' diagnosis based on CXR is correct in only a third of cases. CXR may, however, be helpful in monitoring disease progression and response to treatment
- ***Blood and pleural fluid*** (if available) sampling for microscopy and culture. Consider viral serology (e.g. CMV following transplantation), urinary *Legionella* antigen
- ***Sputum examination*** is often of little diagnostic value in immunocompromised patients, with the possible exceptions of invasive aspergillosis and tuberculosis. Send sputum for acid-fast stain and mycobacterial culture, fungal stain, and culture. Induced sputum has a low yield for PCP in non-HIV patients
- The degree of ***hypoxia*** is often not appreciated; measure oxygen saturations and consider ABGs. Severe hypoxia tends to be more commonly associated with infection due to bacteria, viruses, or *Pneumocystis* than with mycobacteria or fungi.

Is immediate antibiotic treatment required? Immediate empirical treatment with broad-spectrum antibiotics prior to further investigation should be considered, depending on the nature of immunological defect and local hospital policy. In general, neutropenic patients with fever are at significant risk of developing overwhelming sepsis, and should receive prompt antibiotic cover, irrespective of the CXR appearance and presence or absence of respiratory symptoms/signs. More invasive diagnostic procedures can then be reserved for patients who deteriorate or fail to improve within a period of observation (e.g. 2–3 days). In non-neutropenic patients, depending on the clinical circumstances, it is often possible to withhold treatment until definitive investigations have taken place.

Further investigations

More invasive diagnostic techniques are usually required for a definitive diagnosis.

CT chest

- Specific indications not yet defined. Probably not needed in typical cases of bacterial pneumonia or PCP
- Useful in identifying the location and extent of pulmonary disease, and aiding invasive sampling procedures
- Often detects pulmonary disease in the presence of a normal CXR—consider if respiratory symptoms or unexplained fever, but normal CXR
- May be diagnostic, e.g. pulmonary embolism (CTPA), lymphangitis carcinomatosis, invasive aspergillosis ('halo' and 'air crescent' signs).

Bronchoscopy with bronchoalveolar lavage

- First-line investigation; consider early in management. Diagnostic in about 60% of patients overall; up to 70% of patients with infection. Results in change to treatment in around 50% of cases overall. Complications are rare
- Useful in the diagnosis of bacterial pneumonia, PCP (sensitivity 80–90%), cytomegalovirus (sensitivity 85–90%), aspergillosis (sensitivity 50%), tuberculosis, malignant disease, diffuse alveolar haemorrhage, and alveolar proteinosis
- BAL fluid analysis—routine microscopy and culture for bacteria; additional stains and culture for fungi, mycobacteria, *Nocardia*; silver or immunofluorescence stain for *Pneumocystis*; cytology, including flow cytometry, for malignant cells; viral serology; haemosiderin-laden macrophages if alveolar haemorrhage suspected
- Consider additional tests on BAL fluid, such as *Cryptococcus* antigen detection or CMV PCR. *Aspergillus* antigen detection or PCR and *Toxoplasma gondii* PCR are less well validated
- Transbronchial biopsy has a slightly higher sensitivity than BAL for the diagnosis of infection, but carries a risk of bleeding and pneumothorax, which can be serious complications in this patient group; it is not usually performed at initial bronchoscopy, although may be considered, e.g. if lymphangitis is suspected.

Lung biopsy Consider as a second-line investigation if BAL is non-diagnostic. Options include:

- ***Repeat bronchoscopy with transbronchial lung biopsy*** is useful in the diagnosis of malignancy, mycobacteria, fungi, organizing pneumonia, and drug-induced lung disease
- ***VATS or open lung biopsy*** has a greater diagnostic yield than TBB, although it is unclear if this can be directly translated into an improved survival. Results in change to treatment in <50% of patients and complications may be serious
- ***Percutaneous image-guided fine-needle aspiration or biopsy*** for investigation of peripheral nodules.

Causes

Causes of pulmonary disease in the immunocompromised can be broadly divided into infectious and non-infectious; multiple disease processes are common. The nature of immunosuppression may provide clues to the cause(s) of pulmonary disease—solid organ (kidney and liver) transplants are further discussed on p 74, lung transplantation on p 317, HSCT on p 75, and HIV on pp 79-83.

Infectious causes ***(>75% of cases)*** Infection is the commonest cause of respiratory disease in the immunocompromised. The nature of immunological defect may provide clues to the likely infectious agent:

- ***Neutropenia or impaired neutrophil function (e.g. secondary to leukaemia or cytotoxic treatment)*** Bacteria (*Pseudomonas aeruginosa, S. aureus, S. pneumoniae, E. coli, Klebsiella, H. influenzae, Nocardia*), fungi (*Aspergillus, Candida, Mucormycosis*)
- ***Impaired T-lymphocyte function (e.g. secondary to transplantation, cytotoxic treatment, high-dose steroids, lymphoma, AIDS)*** Fungi (PCP, *Cryptococcus neoformans, Candida, Histoplasma, Coccidioides, Blastomyces*), viruses (cytomegalovirus, herpes simplex, varicella-zoster), bacteria (mycobacteria, *Listeria, Legionella, Nocardia*), parasites (*Toxoplasma gondii*)
- ***Hypogammaglobulinaemia or impaired B-lymphocyte function (e.g. secondary to myeloma, acute and chronic lymphocytic leukaemia, lymphoma)*** Encapsulated bacteria (*S. pneumoniae, H. influenzae*).

It should be noted, however, that considerable overlap exists between immune deficiencies, and the pattern of infection will be further modified by prophylactic treatment, e.g. CMV and PCP prophylaxis.

Non-infectious causes ***(<25% of cases)*** Often present with similar, if not identical, clinical and radiological features to infection, and signs such as fever do not reliably differentiate between them. Causes include:

- ***Pulmonary oedema*** Particularly following renal or HSCT transplant
- ***ARDS*** e.g. secondary to sepsis, drugs (e.g. cytarabine, gemcitabine, OKT3 antilymphocyte antibodies, interleukin-2), massive blood transfusion, transfusion-related acute lung injury, aspiration, 'engraftment syndrome' (coinciding with neutrophil engraftment) following HSCT
- ***Drug-induced disease*** Causes include all-trans retinoic acid (ATRA), antithymocyte globulin, azathioprine, bleomycin, busulfan, carmustine, chlorambucil, cyclophosphamide, cytosine arabinoside, hydroxyurea, liposomal amphotericin B, melphalan, mitomycin, methotrexate, sirolimus
- ***Respiratory involvement from the underlying disease*** e.g. lymphoma, leukaemic infiltration, lymphangitis carcinomatosis, connective tissue disease, leucostasis with very high leucocyte counts in leukaemia
- ***Pulmonary embolism*** Often complicated by secondary infection; clinical/radiological features may be confused with invasive aspergillosis; may be more common after kidney transplant
- ***Radiation-induced pulmonary disease*** Pneumonitis (dyspnoea; clear margins on CT; typically follows lung radiotherapy) or organizing pneumonia (cough; extends beyond radiation field on CT; typically follows breast radiotherapy)

- ***Diffuse alveolar haemorrhage*** not uncommon complication of leukaemia, and allogeneic or autologous HSCT; similar clinical presentation to that of pneumonia; haemoptysis is rare; multilobar CXR/CT infiltrates; proposed diagnostic criteria include exclusion of infection, progressively bloodier returns from BAL of three different subsegmental bronchi (although limited sensitivity and specificity), and ≥20% of alveolar macrophages haemosiderin-filled (although may require several days to appear); reported mortality ranges 30–100%
- ***'Idiopathic pneumonia syndrome'*** following allogeneic or autologous HSCT; breathlessness with hypoxia and multilobar CXR/CT infiltrates; infection excluded with BAL and ideally a second later investigation (e.g. repeat BAL or lung biopsy); diffuse alveolar damage or interstitial pneumonitis on biopsy; mortality >70%
- ***Engraftment syndrome*** comprises fever, ARDS, and erythematosus rash during marrow recovery post-HSCT
- ***Chronic airflow obstruction (bronchiolitis obliterans)*** following allogeneic HSCT (from non-identical sibling or unrelated individual; occurs only extremely rarely following autologous procedure); typically associated with chronic graft-versus-host disease (GVHD); gradual onset dry cough, dyspnoea, wheeze, obstructive spirometry; CXR often normal; air-trapping and bronchial dilatation on HRCT; TBB low sensitivity; may be complicated by *Aspergillus* infection; variable course
- ***Post-transplant lymphoproliferative disease*** most common following lung transplant (p 317); may also follow other solid organ or allogeneic HSC transplant
- ***Pulmonary alveolar proteinosis*** (p 630)
- ***Pulmonary veno-occlusive disease***
- ***Pulmonary metastatic calcification*** may complicate chronic renal failure and rarely progress after transplantation; usually asymptomatic, rarely causes restrictive ventilatory defect; CXR shows single or multiple nodules or patches of consolidation, may not appear calcified; CT typically diagnostic, although biopsy occasionally needed
- Right ***hemidiaphragm dysfunction*** is common after liver transplant, and usually not relevant clinically.

Multiple disease processes About 30% of patients have two or more disease processes accounting for their respiratory involvement. Secondary infection with a different infectious agent (commonly *Aspergillus* or Gram-negative bacteria such as *Pseudomonas*) may complicate either a primary respiratory infection or a non-infectious process such as pulmonary embolism. Secondary infection is associated with a poor prognosis; consider particularly in patients who deteriorate after an initial response to treatment, and in patients who are neutropenic.

Pleural effusion Differential diagnosis in non-HIV immunocompromised patients includes cardiac failure and fluid overload, pulmonary embolism, drug-related, parapneumonic (bacterial including *Nocardia*, fungal, e.g. PCP), or related to underlying disease (e.g. leukaemic infiltrates, lymphoma, chylothorax, myeloma). Pleural effusions are common after liver transplant: usually right-sided or bilateral transudates and resolve by third week; may require drainage if symptomatic.

Differential diagnosis of pulmonary complications based on time course after transplantation

Solid organ transplantation

First month post-transplant *(recent surgery ± ITU)*

- Nosocomial bacterial infection (Gram-negative, *S. aureus*—including MRSA, *Legionella*)
- ARDS
- Pulmonary oedema
- Drug-induced
- Pulmonary embolism
- Pleural effusion (especially after liver transplant)
- Right hemidiaphragm dysfunction (after liver transplant).

Months 1–6 *(maximal immunosuppression)*

- Opportunistic infection (CMV, PCP, *Nocardia*, *Aspergillus*, *Scedosporium apiospermum*)
- Drug-induced
- Post-transplant lymphoproliferative disease.

Months >6 *(reduction in immunosuppression, unless rejection)*

- Common community-acquired pathogens (*Haemophilus influenzae*, *Streptococcus pneumoniae*, *Legionella*, tuberculosis, non-tuberculous mycobacteria, PCP, endemic mycoses e.g. *Histoplasma*, viruses e.g. influenza, para-influenza, adenovirus, RSV)
- Opportunistic pathogens (see above)
- Post-transplant lymphoproliferative disease
- Pulmonary metastatic calcification.

Haematopoietic stem cell transplantation (HSCT)

First month post-transplant *(prolonged neutropenia pre-engraftment)*

- Infection (bacteria, e.g. *Pseudomonas aeruginosa*, *Escherichia coli*, *Klebsiella pneumoniae*, *Haemophilus influenzae*, *Staphylococcus aureus*, *Legionella* species; fungi, e.g. *Aspergillus*; viruses e.g. herpes simplex, adenovirus)
- Pulmonary oedema
- ARDS
- Transfusion-related acute lung injury
- Drug-induced
- Diffuse alveolar haemorrhage
- Idiopathic pneumonia syndrome.

Months 1-3 *(impaired cellular immunity post-engraftment, related in part to immunosuppressive drugs and GVHD)*

- Opportunistic infection (Gram-negative bacteria, *Nocardia*, CMV, herpes simplex, PCP)
- Drug-induced
- Diffuse alveolar haemorrhage
- Idiopathic pneumonia syndrome
- Engraftment syndrome
- Post-transplant lymphoproliferative disease
- Pulmonary veno-occlusive disease.

Months >3 *(poor lymphocyte function, particularly following allogeneic HSCT)*

- Infection (Gram-positive bacteria, CMV, herpes, varicella-zoster, tuberculosis, non-tuberculous mycobacteria, PCP, *Aspergillus*, endemic mycoses, e.g. *Histoplasma*)
- Chronic airflow obstruction (bronchiolitis obliterans, associated with GVHD)
- Post-transplant lymphoproliferative disease
- Pulmonary veno-occlusive disease.

Treatment

Antimicrobials Depending on the clinical circumstances, antimicrobials may need to be started prior to definitive investigations (see p 69), although blood cultures should always precede antibiotic treatment. Choice of antimicrobial depends on the underlying condition and local hospital policy.

- In general, most neutropenic patients are treated with broad-spectrum antibiotics providing both Gram-positive and Gram-negative cover, e.g. piperacillin (4.5 g IV qds); antifungals are considered if slow response to treatment or subsequent deterioration. Consider vancomycin if MRSA is a possibility
- Treatment for CMV and PCP is associated with significant side-effects, and ideally should be based on a definitive diagnosis. In unwell patients who are strongly suspected to have PCP, treatment (p 478) can be started immediately, as BAL *Pneumocystis jiroveci* stains remain positive for up to 2 weeks
- Antituberculous treatment should only rarely be administered in the absence of a microbiological diagnosis.

Diuretics Fluid overload and pulmonary oedema are common following renal and HSCT transplantation, and typical clinical and radiological signs may be disguised; consider a trial of diuretics.

Steroids Despite a lack of randomized controlled trials, prednisolone (1–2 mg/kg/day PO, or up to 2 g methylprednisolone IV daily) is often considered in the treatment of drug- or radiation-induced lung disease, engraftment syndrome, diffuse alveolar haemorrhage, and idiopathic pneumonia syndrome following HSCT. Ideally exclude underlying infection prior to starting steroids. Prednisolone (40–80 mg daily PO) is recommended for the treatment of PCP in patients with respiratory failure. Bronchiolitis obliterans following allogeneic HSCT is usually treated with increased immunosuppression.

Supportive treatment Administer oxygen to maintain saturations >95%. Respiratory failure in immunocompromised patients is associated with a poor outcome: mortality following intubation and mechanical ventilation ranges 60–100%. Early intermittent use of non-invasive ventilation in immunocompromised patients with pulmonary infiltrates and hypoxia (defined as breathlessness, respiratory rate >30/min and PaO_2/FiO_2 ratio <200) has been shown to reduce the need for intubation and improve mortality. Before NIV is commenced, a decision regarding suitability for intubation and mechanical ventilation should be made.

Surgery Surgical wedge resection or lobectomy may be considered in the treatment of invasive aspergillosis, either acutely for lesions adjacent to pulmonary vessels that are judged to have a significant risk of massive haemoptysis, or at a later date for residual lesions at risk of reactivation with further chemotherapy.

Further information

Kotloff RM *et al.* Pulmonary complications of solid organ and hematopoietic stem cell transplantation. *AJRCCM* 2004; **170**: 22–48

Shorr AF *et al.* Pulmonary infiltrates in the non-HIV-infected immunocompromised patient. *Chest* 2004; **125**: 260–71

Hilbert G *et al.* Non-invasive ventilation in immunosuppressed patients with pulmonary infiltrates, fever, and acute respiratory failure. *NEJM* 2001; **344**: 481–7

Chapter 13

Pulmonary disease in the immunocompromised (HIV)

Clinical assessment

Widespread use of highly active antiretroviral therapy (HAART) and antimicrobial prophylaxis in HIV has resulted in a longer survival, as well as changes in the nature of respiratory involvement. Respiratory disease remains common in the setting of HIV, and patients should be managed in consultation with an HIV specialist.

Causes of respiratory disease in the HIV-infected patient are listed on p 83. Specific conditions are described separately (e.g. PCP p 476, TB p 487). Key steps in management are as follows.

Clinical assessment

- As with other causes of immunocompromise, clinical features of respiratory disease in HIV-infected patients are non-specific: breathlessness, cough, fever, weight loss, and fatigue are common, although chest symptoms are not always present
- Ask about treatment and compliance with HAART and PCP prophylaxis
- Source of HIV infection may be relevant: Kaposi's sarcoma occurs particularly in homosexual men, and in African men and women; tuberculosis and bacterial pneumonia are more common in IV drug users
- Travel history may be useful: infection with 'endemic mycoses' (e.g. histoplasmosis, blastomycosis, coccidioidomycosis) is well recognized in the USA, but rare in the UK
- Careful examination may provide clues to the respiratory condition. Pulmonary Kaposi's sarcoma is unusual in the absence of disease elsewhere; palatal Kaposi's sarcoma in particular is predictive of pulmonary involvement. Extrapulmonary mycobacterial disease is common, and may involve the liver, lymph nodes, pericardium, and meninges.

Investigations

CXR

- CXR changes are relatively non-specific
- PCP classically appears as bilateral perihilar infiltrates that progress to alveolar shadowing; more unusual patterns include small nodular infiltrates or focal consolidation. CXR is normal in 10% of cases. Pneumothorax is suggestive of PCP
- Appearances of bacterial pneumonia are often atypical, e.g. diffuse bilateral infiltrates mimicking PCP
- Pleural effusion or hilar/mediastinal lymphadenopathy are unusual in PCP, and are more suggestive of mycobacterial infection or Kaposi's sarcoma. CXR cavitation is unusual in tuberculosis occurring late in the course of HIV.

CD4 count Useful in narrowing the differential diagnosis. Bacterial infection, including tuberculosis, occurs at any stage of disease, although infection is more severe at lower CD4 counts; PCP and atypical presentations of tuberculosis occur most commonly at CD4 $<200 \times 10^6$/L; non-tuberculous mycobacteria, Kaposi's sarcoma, and lymphoma occur late in the disease (CD4 $<50 \times 10^6$/L). A recent increase in CD4 count (following the introduction of HAART) may suggest an immune reconstitution inflammatory syndrome (IRIS, see opposite).

Blood cultures should be taken prior to antimicrobial treatment. Bacteraemia is relatively common with bacterial pneumonia in HIV, particularly with *S. pneumoniae* infection. Bacteraemic tuberculosis may occur in advanced disease.

Other blood tests Raised inflammatory markers are a non-specific finding.

Sputum Induced sputum may assist the diagnosis of PCP and mycobacterial disease. Induced sputum has a sensitivity of about 60% for the diagnosis of PCP. Tuberculosis is more likely to be smear-negative in the setting of HIV, as cavitation in these patients is less common. Induced sputum should ideally be obtained in a negative-pressure room.

Other cultures Consider sampling urine, stool, lymph node, or bone marrow in suspected mycobacterial disease, as extrapulmonary disease is common.

CT chest is useful in looking for evidence of respiratory disease in patients with symptoms but a normal CXR, and may be helpful in directing invasive diagnostic procedures. CT is also of benefit in the diagnosis and staging of Kaposi's sarcoma and lymphoma.

Immune reconstitution inflammatory syndrome (IRIS) [immune restoration disease (IRD) or paradoxical reaction] is a fairly poorly defined clinical syndrome resulting from restored immunity to infectious or non-infectious antigens, following the introduction of HAART. The mechanism is uncertain, but probably includes partial recovery of the immune system or an exuberant host-antigen response with host genetic susceptibility. It is more likely in the context of current infection due to mycobacteria, herpes, varicella, and CMV. The clinical features are variable and diverse, and depend on the underlying infectious or non-infectious agent. A clinically silent infection may be 'unmasked' as the CD4 count rises, and may be associated with an excessive inflammatory response.

The commonest clinical features are fever, lymphadenopathy, and worsening respiratory symptoms. New pulmonary infiltrates and pleural effusions are common. TB-IRIS tends to develop within 2 months of the start of HAART, and CNS TB-IRIS is reported up to 10 months after HAART initiation.

Corticosteroids seem to be effective although no RCT data exist. Various regimes are suggested, including methylprednisolone 40 mg bd and prednisolone 20–70 mg od for up to 7 weeks. Infectious agents must also be treated and, in the very unwell, this may mean empirical treatment for PCP and TB, and high-dose steroids, whilst awaiting confirmatory microbiology.

Further investigations and treatment

Bronchoscopy and BAL

- Bronchoscopy and BAL are safe and frequently diagnostic in this patient group, and should be considered early in management, particularly in the presence of a diffuse CXR abnormality or following non-diagnostic induced sputum analysis. BAL should also be considered in patients with a localized CXR abnormality that has not responded to a trial of broad-spectrum antibiotics
- BAL fluid analysis: routine microscopy and culture for bacteria; additional stains and culture for fungi, mycobacteria, *Nocardia*; silver or immunofluorescence stain for *Pneumocystis*; cytology, including flow cytometry for malignant cells; viral serology. Consider additional tests such as *Cryptococcus* antigen detection or CMV PCR
- Both *Nocardia* and *Rhodococcus equi* stain weakly acid-fast, and may be confused with mycobacteria
- Kaposi's sarcoma appears as 'raised bruises' in the trachea or bronchi on bronchoscopy; routine biopsy is not recommended, as diagnostic yield is low and significant haemorrhage may occur.

Lung biopsy If bronchoscopy and BAL are non-diagnostic, consider repeat bronchoscopy with TBB or surgical lung biopsy. TBB has a greater sensitivity than BAL, but potentially serious complications, such as pneumothorax or haemorrhage are significantly more common.

Treatment

- Consider broad-spectrum antibiotics and empirical treatment for PCP (high-dose co-trimoxazole, and steroids if the patient is in respiratory failure p 478). BAL *Pneumocystis* stains remain positive for up to 2 weeks despite treatment, and so empirical treatment for PCP should not be delayed if the patient is unwell and this diagnosis is suspected
- Further antimicrobial treatment can be directed at specific pathogens isolated from BAL or biopsy. CMV is commonly isolated from BAL fluid, but rarely, if ever, causes lung disease in the setting of HIV and the value of antiviral treatment in such cases is unknown
- Supportive therapy with oxygen; consider NIV. ITU admission for invasive ventilation may be required. PCP is the commonest cause of respiratory failure requiring ITU admission in HIV-positive patients. Mortality from PCP requiring mechanical ventilation is about 60%, although it may be significantly higher in patients with low CD4 counts
- Steroids may be effective in the treatment of non-specific interstitial pneumonitis and lymphocytic interstitial pneumonitis.

Causes of respiratory disease in HIV infection

(Commoner causes in bold)

Infectious

Bacteria

- ***Streptococcus pneumoniae***
- ***Haemophilus influenzae***
- ***Staphylococcus aureus***
- ***Gram-negative bacteria, especially Pseudomonas***
- *Nocardia*
- *Rhodococcus equi.*

Mycobacteria

- ***Mycobacterium tuberculosis***
- ***Mycobacterium avium-intracellulare***
- *Mycobacterium kansasii.*

Viruses

- Influenza
- Para-influenza
- Respiratory syncytial virus
- Herpes simplex
- Adenovirus.

Fungi

- ***Pneumocystis jiroveci***
- *Aspergillus* spp.
- *Cryptococcus neoformans*
- Endemic mycoses.

Parasites

- *Strongyloides stercoralis* (hyperinfection syndrome—rare).

Non-infectious

- **IRIS**
- **Kaposi's sarcoma**
- Lymphoma
- Drug-induced lung disease
- Non-specific interstitial pneumonitis
- Lymphocytic interstitial pneumonitis
- Cardiogenic pulmonary oedema
- Increased risk of lung cancer.

Commonest causes of *pleural effusion* in HIV infection are Kaposi's sarcoma, parapneumonic effusion, tuberculosis, PCP, and lymphoma.

Chapter 14
Sleep and ventilation

History

The problem Sleep apnoea and related problems are now a common reason for referral to many respiratory units. This is due to a much better recognition of the syndromes and the increasing prevalence of obesity in the general population. Most respiratory units with sleep services are seeing patients primarily for possible obstructive sleep apnoea (OSA) and, therefore, most patients tend to be sleepy and referrals for insomnia are not usually encouraged.

Patients arrive at a respiratory sleep unit for several different reasons. They are commonly:

- Concerns that the patient may have sleep apnoea, with or without a full house of symptoms
- Loud snoring, with the patient or spouse seeking advice about noise reduction
- Referrals from the ENT department who may be considering offering surgery for snoring and wish to exclude OSA first
- Excessive daytime sleepiness, diagnosis unclear, might just be OSA, might be narcolepsy, etc.
- Assessment pre bariatric surgery as prevalence of OSA very high
- Other nocturnal symptoms such as sleep walking, panic arousals, etc.

Thus in sleep out-patients the issues revolve around making the correct diagnosis of the excessive daytime sleepiness or nocturnal symptoms (and referring on if appropriate), offering simple advice for snoring, or putting the patient through the nasal continuous positive airway pressure (CPAP) induction programme.

Some units perform a sleep study first on the basis of an appropriate referral letter as it is more efficient, others see the patient first and then book a sleep study if indicated. For the purposes of this account it is assumed that the patient is seen first.

History A clear history of the exact presenting complaint is obviously necessary, concentrating on the following points when OSA is suspected (a full discussion is available in the section on OSA, p 567).

- Sleepiness: how severe, what does it interfere with, over how long has it been coming on, and does it reduce quality of life? The Epworth sleepiness scale is useful to assess this (see p 89). This is scored out of 24; 0–9 is considered normal and >9 excessively sleepy. It is only a guide and should be interpreted with the overall history
- Important to differentiate sleepiness (tendency to nod off, due to inadequate sleep) from tiredness (feelings of exhaustion due to many causes, often without a tendency to nod off)
- Snoring and apnoeas. Best assessed from a witness: how loud, continuous, intermittent, and are there recognized 'stopping breathing' or choking episodes during sleep?
- Other OSA symptoms, such as nocturia and restless sleep
- History of weight and neck size increases over the last 5–10 years (recent weight gains common)

- History of nasal or other ENT surgery (previous palate surgery increases discomfort of CPAP)
- Previous medical history (certain risk factors such as mandibular surgery, hypothyroidism, acromegaly, Down's, Prader–Willi, etc.)
- Previous cardiovascular/cerebrovascular history and hypertension history (may influence decision to treat)
- Alcohol and smoking history
- Occupation and shift working
- Driving issues, such as sleepiness while driving and 'near misses' or actual sleep-related accidents
- Does the patient drive for a living and what kind of vehicle or licence?

If OSA seems unlikely, then other causes of sleepiness need to be considered, concentrating on the commonest.

Alternative diagnoses for excessive daytime sleepiness

- Depression, often missed
- Lifestyle issues—alcohol, late night working, shift work, caffeine abuse, family circumstances, etc.
- Drugs—some of the antihypertensives (e.g. β-blockers) and psychoactive drugs (e.g. antidepressants and anxiolytics) can provoke sleepiness
- Narcolepsy—e.g. associated with cataplexy (sudden loss of muscle tone in response to excitement or anticipation), sleep paralysis (frightening paralysis on wakening for a few seconds or minutes), and prolific vivid dreaming, often at sleep onset or during daytime naps
- Periodic limb movements during sleep (associated with restless legs during the day, especially in renal failure)
- Post-severe head injury or cranial irradiation (hypothalamic damage)
- Post-infectious (e.g. Epstein–Barr virus)
- Idiopathic (sometimes hereditary)
- Certain neurological disorders such as myotonic dystrophy, Parkinson's, and previous stroke
- Simply being at the sleepier end of the normal spectrum
- The symptom may really be tiredness, such as in 'ME' or insomnia, when the ESS is usually low
- Blind insomnia/sleepiness—circadian problem when 24-h cycle not linked with the real world through blue light exposure and melatonin production.

Examination and investigations

Examination of these patients is often relatively unhelpful.

In OSA the main features to look for are:

- Neck circumference (best measure of the obesity contribution to the cause of OSA, >17 in) and BMI
- Oropharynx, usually crowded with boggy mucosa, with perhaps large tonsils
- Teeth, crowding suggests retrognathia/micrognathia (and mandibular advancement devices require sound teeth)
- Nasal patency (how easy will nasal CPAP be?).

Also:

- Assessment of respiratory function, signs of cor pulmonale, FEV_1/VC ratio and SaO_2 (COPD increases likelihood of being in type II ventilatory failure, so-called 'overlap syndrome')
- Blood pressure (may influence decision to treat OSA)
- Evidence of endocrine abnormalities: hypothyroidism, acromegaly, Cushing's, diabetes.

It may also be appropriate to look for:

- Evidence of a neuromuscular disorder, including a previous stroke
- Evidence of heart failure (central sleep apnoea, or Cheyne–Stokes respiration, which can produce overnight oximetry traces similar to those of OSA).

Clinic tests to perform

- Blood gas estimation if respiratory failure suspected (these OSA patients require more urgent treatment)
- Thyroid function (hypothyroidism not always clinically obvious) plus other hormones if indicated
- Routine haematology and biochemistry (prevalence of type II diabetes will be high in this overweight population)
- Some would recommend a fuller cardiovascular risk assessment including cholesterol, fasting triglycerides, glucose, and folate since these patients are often in a high risk group (untreated 10-year cardiovascular event risk typically predicted to be about 35%).

Other scenarios If it is known already from a prior sleep study that the patient has OSA, then the clinic appointment will revolve around a joint decision between the doctor and the patient as to whether a trial of treatment is indicated (usually nasal CPAP). This will depend mainly on the severity of symptoms vs. the perceived inconvenience of the treatment. An abnormal sleep study is not a reason in its own right to prescribe CPAP. Weight loss is important, but rarely achievable, and other treatable causes of OSA must not be missed (e.g. hypothyroidism, tonsillar hypertrophy) simply because nasal CPAP is available.

If the patient has come via ENT and is being considered for pharyngeal surgery, then the respiratory physician's role is to dissuade the patient from this route as the objective success rate is poor and the hazards significant. The presence of significant OSA is a contraindication to surgery. All other approaches to snoring, such as the use of mandibular advancement devices, should be considered first, and pharyngeal surgery regarded as the last resort of the totally desperate.

EPWORTH SLEEPINESS SCALE

Name:..........................Hospital number....................... Date:.......................

Your age (Yrs)...........Your sex (Male = M / Female = F).................

- How likely are you to doze off or fall asleep in the situations described in the box below, in contrast to feeling just tired?
- This refers to your usual way of life in recent times.
- Even if you haven't done some of these things recently try to work out how they would have affected you.
- Use the following scale to choose the most appropriate number for each situation:-

0 = Would never doze
1 = Slight chance of dozing
2 = Moderate chance of dozing
3 = High chance of dozing

Situation	Chance of dozing
Sitting and reading	❑
Watching TV	❑
Sitting, inactive in a public place (e.g. a theatre or a meeting)	❑
As a passenger in a car for an hour without a break	❑
Lying down to rest in the afternoon when circumstances permit	❑
Sitting and talking to someone	❑
Sitting quietly after a lunch without alcohol	❑
In a car, while stopped for a few minutes in the traffic	❑
Thank you for your cooperation Total score =	❑

Fig 14.1 Epworth Sleepiness Scale questionnaire.

Chapter 15

Unexplained ventilatory failure

Causes

Definition Ventilatory failure is conventionally divided into type I (hypoxia only, PaO_2 <8 kPa) and type II (hypoxia and hypercapnia, $PaCO_2$ >6 kPa): they are conceptually quite different. Type I is an increased alveolar-to-arterial (A–a) oxygen gradient (implying increased ventilation/perfusion mismatch, V/Q), with adequate alveolar ventilation to maintain a normal $PaCO_2$. The number of causes is vast, including most of respiratory medicine, and requires the usual 'history, examination, and investigations'.

A more difficult, less common, clinical scenario is an unexplained rise in $PaCO_2$ (>6 kPa, type II), with no obvious cause following a standard assessment. This may occur in the out-patient, ward, A&E, or ICU setting.

Pathophysiology A rise in $PaCO_2$ can be due to V/Q mismatch with inadequate compensatory hyperventilation, e.g. overwhelming asthma, when there will also be a large A–a gradient indicating this increased V/Q mismatch. However, it can also be due to inadequate ventilatory drive, or primary ventilatory pump failure, where the A–a gradient will usually be normal. The list below contains mainly the causes that might not have been suspected from the initial assessment, but for completeness also includes more obvious causes. The conditions with asterisks are the ones most commonly discovered when the cause is not immediately obvious.

Failure of drive

Brainstem abnormality

- Polio and post-polio syndrome* (exact mechanism unclear)
- Brainstem stroke (involvement of respiratory centres bilaterally)
- Arnold–Chiari malformation—herniation of cerebellum into foramen magnum compressing the brainstem
- Syringobulbia—expansion of a fluid compartment in the middle of the spinal cord extending up into the medulla (can be associated with Arnold–Chiari malformation)
- Surgical damage during operations for Arnold–Chiari and syringobulbia
- Encephalitis
- Brainstem tumour
- Congenital—usually presents soon after birth, can be later; abnormalities of neural crest development due to increased number of 'alanine repeats' in one of the homeobox genes (PHOX2B)

Suppression

- Sedative drugs, including alcohol, opiates, etc.*
- Metabolic alkalosis (hypokalaemic alkalosis, diuretic-induced, prolonged vomiting)

Pump failure

Neurological (particularly if diaphragm involved)

- Myopathies
    - Acid maltase deficiency (Pompe's), diaphragm paralysis commonly occurs early on*
    - Duchenne muscular dystrophy
    - Myotonic dystrophy
    - Several other very rare primary or secondary myopathies, e.g. limb girdle, hypothyroid, drugs (hydroxychloroquine)
- Neuropathy
    - Motor neuron disease (MND)* can affect diaphragm early on
    - Bilateral diaphragm paralysis*, e.g. trauma, bilateral neuralgic amyotrophy (also known as 'brachial neuritis', inflammatory damage to nerves of lower brachial plexus—cause unknown)
    - Guillain–Barré
    - Spinal muscular atrophy, autosomal recessive, spinal cord motor neurons
    - High cord transection
- Neuromuscular junction abnormalities
    - Myasthenia gravis*
    - Lambert–Eaton Myasthenic syndrome (LEMS)
    - Anti-acetylcholine esterase poisoning (usually from organophosphate insecticides)
- Mixed
    - Post- ITU ('critical care neuropathy'), post muscle relaxant drugs*

Chest wall

- Obesity*
- Scoliosis*
- Post thoracoplasty (usually 'three stage', many ribs caved in starting from the top down—done for tuberculosis prior to effective chemotherapy)
- Flail chest
- Pneumothorax/large effusion
- Severe ankylosing spondilitis

Airways obstruction/mixed

- Unrecognized COPD/severe asthma*
- Obstructive sleep apnoea and additional COPD/obesity/muscle weakness*, sometimes called 'overlap syndrome'.

The ventilatory loading effects of obesity, COPD, and OSA can summate to produce ventilatory failure, when on their own they would not be regarded as of sufficient severity. Estimating the contribution each is making to an individual's ventilatory failure can influence therapy, and expectations of success: e.g. if OSA dominant (>4% SaO_2 dips/h >30) the ventilatory failure is likely to respond to CPAP; dominant COPD (FEV_1 <25% predicted) will need maximal lower airways dilator therapy (thresholds only for general guidance); but the likely poor response of the lower airways obstruction will mean that even limited additional weight reduction, and/or treatment of milder OSA, may be useful in the latter situation.

Clinical presentation

Slow onset

In several of the above conditions, e.g. acid maltase deficiency, MND, and scoliosis, the onset of ventilatory failure can be insidious and include:

- General fatigue and/or hypersomnolence
- Headaches on awakening
- Morning confusion
- Morning cyanosis
- Ankle oedema (fluid retention, cor pulmonale, from the hypoxia).
- Dyspnoea standing in the swimming pool (this usually indicates diaphragm paralysis, as pressure of water, even at 1 m depth, pushes unopposed diaphragm further up into the chest)
- Swallowing difficulties (often MND), or other evidence of a more generalized proximal neuromuscular problem.

Rapid onset

Sometimes the significance of these symptoms is missed for a while and a relatively trivial respiratory tract infection tips the balance and the patient goes into severe ventilatory failure with coma. These individuals will end up ventilated on ICU and may be difficult to wean, or present again with ventilatory failure a few weeks after discharge.

Further information

Resta O *et al.* Sleep-related breathing disorders, loud snoring and excessive daytime sleepiness in obese subjects. *Int J Obes Relat Metab Disord* 2001; **25**: 669-75

Clinical assessment and management

History, examination, and investigations

History Carefully taken history, e.g. symptoms of subtle weakness prior to presentation, episode of shoulder pain (neuralgic amyotrophy), past history of polio, orthopnoea (diaphragm weakness), drug history. Often this is not available as the patient may present unconscious.

Examination Thorough examination, particularly neurological, e.g. fasciculation, diaphragm weakness (inward drawing of abdomen on inspiration or sniffing—masked if on positive pressure ventilation), myotonia, as well as rarer signs seen in some of the conditions listed previously.

Blood gases taken breathing air (following >20 min off extra O_2)

- Degree of CO_2 retention
- Presence of a base excess indicating chronicity of CO_2 retention
- Calculate A–a gradient to detect any V/Q mismatch (p 792)
- In pure hypoventilation there should be no significant A–a gradient (<2 kPa), unless there is associated basal atelectasis from poor lung expansion and/or obesity.

Pulmonary function tests (p 827)

- Presence of unexpected severe airways obstruction
- Reduced vital capacity (neurological or chest wall)
- Further fall of VC (>20% definitely abnormal) on lying down—indicative of diaphragm paralysis. A supine VC of <25% predicted is most predictive of this being the main cause of the raised $PaCO_2$.
- Mouth pressures, sniff pressures, or trans-diaphragmatic pressures; not much more helpful than lying and standing VC.

Specific tests—for some of the conditions listed above such as:

- EMG studies–MND, myotonia
- MRI–Gadolinium enhanced: Arnold–Chiari, brainstem lesion, syrinx
- CPK–Some myopathies
- Sleep study–E.g. (i) REM hypoxia (early marker of ventilatory failure when supine VC usually has dropped below 60% predicted normal), (ii) continuous nocturnal hypoventilation (when supine VC has dropped below 40% predicted), and (iii) obstructive sleep apnoea
- Blood film for abnormal lymphocyte cytoplasmic vacuolation (mainly acid maltase deficiency)
- Muscle biopsy–acid maltase deficiency (glycogen-containing vacuoles and low enzyme levels).

Management of the underlying condition, if available, is paramount. Weak expiratory muscles and weak laryngeal adduction prevent effective coughing with an increased incidence of serious chest infections. Clearing retained secretions can be a major problem. Physiotherapists can help teach patients and their carers sputum clearance techniques. Increasing the lung volume with positive pressure devices (e.g. the Bird device) and 'breath stacking' allows a higher expiratory flow with improved clearance. Mechanical insufflator/exsufflator devices are available that both increase inspiratory volume and speed expiratory flows. Their role is still being evaluated.

Lying down and sleeping with the ***whole bed tipped head up*** by about 20° greatly improves ventilation in the presence of bilateral diaphragm paralysis. Just elevating the top half of the bed, leaving the abdomen and legs horizontal, does not work. The abdominal contents have to descend into the pelvis to effectively 'offload' the diaphragm. This posture will also improve the ability to wean from assisted ventilation.

In the situation of irreversibility, the decision will need to be taken as to whether non-invasive ventilation is appropriate (p 693).

Part 2

Clinical conditions

Chapter 16

Acute respiratory distress syndrome

Pathophysiology and diagnosis

Definition and epidemiology ARDS (previously shock lung) is not a single entity, but represents the severe end of a spectrum of acute lung injury due to many different insults. Essentially it is:

- Acute, persistent, lung inflammation, increased vascular permeability
- Bilateral and extensive infiltrates on the CXR
- Very poor oxygenation despite PEEP with variable ways of defining the severity of this. PaO_2/FiO_2 ratio <27 using kPa, or <200 using mmHg.
- e.g. PaO_2 only 10 kPa on 0.60 (60%) O_2, ratio = 16.7, therefore <27
- Not due to clinical left ventricular failure or associated with a wedge pressure of over 18 mmHg (i.e. non-cardiogenic)
- Most commonly seen on the ITU where about 10% of such patients will have ARDS depending on the definition.

The Murray lung injury score, grading ARDS, is based on plain CXR findings, oxygenation, PEEP level, and respiratory system compliance (see p 105).

Pathophysiology Inflammatory damage to the alveoli, either by locally produced pro-inflammatory mediators, or remotely produced and arriving via the pulmonary artery. The change in pulmonary capillary permeability allows fluid and protein leakage into the alveolar spaces with pulmonary infiltrates. The alveolar surfactant is diluted with loss of its stabilizing effect, resulting in diffuse alveolar collapse and stiff lungs. This leads to:

- Gross impairment of V/Q matching with shunting causing arterial hypoxia and very large A–a gradients. There are usually enough remaining functioning alveoli such that a degree of hyperventilation maintains CO_2 clearance; thus hypercapnia is infrequently a problem
- Pulmonary hypertension will develop secondary to the hypoxia, but this is probably helpful (aids V/Q matching), rather than deleterious
- Reduced compliance (stiff lungs) due to loss of functioning alveoli (alveolar collapse, filled with fluid and protein) and hyperinflation of remaining alveoli to their limits of distension.

There are many causes of pro-inflammatory mediator release sufficient to cause ARDS and there may be more than one present. Common causes in order of prevalence:

- Sepsis/pneumonia; secondary risk factors for developing ARDS, when septic, are alcoholism and cigarette smoking
- Gastric aspiration (even if on a proton pump inhibitor, indicating that a low pH is not the only damaging component)
- Trauma/burns, via sepsis, lung trauma, smoke inhalation, fat emboli, and possibly direct effects of large amounts of necrotic tissue.

Less common causes

- Transfusion-related acute lung injury (TRALI), caused by any blood product (possibly due to HLA/white blood cell antibodies, commoner with older blood products, >6 units); usually occurs within a few hours of transfusion. No specific therapy or evidence of steroid response
- Transplanted lung—worse if the lung poorly preserved

- Post-bone marrow transplant as bone marrow recovers
- Drug overdose, e.g. tricyclic antidepressants, opiates, cocaine, aspirin
- Acute pancreatitis
- Near drowning
- Following upper airway obstruction; mechanism unclear
- Acute form of UIP/CFA. Also called AIP and used to be known as acute Hamman–Rich syndrome (p 272).

The course of ARDS is fairly characteristic

Phase 1 is the early period of alveolar damage and hypoxaemia with pulmonary infiltration.

Phase 2 develops after a week or so as the pulmonary infiltrates resolve, and on histology seems to be associated with an increase in type II pneumocytes (surfactant producers), myofibroblasts, and early collagen formation.

Phase 3 if the patient survives, is the fibrotic stage that leaves the lung with cysts, deranged micro-architecture, and much fibrosis on histology.

Clinical features ARDS should be considered in any patient with a predisposing risk factor who develops severe hypoxaemia, stiff lungs, and a widespread diffuse pulmonary infiltrate. Approximately 1–2 days following the clinical presentation of the precipitating cause (sepsis, aspiration, etc.), there is rapidly worsening dyspnoea (± a dry cough) and hypoxaemia, requiring rapidly escalating amounts of supplemental oxygen up to 100% via a non-rebreathe system (p 704). Coarse crackles in the chest. Intubation and ventilation are nearly always required, although initiating CPAP via a face-mask at 5–10 cmH_2O with 100% O_2 can improve oxygenation temporarily.

Diagnosis There are no specific tests that allow a confident diagnosis, and exclusion of other more specifically treatable diagnoses is required. The cause for the ARDS needs to be established and prevented from continuing or reccurring if possible. The CXR or CT show diffuse alveolar infiltrates and air bronchograms, similar in appearance to cardiogenic pulmonary oedema or diffuse pulmonary haemorrhage. Left ventricular failure may be excluded on clinical grounds or by echocardiography, but confident exclusion requires a wedge pressure measurement less than 18 mmHg. Diffuse alveolar haemorrhage can occur in Goodpasture's, Wegener's, and SLE; clues will include a drop in haemoglobin, blood in the airways and pulmonary secretions, and other clinical features of one of these disorders. Some pulmonary infections (e.g. mycobacteria, *Legionella*, PCP, viral pneumonia) may mimic ARDS and lavage fluid may reveal these. Some centres advocate lung biopsy to exclude alternatives, although the diagnostic yield is very low if a lavage is negative. Occasionally, cancer and lymphangitis carcinomatosa can also mimic ARDS, and these will show on a lung biopsy.

Management and complications

Management The essential aspects of management are to treat the precipitating cause, provide best supportive care with adequate oxygenation, and avoid further damage from barotrauma, hyperoxia, and nosocomial infections. Mechanical ventilation with PEEP and high inflation pressures are almost always required to maintain oxygenation (%SaO_2 values in the low 90s are entirely adequate). There is some evidence that high inflation pressures may worsen ARDS directly (micro-barotrauma); therefore, try to maintain plateau pressures <30 mmHg.

Many special ventilation techniques have been tried to reduce the high inflation pressures that result from the stiff lungs (low compliance). For example, using low tidal volumes to reduce inflation pressures (6 mL/kg ideal body weight compared with 12 mL/kg) reduces mortality by 10%. Reducing the minute ventilation and allowing the $PaCO_2$ to rise (permissive hypercapnia), also reduces the inflation pressures.

Prone ventilation has been tried in an attempt to improve V/Q matching and initial increases in PaO_2 are observed, but with no apparent effect on survival.

Several different artificial surfactants have been tried to try and improve lung compliance, although good delivery to the abnormal areas is unlikely. Although effective in animal models, the RCTs have been negative in humans.

Different degrees of hydration have been compared, with reduced fluid balances improving gas exchange, but again with no impact on survival (but no harm either).

High-dose steroids have been used, but there is evidence of harm as well as benefit, and minimal evidence of overall improved survival. A recent meta-analysis concluded there was no overall significant benefit, but certain subgroups may do slightly better and others worse: e.g. steroids are possibly beneficial during the first 14 days, but detrimental thereafter. A recent RCT (total $n = 91$) on prolonged methylprednisolone infusion (1 mg/kg/day) for early ARDS (<72 h) showed improvement in a number of outcomes and halved mortality.

Extracorporeal oxygenation/CO_2 removal will buy time and allow the lung to 'rest', but these techniques are very expensive and it is difficult to demonstrate any long-term benefit.

Complications of ARDS include:

- The high ventilation pressures lead to barotrauma: pneumothorax, surgical emphysema, pneumomediastinum. Pneumothorax may be lethal, but difficult to detect on a CXR in the supine patient
- Nosocomial infections occur in about half the patients, making surveillance bronchoalveolar lavage important
- Myopathy associated with long-term neuromuscular blockade, high steroid doses, and poor glycaemic control
- Non-specific problems of venous thromboembolism, GI haemorrhage, inadequate nutrition.

Prognosis has improved over the last 20 years, probably due to improvements in supportive care rather than an ability to modify the inflammatory process and its subsequent repair. Prognosis is worse with intra-pulmonary causes. Early deaths are usually due to the precipitating condition, and later deaths to complications. Over half the patients will survive with varying residual lung damage, although the pulmonary function tests often show only minor restrictive abnormalities (and reduced kCO), indicating the considerable capacity of the lung to recover.

Future developments

- The optimal level of PEEP in a particular patient is difficult to predict. Inadequate PEEP allows more atelectasis, but too high PEEP contributes to over-distension of remaining alveoli and further barotrauma when there are no more 'recruitable' alveoli. Ways to estimate the best PEEP are under investigation. High-frequency ventilation has been around a long while, but its place in ARDS is still unclear. More recently, liquid ventilation with perfluorocarbons has been tried. These dense oxygen-carrying liquids reduce the heterogeneity of ventilation by nullifying the requirement for surfactant, thus recruiting the collapsed alveoli. There are improvements in oxygenation but no evidence yet of increased long-term survival.
- Nitric oxide (NO) has been tried with clear improvements in oxygenation, but very little effect on survival. The mode of action is not clear and may be more than just vasodilatation. Inhaled prostacyclin is similarly unconvincing. Anti-inflammatory and anti-oxidant therapies are still very much in the experimental phase. There are current trials looking at low-dose inhaled carbon monoxide as an anti-inflammatory.
- Biomarkers from either blood or bronchoalveolar lavage are being investigated as to their potential to predict steroid responsiveness (e.g. procollagen).
- 'Off the shelf' artificial lung systems are now becoming clinically useful to buy time while the lungs recover. The Novalung is an example, but such therapy is very expensive.

Further information

Murray ARDS score calculation, *www.cesar-trial.org* (Scroll down to just above 'Cesar site contents')

Efficacy and safety of corticosteroids for persistent acute respiratory distress syndrome. NHLBI ARDS clinical trials network. *NEJM* 2006; **354**: 1671–84

Slutsky AS and Hudson LD. PEEP or no PEEP. *NEJM* 2006; **354**: 1839–41

Wheeler A and Bernard G. Acute lung injury and the acute respiratory distress syndrome: a clinical review. *Lancet* 2007; **369**: 1553–64

Meduri GU *et al.* Methylprednisolone infusion in early severe ARDS: results of a randomized controlled trial. *Chest* 2007; **131**: 945–6

http://medgadget.com/archives/2007/02/novalung_ila_me.html (Novalung)

Chapter 17

Asbestos and the lung

Asbestos

Asbestos consists of a family of naturally occurring hydrated silicate fibres that may be subdivided into two groups:

- Curly *serpentine* fibres, of which chrysotile (white) is the only fibre currently in commercial use
- Straight needle-like *amphiboles*, which comprise crocidolite (blue), amosite (brown), anthophyllite, tremolite, and actinolite

Fibres differ in their lung clearance kinetics and pathogenic potential; amphibole fibres clear more slowly from the lung and are more carcinogenic than chrysotile. Whilst asbestos usage in developed countries is restricted, the use of chrysotile asbestos in developing economies continues to rise.

Mechanisms of exposure

Occupational exposure accounts for the majority of cases of asbestos-related disease and includes:

- Mining, milling, and transport of asbestos
- Use of asbestos products, e.g. in construction and demolition, floor tiling, insulation, fireproofing, textiles, friction materials (brake linings), ship building, pipefitting, electrical repair, boiler fitting and lagging, carpentry, plumbing, and welding.

Domestic exposure may include:

- Relatives of asbestos workers exposed to 'carry home' asbestos in hair or clothes
- Following remodelling or renovation in contaminated buildings
- Local geological exposure from natural deposits, e.g. areas of central and south-east Turkey, north-west Greece, and Corsica
- Urban environment (although undisturbed and non-friable asbestos building insulation is not considered hazardous).

A complete occupational history is essential if asbestos-related disease is suspected, and should include the method of exposure with dates and names of employers. This information may be of medico-legal importance and ideally should be elicited during the first consultation.

Asbestos-related lung disease comprises:

- Benign asbestos-related pleural disease
  - Pleural plaques
  - Benign asbestos-related pleural effusion
  - Diffuse pleural thickening
  - Rounded atelectasis
- Asbestosis
- Mesothelioma
- Lung cancer.

Other diseases linked to asbestos exposure include pericarditis and, perhaps, head and neck, and gastrointestinal cancers. Whether asbestos exposure truly leads to an increased risk of lung cancer in the absence of asbestosis remains controversial.

Asbestos-related disease typically exhibits a long latency period of 20–40 years from exposure. Peak industrial asbestos use in the UK occurred in the early 1970s, and asbestos-related disease is likely to remain common for at least the next 20 years. The incidence of mesothelioma is forecast to peak in 2015–2020 in Europe.

All deaths should be notified to the coroner if asbestos-related disease is suspected or proven.

Benign asbestos-related pleural disease

Pleural plaques

- Most common manifestation of asbestos exposure
- Discrete areas of white or yellow thickening on the parietal pleura; may calcify
- Bilateral and occur particularly on the posterolateral chest wall, over the mediastinal pleura, and on the dome of the diaphragm
- Develop 20–30 years after exposure; incidence (but not the extent of plaques) increases with longer duration of exposure; found in up to 50% of asbestos-exposed workers and may also occur after low-dose exposures
- Usually asymptomatic, although if extensive may be associated with mild breathlessness due to pleural restriction
- Effect on pulmonary function is uncertain: most studies have failed to demonstrate abnormal lung function, although otherwise unexplained mild airways obstruction or restriction has been described in some populations of asbestos workers with pleural plaques—the mechanism of this is unclear, although it may reflect asbestos-induced small airway disease or early interstitial fibrosis, respectively
- HRCT is more sensitive than CXR in detecting pleural plaques
- There is no evidence that plaques are pre-malignant
- No longer eligible for compensation (p 118)
- Tuberculosis, trauma, and haemothorax may each cause single pleural plaques; multiple plaques are highly suggestive of asbestos exposure, however.

Benign asbestos-related pleural effusions

- Relatively early manifestation of asbestos pleural disease; usually occurs within 10 years of exposure
- Development is considered to be dose-dependent, although can occur after minimal exposure
- Typically small and unilateral, and may be asymptomatic or occasionally associated with pleuritic pain, fever, and dyspnoea
- Usually resolve spontaneously over a few months, although some recur
- The pleural effusion is an exudate, often bloodstained, with no characteristic findings on pleural fluid analysis
- Diagnosis depends on a history of asbestos exposure and the exclusion of other causes, including mesothelioma
- Benign asbestos pleurisy may precede the development of diffuse pleural thickening; there is no clear association with mesothelioma
- Treat symptomatically, with pleural aspiration for breathlessness and NSAIDs for pain.

Diffuse pleural thickening (DPT)

- Consists of extensive fibrosis of the visceral pleura with areas of adhesion with the parietal pleura and consequent obliteration of the pleural space
- Unlike pleural plaques, its margins are ill-defined, and it may involve the costophrenic angles, apices, and interlobar fissures
- Development appears to be dose-related and may follow recurrent asbestos pleurisy
- On CXR, it may be defined as a smooth uninterrupted pleural opacity extending over at least a quarter of the chest wall, with or without obliteration of the costophrenic angles; on CT, the pleural density extends more than 8 cm craniocaudally, 5 cm laterally, and is more than 3 mm thick
- Symptoms are relatively common and comprise exertional breathlessness and chest pain, which can be chronic and severe
- May lead to significant restrictive pulmonary function impairment, especially if the costophrenic angle is obliterated; hypercapnic respiratory failure has been described
- Pleural biopsy may be required to distinguish it from mesothelioma
- Treatment is difficult; decortication often fails to result in clinical or functional improvement
- Patient may be eligible for compensation (see p 118).

Rounded atelectasis

(also known as folded lung, Blesovsky syndrome, or shrinking pleuritis with atelectasis)

- Develops as contracting visceral pleural fibrosis; ensnares and then twists the underlying lung, resulting in the distinctive radiological appearance of a rounded or oval pleural-based mass of 2.5–5 cm in diameter
- Asbestos exposure is the most common cause, although any cause of pleural inflammation may result in rounded atelectasis
- CT is often diagnostic, demonstrating a 'comet tail' of vessels and bronchi converging toward the lesion, adjacent thickened pleura, and volume loss in the affected lobe
- An atypical appearance may require biopsy to exclude malignant disease
- Typically asymptomatic, although breathlessness or dry cough may occur
- Usually stable or slowly progressive, and no specific treatment is required
- Surgical decortication may improve symptoms, but frequently results in reduced lung volumes and is not generally recommended.

Further information

American Thoracic Society Statement:. Diagnosis and initial management of non-malignant diseases related to asbestos. *AJRCCM* 2004; **170**: 691–715.

Asbestosis

Definition Chronic interstitial fibrosis resulting from asbestos inhalation.

Causes Factors affecting disease development include:

- ***Degree and length of asbestos exposure***—a clear dose–response relationship exists; usually seen in workers with many years of high exposure, although may follow a very high exposure of short duration, resulting in a shorter latency period
- ***Fibre type***—amphibole fibres are probably more fibrogenic than chrysotile, although most exposures are mixed fibre types
- ***Cigarette smoking*** increases the severity and rate of progression of asbestosis.

Latency period from first exposure to clinical disease is usually at least 15–20 years and may be >40 years.

Clinical features Insidious onset of breathlessness, dry cough. Bibasal late-inspiratory crackles, clubbing in 40% of cases. May progress to respiratory failure, cor pulmonale.

Differential diagnosis includes other causes of interstitial fibrosis, particularly usual interstitial pneumonitis (UIP).

Investigations

- ***CXR*** Bilateral symmetrical reticulonodular pattern, primarily affecting the lower lobes peripherally, which may extend upwards to involve the mid and upper zones; may progress to honeycomb lung. Massive bilateral upper lobe fibrosis (without lower lobe involvement) is rare, but well described. Associated pleural thickening or plaques may be seen, and suggest a diagnosis of asbestosis, rather than UIP. Classification is based on size, thickness, and profusion of opacities. CXR insensitive to early disease; may be normal in 15–20% of symptomatic biopsy-proven asbestosis
- ***HRCT*** is more sensitive than CXR and is abnormal in 10–30% of cases with a normal CXR. Features include basal 'ground-glass' opacities (seen early in the disease), parenchymal bands, subpleural curvilinear lines and opacities, interlobular septal thickening, and signs of fibrosis (traction bronchiectasis, loss of lobular architecture, honeycombing in advanced disease)
- ***PFTs*** are classically restrictive with reduced lung volumes and transfer factor, although obstructive or mixed patterns may also occur (perhaps reflecting asbestos-induced small airway disease)
- Positive ***gallium scan*** may be seen with normal CXR; correlates poorly with lung function
- Analysis of ***sputum*** or ***bronchoalveolar* lavage** may demonstrate asbestos bodies, although sensitivity is limited. The finding of interstitial fibrosis in the absence of asbestos bodies on ***lung biopsy*** *makes* asbestosis unlikely. Analysis of material for asbestos bodies is only very rarely indicated, usually for research or litigation purposes.

In general, CXR and HRCT show only limited correlation with physiological disease severity.

Diagnosis Gold standard is pathological demonstration of fibrosis with mineralogical quantification of asbestos bodies; in practice this is rarely required and a diagnosis can be made on the basis of a history of significant asbestos exposure with appropriate delay between exposure and disease, and radiographic evidence of fibrosis.

Treatment

- No pharmacological treatment is of proven benefit
- Supportive management, including supplementary oxygen as required, influenza and pneumococcal immunization, smoking cessation, compensation if exposure was occupational (p 118).

Prognosis varies widely. After removal from exposure, progression occurs in 5–40% of patients over 10 years; progression is faster following greater exposure, although rapid progression over 1–2 years is unusual and more in keeping with UIP. Fewer CXR opacities after exposure are associated with better prognosis. Increased risk of developing lung cancer.

Mesothelioma: diagnosis

Definition Malignant tumour of serosal surfaces (most commonly the pleura) usually resulting from asbestos exposure.

Causes Asbestos is the major single cause and there is a history of occupational asbestos exposure in up to 90% of cases. All types of asbestos can cause mesothelioma—amphibole is the most potent, but also evidence for chrysotile. Mean latent interval between first exposure and death is around 40 years; cases with latency <15 years are rare. Not dose-related (unlike asbestosis or bronchogenic cancers) and no evidence for a threshold asbestos dose below which there is no risk, although the risk at low exposure levels is small. No significant association with smoking. The mechanism through which asbestos fibres result in mesothelioma is unclear; possibilities include direct irritation of the parietal pleura, disruption of mitosis, generation of toxic oxygen radicals, and stimulation of mitogen-activated kinases leading to proto-oncogene activation.

Other causes of mesothelioma include non-asbestos fibres, such as erionite, which is found in rocks in Cappadocia, Turkey—mesothelioma accounts for up to a quarter of all adult deaths in local villages. Evidence for simian virus 40 (contaminated polio vaccine in 1950s/60s) is limited. Rare cases of mesothelioma caused by ionizing radiation or chest injury are described. 'Spontaneous' mesothelioma in children is also documented.

Clinical features of pleural mesothelioma:

- Chest pain (typically dull ache, 'boring', diffuse, occasionally pleuritic), breathlessness; a small proportion are asymptomatic. Profuse sweating may occur
- Consider in any patient with a pleural effusion or pleural thickening, particularly if chest pain is present
- Rarely may present with persistent chest pain and a normal CXR
- Weight loss and fatigue uncommon at presentation (<30% of cases)
- Clubbing is very rare (<1%)
- Chest wall invasion may be seen (especially at thoracentesis sites)
- Bilateral pleural involvement is unusual at presentation
- Paraneoplastic syndromes are described, e.g. disseminated intravascular coagulation.

Differential diagnosis includes benign asbestos pleural effusion, diffuse pleural thickening, and adenocarcinoma involving the pleura.

Investigations

1. Pleural fluid aspiration typically reveals an exudative straw-coloured or bloody effusion. Cytological analysis may provide the diagnosis (sensitivity ranges 32–84%), and is often useful in excluding other pathology, e.g. adenocarcinoma. Pleural fluid glucose and pH may be low in extensive tumours. Mesothelioma may track through the chest wall along thoracocentesis sites; avoid repeated pleural aspiration if the diagnosis is suspected, and 'tattoo' aspiration sites with indelible ink to guide subsequent prophylactic radiotherapy.

*2. **Imaging*** CXR and CT features include:
- Moderate to large pleural effusion, usually with pleural nodularity and enhancement following pleural contrast and involvement of mediastinal pleura
- Localized pleural mass or thickening without free fluid
- Uniform encasement of lung resulting in small hemithorax
- Local invasion of chest wall, ribs, heart, mediastinum, hilar nodes, and diaphragm; transdiaphragmatic spread and invasion of contralateral pleura
- Associated pleural plaques or interstitial fibrosis in a minority of cases.

The role of MRI is unclear—it may provide additional information in some cases, e.g. chest wall invasion, although is rarely required. PET may have a role in distinguishing benign and malignant pleural disease as well as identifying lymph node spread for staging, although it is not widely used.

*3. **Biopsy*** The diagnosis should be confirmed histologically except when the patient is too unwell or too frail for biopsy. Ultrasound- or CT-guided cutting needle biopsy and thoracoscopic biopsy of pleural masses have a high diagnostic yield and should be used in preference to blind (Abrams') biopsy techniques. Early use of thoracoscopy may both provide a diagnosis and enable treatment of large effusions with talc pleurodesis, thereby avoiding repeated non-diagnostic procedures with attendant problems of needle-track spread.

Histological subtypes

- Epithelioid (50% of cases; may be confused with adenocarcinoma; better prognosis)
- Sarcomatoid (or fibrous)
- Mixed (biphasic).

Immunohistochemistry is key to making the diagnosis. Positive staining for calretinin indicates mesothelial origin (as opposed to adenocarcinoma), and staining for epithelial membrane antigen (EMA, also called CA15-3 and mucin-1) in a peripheral distribution strongly suggests mesothelioma. CEA staining is almost always negative in mesothelioma. Electron microscopy of histopathological specimens may also help to distinguish mesothelioma from adenocarcinoma.

Staging No widely accepted staging system. Proposed schemes include Stage I–IV scheme and TNM classification; surgery is required for final staging. Poor prognostic features include transdiaphragmatic muscle invasion and involvement of mediastinal lymph nodes, male gender, poor performance status, and sarcomatoid histology.

Further information

BTS Statement on malignant mesothelioma in the United Kingdom. *Thorax* 2007; **62**: ii1–ii19.

Robinson BW, Lake RA. Advances in malignant mesothelioma. *NEJM* 2005; **353**: 1591–1603.

Mesothelioma: treatment and outcome

Treatment

Management of pleural effusions Talc pleurodesis is the treatment of choice, and early pleurodesis is preferable to repeated pleural aspirations. This can be achieved either medically or at thoracoscopy, depending on local resources. Pleurodesis is not possible if the lung does not re-expand following drainage of pleural fluid ('trapped lung'), and the resulting recurrent pleural effusions are difficult to manage; indwelling pleural catheters allow fluid drainage without needle aspiration and are useful in this situation. The value of pleuroperitoneal shunts remains uncertain.

Radiotherapy Prophylactic radiotherapy appears to reduce chest wall invasion by tumour following pleural aspiration or biopsy: three fractions reduced the risk of tracking from 40% to 0 in a randomized study of 40 patients, although a more recent study failed to demonstrate a benefit. Recurrence may follow delayed prophylactic radiotherapy, so it is usually administered within 4 weeks. Palliative radiotherapy provides pain relief in a proportion of patients with chest wall pain, but is less useful in the treatment of breathlessness or SVCO.

Surgery There are currently no reported randomized controlled trials assessing the outcomes of radical surgery, and its use is controversial. It should be considered only in centres with experience and if there is a firm diagnosis of epithelioid mesothelioma, the patient is otherwise fit, and there is no radiological evidence of lymph node involvement. Avoid chemical pleurodesis in such cases. Operative mortality is approximately 6%. Trimodality therapy (extrapleuropneumonectomy followed by radiotherapy and chemotherapy) may have a role; trials are pending.

Chemotherapy Patients with good performance status should have the option of discussing chemotherapy with an appropriate specialist. Studies have suggested limited benefits with two different regimes. Pemetrexed (an inhibitor of certain DNA synthesis proteins, e.g. thymidylate synthase) plus cisplatin has an objective response rate (tumour shrinkage of >50%) of 41% and appears to convey a survival advantage of just under 3 months when compared with cisplatin alone; pemetrexed has recently been approved by NICE, although it is expensive and ongoing treatment of an individual may be dependent upon objective metabolic responses based on CT-PET scanning. Gemcitabine plus cisplatin led to objective response rates of 33 and 48% in two trials, with quality-of-life benefits. Trials are ongoing.

General management Early involvement of a pain relief and palliative care service is required. Ensure adequate analgesia: opiates and NSAIDs for chest wall pain; consider carbamazepine or sodium valproate for neuropathic pain (from intercostal nerve or vertebral involvement); nerve blocks or cordotomy may be required. Breathlessness may be multifactorial, e.g. pleural effusion, lung compression, chest wall restriction, pericardial involvement, anaemia, pain, anxiety, and fear. Liaise with GP, specialist nurse, palliative care teams. Remind GP that all deaths have to be reported to the coroner. Discuss compensation issues (p 118).

Clinical course Median survival is 9–12 months from diagnosis. Typically progresses by local extension, sometimes leading to involvement of the contralateral lung or peritoneum, SVCO, cardiac tamponade, or spinal cord compression. Distant metastases are common (50% at autopsy), although occur late and are rarely clinically apparent.

Peritoneal mesothelioma is rarer than pleural mesothelioma, and may be associated with more prolonged asbestos exposure. Remains intra-abdominal in most cases. Clinical features include abdominal discomfort, weight loss, ascites, and in some cases organ involvement (e.g. intestinal obstruction). Fine-needle aspiration of omental masses may provide a diagnosis, although laparoscopy is often required. Prognosis is worse than for pleural mesothelioma, with median survival 7.4 months. No treatment is of proven benefit.

Mesothelioma has also been described affecting *other serosal surfaces*, such as pericardium and tunica vaginalis.

Future developments

- Measurement of serum mesothelin-related protein (SMRP; a soluble product of the surface protein mesothelin) may have a diagnostic role: SMRP is frequently raised in patients with mesothelioma, but only very rarely in healthy controls or patients with other malignant or inflammatory lung or pleural disease
- Microarray studies of gene expression in tumour samples may prove to be useful in both distinguishing mesothelioma from adenocarcinoma and in predicting prognosis
- Novel therapeutic strategies using immunotherapy (e.g. recombinant interferon-alpha), gene therapy, anti-angiogenic agents, and photodynamic therapy are in development. Combinations of immunotherapy with chemotherapy appear particularly promising.

Compensation for asbestos-related diseases

Identification of asbestos exposure is essential for the patient to be able to claim compensation. Patients are not eligible for compensation if their exposure occurred whilst they were self-employed. There are two principal sources of compensation.

From the Government: apply to the ***Benefits Agency*** (Department of Social Security) for industrial injuries disablement benefit, using form BI100PN. Available for the following diseases:

- Diffuse pleural thickening
- Asbestosis
- Lung cancer associated with diffuse pleural thickening or asbestosis
- Mesothelioma.

There must be a clear history of asbestos exposure at work. Compensation is not available for pleural plaques alone. If successful, may then apply for a single payment from the government under the Pneumoconiosis, etc. (Worker's Compensation) Act 1979. The value of compensation reflects the degree of disability from which the patient is considered to suffer and their age at diagnosis. Next-of-kin may also claim within 6 months posthumously. The War Pensions Scheme may provide compensation for disease resulting from asbestos exposure with HM forces (form WPA1).

*From the Courts: **Common law*** compensation directly from a previous employer. Can be claimed from the employer's insurer, even if the employer is now out of existence. Advise patient to seek advice as soon as possible from a solicitor with relevant experience. Claims must be initiated within 3 years of the individual's first awareness that they have an asbestos-related disease attempts to initiate claims after 3 years may be statute barred. Inform the patient of this and document the conversation in the medical notes. A Court of Appeal ruling in March 2006 concluded that pleural plaques alone should now no longer be considered an indication for compensation, and a subsequent appeal failed to overturn this ruling in the House of Lords. Awards for asbestosis range from £15,000 to £50,000, depending on symptoms and the degree of disability; such patients may accept a greater 'once and for all' award and forego their right to further claims in the event of mesothelioma developing. Typical awards for mesothelioma are £45,000–£50,000 and additional amounts may be claimed for care and future loss of wages; total compensation may exceed £100,000. Successful claims have also been made for mesothelioma occurring in relatives who were exposed to asbestos whilst washing work clothes.

Further information

DSS Benefits Agency enquiry line 0800 882200 or 0800 2792322. Advice on available benefits and completing claim applications. Leaflets SD5 'Ill or Disabled Because of Work' and NI12 'If you have an Industrial Disease' may be helpful. Website www.dwp.gov.uk/index.asp contains further information on the Pneumoconiosis etc. (Worker's Compensation) Act 1979, as well as many useful contacts and links

London Hazards Centre. http://www.lhc.org.uk/members/pubs/books/asbestos/asb_toc.htm

Occupational and Environmental Diseases Association offers support and advice to patients and their relatives including information on solicitors and the process of compensation. PO Box 26, Enfield, Middlesex EN1 2NT. Telephone 020 8360 8490. Website www.oeda.demon.co.uk

http://www.mesoinfo.com

http://www.mesothelioma-facts.com

Chapter 18

Asthma

Definition, epidemiology, pathophysiology, aetiology

Definition There is no universally agreed definition; it is usually a clinical diagnosis—a chronic airway inflammatory disorder with inflammation due to complex interactions between inflammatory cells, mediators, and airway cells. This is characterized by airway hyperreactivity to a variety of non-specific stimuli, leading to a variable degree of airway obstruction, some of which may become irreversible over many years.

In susceptible individuals this leads to recurrent episodes of wheeze, chest tightness, breathlessness, and cough (particularly at night).

- The disease is associated with widespread and variable airflow obstruction, which may reverse spontaneously or with treatment
- Airway inflammatory changes lead to increased bronchial responsiveness to a variety of non-specific stimuli

Epidemiology It is the commonest chronic respiratory disease in the UK, with a prevalence of 10–15%. There is a wide variation in disease prevalence, with highest levels seen in English-speaking countries (where there is also a high prevalence of sensitization to common aeroallergens). The reason for the increasing worldwide prevalence over the last few decades is unclear.

Pathophysiology Best described as chronic eosinophilic bronchitis/bronchiolitis. Airway inflammation is seen, with cellular infiltration by T helper-2 (Th2) cells, lymphocytes, eosinophils, and mast cells. There is large and small airway involvement, and cytokine production (platelet activating factor and leukotrienes).

Airway obstruction occurs due to a combination of:

- Inflammatory cell infiltration
- Mucus hypersecretion with mucus plug formation
- Smooth muscle contraction

This may become irreversible over time due to:

- Basement membrane thickening, collagen deposition, and epithelial desquamation
- Airway remodelling occurs in chronic disease, with smooth muscle hypertrophy and hyperplasia. This is now recognized as increasingly important in the pathophysiology of the most difficult to treat chronic asthma

Aetiology This is due to a combination of genetic and environmental factors, with many different genes identified.

Immunological mechanisms A subgroup of asthmatics are atopic, and therefore react to antigen challenge by producing specific IgE from B lymphocytes. This leads to the formation of IgE–antigen complexes that bind to mast cells, basophils, and macrophages, leading to the release of preformed mediators, such as histamine, and eosinophil chemotactic factor. These factors cause bronchoconstriction and airway oedema.

Prostaglandins, leukotrienes, kinins, and platelet activating factor (PAF), are all important secondary messengers involved in the inflammatory response.

A subgroup of asthmatics (up to 25%) are now recognized to have non-eosinophilic disease, which may be associated with a poorer short-term response to inhaled corticosteroids, and is associated with neutrophilic airway inflammation and innate immunity.

Genetic factors A hereditary component to asthma and atopy is well established, and a number of chromosomes and linkages are implicated. The multiple mechanisms and second messengers involved in asthma make the contribution of the effects of specific genes difficult to determine. Established susceptibility loci include the genes ADAM33, GPRA (G-protein related receptor for asthma), and ORMDL3, a member of a gene family that encodes transmembrane endoplasmic reticulum proteins. The latter was very recently identified by a genome-wide screen, and its function and role in the pathogenesis of asthma is not yet clear.

Hygiene hypothesis This suggests that early life exposure to endotoxin switches off the allergic response (by reducing Th2-mediated responses), leading to reduced allergen sensitivity later in life, therefore reducing allergen-driven diseases such as asthma. Large epidemiological studies support this hypothesis.

Environmental factors The increasing prevalence of asthma appears to be associated with a rising standard of living worldwide, and not just in westernized societies. This has implicated a number of environmental factors. A number of explanations are speculated (but not proven), including dietary changes, a reduction in childhood infections, increased immunization, or a combination of all three.

Phenotypic differences It is increasingly recognized that 'asthma' is likely to represent a number of different 'diseases' or subphenotypes, rather than one disease with a unifying pathological mechanism. Subphenotypes may differ in underlying pathophysiology, clinical features, and disease course, and research aimed at clearly identifying such disease groups (for example, through the use of biomarkers or the host genetic profile) is ongoing.

Clinical features

- Cough
- Shortness of breath
- Wheeze
- Chest tightness.

Classically these are variable, intermittent, worse at night, associated with specific triggers, e.g. pollens, cat and dog dander, and non-specific triggers, e.g. cold air, perfumes, and bleaches, due to airway hypersensitivity. Asthma may be labelled 'cough variant' or 'cough predominant', when cough is the major symptom.

Examination

- May be entirely normal
- Classically expiratory wheeze is heard
- Chest deformity/hyperinflation - longstanding/poorly controlled asthma
- Severe life-threatening asthma may have no wheeze and a silent chest.

Diagnosis

This is often a clinical diagnosis but should be supported by objective measurements. Important to:

- Identify provoking factors, e.g. cold air, bleach, perfume, and environmental aeroallergens (grasses, pollen, hay), and any occupational exposures
- Assess disease severity. Longitudinal studies show greater decline in lung function in asthmatics than non-asthmatics—greater still in asthmatics who smoke.

Don't forget to look for/ask about:

- Nasal symptoms–obstruction, rhinorrhoea, hyposmia
- Atopic dermatitis/eczema/hay fever
- Allergies including food allergy
- Reflux/GORD disease (treating reflux may improve asthma control)
- Laryngo/pharyngeal reflux (hoarse voice, throat clearing, acid in throat)
- Triggers—including exercise, menstruation
- Social situation/stresses
- Aspirin sensitivity (associated with later onset asthma and nasal polyps)
- Family history.

The diagnosis is based on the presence of:

- Symptoms (cough, wheeze, breathlessness)
- Day-to-day peak flow variability (>15% variability or reversibility to inhaled β_2 agonist)
- Airway hyperresponsiveness.

Consider the diagnosis of asthma in:

- Recurrent cough, episodic breathlessness, and wheeze
- Chest tightness
- Isolated or nocturnal cough
- Exercised-induced cough or breathlessness
- Hyperventilation syndrome (p 255).

Aspirin-induced asthma (AIA)

- Defined as chronic rhinoconjunctivitis, nasal polyps, and asthma
- Asthma is precipitated by ingestion of aspirin or other NSAIDs
- Occurs in up to 20% of asthmatics, and is commoner in women
- The mechanism is thought to be via aspirin inhibition of the cyclo-oxygenase pathway, with excess leukotriene production via the lipo-oxygenase pathway
- BAL and urine in AIA patients show excess leukotrienes post aspirin exposure
- Loss of anti-inflammatory prostaglandin E2 may also be important.

Oral allergy syndrome

A subset of patients sensitized to aeroallergens, such as tree and grass pollens, develop localized lip angioedema after ingestion of specific fruits that share cross-reactive epitopes with pollen allergens. The reaction occurs immediately after ingesting the fruit. Cooked fruit is usually tolerated, presumably because the culpable proteins are denatured with cooking. Birch pollens cross-react with apples, hazelnuts, and potato. Ragwort shares epitopes with melon and bananas.

Investigations

The number of investigations required depends on the certainty of the diagnosis from the history, simple spirometry, and peak flow recordings. Most patients referred for a respiratory opinion will already have completed home peak flow recordings and have had a CXR. Repeating PEFs may still be of benefit. Objective evidence of asthma is important before starting long-term therapy with potentially harmful drugs, such as inhaled steroids.

Essential investigations (on which the diagnosis is based)

- *Peak flow recording/simple spirometry* to look for variability and response to treatment. Airway obstruction leads to decreased peak expiratory flow rate (PEFR) and forced expiratory volume in one second (FEV_1), but these may be normal between episodes of bronchospasm. If they are persistently normal, the diagnosis must be in doubt. The diagnosis is certain if:
  - 20% diurnal PEF variation on >3 days per week, in a week of peak flow diary measures
  - FEV_1 >15% decrease after 6 min exercise
  - FEV_1 >15% (or 200 mL) increase after 2 week trial of oral steroid (30 mg prednisolone od)
- *Bronchodilator reversibility testing* FEV_1 >15% (or 200 mL) increase after short-acting β_2 agonist therapy (e.g. salbutamol 400 μg by MDI with spacer or 2.5 mg by nebulizer)

Non essential/optional investigations

- *Blood tests*
  - FBC (eosinophilia—question the diagnosis if high total eosinophil count; consider Churg–Strauss syndrome)
  - IgE (associated atopy, i.e. positive skin prick tests to common allergens, often with associated allergic rhinitis and eczema)
- *Aspergillus precipitins* (*Aspergillus* sensitivity, ABPA) see Chapter 41
- Specific IgE if other environmental triggers suspected
- *CXR* if atypical symptoms. May show hyperinflation or evidence of localized abnormality simulating wheeze, e.g. adenoma (rare)
- *Skin tests* to define atopic constitution, or identify potential triggers
- *Metacholine/histamine challenge* measures bronchial hyperresponsiveness (BHR) as a PC_{20}, the dose of agent provoking a 20% fall in FEV_1.
- Asthma is suggested by a PC_{20} below 8 mg/mL. Normal subjects have a PC_{20} >16 mg/mL. The absence of BHR virtually excludes the diagnosis of asthma; however, the presence of BHR does not prove asthma.
- *Bronchial provocation tests* aim to demonstrate bronchospasm to an inhaled agent, usually occupational. The response to an aerosolized sample of a suspected agent may be useful if the diagnosis of occupational asthma is suspected, but PEF recordings at home, work, and on holiday may be more useful. Should only be carried out in a tertiary referral centre, under expert supervision

- *Sputum analysis* Sputum eosinophilia may help confirm the diagnosis
- *Laryngoscopy/ENT examination* Useful if concerns about nasal symptoms or obstruction, e.g. from polyps, or to exclude upper airway obstruction, or a vocal cord abnormality
- *Bronchoscopy* Rarely needed. Its main use is to exclude an obstructing airway tumour, e.g. carcinoid
- *Lung biopsy* is very occasionally needed in those in whom no adequate explanation for persistent and minimally reversible air flow obstruction is seen, to exclude another cause, e.g. bronchiolitis obliterans
- *Biomarkers* Studies support the use of exhaled NO to determine optimum inhaled corticosteroid dose in moderate asthma. This may also be useful in diagnosis.

Main differential diagnoses in asthma

Consider especially if unusual features in the history, or poor correlation between objective measures and symptoms, or poor treatment response:

- Upper airway obstruction (breathlessness, noisy, stridulous breathing, low peak flows out of proportion to FEV_1)
- Foreign body aspiration
- Tumour, especially tracheal (but can respond to steroids)
- CCF (young patient with a murmur)
- Vocal cord dysfunction
- Hyperventilation syndrome
- Chronic thromboembolic disease or primary pulmonary hypertension
- Interstitial lung disease
- Churg–Strauss syndrome (and other eosinophilic lung diseases)
- Bronchiolitis (p 159)
- Gastro-oesophageal reflux disease.

Acute severe asthma

Most asthma deaths occur outside hospital and are:

- In patients with chronic severe disease
- In those receiving inadequate medical treatment
- In those who have been symptomatically deteriorating and may have already sought medical help
- Associated with adverse behavioural and psychosocial factors.

Fatality in asthma is due to cardiac arrest secondary to hypoxia and acidosis—reversal of hypoxia is paramount

Give high flow oxygen

Risk factors for fatal or near fatal asthma

- Previous near fatal asthma, e.g. previous ventilation or respiratory acidosis
- Three or more classes of asthma medication
- Repeated A&E attendances
- Large β_2 agonist use
- Adverse psychosocial features
- Brittle asthma.

Brittle asthma—appears to be a particular subtype or 'phenotype'

- *Type 1*—wide PEF variability (>40% diurnal variation for >50% of the time over >150 days), despite appropriate therapy
- *Type 2*—sudden severe attacks on background of apparently good control.

Severity of acute asthma

Moderate

- Increasing symptoms
- PEFR 50–75% predicted or best
- No features of acute severe asthma
- One hour following treatment in A&E, patients with PEF >75% predicted or best may be discharged home with appropriate changes to their asthma medication in the absence of concerns, e.g.
  - Significant ongoing symptoms
  - Compliance concerns
  - Living alone
  - Psychological problems or learning difficulties
  - Previous near fatal or brittle asthma
  - Nocturnal presentation
  - Pregnant
  - Exacerbation despite adequate oral steroid pre-presentation.

Severe asthma

Defined as any of:

- PEFR 33–50% predicted or best
- RR >25
- HR >110
- Inability to complete sentence in one breath.

Life-threatening asthma

Any one of:

- PEFR <33%
- SaO_2 <92% (NB needs ABG)
- PaO_2 <8 kPa
- Normal CO_2 (4.6–6 kPa)
- Silent chest
- Cyanosis
- Poor respiratory effort
- Bradycardia/arrhythmia/hypotension
- Exhaustion
- Confusion
- Coma.

Near fatal asthma

- Raised $PaCO_2$ and/or
- Needing mechanical ventilation with raised inflation pressures.

►► Hospital treatment of acute asthma

Airway—ensure no upper airway obstruction
Breathing—give high flow oxygen
Circulation—gain IV access

Monitoring

- Record PEF on arrival in A&E, 15–30 min after starting treatment, and regularly thereafter according to response
- Record O_2 saturation and maintain ≥92%
- ABG for pH and $PaCO_2$ if saturation <93% or other severe features
- Record and document heart rate and respiratory rate
- Measure glucose and potassium
- Oxygen—high concentration (40–60%) and high flow mask, e.g. Hudson
- CXR to exclude infection/pneumothorax.

NB CO_2 retention following administration of high-flow oxygen is not a problem in acute asthma. *A high CO_2 indicates a life-threatening attack and should precipitate urgent ITU review for ventilatory support, not controlled oxygen therapy.* CO_2 is often low (due to hyperventilation). A normal CO_2 may indicate a tiring patient.

►► Hospital treatment of acute asthma (*cont.*)

Treatment

β_2 *agonist*—inhaled or nebulized, e.g. nebulized salbutamol 2.5–5 mg, driven by oxygen.
Give repeated doses, or continuous, e.g. 5–10 mg per hour.
Use IV only if inhaled therapy cannot be used reliably (rarely the case).
NB risk of hypokalaemia with β_2 agonist and steroids.

Anticholinergic—nebulized ipratropium bromide added to β_2 agonist therapy may improve bronchodilatation in acute severe asthma, if poor initial β_2 agonist response.

Steroids—the earlier given in an attack, the better the outcome.
Oral is as effective as intravenous.
Dose 40–50 mg oral prednisolone, continuing for at least 5 days or until recovery. There is no agreed definition of recovery, but sensible to continue oral steroids until peak flow is maintained for 5–7 days. The dose can be stopped abruptly (assuming the patient continues on inhaled steroid). This does not apply to patients on repeated doses, or long-term steroids, where a longer course may be appropriate.
Inhaled corticosteroids should be continued (or started as soon as possible) as part of the chronic disease management plan.

IV magnesium sulphate—immediately if very severe, and if poor response to above therapies, 1.2–2 g IV infusion over 20 min. The safety and efficacy of repeated doses has not been assessed. Recent data suggest nebulized magnesium may also be of benefit, though must be adequately diluted. Further data are awaited.

IV aminophylline—some patients may respond, give if poor response to initial therapy, in acute severe or life-threatening disease.
Dose 5 mg/kg loading dose over 20 min, followed by continuous infusion of 0.5–0.7 mg/kg (500 mg in 500 mL normal saline or 0.5% dextrose at (0.5 x body weight in kg) mL/h). If on maintenance therapy, do not give loading dose but start continuous infusion.
NB Needs therapeutic drug monitoring. Side-effects: nausea, arrhythmias, palpitations.

Antibiotics—only if infective element to the exacerbation. Most exacerbations are due to viruses, especially the common cold. *C. pneumoniae* and *M. pneumoniae* are also implicated.

IV fluids—patients are often dehydrated. Hypokalaemia (due to β_2 agonists) must be corrected.

IM adrenaline—may be useful if near arrest, whilst waiting for ITU support.

ITU referral

Liaise with ITU early! Better to discuss early a patient who does not subsequently need ITU input, than to find you and your patient in difficulty, with no ITU bed.
There is no evidence to support the use of NIV in the management of asthma. Hypercapnic respiratory failure in acute severe asthma is an urgent indication for endotracheal intubation.

When to discuss with ITU

- Worsening PEF despite treatment
- Worsening hypoxia
- Hypercapnia
- Falling pH
- Exhaustion/poor respiratory effort
- Drowsiness/confusion
- Respiratory arrest.

Discharge

Consider discharge when:

- Reduced β_2 agonist dose
- Off nebulized drugs and on inhalers ≥24 h
- PEF ≥75% predicted or best
- Minimal PEF diurnal variation
- Appropriate education has been given.

Prior to discharge consider

- Reason for the exacerbation. Could it have been avoided?
- Check patient's self-management plan/asthma action plan
- Check inhaler technique (p 686)
- Book an appointment with GP or practice nurse for within 24 h
- Book chest clinic appointment.

Chronic asthma: management

Aim to minimize symptoms and prevent exacerbations, prevent the potential consequences of longstanding airway inflammation leading to airway remodelling and chronic unresponsive airway obstruction, and improve quality of life.

The emphasis should be on education, self-management, and personal asthma action plans. Aim for:

- Minimal day and night symptoms
- No exacerbations
- Normal lung function and prevention of lung function decline with the development of fixed airflow obstruction
- No limit to physical activity
- Minimum steroid dose.

Treatment is based on disease severity using a step up/step down approach, starting treatment at the level appropriate to disease severity, based on the history, spirometry, and medication usage.

The main aims during out-patient review are:

- Ensure the diagnosis is correct and that symptoms are due to asthma and not coexistent/alternative pathology (e.g. reflux, hyperventilation syndrome, etc.)
- Aim for no symptoms/normal lung function on minimal treatment
- Ensure an action plan is in place for exacerbations
- Identify patients at risk of an adverse outcome.

Pharmacological management

British Thoracic Society Guidelines for the Management of Asthma

Step 1—mild intermittent asthma

- Short-acting β_2 agonist
- Check compliance, inhaler technique (including Volumatic or other spacer), and eliminate potential triggers
- 10 puffs per day (2 or more canisters/month) is a marker of poorly controlled disease.

Step 2—regular preventer therapy

- Start at 400 μg/day beclomethasone (BDP) in a twice daily dose
- Titrate steroid dose to symptoms, aiming for lowest effective dose
- Local steroid side-effects only (oral candida, dysphonia) from BDP ≤ 800 μg per day
- Possible dose-related bone density effects at this dose or above
- Fluticasone (Flixotide®) provides equal clinical activity to budesonide (e.g. Polemicist®) at half dosage. Mometasone (Asmanex®) is a new inhaled steroid; the current limited evidence suggests it is equivalent to twice the dose of BDP. Ciclesonide (Alvesco®) is another new inhaled steroid. It is a pro-drug, and the available evidence suggests it may have fewer local oropharyngeal side effects and less systemic activity than conventional inhaled steroids. The clinical benefit and efficacy to safety ratio data have not been fully established.

- Qvar® (beclomethaosne diproprionate) has a smaller particle size and may be of benefit in some, 400 μg bd is as effective as fluticasone 500 μg bd

Step 3—add on therapy

- If taking 200–800 μg/day inhaled steroid, consider long-acting β_2 agonist. A combination preparation may be appropriate
- If there is no response to a LABA, stop it and increase the inhaled steroid
- The combination of an inhaled corticosteroid and LABA is now licensed as maintenance ***and*** reliever therapy, if a rapid onset LABA, e.g. formoterol (Oxis®) is used, in the context of a personal asthma action plan. It is not clear if this is superior to more conventional doses of inhaled steroid and LABA.

Step 4—Poor control on moderate dose inhaled steroid and add on therapy: addition of fourth drug

- Ensure definite benefit is obtained from any of these subsequent drugs before continuing
- Leukotriene receptor antagonist—about a third of patients respond. May be useful if atopic or for exercise-induced asthma. Trial for 1 month and stop if there is no response. Also indicated in allergic rhinitis—so consider if this is present as well
- Theophylline (has side-effects, e.g. nausea, and needs therapeutic drug monitoring)
- Slow-release oral β_2 agonist.

Step 5—Continuous or frequent use of oral steroids

- NB Risk of side-effects if on oral steroids for >3 months or 3–4 courses per year
- Warn patient of potential side-effects (hypertension, diabetes, cataracts, gastric erosions) and ask GP to monitor. Start osteoporosis prophylaxis with calcium and vitamin D, or a bisphosphonate. Document baseline bone densitometry in those receiving prednisolone for more than 3 months (see p 678). See www.rcplondon.ac.uk
- Aim for the lowest possible dose steroid.

Chronic asthma: additional treatment options

Steroid-sparing drugs, e.g. methotrexate, oral gold, and ciclosporin—may be useful if other treatments are unsuccessful. They may reduce long-term steroid requirements, but all have side-effects and need haematological surveillance. There are very few data to support their use, and significant variability in response. Guidelines suggest a 3-month trial, once other drugs have proven unsuccessful, with treatment in a centre with experience of their use.

Continuous subcutaneous terbutaline infusion via a portable syringe driver may be useful. Standard dose is 5 mg over 24 h, but up to 15 mg/24 h may be given. Use terbutaline nebulizer solution (2.5 mg/mL) e.g. for 10 mg/24 h, use 4 ml of nebulizer solution, with 6 ml of saline, infuse the 10 ml over 24 h. Beneficial effects have been reported in severe asthma, but safety and efficacy have not been assessed in RCTs. Best responders may be those with marked PEFR variability ('type 1 brittle asthmatics') to allow steroid reduction.

Omalizumub Recombinant humanized monoclonal antibody against IgE has been shown to reduce early and late asthmatic responses after allergen challenge, and is now licensed for atopic individuals with difficult to control disease, in combination with other standard treatments. The drug removes circulating and tissue IgE by promoting loss of high affinity IgE receptors on mast cells, basophils, and dendritic cells, leading to reduced airway inflammation. Compared with placebo, it has been shown to reduce exacerbation rates, with improvement in asthma symptoms and quality of life scores, but with no overall change in lung function. Meta-analyses suggest a reduction of around 100 µg of inhaled corticosteroid is achieved per day compared with placebo.

Omalizumub is given as a subcutaneous injection every 2–4 weeks. The dose depends on the patient's weight and serum IgE concentration; the peak response is at 12–16 weeks and two-thirds of patients respond. The serum IgE should be 30–700 IU (there is a high risk of anaphylaxis at higher IgE levels).

There is some debate as to whether the high cost of the drug can be justified. The 2007 NICE guidelines suggest its use for severe persistent allergic asthma, which is unstable despite optimized standard therapy, and should be used for a trial period of a maximum of 16 weeks, ceasing if there is no clinical response.

Additional points

- ***Regular review***—to ensure patients are on appropriate treatment for their disease severity, and are maintained on the lowest possible inhaled steroid dose. Step down treatment if patient stable for 3 months or more. Step down inhaled steroid by reducing dose by 25% at 3-monthly intervals.

- ***Asthma action plan***—all patients with severe asthma should have an agreed written asthma action plan (self-management plan), their own peak flow meter, and regular checks on compliance and inhaler technique. A self-management plan should include specific advice about recognizing loss of asthma control and action to take if asthma deteriorates. Patients on low dose inhaled steroids (200 μg) should have their dose increased five-fold at the start of an exacerbation. This should not be extrapolated to higher inhaled steroid doses. The previous recommendation of doubling the dose of inhaled steroid at the start of an exacerbation is unproven.

Monitoring morbidity—the 3 RCP questions

In the last week or month:
- Have you had difficulty sleeping because of your asthma symptoms (including cough)?
- Have you had your usual asthma symptoms during the day (cough, wheeze, chest tightness, or breathlessness)?
- Has your asthma interfered with your usual activities (e.g. work, housework)?

Further information

Walker S. Anti-IgE for chronic asthma. Cochrane Database Syst Review 2003; **3**: CD003559.

Holgate ST. Efficacy and safety of anti-immunoglobulin-E antibody (omalizumab) in severe allergic asthma. *Clin Exp Allergy* 2004; **34**: 632.

Non-pharmacological management

Allergen avoidance may reduce severity of disease in sensitized individuals. House dust mite control measures need to be comprehensive—there is no current evidence to support it, although trials are ongoing. Pet removal may be useful, if the history is suggestive, and sensitivity has been demonstrated by skin prick testing or raised specific IgE levels.

Smoking cessation may reduce asthma severity. Current and previous smoking reduces the effect of inhaled steroid; these individuals may need higher steroid doses.

Complementary therapies No current evidence exists.

Dietary manipulation No consistent evidence and none supported by interventional trials. Low magnesium intake is associated with increased asthma prevalence. Fish oils may be beneficial.

Weight reduction in obese asthmatics leads to improved control.

Immunotherapy Desensitization using allergen-specific immunotherapy may be beneficial in a small subgroup of patients.

Buteyko breathing technique is a series of breathing exercises that mimic yoga breathing techniques. One study showed a reduction in the use of inhaled bronchodilator and steroid use in asthmatics carrying out these exercises, with no change in lung function or bronchial hyperresponsiveness. Cochrane review of breathing exercises concluded that there was no evidence of improvement in lung function, but improved quality of life scores.

Future developments

New steroids Research for 'dissociated steroids' is ongoing. These are steroids in which the useful anti-inflammatory effects (mediated by transcription factor inhibition) are dissociated from the side-effects (mediated via glucocorticoid DNA binding). Safer steroids, e.g. ciclesonide, a new once-a-day inhaled steroid, appear to have an improved side-effect profile. Ciclesonide is a pro-drug, activated by airway esterases, with fewer side-effects due to high degrees of protein binding.

Eosinophil inhibitors A variety of approaches to inhibit eosinophil recruitment are under investigation, including adhesion molecule inhibition and eosinophil chemotactic receptor inhibition.

Phosphodiesterase-4 inhibitors New generation phosphodiesterase (PDE)-4 inhibitors, e.g. roflumilast, are being investigated in clinical trials. These drugs have a broad anti-inflammatory action, with neutrophil inhibitory effects. Early clinical trial data looks promising.

Cytokine modulators Tumour necrosis factor (TNF)–alpha plays an important role in the pathogenesis of asthma. Anti-TNF antibodies have been beneficial in the treatment of inflammatory bowel disease and rheumatoid arthritis. Anti-TNF may be useful in the treatment of severe asthma, as it may block other important leukotrienes, e.g. IL-13.

Bronchial thermoplasty This is the application of controlled radiofrequency energy to the airway wall, using a specialized catheter at bronchoscopy. It heats the tissue to about 65°C, reducing muscle mass in the small and medium-sized airways, with several airways treated under direct vision at each session. Three separate sessions are required to treat all accessible airways. This has been assessed in a small non-randomized study and is well tolerated. Improved asthma quality of life scores, reduced airway hyperresponsiveness, and reduced oral steroid doses are reported, with no reduction in hospital admissions. The mechanism of action is unlikely to be improved airway contractility alone, and neurohumoral effects are postulated. A small placebo controlled trial in 32 patients has shown significantly worse initial symptoms and side-effects, but a small longer-term improvement at 22 and 52 weeks.

Further information

British Guideline on the management of asthma. Thorax 2003; 58: S1, updated 2007

Pavord ID *et al*. Safety and efficacy of bronchial thermoplasty in symptomatic severe asthma. *AJRRCM* 2007; 176(12): 1185–91

http://www.brit-thoracic.org.uk/iqs/sid.06309940811162053801561/asthma.html —a good site from which to download copies of the asthma guidelines in various formats and to obtain training information

www.occupationalasthma.com

www.ginasthma.com

Difficult/refractory asthma

Patients with refractory asthma are a small subgroup of asthma patients (5–10%). They have difficult to treat disease, reflected by high maintenance medication requirements, or persistent symptoms and air flow obstruction, with multiple exacerbations, despite high medication use. They have high numbers of admissions, and cause significant anxiety to their families and medical staff. There is a wide range of disease severity, including those with highly labile disease and those with severe, more chronic air flow obstruction. No consensus definition.

The disease is usually 'defined' on the basis of:

- Medication requirements (typically continuous or near continuous oral steroids)
- Asthma symptoms
- Frequency of exacerbations
- Severity of airflow limitation

Patients exhibit the features of asthma, and it is thought that the airflow obstruction, airway hyperresponsiveness, and PEF diurnal variability are more severe in refractory disease, though the physiological reasons for this remain unclear.

These patients typically fail to completely reverse their airflow obstruction following a 2-week course of oral prednisolone and demonstrate a poor bronchodilator response to inhaled β_2 agonists.

The pathological mechanism is likely to be ongoing airway inflammation, with increasing airway fibrosis, but this is not proven. Other possibilities include steroid resistance (see opposite), β_2 receptor down-regulation, or a different disease process altogether. Whether they represent a different asthma 'phenotype' is unclear.

Diagnosis of refractory asthma

- Confirm the diagnosis is correct—this will mean going back through the notes and retaking a thorough history
- Confirm reversible airflow limitation now or in the past (as for non-refractory asthma; see p 126)
- Consider other diagnoses for cough, breathlessness, and wheeze, and investigate for potential exacerbating diseases:
  - COPD/smoking
  - Bronchiectasis/cystic fibrosis
  - Sinus disease—consider ENT review
  - Churg–Strauss syndrome/eosinophilic syndromes—consider ANCA
  - Systemic disease—thyroid disease or vasculitis
  - Allergic bronchopulmonary aspergillosis—consider *Aspergillus* precipitins/skin tests/IgE
  - Vocal cord dysfunction—consider laryngoscopy
  - Hyperventilation syndrome
  - Gastro-oesophageal reflux—consider OGD/24 h pH
  - Upper airway obstruction—consider CT or bronchoscopy
  - Obstructive sleep apnoea—consider sleep study
  - Obesity
  - Cardiac dysfunction—consider echo and/or cardiological opinion

- Psychiatric/emotional issues/depression/secondary gain—consider psychiatry or psychology review
- Functional wheeze by breathing near residual volume

Refractory asthma

Before labelling a patient as 'refractory', compliance must be confirmed. This may be by checking pharmacy prescription records, using inhaler devices monitoring medication usage, or by measurement of plasma prednisolone or early morning cortisol levels.

Treatment is that of non-refractory asthma, with inhaled long-acting β_2 agonists and high-dose inhaled corticosteroids (see pp 132–136). Ensure treatment trials are adequate and adhered to.

- In patients unable to tolerate a prednisolone dose <20 mg per day, corticosteroid pharmacokinetic studies may be useful. However, <25% of patients with severe asthma show clinically significantly increased prednisolone clearance (usually a specific reason can be identified, such as concomitant use of enzyme inducing medication). IM steroid, e.g. triamcinolone 120 mg, may be useful if compliance is a major problem.
- Nebulized budesonide (Respules®, 1–2 mg bd) may be of benefit.
- Inflammatory markers, e.g. sputum or plasma eosinophil counts or exhaled nitric oxide levels, may be useful to assess medication response, although no trials have demonstrated their use clinically in this group of patients.
- Anti-inflammatory and immunomodulating drugs (specialized centre only). Include methotrexate, cyclosporin, oral gold, and intravenous gammaglobulin. None of these have been studied in a randomized controlled trial in this group of patients and none have demonstrated improvement in airway hyperresponsiveness.
- Macrolide antibiotics have anti-inflammatory and immune modulatory effects, reducing airway reactivity, and eosinophilic inflammation, and have been shown to reduce oral steroid requirements. Persistence of airway infection by *C. pneumoniae and Mycoplasma* is increasingly recognized as a contributory factor in persistent airflow obstruction, and recurrent exacerbations and macrolide antibiotics may act in this situation to clear persistent infection. Use, e.g. azithromycin, 250 mg, on alternate days, or 3 times a week, or 500 mg twice weekly. Six-weekly LFT monitoring is required. Risk of hearing loss.

'Steroid-resistant' asthma This subgroup of patients represents a very small proportion of refractory asthma patients. Middle-aged obese women, often with other additional diagnoses, are overrepresented in this group. They require supportive treatment, without high doses of glucocorticoids. Diagnoses other than asthma are likely and investigation should be directed towards these. Whether they represent a further 'asthma phenotype' is not clear.

Further information

Robinson DS *et al.* Systematic assessment of difficult-to-treat asthma. *ERJ* 2003; **22**: 478–83

Thomas PS *et al.* Pseudo-steroid resistant asthma. *Thorax* 1999; **54**: 352–6

Asthma in pregnancy

- Pregnancy can affect asthma
- Asthma can affect the outcome of pregnancy
- Prognosis—1/3 worsen, 1/3 improve, 1/3 no change
- Asthma course is likely to be similar in successive pregnancies
- Severe asthma is more likely to deteriorate than mild asthma
- Most exacerbations occur late, in the second and third trimester, and are due to viral infections and non-adherence to inhaled corticosteroid

Pre-pregnancy counselling

- Asthmatics must continue normal asthma medication
- Give smoking cessation advice
- Monitor the pregnant asthmatic closely
- Severe exacerbations in pregnancy are associated with low birth weight infants, an effect similar to maternal smoking in pregnancy

Acute asthma in pregnancy

- Risk to fetus of uncontrolled asthma outweighs any small risk of drugs
- Asthma medications are generally safe in pregnancy
- Steroids should be continued

- Drug therapy as for non-asthmatics, including inhaled and oral corticosteroids
- Maintain oxygen saturation >95%
- Continuous fetal monitoring for acute severe asthma
- Liaise with obstetrician if acute severe asthma

Leukotriene receptor antagonists

Limited safety data available for use in pregnancy and it is recommended not to start using whilst pregnant. Continue in women who have previously demonstrated significant improvement in disease control prior to pregnancy.

Management during labour

- Acute asthma is rare in labour (probably due to high sympathetic drive)
- Close liaison between the respiratory and obstetric teams is paramount, with close fetal monitoring
- Management should be as for non-pregnant individuals, see pp 132–136), maintaining the oxygen saturation >95%. There is no RCT data for magnesium sulphate, although it is used in eclampsia
- Regional anaesthetic blockade is preferable to general anaesthesia
- Prostaglandin E_2 may be safely used for induction of labour
- Prostaglandin F_2 alpha (for post-partum bleeding) may cause bronchospasm
- Give parenteral hydrocortisone 100 mg 6–8-hourly during labour if on oral prednisolone at >7.5 mg daily for >2 weeks prior to delivery

Breast-feeding

- An asthmatic mother may reduce the chance of atopy in her child by breast-feeding; current opinion is divided
- Prednisolone is secreted in breast milk, but the infant is exposed to only tiny and clinically irrelevant doses.

Occupational asthma

- This is asthma due to specific workplace sensitizers and may account for 10% of adult onset asthma
- The diagnosis is often difficult to make
- Early diagnosis is important, as earlier removal from the workplace in affected individuals leads to a better outcome
- It is different to asthma exacerbated by irritants in the workplace, and can occur in individuals with or without prior asthma.

- Agents induce asthma through immunological and non-immunological mechanisms. Immunological disease appears after a latency period of exposure; thus it is necessary for the worker to be sensitized to the casual agent (e.g. acid anhydride—baker's asthma). Non-immunological disease is characterized by the absence of a latent period and occurs after accidental exposure to high concentrations of a workplace irritant. This is irritant induced asthma (previously named reactive airways dysfunction syndrome), usually caused by exposure to, e.g. smoke, vapours, or fumes, with a strong temporal relationship between irritant exposure and the development of asthma type symptoms.
- The latency between first exposure and symptom onset can be long, and depends on the sensitizing agent—an accurate history therefore includes current and past exposures
- Once sensitized, re-exposure to very low concentrations can provoke symptoms
- May be associated with rhinitis and urticaria
- Improves away from work, but can take several days to settle.

Risk factors

- Atopy
- HLA type (e.g. HLA-DQB1*0503 associated with isocyanate allergy)
- Smoking (especially for high molecular weight agents).

Diagnosis

- Confirm the diagnosis of asthma
- Confirm the relationship between asthma and work exposures
- Find the specific cause

There are two useful screening questions:

- Is your asthma worse when at work?
- Does your asthma improve when away from work or on holiday?

Document lung function deterioration in the workplace, usually by serial peak flow recording at work, at home, and on holiday.

Bronchial provocation/challenge testing using suspected agent—only in specialized centres, but difficulties with testing and producing a valid test substance mean that a negative specific bronchial challenge in a worker with otherwise good evidence of occupational asthma is not sufficient to exclude the diagnosis.

Skin prick testing/specific IgE for certain sensitizers (although a positive test only indicates sensitization which can occur with or without disease).

Document

- The range of chemicals used
- Working practices
- Use of personal protective equipment.

Serial PEF recording in occupational asthma

- Record every 2 h from waking to sleep
- For 4 weeks, whilst no changes to treatment
- Document home/work periods and any holidays
- Analysis is best made by experts, usually using a criterion-based analysis system, e.g. OASYS (a computer program that plots and interprets serial peak flow recordings; see www.occupationalasthma.com)
- Patients may be sensitized to more than one agent and over 300 agents are identified. See wwww.asmanet.com

Table 18.1 Causes of occupational asthma

Sensitizing agent	Occupational exposure
Low molecular weight agents (act as haptens)	
Isocyanates	Paint spraying, adhesives, polyurethane foams
Acid anhydrides	Epoxy paint, varnish, resins, baking
Metals	Welding, plating, metal refining
Glutaraldehyde and other disinfectants	Health care workers
Drugs	Pharmaceutical industry
High molecular weight agents	
Amine dyes	Cosmetics, hair dyes, rubber workers
Wood dusts, bark	Textile workers, joiners, carpenters
Animal-derived antigens	Vets, laboratory workers (20% affected)
Biological enzymes	Detergent industry, pharmaceuticals
Plant products	Bakers, hairdressers
Fluxes, colophony	Solderers, electronics industry

Management of occupational asthma

- Identify the cause
- Remove the worker from exposure
- Continue employment if at all possible
- Early diagnosis and removal from exposure are important factors for a good outcome
- Improvement in FEV_1 may be maintained for one year following last exposure, and for up to 2 years for non-specific responsiveness
- The decision to remove the patient from the workplace should not be taken lightly, and should be made by a consultant with experience of occupational lung disease.
- The employee may be eligible for Disablement Benefit (no proof of negligence is required).

Latex allergy is seen in up to 18% of health care workers, and is the leading cause of occupational asthma in this group due to the widespread use of latex gloves. It is potentially serious, with avocado, bananas, kiwi, and chestnuts cross-reacting to give a similar clinical picture. Treatment is absolute avoidance; those affected should wear a MedicAlert bracelet and always use non-latex gloves.

Vocal cord dysfunction

A proportion of patients labelled as having severe asthma, will have symptoms originating from the upper airway. This can be due to vocal cord dysfunction (VCD) and/or so-called 'upper airway hyperresponsiveness'; these are different, but overlap. VCD is likely to arise from interrelationships between laryngeal hyperresponsiveness and autonomic imbalance, with inputs from potential aetiological/aggravating factors, such as reflux, psychological stress, hypocapnia (hyperventilation). Increased laryngeal hyperresponsiveness can occur following respiratory tract infections and possibly asthma itself. Upper airway hyperresponsiveness may include more than just the larynx, but this is not clear.

Patients will typically present with asthma symptoms, with associated triggers, e.g. odours, cold air. They typically have no reduction in peak flow or response to asthma medications (though this is possible).

A careful history will reveal shortness of breath that is of short duration, worse on inspiration, and extremely sudden in onset, with symptom-free periods.

Pathogenesis

- Recent URTI, may take months to settle
- Post-nasal drip/chronic sinusitis
- Gastro-oesophageal reflux disease with micro aspiration
- Chronic laryngitis
- Hyperventilation in association with anxiety/panic
- It is postulated that the origin of the vocal cord closure may stem from a reflex airway protective mechanism.

Diagnosis is based on excluding other causes of cough and breathlessness. It may be suggested by hearing a more stridulous noise and lack of basal wheeze. The gold standard is visualization of abnormal vocal cord movement at laryngoscopy, where there is excessive adduction of the anterior two-thirds of cords with the creation of a posterior 'glottic chink'; although this finding may not always be present at the time of study. The flow volume loop should show inspiratory flow limitation, with 'stuttering' of the flow.

Treatment (for which there are no randomized controlled trials)

- Speech therapy
- Panting (autopeep)
- Coughing and cough suppression techniques
- Inspiratory resistance devices
- HELIOX/nebulized saline/lidocaine spray
- Sedatives
- Exercise.

Further information

Newman KB *et al.* Clinical features of vocal cord dysfunction. *AJRCCM* 1995; **152**: 1382–6

Stanton AE, Bucknall CE. Vocal cord dysfunction. A review. Breathe 2005; **2**: 31–5 (http://www.ersnet.org/ers/LR/browse/viewPDF.aspx?id_attach=10896)

Allergic rhinitis (hay fever)

This is the syndrome of nasal discharge or blockage with nasal and/or eye itching, and sneezing. It is often associated with post-nasal drip, cough, fatigue, and with significant morbidity. Allergic rhinitis is defined as perennial if the symptoms occur year round and seasonal if occurring at a particular time of year. The prevalence is increasing and affects up to 15% of the UK population. Up to 30% of patients with persistent allergic rhinitis have asthma.

Aetiology The lining of the nose is in continuum with the lower respiratory tract, and inflammation of the upper and lower airways often co-exists. Common aeroallergens provoking seasonal allergic rhinitis are tree pollen in the spring, and grass pollen in the summer months. Perennial rhinitis usually reflects allergy to indoor allergens, such as house dust mite (the provoking allergen is a digestive enzyme that is shed in the faeces), cat salivary protein, cockroaches, or animal dander.

Pathophysiology Symptoms occur following the inhalation of allergen to which the subject is sensitized, and against which they have IgE antibodies. These antibodies bind to mast cell IgE receptors, with the release of mediators, including tryptase and histamine, causing symptoms immediately after exposure.

Diagnosis is usually made from the history, which should identify the triggers to the disease. The main differential diagnosis is with sinusitis due to bacterial infection and upper airway involvement due to vasculitis. Asthma is common in association with rhinitis and treatment of rhinosinusitis in association with asthma leads to improved asthma control. Up to 50% of asthma patients will have allergic rhinitis.

Treatment

- Allergen avoidance This may be easier said than done. It can take up to 20 weeks to remove cat allergen from a house. Keeping car and house windows shut and wearing sunglasses may help avoid pollen. Pollen counts are highest in the afternoon and early evening
- Non-sedating antihistamines, improve sneezing and itching, but have no effect on nasal blockage
- Topical intranasal steroid, e.g. budesonide triamcinolone
- Topical anticholinergics, e.g. ipratropium, may be useful for rhinorrhea, if uncontrolled with topical nasal steroids
- Topical sodium cromoglycate may be beneficial, particularly for allergic conjunctivitis
- Decongestants, e.g. oxymetazoline, may help, but rebound nasal blockage and tachyphylaxis are a potential problem if used regularly.
- Leukotrene receptor antagonists (e.g. montelukast) may be beneficial.

Chapter 19

Bronchiectasis

Epidemiology, pathophysiology, and causes

Definition Irreversible abnormal dilatation of one or more bronchi, with chronic airway inflammation. Associated chronic sputum production, recurrent chest infections, and airflow obstruction.

Epidemiology The prevalence of bronchiectasis is unknown, but is probably falling due to vaccinations and the improved and earlier treatment of childhood infections. However, the advent of HRCT scanning may now lead to the diagnosis of more subtle (and possibly subclinical) disease.

Pathophysiology An initial (usually infectious) insult is needed to damage the airways. Disordered anatomy leads to secondary bacterial colonization, perpetuating inflammatory change and damaging the mucociliary escalator. This prevents bacterial clearance and leads to further airway damage. Major airways and bronchioles are involved, with mucosal oedema, inflammation, and ulceration. Terminal bronchioles become obstructed with secretions, leading to volume loss. A chronic host inflammatory response ensues, with free-radical formation and the production of neutrophil elastase, further contributing to the inflammatory process. Bronchial neovascularization occurs with hypertrophy and tortuosity of the bronchial arteries (which are at systemic pressure), which may lead to intermittent haemoptyses.

Aetiology The causes of bronchiectasis are many and varied (see Table 19.1). In general, the aetiology is either a one-off infectious insult, or an underlying immune deficiency. Determining the aetiology of the condition may lead to different management if, for example, the underlying cause is found to be cystic fibrosis or an immune deficiency. The cause is idiopathic in around 50% of cases and these are likely to be due to an (as yet unidentified) impairment in host defence.

The most important cause to exclude is cystic fibrosis (see p 205). Even relatively mild bronchiectasis diagnosed in middle age can be due to CF. The diagnosis can alter management, with:

- Involvement of the multidisciplinary CF team
- Attention to other potential problems, e.g. gastrointestinal disease, sinus disease, diabetes
- Inheritance (relevant to the rest of the family)
- Fertility issues.

Consider genotyping for CF if:

- Predominantly upper lobe disease
- *Haemophilus influenzae* or *Pseudomonas aeruginosa* colonization
- Malnutrition ± malabsorption, diabetes
- Family history of cystic fibrosis or bronchiectasis
- Associated subfertility or infertility.

A normal chloride sweat test does not exclude CF, as some mutations are associated with normal sweat chloride levels. The test is also difficult and subject to a number of technical errors. Only 90% of CF sufferers have a recognizable gene defect (there are over 1000 CFTR mutations).

Table 19.1 Causes of bronchiectasis

Genetic	Cystic fibrosis
Congenital	Pulmonary sequestration
Post-infective	Tuberculosis
	Whooping cough (if infection in a localized area)
	Severe pneumonia
	Non-tuberculous mycobacteria (NTM)—there is some debate as to whether the bronchiectasis seen in association with NTM (classically in elderly females) is caused by or secondarily infected by NTM
Immune deficiency	Primary—hypogammaglobulinaemia
	Secondary—HIV, CLL, nephrotic syndrome
	(Excessive immune response—ABPA)
Mucociliary clearance abnormalities	
	Primary ciliary dyskinesia (see p 628)
	Kartagener's syndrome
	Young's syndrome (bronchiectasis, sinusitis, and azoospermia—i.e. clinical features identical to those of CF)
Toxic insults	Aspiration
	Inhalation (toxic gases, chemicals)
Mechanical insults	Foreign body aspiration
	Extrinsic lymph node compression
	Intrinsic (intraluminal) obstructing tumour
Associations	Bronchiectasis is associated with a number of systemic diseases, so cough and sputum production in these conditions should trigger referral to determine the cause:
	Rheumatoid arthritis (up to 35% of RA patients have bronchiectasis)
	Connective tissue diseases, e.g. Sjögren's syndrome, SLE
	Ulcerative colitis and Crohn's disease (see p 248)
	Chronic sinusitis
	Yellow nail syndrome
	Marfan's syndrome

Clinical features and diagnosis

Suspect bronchiectasis in a patient with recurrent episodes of 'bronchitis' over several years prior to presentation.

The clinical picture is one of:

- *Symptoms*
  - Cough
  - Chronic sputum production (typically tenacious, purulent, and daily)
  - Intermittent haemoptyses
  - Breathlessness
  - Intermittent pleuritic pain (usually in association with infections)
  - Lethargy/malaise.
- *Signs*
  - Coarse inspiratory and expiratory crackles on auscultation
  - Airflow obstruction with wheeze.

Diagnosis is usually made clinically, with high resolution CT chest for confirmation.

Investigations are aimed at:

- Confirming the diagnosis
- Identifying a treatable underlying cause for the bronchiectasis (possible in about 40%)
- Optimizing management to prevent exacerbations and further lung damage

Essential investigations

- ***CXR*** sensitivity is only 50%, classically shows 'ring shadows' and 'tramlines'—indicating thickened airways, and the 'gloved finger' appearance. consolidation around thickened and dilated airways
- ***HRCT*** chest is 97% sensitive in detecting disease. Expiratory scans may be useful to demonstrate post-obstructive air trapping, indicative of small airways disease. Typically shows airway dilatation to the lung periphery, bronchial wall thickening, and the airway appearing larger than its accompanying vessel (signet ring sign). If the bronchiectasis is localized to a single lobe, CT is useful to determine whether a central obstructing lesion is present. Contiguous 3-mm slices are needed to exclude a central airway lesion if there is associated haemoptysis. Symptoms correlate with wall thickening and mucous plugging on CT scan. Traction bronchiectasis seen in UIP is airway dilatation secondary to airway distortion, seen with chronic severe interstitial fibrosis
- **Sputum microbiology** Standard M, C & S (including for atypical organisms), acid-fast bacilli, and *Aspergillus*
- **Pulmonary function tests** with reversibility testing
- **Immunoglobulins A, M, E, G** (including IgG subclasses, if total IgG is low)
- ***Aspergillus precipitins*** See p 467.

Second-line investigations

- **CF genotyping** (see p 206)
- **Autoantibodies** (ANA, RhF, dsDNA) if associated arthritis/connective tissue disease
- **Vaccination response** to tetanus, *Haemophilus influenzae*, and pneumococcal antibodies, if underlying immunosuppression suspected
- **Skin tests/RAST** to identify specific sensitizers (usually *Aspergillus*)
- **Detailed immunological investigation** (including neutrophil and lymphocyte function studies)
- **Bronchoscopy** to exclude a foreign body if suggested by CT; obtain microbiological samples if unusual clinical presentation, or failure to respond to standard antibiotics
- **Nasal brushings/biopsy** (in tertiary centre) to assess ciliary beat frequency with video microscopy
- **Saccharin test** The time for saccharin to be tasted in the mouth after deposition of a 0.5-mm particle on the inferior turbinate of the nose. Normal is less than 30 min. A poor man's cilial function test
- α_1-**antitrypsin levels** if deficiency is suspected
- **Barium swallow/oesophageal imaging** if recurrent aspiration suspected.

General management

The main aims of management are:

- Treatment of any underlying medical condition
- Prevention of exacerbations and progression of underlying disease by physiotherapy. The options for airway clearance include:
  - Postural or autogenic drainage
  - Active cycle of breathing technique—this involves breathing control with forced expiration (huffing) using variable thoracic expansion
  - Cough augmentation—using flutter valves/cough insufflator/ high-frequency oscillation
  - Exercise regimes—important to prevent general deconditioning
  - The physiotherapist is also vital during admission for exacerbations to help clear tenacious sputum
  - Nebulized hypertonic saline may improve airway clearance, although there is no RCT data to support its use
- Reduction of bacterial load and prevention of secondary airway inflammation and damage, with antimicrobial chemotherapy
- Supportive treatment—treatment of associated airflow obstruction
- Optimize nutrition
- Refer for surgery if necessary—localized resection of affected area
- Refer for transplantation if indicated.

Antimicrobial chemotherapy

- This may be intermittent for exacerbations only (for mild disease) or long term for more severe disease. Antibiotics may be oral, nebulized, or intravenous
- Regular sputum surveillance will ensure the likely colonizing organism is known
- *In vivo* sensitivity may be different to *in vitro* sensitivity
- Patients need a higher antibiotic dose and for a longer time period (usually 2 weeks minimum) than people without bronchiectasis
- Antibiotic treatment choice depends on the severity of the underlying disease
- Treatment response is usually assessed by a fall in sputum volume, and change to mucoid from purulent or mucopurulent sputum, with an improvement in systemic symptoms, spirometry, and CRP
- *Pseudomonas*-colonized patients have more frequent exacerbations, worse CT scan appearances, and a faster decline in lung function.

Progressive bacterial colonization Different bacteria colonize the airways at different stages of the disease, and their attempted eradication and suppression is vital to the treatment of bronchiectasis. The usual order of colonization is:

- *Staphylococcus aureus*
- *Haemophilus influenzae*
- *Moraxella catarrhalis*
- *Pseudomonas species.*

Exacerbation treatment An exacerbation is usually a clinical diagnosis, with an increase in sputum volume and tenacity, with discoloration. It may be associated with chest pain, haemoptysis and wheeze, and systemic upset—fevers, lethargy, and anorexia. The CRP may be elevated. Treatment depends on the potential pathogens and resident flora. Nebulized bronchodilators and regular physiotherapy (as an in- or out-patient) may also be needed.

Exacerbation of mild bronchiectasis

- Antibiotics for exacerbations only (tailored to the colonizing organism)
- 2-week course of oral ciprofloxacin at 750 mg bd if *Pseudomonas aeruginosa* colonized
- If early relapse, with a return to purulent sputum within 6–8 weeks, consider long-term oral antibiotics, e.g. amoxicillin 500 mg bd or doxycycline 100 mg od. If treatment failure, change to appropriate intravenous antibiotics, until clinical improvement.

Exacerbation of more severe bronchiectasis

Chronic suppressive antibiotics aim to prevent progression of disease, by reducing bacterial load and preventing ongoing inflammation, thereby reducing morbidity and improving quality of life.

- Antibiotics are usually given for at least 2 days after the sputum has cleared—often for 2 weeks
- If oral antibiotics fail, intravenous treatment is required. This may mean in-patient admission, or could involve long-line insertion, patient education in self-administration of intravenous antibiotics, and involvement of a home care team.

First isolate of Pseudomonas aeruginosa (see also p 211)

- Initial treatment is often aggressive with a 4–6 week course of oral ciprofloxacin 500–750 mg bd, and concurrent nebulized aminoglycoside, such as colistin 1–2 mega units bd
- If this fails and the patient still has *Pseudomonas* on sputum culture, intravenous antibiotics, usually an aminoglycoside and anti-pseudomonal penicillin (minimum 2 weeks), is required
- Consider long-term therapy with regular nebulized aminoglycoside to reduce levels of *Pseudomonas* and reduce subsequent exacerbations and airway inflammation.

Macrolide antibiotics have both anti-bacterial and immunomodulatory properties and have greater immunosuppressive effects than corticosteroids. They decrease mucous production, alter inflammatory mediator release, and inhibit *Pseudomonas* virulence factors and biofilm formation. Five small trials have reported beneficial effects of macrolides in bronchiectasis, with reduced sputum volume, improved lung function, and symptoms. The drugs are well tolerated, though concerns have been raised about non-tuberculous mycobacterial resistance with long-term use. Azithromycin 250 mg on alternate days or 3 times weekly, or 500 mg twice weekly (with LFT monitoring) are possible regimes. Risk of hearing loss. See p 162 (bronchiolitis).

Further management

- **Self-management plan**—patients need an individual plan for exacerbations, which usually involves having a supply of home antibiotics
- Treatment of associated **airflow obstruction/wheeze** with inhaled steroids and/or bronchodilators
- There is no specific treatment for abnormalities of mucociliary function, although β_2 agonists may enhance airway clearance
- **Nebulized DNase** (Dornase alpha)—no evidence for the use of this in non-CF bronchiectasis, but it may be useful in severe exacerbations if the sputum is very tenacious and expectoration is difficult
- **Nebulized hypertonic saline** (7%) may aid sputum clearance
- ***N*-acetylcysteine**
- **Annual influenza and pneumococcal vaccinations**
- **Osteoporosis prophylaxis** (if on long-term steroids)
- **Reflux** treatment if aspiration
- **Immunoglobulin replacement therapy** Patients found to have immunoglobulin deficiency should be referred to an immunologist for further assessment. Intravenous immunoglobulin replacement therapy is usually given once or twice monthly, as a day case
- **Surgery** This is the only potential curative treatment, with resection of a single chronically infected lobe occasionally being of benefit. It is less commonly needed now, as the incidence of single-lobe disease related to previous severe childhood pneumonia is falling. Surgery may be indicated for life-threatening haemoptysis
- **Transplant** is most commonly performed for CF bronchiectasis, but referral may be warranted for severe non-CF-related disease.

Complications of bronchiectasis

- Infective exacerbation
- Haemoptysis—small volume haemoptysis (increasing during exacerbations) is common
- Massive haemoptysis (usually from tortuous bronchial arteries around damaged lung, e.g. bulla) is a life-threatening emergency (see p 40)
- Pneumothorax
- Respiratory failure
- Brain abscess (now very rare)
- Amyloidosis.

Bronchiectasis and *Aspergillus*

- Allergic bronchopulmonary aspergillosis (ABPA)—excessive immune response to environmental fungus *Aspergillus* (most commonly *Fumigatus species*); may be the cause of bronchiectasis (suspect particularly if upper lobe disease), as mucus plugs become impacted in distal airways, causing airway damage and subsequent dilatation. See p 468
- Aspergilloma—*Aspergillus* may colonize damaged airways with formation of a fungus ball (mycetoma) within a previously formed cavity. This is extremely difficult to treat. Most commonly it causes systemic upset and haemoptysis. See p 474.

Further information

Prolonged antibiotics for purulent bronchiectasis in children and adults. *Cochrane Database Syst Rev* 2007/; **2**: CD001392

Chapter 20

Bronchiolitis

Pathophysiology and causes

Definition and epidemiology Bronchioles are small airways of diameter <2 mm, lined by bronchial epithelium and with no cartilage in their walls. Terminal bronchioles lead to alveoli. Many bronchioles need to be affected by disease before a patient becomes symptomatic, when there will be increased airway resistance unresponsive to β_2 stimulants. Bronchiolitis is poorly understood and is a mixture of conditions.

Disease seems to affect bronchioles in two main ways:

- Affecting the bronchioles in isolation, with non-specific injury causing subsequent epithelial damage and inflammation, e.g. viral bronchiolitis
- As a bronchiolitis associated with other airway disease, where the bronchiolitis may be more of an incidental finding along with other pathologies, e.g. COP, hypersensitivity pneumonitis, RB-ILD, Langerhans cell histiocytosis

Pathophysiology is unclear. There is probably an initial injury to the epithelium of the bronchioles with subsequent inflammation. Adjacent alveoli are often also involved. There are two main pathological patterns of bronchiolitis. Both can exist in the same patient.

- ***Proliferative bronchiolitis*** More common of the two patterns. Non-specific reaction to bronchiolar injury, with organizing exudate within the bronchiolar lumen. Proliferation of intraluminal fibrotic buds, called Masson bodies, seen in bronchioles, alveoli, and alveolar ducts. Associated alveolar wall inflammation and foamy macrophages in alveolar spaces. May completely or partially resolve. Tends to be more responsive to steroids. The pathology merges with that of COP (see p 270)
- ***Constrictive bronchiolitis*** Less common. Concentric narrowing of the bronchiolar wall due to cellular infiltrates ± smooth muscle hyperplasia, which may cause extrinsic compression, obliteration, distortion, mucus collection, peribronchiolar fibrosis, and scarring. Patchy in distribution. Typically progressive and unresponsive to steroid therapy. Usually leads to respiratory failure and death.

In practice, these are the commonest situations in which a diagnosis of bronchiolitis is useful:

- Viral bronchiolitis (RSV)
- Post-lung transplant (obliterative bronchiolitis)
- Post-bone marrow transplant
- Connective tissue disease (usually rheumatoid arthritis)
- In association with interstitial lung disease and airways disease
- Diffuse panbronchiolitis (including Japanese panbronchiolitis).

Causes of bronchiolitis

Proliferative bronchiolitis (associated with organizing pneumonia)

Commoner causes

- COP (see p 270)
- Hypersensitivity pneumonitis (see p 249)
- Chronic eosinophilic pneumonia (see p 232)
- Connective tissue disease—rheumatoid arthritis, polymyositis, dermatomyositis (see p 185)
- Post bone marrow, heart, and lung transplant
- Organizing acute infection—mycoplasma, *Legionella*, influenza, CMV, HIV, PCP.

Rarer causes

- ARDS (see p 101)
- Vasculitides, including Wegener's granulomatosis (see p 649)
- Drug-induced reactions, such as L-tryptophan, busulfan, cocaine
- Chronic thyroiditis
- Ulcerative colitis
- Radiation or aspiration pneumonitis
- Distal to bronchial obstruction
- Common variable immunodeficiency syndrome.

Constrictive bronchiolitis

Commoner causes

- Connective tissue disease, particularly rheumatoid arthritis, especially women in their 50s and 60s, with longstanding rheumatoid arthritis May be related to penicillamine therapy
- Infection—viral (adenovirus, RSV, influenza, para-influenza), mycoplasma.

Rarer causes

- 'Chronic rejection phenomenon' in heart, lung, bone marrow transplants—affects up to 65% of lung transplant patients after 5 years post-transplant and is the primary cause of late death, bronchiolitis obliterans syndrome (see p 328). Patients taking statins post-transplant have a lower incidence of this; reasons unclear
- Diffuse panbronchiolitis (including Japanese panbronchiolitis).
- Following inhalation injury: mineral dusts, such as asbestos, silica, iron oxide, aluminium oxide, talc, mica, coal, sulphur dioxide, nitrogen oxide, ammonia, chlorine, phosgene—may develop cough days to weeks after exposure
- Drug reaction
- Hypersensitivity reactions
- Ulcerative colitis
- Cryptogenic. Rare, mostly women >40. Cough and dyspnoea. PFT: progressive airflow obstruction and air trapping. KCO decreased, no bronchodilator response.

Management

Clinical features Insidious onset of cough and dyspnoea over weeks to months. There may be an associated medical history, such as a transplant, connective tissue disease, or vasculitis, or a history of mineral dust or drug exposure. Possible history of recent viral illness.

Investigations

- ***PFTs*** Obstructive defect may be found, with no bronchodilator reversibility, particularly in constrictive bronchiolitis. Proliferative bronchiolitis can cause a restrictive or mixed defect
- ***CXR*** can be normal or may show hyperinflation, especially with constrictive bronchiolitis, diffuse infiltrates with proliferative bronchiolitis, which may be migratory
- ***HRCT*** is helpful and may be performed prone in full expiration. (Prone CT is used to minimize any gravity-dependent changes.) Normal bronchioles are too small to be seen; indirect signs of disease may be hyperinflation, air trapping, causing a mosaic pattern and subsegmental atelectasis. Bronchioles with thickened walls due to inflammation and dilatation may be seen. CT is also useful to assess for signs of associated interstitial lung disease
- ***Open or thoracoscopic lung biopsy*** may be required to make the diagnosis, as transbronchial biopsies are usually inadequate. The small airways need particularly carefully examination.

Management

- Treat any underlying disorder
- Cough suppressants
- Long-term macrolide antibiotics, such as erythromycin 200–600 mg/day may improve symptoms, lung function, and mortality, especially in those with *diffuse panbronchiolitis* and *cryptogenic bronchiolitis*. Erythromycin lowers the neutrophil count by an unknown mechanism and reduces the number of lymphocytes
- Steroids are effective in cases of proliferative bronchiolitis and can treat the associated organizing pneumonia. They may also be beneficial in bronchiolitis due to inhalation injury, both in early and later stages. Relapses of the bronchiolitis may occur on stopping the steroids.

Bronchiolitis: specific conditions

Diffuse panbronchiolitis/Japanese panbronchiolitis This is a distinct condition and used to be thought of as rare outside Japan. Described 30 years ago in Japan, it is recognized there as a condition involving both the upper and lower respiratory tracts, with bronchiolar inflammation and chronic sinusitis. An infectious aetiology was postulated as the cause of this disease, but no particular organism has been consistently found. It can be familial and is associated with HLA-B54 (specific to East Asians) and A11. More prevalent in men, mean age at presentation 45, occurs particularly in non-smokers, and chronic sinusitis can precede the chest symptoms often by years. More recently, a very similar clinical condition has been increasingly described outside Japan and where sinusitis is less commonly found. This diffuse version is also an idiopathic inflammatory and suppurative disorder of the respiratory bronchioles causing progressive and severe airways obstruction. It is presumably very similar to the Japanese variety and probably under-recognized. Most of these patients have a productive cough with purulent sputum, exertional dyspnoea, wheeze, and weight loss. There may be signs of progressive respiratory failure and cor pulmonale with crackles and wheezes on auscultation.

- ***PFTs*** are obstructive, although may show a mixed pattern, with minimal airway hyperresponsiveness. kCO is reduced
- ***CXR and CT*** may show diffuse ill-defined nodules (sometimes 'tree-in-bud'), bronchiectasis, and air trapping
- ***Sputum cultures*** may repeatedly show growths of *Haemophilus influenzae, Pseudomonas aeruginosa,* and less commonly *Streptococcus pneumoniae, Klebsiella pneumoniae*, or *Staphylococcus aureus*. These should be treated, but can be hard to eradicate
- ***Cold agglutinins*** may be positive, mycoplasma tests are negative
- ***BAL*** shows marked neutrophilia
- ***Open or thoracoscopic lung biopsy,*** although this may not be considered necessary in areas where panbronchiolitis is prevalent. Bronchiolar histology is characteristic, although not pathognomonic, with transmural infiltrate of lymphocytes, plasma cells, and foamy macrophages. The intraluminal exudates may be organized to form a polypoid plug.

Treatment with low-dose erythromycin 400–600 mg/day for 2–6 months, and in some Japanese studies over 2 years, confers a significant survival benefit, most likely related to its anti-inflammatory and immunomodulatory effects (inhibits many cytokines), as well as reducing mucin secretion, rather than through its antibacterial effects. Untreated, 50% 5-year mortality. Azithromycin 250 mg three times a week may be a suitable alternative. Relapses occur, but usually respond to macrolides again.

Acute bronchiolitis This is a seasonal epidemic infective illness, common in infants <1 year, who present with coryza, low grade fever, cough, wheezing, tachypnoea, respiratory distress, hyperinflation, and tachycardia. It is most commonly caused by respiratory syncytial virus (RSV), but also adenovirus, influenza, para-influenza, rhinovirus, human metapneumo virus, mycoplasma, and *Chlamydia*. In adults, acute bronchiolitis is caused by the same organisms, but is less severe.

- ***CXR*** may be normal or show hyperinflation, occasionally with patchy opacities, consolidation, and collapse
- ***Histologically*** there is acute and chronic inflammation of bronchioles, with necrosis, sloughing, oedema, and inflammatory exudates in the bronchiolar lumen.

Treatment is supportive, with oxygen, fluids. Steroids and bronchodilators may be given if severe, but systematic reviews in children show no significant outcome benefit.

Further information

Ryu JH *et al.* Bronchiolar disorders. *Am J Respir Crit Care Med* 2003; **168**: 1277–92

Smyth RL, Openshaw PJ. Bronchiolitis. *Lancet* 2006; **368**: 312–22

Poletti V *et al.* Diffuse panbronchiolitis. *Eur Respir J* 2006; **28**: 862–71

Chapter 21

Chronic obstructive pulmonary disease (COPD)

Definition, aetiology, pathology, and clinical features

COPD is common and is mostly due to smoking. Patients with COPD represent a large proportion of in-patient (approximately 12% of all general medical admissions) and out-patient work for the chest physician.

Definition

- Fixed airflow obstruction
- Minimal or no reversibility with bronchodilators
- Minimal variability in day-to-day symptoms
- Slowly progressive and irreversible deterioration in lung function, leading to progressively worsening symptoms.

Aetiology 95% of cases are smoking-related, typically >20 pack years. COPD occurs in 10–20% of smokers, indicating that there is probable genetic susceptibility. COPD is increasing in frequency worldwide, particularly in some developing countries, due to high levels of smoking. It can also be caused by environmental and occupational factors such as dusts, chemicals, and air pollution.

Pathology

- ***Mucous gland hyperplasia*** particularly in the large airways, with mucous hypersecretion and therefore a chronic productive cough. Other mucosal damage from smoke:
  - ***Squamous metaplasia*** Replacement of the normal ciliated columnar epithelium by a squamous epithelium
  - ***Loss of cilial function*** This leads to impairment of the normal functioning of the mucociliary escalator, another reason for the chronic productive cough
- ***Chronic inflammation and fibrosis*** of small airways, characterized by CD8 lymphocyte, macrophage, and neutrophil infiltration, with release of pro-inflammatory cytokines. Recurrent infections may perpetuate airway inflammation
- ***Emphysema*** due to alveolar wall destruction causing irreversible enlargement of air spaces distal to the terminal bronchiole (the acinus), with subsequent loss of elastic recoil and hyperinflated lungs
  - Panacinar emphysema can occur with dilated air spaces evenly distributed across acinii
  - Centriacinar or proximal emphysema can occur with dilated air spaces found in association with the respiratory bronchioles
  - Periacinar or paraseptal emphysema can occur with dilated air spaces at the edge of the acinar unit and abutting a fixed structure, such as the pleura or a vessel
- ***Thickened pulmonary arteriolar wall and remodelling*** occur with hypoxia. Leads to increased pulmonary vascular resistance, pulmonary hypertension, and impaired gas exchange.

The cause of the increase in airways resistance and hence expiratory flow limitation is multifactorial. Small airway inflammation reduces the airway lumen. Emphysema destroys the radial attachments to the small airways, which normally hold them open and resist dynamic compression.

COPD is increasingly being recognized as having features not only of pulmonary, but also systemic inflammation and this may be the cause of the comorbidities found in patients with COPD. Daily activities are often modified to avoid dyspnoea, which can lead to deconditioning, muscle weakness, and wasting, meaning standing and walking become even harder. This leads to a vicious cycle of inactivity.

Clinical features

- Dyspnoea
- Productive cough
- Decreased exercise tolerance
- Wheeze.

Significant airflow obstruction may be present before the patient is aware of it.

Signs depend on the severity of the underlying disease.
- Raised respiratory rate
- Hyperexpanded/barrel chest
- Prolonged expiratory time >5 s, with pursed lip breathing
- Use of accessory muscles of respiration
- Quiet breath sounds (especially in the lung apices) ± wheeze
- Quiet heart sounds (due to overlying hyperinflated lung)
- Possible basal crepitations
- Signs of cor pulmonale and CO_2 retention (ankle oedema, raised JVP, warm peripheries, plethoric conjunctivae, bounding pulse, polycythaemia. Flapping tremor if CO_2 acutely raised).

Further information

NICE guidelines for COPD. February 2004. www.nice.org.uk

ERS Consensus Statement—optimal assessment and management of COPD. *ERJ* 1995; **8**: 1398–420

MacNee W, Calverley PMA. Management of COPD. *Thorax* 2003; **58**: 261–5

www.copd-international.com, www.lunguk.org/copd. Patient information websites

Investigations

Pulmonary function tests

- Obstructive spirometry and flow-volume loops
- Reduced FEV_1 to <80% predicted (FEV_1 is the measurement of choice to assess progression of COPD, but it correlates weakly with the degree of dyspnoea. Changes in FEV_1 do not reflect the decline in a patient's health)
- FEV_1/FVC <0.7
- Minimal bronchodilator reversibility (<15%, usually <10%) and minimal steroid reversibility (how to perform these, see p 175). It is not necessary to test these in most patients, but is useful if there is diagnostic uncertainty or if the patient is thought to have both COPD and asthma
- Raised total lung volume, FRC, and residual volume because of emphysema, air trapping, and loss of elastic recoil
- Decreased TLCO and kCO because presence of emphysema decreases surface area available for gas diffusion.

CXR is not required for diagnosis and repeated CXR is unnecessary unless other diagnoses are being considered (most importantly lung cancer or bronchiectasis).

- Hyperinflated lung fields with attenuation of peripheral vasculature—'black lung sign'. More than 7 posterior ribs seen
- Flattened diaphragms (best CXR correlate of post-mortem degree of emphysema)
- More horizontal ribs
- May see bullae, especially in the lung apices, which if large can be mistaken for a pneumothorax due to the loss of lung markings (CT can differentiate).

Consider checking α_1-antitrypsin levels (see p 182), FBC to ensure not anaemic, TFT if unduly breathless. CRP is slightly increased in COPD, but decreases after steroid treatment. It may be related to the presence of comorbidities and may aid the assessment of the systemic effects of COPD, particularly in the research setting.

Diagnosis is based on the history of smoking and progressive dyspnoea, with evidence of irreversible airflow obstruction on spirometry. Asthma is the most important differential diagnosis. Asthma is steroid and bronchodilator responsive. Nearly all patients with COPD will have a smoking history; this is not universal in asthma. Symptoms are common under the age of 35 in asthma; rare in COPD. Chronic productive cough is common is COPD and uncommon in asthma. Breathlessness is progressive and persistent in COPD, but variable in asthma. In asthma there is significant diurnal or day-to-day variability of symptoms, and night-time waking with SOB or wheeze are common; these symptoms are uncommon in COPD. Some patients have both.

COPD severity according to NICE guidelines 2004

(which differ slightly from the GOLD guidelines)

Mild	FEV_1 50–80% predicted. May or may not be symptomatic with cough or sputum
Moderate	FEV_1 30–49% predicted. Increased FRC, reduced TLCO Likely to be symptomatic (cough, sputum, dyspnoea), often managed by patient's GP
Severe	FEV_1 <30% predicted. Marked hyperinflation, TLCO usually low. Usually hypoxic, with signs of cor pulmonale. Symptomatic, often needing hospital admissions

MRC dyspnoea scale

1. Not troubled by breathlessness except on strenuous exercise
2. Short of breath when hurrying or walking up a slight hill
3. Walks slower than contemporaries on level ground because of breathlessness or has to stop for breath when walking at own pace
4. Stops for breath after walking about 100 m or after a few minutes on level ground
5. Too breathless to leave the house, or breathless when dressing or undressing.

BODE Index

Variable	**Points on BODE index**			
0	1	2	3	
FEV_1, (% predicted)	≥65	50–64	36–49	≤35
Distance walked in 6 min (m)	≥350	250–349	150–249	≤149
MRC dyspnoea scale	0–1	2	3	4
Body mass index	≥21	≤21		

This is a simple multidimensional grading system for COPD, using **B**MI, airflow **O**bstruction, **D**yspnoea and **E**xercise capacity as its scoring variables. It has been shown to be better than FEV_1 at predicting risk of hospitalization and death in patients with COPD. Patients are scored as having a BODE index of between 0 and 10, with higher scores indicating a higher risk of death. It is being widely used, particularly in research studies (Celli BR *et al. NEJM* 2004; **350:** 1005–12).

Non-pharmacological management of stable COPD

Aims of COPD management should include:
- Ensuring the diagnosis is correct
- Stopping smoking
- Optimizing treatment by minimizing symptoms where possible
- Helping the patient maintain their quality of life.

Management should be delivered by a multi-disciplinary team.
No treatment has yet been shown to modify disease progression in the long term, except for stopping smoking.

Smoking cessation is the only intervention that is proven to decrease the smoking-related decline in lung function. All patients with COPD who smoke should be encouraged to stop at every opportunity. Figure 21.1 shows the accelerated decline in FEV_1 in susceptible smokers and the delay in this acceleration from stopping smoking; susceptible smokers, however, never regain the original curve. Nicotine replacement therapy should be used to aid smoking cessation (see p 730).

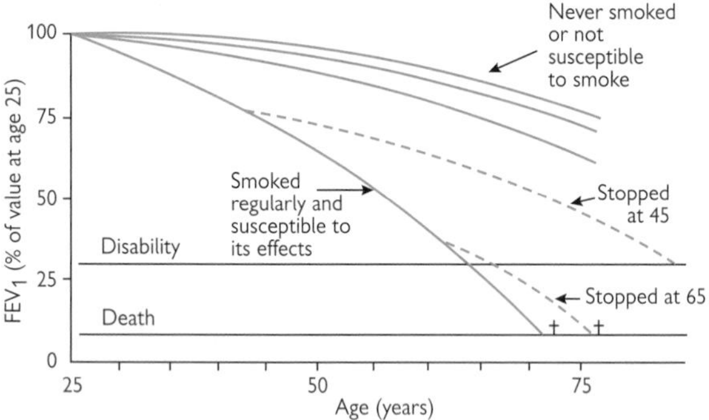

Fig. 21.1. Modification of the Fletcher–Peto diagram of FEV_1 decline in susceptible smokers

Education can improve ability to manage illness and stop smoking.

Pulmonary rehabilitation is a multidisciplinary programme, with RCT evidence that it improves exercise tolerance, quality of life, and reduces hospital admissions. Muscle mass, particularly in the lower limbs, is reduced in people with COPD compared with age-matched healthy controls. This is an independent predictor of mortality and disability, independent of the severity of the underlying lung disease and may reflect the systemic nature of COPD. The mainstay of rehabilitation is graded exercise to improve muscle function, but also includes breathing techniques and education.

Programmes vary, but are usually run on an out-patient basis over several weeks, with multidisciplinary involvement (see p 723). Should be made available to all appropriate patients with COPD.

Diet Weight loss is recommended if the patient is obese, to minimize respiratory effort. If the patient is very breathless, calorific intake may be low and a catabolic state may exist. A low BMI is associated with impaired pulmonary status, decreased diaphragm mass, lower exercise capacity and increased mortality rate compared with people with a normal BMI. Nutritional supplementation may therefore be necessary. Maintaining body weight and muscle mass correlates well with survival.

Psychosocial support Practical support at home, day centres; car disability badge; assess for signs of anxiety and depression.

Pharmacological management of stable COPD

Pharmacological management aims to relieve symptoms and reduce exacerbations, but will not modify disease. Increase treatment in a stepwise fashion. Exacerbations require additional therapeutic support (see p 176).

Bronchodilators Simple pulmonary function testing may not show significant bronchodilator reversibility of FEV_1, but bronchodilators provide therapeutic benefit in the long term by reducing dyspnoea, perhaps by decreasing chest hyperinflation.

- Initially prescribe short-acting β_2-agonists as required for symptom relief
- If the patient remains symptomatic, prescribe short-acting β_2-agonist with short acting anti-cholinergic
- If symptoms persists, try therapeutic trial of regular long-acting bronchodilator, with or without an anti-cholinergic. Stop if no benefit (expensive). Continue if the patient has 2 or more exacerbations per year, as there is evidence for a reduction in exacerbation frequency and hence decreased health resource utilization
- Oral methylxanthines, such as theophyllines, can be used as a maintenance therapy and may improve symptoms. Add after inhaled bronchodilators and trial of inhaled steroids; continue only if symptoms improve. Their method of action is unclear, but they may have an anti-inflammatory effect. Take care regarding therapeutic/toxic levels, especially in elderly patients
- Inhaler therapy provides adequate bronchodilator doses for most patients, especially when used with a spacer device. It is important to check the patient's inhaler technique
- Nebulizer therapy is indicated if the patient is unable to use inhalers, or if they are disabled or distressed with breathlessness despite maximal inhaler therapy. Only those with a clear response, with reduction in symptoms or improvement in activities of daily living, should continue with long-term domiciliary nebulized treatment (usually with salbutamol and ipratropium), as there is a significant placebo effect.

Inhaled steroids should be prescribed to all patients with an $FEV_1 \leq 60\%$ predicted, who have had 2 or more exacerbations per year requiring treatment with antibiotics or oral steroids. Clinical trials of inhaled steroids have shown a reduction in exacerbation frequency and severity in severe COPD, but no slowing in the decline in lung function. Warn patients regarding steroid side-effects and document. Use in combination with bronchodilator.

Oral steroids are not recommended as a maintenance therapy in COPD. It may, however, be difficult to withdraw them in patients with severe COPD following an exacerbation. If so, keep the dose as low as possible and prescribe osteoporosis prophylaxis if indicated. Warn regarding steroid side-effects and document.

Oxygen can be administered via a cylinder for short burst oxygen therapy as required for symptomatic relief, such as after climbing stairs (there is little trial evidence to support this use—only continue if improvement in breathlessness documented), or as long-term oxygen therapy (LTOT) via an oxygen concentrator. The latter is for patients in respiratory failure, with a PaO_2 <7.3 kPa or PaO_2 of 7.3–8 kPa with any of secondary polycythaemia, peripheral oedema, or pulmonary hypertension present, to use for a minimum of 15 h per day (including sleep). Additional ambulatory cylinders can be provided. Low flow oxygen, such as 2–4 L/min via nasal prongs, is usually adequate. Small changes in CO_2 retention with oxygen administration can be tolerated if asymptomatic and no respiratory acidosis. Associated OSA is a risk factor for CO_2 retention. (For further information on prescribing oxygen, see p 703.)

Vaccination Influenza vaccine annually and pneumococcal vaccine. Meta-analysis showed a decrease in exacerbations occurs 3 weeks after receiving influenza vaccine and there is no evidence of an earlier increase in exacerbations due directly to vaccination.

Antibiotics No trials of antibiotic prophylaxis have been done. Many respiratory physicians prescribe low-dose rotating antibiotics, particularly over the winter. Trials are urgently required. It is likely that this strategy would be more effective than inhaled steroids.

Mucolytics (carbocisteine, mecysteine hydrochloride) may benefit some patients with chronic productive cough to facilitate expectoration by reducing sputum viscosity. Prescribe for a 4-week trial period and only continue if there is evidence of improvement. Meta-analyses show mucolytics cause a significant decrease in the number of COPD exacerbations and decrease the number of days of disability, although the benefit may only apply if the patient is not taking inhaled steroids. Worth trying in those with moderate to severe COPD, with frequent or prolonged exacerbations, or those repeatedly in hospital with COPD exacerbations. Caution if known peptic ulcer disease.

Palliative care/respiratory sedation Use of low-dose sedatives, such as morphine sulphate solution 10 mg as required or diazepam 2 mg bd, can be used as a palliative measure (see pp 720–21), aiming to relieve the sensation of dyspnoea and associated anxiety, in those with severe COPD. Dose may need to be titrated against any rise in CO_2 (surprisingly uncommon).

New anti-inflammatory drugs

Erdosteine is a thiol compound with effects on bacterial adhesiveness as well as anti-oxidant and mucoactive properties. RCT in moderate COPD showed decreased exacerbations vs. placebo over 8 months, no loss of lung function, and improved health-related quality of life.

Roflumilast and cilomilast are phosphodiesterase 4 inhibitors, which elicit anti-inflammatory effects. RCT of roflumilast in moderate to severe COPD showed a significant improvement in FEV_1 over 24 h vs. placebo and a reduction in the rate of mild exacerbations. Long-term studies are required to evaluate its efficacy and role further. Cilomilast has shown similar results.

An approach to COPD in the out-patient clinic

- Establish diagnosis and severity—pulmonary function tests, CXR
- Ensure there are no other causes for symptoms, e.g. anaemia, pulmonary emboli, heart failure, interstitial lung disease, thyroid dysfunction, pneumothorax, large bulla, arrhythmia, depression
- Encourage the patient to stop smoking
- Review current treatment—optimize bronchodilatation and inhaled steroids
- Assess whether there is any need for a nebulizer
- Check oxygen saturation and perform blood gas if <92%. Consider LTOT
- Consider pulmonary rehabilitation
- Check vaccinations are up to date
- Involve respiratory nurse specialist for input in the community if appropriate
- Follow up in clinic if ongoing medical issues, including whether patient may be a lung transplant candidate (see p 318). Otherwise discharge back to GP
- Inform GP of all the above decisions.

Further information

Poole PJ *et al.* Influenza vaccination for patients with COPD. *Cochrane Database Syst Rev* 2006; **1**: CD002733

Poole PJ, Black PN. Mucolytic agents for chronic bronchitis or COPD. *Cochrane Database Syst Rev* 2006; **3**: CD001287

Black P *et al.* Prophylactic antibiotic therapy for chronic bronchitis. *Cochrane Database Syst Rev* 2003; **1**: CD004105

How to perform a steroid trial to help distinguish asthma from COPD (if diagnosis unclear)

Measure FEV_1 and slow VC before and after:

- either a high-dose inhaled steroid for 6–8 weeks
- or a 2-week course of oral prednisolone, 30 mg/day

>15% increase in FEV_1 implies steroid reversibility and patient is likely to have asthma.

>15% increase in slow VC suggests significantly reduced air trapping and may indicate significant asthma. May occur with a significantly smaller change in FEV_1.

Document results of trial clearly in notes.

Testing for bronchodilator reversibility to help distinguish asthma from COPD

- Check FEV_1. Give patient a short acting β_2 agonist, either nebulized or inhaled via spacer. 15–30 min after this, recheck the FEV_1.
- Subtract the pre-test value from the post-test value, divide the difference by the pre-test value, and express as a percentage increase from baseline. >15% increase or >200 ml indicates bronchodilator reversibility
- Avoid short-acting bronchodilator in the preceding 6 h, a long-acting bronchodilator in the preceding 12 h, or a long-acting anticholinergic or slow release theophylline in the preceding 24 h.

COPD exacerbations

Exacerbations may cause mild symptoms in those with relatively preserved lung function, but can cause considerable morbidity in those with limited respiratory reserve. It has been increasingly recognized that significant numbers of patients do not regain their premorbid lung function or quality of life following an exacerbation, and those with frequent exacerbations experience a more rapid FEV_1 decline than those with fewer exacerbations. Exacerbation frequency increases with COPD severity. Exacerbations are 50% more likely in winter (possibly viruses survive better in the cold and people crowd together indoors). An exacerbation is essentially a clinical diagnosis.

Causes may be infective organisms, either viral or bacterial, or non-infective causes, such as pollution or temperature fall. Common bacterial pathogens are *Haemophilus influenzae*, *Streptococcus pneumoniae*, and *Moraxella catarrhalis*, and the commonest viral pathogens are rhinovirus, RSV, influenza, coronavirus, and adenovirus. Consider the possibility of PE or pneumothorax.

Symptoms include increased sputum volume and/or purulence, increasing dyspnoea or wheeze, chest tightness, fluid retention.

Pathophysiology There is increased airway resistance due to bronchospasm, mucosal oedema, and increased sputum. This worsens expiratory flow limitation and expiration takes longer. Shallow rapid breathing further limits the time for expiration. This promotes dynamic hyperinflation and this itself causes mechanical compromise within the lung and the airway. Maximal recruitment of the accessory muscles is required and thoraco-abdominal dysynchrony is often present.

▶▶ Management summary: acute exacerbation of COPD

- Assess the severity of the exacerbation by measuring respiratory rate, oxygen saturations, degree of air entry, tachycardia, BP, peripheral perfusion, conscious level, mental state
- Exclude a pneumothorax clinically
- If hypoxic, give controlled 24–35% oxygen via Venturi facemask to aim for SaO_2 88–92%, salbutamol nebulizer, establish venous access
- Check blood gas
- Request a CXR
- Perform ECG
- Check bloods for WCC, CRP, potassium, etc.
- Optimize volume status
- Take a brief history if possible. Important to know what patient's normal functional status is like, such as exercise tolerance and the need for help with activities of daily living. Old hospital notes are helpful regarding severity of disease, and whether previous decisions have been made regarding ventilation or resuscitation
- Nebulized bronchodilators—salbutamol 2.5–5 mg and ipratropium 500 μg on arrival and 4–6-hourly. Run nebulizer with air not oxygen
- Continued oxygen therapy, aiming to maintain saturations between 80% and 90%. Repeat blood gases after 60 min to ensure improvement if hypoxic or acidotic. Repeat if clinical deterioration
- Consider antibiotics
- Oral steroids
- Consider intravenous aminophylline if not improving with nebulizers
- Consider intensive care—ideally consultant-led decision with the patient, their family, and ITU regarding invasive mechanical ventilation. Document in the medical notes. Consider resuscitation status
- Consider non-invasive ventilation—pH 7.3 or less, hypoxia, hypercapnia, conscious. Decide if this is the ceiling of therapy
- Consider doxapram if NIV not available or not tolerated
- DVT prophylaxis
- Early mobilization
- Nutrition.

Further information

Intermediate care Hospital-at-Home in COPD: BTS guideline. *Thorax* 2007; **62**: 200-210

Ram FSF *et al.* Hospital at home for patients with acute exacerbations of COPD: systematic review of the evidence. *BMJ* 2004; **329**: 315–18

Review series: COPD exacerbations. *Thorax* 2006; **61**: 164–8, 250–8, 440–7, 535–44, 354–61

Management of exacerbations

- Assess the severity of the exacerbation: increase in dyspnoea, tachypnoea, use of accessory muscles, new cyanosis, pedal oedema, or confusion
- Exclude alternative diagnoses, such as pneumothorax, PE, pulmonary oedema)
- Can the patient self-care and self-medicate? In the presence of severe symptoms, with possible comorbid disease and decreased functional activities, the patient is likely to need hospital management
- Investigate with CXR, ABGs, ECG, FBC, and U&Es. *Admission arterial pH is the best predictor of survival.* A pH <7.25 is associated with a rapidly rising mortality. A *raised* pH may imply an alternative diagnosis, not associated with worsening airways obstruction. Check theophylline level if patient is taking regularly; consider sending sputum for culture if it is purulent.

Treatment

- ***Antibiotics*** if sputum purulent, pyrexial, high CRP, new changes on CXR
- ***Systemic steroids*** for all patients with exacerbations of COPD who are admitted to hospital or are significantly more breathless than usual. Give prednisolone 30 mg/day for 1 to 2 weeks, unless there are specific contraindications. Optimum dose and length of steroids not established. This improves FEV_1, improves symptoms, and shortens recovery time. Long-term steroid treatment should be avoided due to side-effects. If the patient has a longer course of steroids, or repeated courses due to repeated exacerbations, the dose will need to be tailed off slowly
- ***Inhaled or nebulized bronchodilators*** Breathless unwell patients may benefit from nebulizer therapy in the acute period to reduce symptoms and improve airflow obstruction
- ***Controlled oxygen therapy*** 24–35% via Venturi facemask, with oximetry, arterial blood gases, or capillary gas monitoring. Guidelines suggest maintaining saturations between 88% and 92%, balancing hypoxia, hypercapnia, and pH. Too little oxygen causes anaerobic metabolism and metabolic acidosis (probably SaO_2 >80% would prevent this); too much oxygen (SaO_2 >92%) can cause hypercapnia and a respiratory acidosis. A deteriorating pH to below 7.25 has a much poorer prognosis. Make sure your instructions to the ward staff are clear as to the need to keep the SaO_2 within this window by changing the % O_2 delivered as necessary. Falling conscious level is the best clinical marker of significant CO_2 retention and acidosis
- ***Intravenous aminophylline*** Evidence is lacking regarding the effectiveness of IV aminophylline, but it may be beneficial, particularly if the patient is wheezy and has not improved with nebulizers alone. Give a loading dose, unless the patient is on regular oral aminophylline, followed by a maintenance infusion. Need to monitor aminophylline levels daily. Main side-effects are tachycardia and nausea.

- ***Non-invasive ventilation (NIV)*** Effective in supporting patients during an exacerbation, when maximal medical treatment has not been effective. Appropriate for conscious patients with ongoing respiratory acidosis (pH 7.35 or less), hypoxia, and hypercapnia. May avoid intubation. Ceiling of treatment should be determined **before** its use (See p 693.).
- ***Doxapram*** Intravenous respiratory stimulant. Can be used to drive respiratory rate (if below 20 /min) and depth in COPD exacerbation and hence improve hypoxia, hypercapnia, and respiratory acidosis, particularly when induced by oxygen therapy. It can overdrive breathing to the point of respiratory muscle fatigue, collapse, and death, and causes metabolic acidosis, agitation, and cardiac arrhythmias. It should only be used at the lowest possible dose (0.5–3 mg/min) in the short term (usually 24–36 h), aiming to reduce $PaCO_2$ (and raise pH) by only a small amount. Its use has largely been replaced by NIV, but may be used if NIV is not available or not tolerated.
- ***Acetazolamide*** generates a metabolic acidosis by reducing the kidney's ability to secrete [H+] into urine (blocks carbonic anhydrase that interconverts CO_2 and H^+/HCO_3^-). There is only one situation in which provoking a metabolic acidosis might be appropriate: following a transient period of hypoventilation (perhaps due to pump failure/increased airways obstruction) or after permissive hypercapnia on the ICU, the previous appropriate compensatory rise in blood [HCO_3^-] can now be too high for the improving $PaCO_2$. This generates a blood alkalosis (pH>7.4), which itself depresses ventilation, and delays the return of PaO_2 and $PaCO_2$ to normal. The judicious use of a few doses of acetazolamide (250 mg OD), but only safe when the pH is alkaline, can hasten the recovery.
- ***Intubation/intensive*** care If the patient is not responding to medical therapy, a decision regarding invasive mechanical ventilation needs to be made. This may be considered to be appropriate if the patient usually has a good functional status, with minimal other comorbidity. These decisions should ideally be discussed with the patient, their family, their consultant, and the ITU consultant, and documented in the medical notes. Resuscitation decisions should also be made.
- ***Early rehabilitation*** to prevent muscle wasting and deconditioning
- ***Nutrition***
- ***Acute respiratory assessment service (ARAS)/'Hospital at home'*** Respiratory nurse-led service supporting early discharge of COPD patients after hospital assessment and providing ongoing respiratory care at home. CXR, SaO_2, and baseline spirometry (if this is first presentation) should be performed prior to discharge. Reduces length of in-patient stay and hence is an economic alternative. Unsuitable patients are those with impaired GCS, acute confusion, pH<7.35, acute changes on CXR, concomitant medical problems requiring in-patient stay, insufficient social support (including living far from the hospital and not having a telephone), new hypoxia with SaO_2 <90%, and unable to provide oxygen at home.

Surgical treatment

Lung transplant In young patients (below 60–65) with severe disease, often due to α_1-antitrypsin deficiency, single lung transplant may be an option. Local transplant teams will advise regarding local criteria.

Bullectomy Suitable for selected patients who are breathless, have FEV_1 <50% predicted, and isolated large bulla seen on CT. Improves chest hyperinflation.

Lung volume reduction surgery (LVRS) Resection of areas of bullous emphysema to reduce chest hyperinflation and improve diaphragmatic function, elastic recoil, physiology of the lungs, and hence functional status of the patient. Patients who may be considered are those with FEV_1 20–30% predicted, with symptomatic dyspnoea despite maximal medical therapy, and with upper lobe predominant emphysema on CT, giving target areas to resect. $PaCO_2$ should be less than 7.3 kPa and TLCO >20% predicted. Pre-operative assessment: PFTs, 6 min walk test, quality of life, and dyspnoea indicators. Surgery is performed in specialist centres via median sternotomy or by thoracoscopy. Usually the upper lobe is stapled below the level of the emphysema and then removed. Improvements are seen in FEV_1 and RV, dyspnoea, and quality of life scores. These effects are maximal between 2 and 6 months post-surgery. Symptomatic improvement is sustained for about 2–4 years. Post-operative complications: persistent air leak >7 days in 30–40%, pneumonia in up to 22%, respiratory failure in up to 13%. Post-operative mortality 2.4–17% reported.

The National Emphysema Treatment Trial (Michigan, USA) randomized 1218 patients to receive medical treatment or LVRS. Mean airflow limitation of the subjects was 27% predicted. The most recent analysis, published after 4 years of follow-up, has shown LVRS demonstrates an overall survival advantage compared with medical therapy alone. Improvements in maximal exercise and health-related quality of life were also found over 3 and 4 years, respectively. The greatest survival benefits, improved exercise and symptoms over 5 years, were in those with both low exercise capacity and upper-lobe-predominant emphysema. Those with high exercise capacity and upper-lobe-predominant emphysema obtained no survival advantage, but exercise and health-related quality of life improved. Interim analysis had shown increased mortality from LVRS for patients with FEV_1 or TLCO <20% predicted, or with homogeneous emphysema. Surgery is not, therefore, recommended for these groups.

Bronchoscopic lung volume reduction is under evaluation, with one-way valve implants placed within the segmental and sub-segmental bronchi that supply the hyperinflated lobes. It is a minimally invasive variation on lung volume reduction surgery, with the aim of improving lung function and quality of life. Pilot studies in end-stage emphysema (mean FEV_1 30% predicted) have shown the procedure to be safe, although a small subset of patients developed pneumothorax and one death (in 98 patients) has been reported. Significant improvements in RV, FEV_1, FVC and 6 min walk were found at 30 and 90 days. A multi-centre RCT (the VENT trial) has been completed of best medical care (including pulmonary rehabilitation) vs.

best medical care plus unilateral endoscopic bronchial valve. Early presented results (ERS 2007) of 321 patients after 6 months of follow up (220 in the valve group) showed a significant improvement in FEV_1 and 6 min walk test in the valve group. Knowledge and skill is improving in this area and further studies are planned.

Airway bypass aims to improve respiratory mechanics by creating new exit pathways for air trapped in emphysematous lungs. The wall of a segmental bronchus is punctured under bronchoscopic guidance and a stent is inserted, creating an internal bronchopulmonary communication for expiration. Hence, hyperinflation decreases and lung mechanics are improved. This is at an early stage of research.

Further information

Naunheim KS *et al.* Long term follow-up of patients receiving LVRS vs. medical therapy for severe emphysema by the NETT research group. *Ann Thoracic Surg* 2006; **82**: 431–43

Fishman A *et al.* A randomized trial comparing lung-volume-reduction surgery with medical therapy for severe emphysema. *N Engl J Med* 2003; **22**: 2059–73.

Criner GJ *et al.* Prospective randomised trial comparing bilateral LVRS to pulmonary rehabilitation in severe COPD. *Am Resp Crit Care Med* 1999; **160**: 2018–27

Geddes D *et al.* Effect of LVRS in patients with severe emphysema. *NEJM* 2000; **343**: 239–45

Toma TP *et al.* Bronchoscopic volume reduction with valve implants in patients with severe emphysema. *Lancet* 2003; **361**: 931–3

Benditt JO. Surgical therapies for COPD. *Respir Care* 2004; **49**: 53–63

α_1-antitrypsin (α_1-AT) deficiency

This is an inherited condition that is associated with the early development of emphysema. It is common (estimated 1 in 2000–5000 individuals) and is probably under-diagnosed, as it is often asymptomatic in non-smokers.

Pathophysiology α_1-AT is a glycoprotein protease inhibitor produced by the liver. It is secreted via the bloodstream into the lungs and opposes neutrophil elastase, which destroys alveolar wall connective tissue. Elastase is produced in increased levels by pulmonary neutrophils and macrophages in response to smoking and lung infections. If α_1-AT is deficient, the elastase cannot be opposed, and subsequently basal emphysema develops. The disease is worse in smokers and can cause COPD at a young age (40s and 50s). There may also be associated liver dysfunction, chronic hepatitis, cirrhosis, and hepatoma, as abnormal protein secretion accumulates in the liver. Predisposition also to skin disease (panniculitis) and vasculitis (especially ANCA +).

Genetics α_1-AT deficiency is inherited as an autosomal co-dominant disorder. So far more than 100 different alleles have been identified for this gene (SERPINA 1) on the long arm of chromosome 14. The commonest alleles are the *M* allele (normal), the partially defective *S* allele, and the almost fully defective *Z* allele (lysine is substituted for glutamic acid at position 342, leading to abnormal folding, preventing post-translational processing with retention within cells), commonest in Scandinavia.

- MM, the normal phenotype. Background population risk of emphysema
- MS, MZ have 50–70% of normal α_1-protease inhibitor (Pi) levels. Background risk of emphysema
- SZ, SS have 35–50% of normal levels. 20–50% risk of emphysema
- Homozygous ZZ has only 10–20% of normal levels. 80–100% risk of emphysema

Screening for the defect should be carried out especially in patients <40 with COPD. Also patients with unexplained liver disease should be screened. Send blood for α_1-AT concentrations and genotyping if levels are low. Siblings should be screened and the particular importance of not smoking and avoiding passive smoking emphasized. Non-smokers are usually asymptomatic.

Treatment includes usual therapy for COPD. Specific treatment is known as augmentation therapy, with weekly/2-weekly/monthly infusions of purified α_1-AT from pooled human plasma. This raises concentrations in serum and epithelial-lining fluid above the protective threshold. It appears to be safe, with minimal side-effects. A large cohort study showed reduced mortality amongst infusion recipients, with a slowing of lung function decline (by 27 ml/year, $p = 0.03$) in a subgroup with moderate emphysema. An RCT showed no significant differences between augmentation and control groups, although there was a trend towards slower loss of lung tissue on CT scan in the augmentation group ($p = 0.07$). It has, however, been recommended as a treatment by groups including the ATS and ERS for those with moderate (FEV_1 35–60% predicted) emphysema due to α_1-AT deficiency, but not those with mild or severe disease or those post lung transplant for α_1-AT deficiency, except during episodes of acute rejection and infection (when inflammation causes free elastase activity). It is expensive and its cost-effectiveness in terms of cost per year of life saved is high. It is, however, the only specific therapy available at present.

Future developments Inhaled α_1-AT may provide a way of delivering the enzyme to the lower respiratory tract to have its action locally and potentially reduce inflammation. Gene therapy is under development, finding ways of delivering the α_1-AT gene into the cell. Other strategies include inhibition of hepatic polymerization of α_1-AT, promotion of hepatic secretion, inhibition of neutrophil elastase by synthetic inhibitors to avoid the use of human plasma, and pegylation of α_1-AT to prolong its serum half-life.

Further information

ADAPT programme (Antitrypsin deficiency Assessment and Programme for Treatment) www.aatregistry.org/ukusa.html headed by Prof R Stockley, Queen Elizabeth Hospital Birmingham. Aims to have a comprehensive database of all patients with α1-antitrypsin deficiency in the UK, as well as offering assessment and treatment in a single UK centre.

Stoller JK, Aboussouan LS. α1-antitrypsin deficiency. *Lancet* 2005; **365**: 2225–36

Review series: α1-antitrypsin deficiency. *Thorax* 2004: **59**: 64–9, 259–64, 441–5,529–35, 708–12, 904–9

UK alpha1 antitrypsin deficiency support group www.alpha1.org.uk/index.html

Chapter 22

Connective tissue disease and the lung

Differential diagnosis and standard tests

Patients with connective tissue diseases can develop pulmonary complications, for which they might be referred to a chest physician. Patients typically present with symptoms of dyspnoea, cough, fever, or chest pain. They may often be on immunosuppressive drugs.

Differential diagnosis

In practice, the main differential diagnosis lies between:

Opportunistic pulmonary infection

- May be in those on immunosuppressive drugs, or functionally immunosuppressed from underlying disease
- Any usual organism, also TB, non-tuberculous mycobacteria, PCP, fungi, cytomegalovirus
- Often acute onset with non-specific features of low-grade fever, productive cough, raised inflammatory markers
- Can be very unwell and need full supportive treatment with ITU.

Original connective tissue disease now affecting the lung

- Often inflammation or fibrosis
- Usually more indolent presentation, with dry cough and dyspnoea, but can become acutely unwell with background of chronic lung disease
- Fine inspiratory crackles on auscultation
- Consider development of pulmonary hypertension in patients with systemic sclerosis.

New pulmonary pathology

- Unrelated to the original condition, including pulmonary thromboembolic disease.

Drug side-effects

- Methotrexate—pneumonitis occurs in 5% of patients receiving methotrexate. Potentially life-threatening. Mortality 15–20%. Cough, fever, dyspnoea, widespread crackles, restrictive defect, and pulmonary infiltrates on CXR and CT. Peripheral eosinophilia in 50%. BAL lymphocytosis. Usually subacute onset, but may be sudden. Usually within 4 months of starting methotrexate. Non-specific histological findings. No more common in those with pre-existing lung disease. Treatment: stop the drug, commence steroids, and avoid methotrexate in the future. Can be reversible. Can get mild intractable cough with methotrexate
- Gold—alveolar opacities seen on HRCT, with associated fever and skin rash. BAL lymphocytosis. Treatment: stop the drug and commence steroids. Usually reversible
- Penicillamine—causes obliterative bronchiolitis in rheumatoid arthritis. Can also cause a hypersensitivity pneumonitis and a pulmonary–renal syndrome causing alveolar haemorrhage. May respond to stopping the drug.

Standard tests to consider for the investigation of these patients

- Oxygen saturations and blood gas
- CXR ± HRCT
- Culture of respiratory secretions
- Pulmonary function tests, including KCO
- Autoantibody and inflammatory marker levels
- Bronchoscopy and bronchoalveolar lavage
- Transbronchial or open lung biopsies.

For an approach to:

- Diffuse lung disease, see p 29
- Diffuse alveolar haemorrhage, see p 25
- Pulmonary disease in the immunocompromised host (non-HIV), see p 67.

Rheumatoid arthritis (RA)

- Persistent deforming symmetrical peripheral arthropathy
- Pulmonary disease is commoner in men and occasionally occurs before the development of joint problems
- Pneumonia is a common terminal event, causing 15–20% of rheumatoid arthritis deaths

Pleuritis Frequent, occurring in more than 30% of patients and usually mild. Pleuritic pain, with no obvious other cause.

Pleural effusion Usually asymptomatic. Fluid is typically exudative with a low glucose and low pH and usually a lymphocytosis. Need to exclude other causes for effusion, such as empyema or malignancy. If problematic, may require drainage and steroids. (See p 360.)

Pulmonary fibrosis Minor pulmonary fibrosis found in up to 60% of patients in lung biopsy studies, but CXR changes only seen in 1–5%. Hence symptomatic disease is unusual. Tends to occur in patients who have multi-system disease, including vasculitis, and those with nodules, seropositive disease, and high ANA titres. More common in men, and smoking is a risk factor for fibrosis development.

- *Presents* with progressive dyspnoea
- *Examination*: clubbing and bilateral basal crepitations
- *PFTs*: low kCO, restrictive pattern
- Radiologically and histologically similar to usual interstitial pneumonitis (UIP), with subpleural basal reticular pattern, but can be like non-specific interstitial pneumonitis (NSIP)
- *Treatment*: steroids or immunosuppressants do little to change the course, but should be tried

Acute pneumonitis also recognized, which presents with rapidly deteriorating dyspnoea and development of respiratory failure, or acute deterioration on a background of chronic fibrosis. Acute pneumonitis tends to be more steroid responsive.

Pulmonary nodules occur in less than 5% of patients with RA. Usually found incidentally on CXR. Only occur in seropositive disease, and patients may have other nodules elsewhere, such as elbows and fingers. Single or multiple; may measure up to 7 cm. May cavitate and cause haemoptysis or pneumothorax. Mostly asymptomatic. Main differential diagnosis is lung cancer. Usually followed on CT to ensure they are of stable size. They typically show mild uptake on PET, consistent with other benign lesions. May need biopsy to exclude malignancy.

Bronchiectasis is often subtle with minimal clinical features, but may be found in 30%. May be seen in association with pulmonary fibrosis. Diagnosis made on HRCT.

Organizing pneumonia The clinical syndrome of pneumonia with fever, dyspnoea, and multifocal consolidation, which do not respond to antibiotics. Can be disease- or drug-induced (gold), or have no obvious cause, and is then known as cryptogenic (see p 270). Confirmed by trans-bronchial or open lung biopsy showing acini filled with loose connective tissue and a variable inflammatory infiltrate. Often a dramatic response to steroids. May need long-term immunosuppression.

Obliterative bronchiolitis Rare. Terminal bronchioles progressively obliterated by inflammatory connective tissue.

- May present with dyspnoea and hyperinflated chest, with basal crepitations
- *PFTs*: irreversible obstructive pattern
- *CXR*: hyperinflation, no infiltrates
- *HRCT*: mosaic pattern
- *Biopsy* shows destruction of terminal bronchiolar wall by granulation tissue, effacement of the lumen, and replacement of the bronchiole by fibrous tissue. Irreversible pathology, usually unresponsive to treatment
- May be rapidly progressive
- Can give trial of oral steroids, continuing with high-dose inhaled steroids if any response. Consider transplant. Penicillamine was thought to be a causative factor, but the evidence for this is now weaker.

Vasculitis and rarely pulmonary haemorrhage.

Cricoarytenoid arthritis Seen in studies in up to 75% of patients with rheumatoid arthritis by fibre-optic laryngoscopy and HRCT, but rarely symptomatic. Unrelated to lung fibrosis. Can cause sore throat, hoarse voice, upper airways obstruction with stridor, or OSA. Flow–volume loop may be abnormal. This may need tracheostomy and steroids—oral and joint injection.

Caplan's syndrome Rheumatoid arthritis, single or multiple chest nodules, and coal-worker's pneumoconiosis.

Systemic lupus erythematosus (SLE)

- Multi-organ autoimmune disease, mainly affecting women
- Double-stranded DNA antibodies present in high titres and these may be the causative agent
- Can also get a drug-induced lupus syndrome, which improves when the drug is stopped
- Pulmonary disease often seen and may be a presenting feature of the disease

Pleural disease Most common manifestation of pulmonary disease. Often asymptomatic, but may have pain due to pleuritis. Pleural effusions found in 50% of patients, which cause breathlessness. These are often bilateral and exudative, with a neutrophilia or a lymphocytosis if the effusion is chronic. Can be haemorrhagic. Pleural biopsy findings are non-specific. Need to exclude other causes for effusion, such as empyema or malignancy. If symptomatic, may need treatment with non-steroidal anti-inflammatory drugs or steroids.

Atelectasis associated with pleurisy or effusion.

Diffuse lung disease Occurs in up to 70% of patients, but usually mild and asymptomatic. Radiologically similar to rheumatoid lung fibrosis. Only 5% develop clinical disease similar to UIP with dyspnoea, cough, and basal crackles. May be associated with pleuritic pain. PFTs show restrictive defect with reduced kCO. Rarely, progressive and severe.

Acute lupus pneumonitis In <2%, severe illness with high mortality rate of over 50%. Cough, dyspnoea, fever, pleuritic pain, hypoxia. Widespread crackles. CXR shows infiltrates, which may be widespread. Histologically non-specific. Need to exclude infection, pulmonary oedema. Treatment with steroids and cytotoxic drugs may be necessary and may have dramatic response. Can progress to chronic interstitial pneumonitis.

Bronchiolitis obliterans See p 161.

Pulmonary nodules See p 312.

Pulmonary hypertension due to pulmonary vasoconstriction, rather than pulmonary vasculitis. Commoner in those with Raynaud's phenomenon. Associated with poorer prognosis: 50% 2-year mortality. Diagnosed on echocardiography. Need to exclude pulmonary emboli as a cause, especially in those with antiphospholipid antibodies. Treatment as for idiopathic pulmonary hypertension (see p 394).

Pulmonary emboli Commoner in the 20–30% with antiphospholipid antibodies.

Shrinking lung syndrome Dyspnoea caused by reduced lung volumes and poor respiratory reserve due to diaphragmatic muscle weakness. Small lungs on CXR. Normal lung parenchyma on CT. Restrictive lung function tests, with high kCO. May improve with steroids.

Alveolar haemorrhage Rare. May be life-threatening. Can have associated glomerulonephritis. Acute dyspnoea with infiltrates on CXR. Raised kCO. Treat with high-dose steroids + cyclophosphamide.

Criteria of the American College of Rheumatology for the classification of SLE

SLE if 4 or more criteria present, serially or simultaneously, during any interval

- Malar rash
- Discoid rash
- Photosensitivity
- Oral ulcers
- Arthritis
- Serositis
- Pleuritis or pericarditis
- Renal disorder: proteinuria >0.5 g/24 h or 3+ persistently, or cellular casts
- Neurological disorder: seizures or psychosis (having excluded drugs or other causes)
- Haematological disorder: haemolytic anaemia or leucopenia (<4.0 x 10^9/L on two or more occasions), lymphopenia (1.5 x 10^9/L on two or more occasions), thrombocytopenia (<100 x 10^9/L)
- Immunological disorder: raised anti-dsDNA antibody, anti-Sm antibody, positive finding of antiphospholipid antibodies
- Antinuclear antibody in raised titre (in the absence of drugs known to be associated with drug-induced lupus).

Drug-induced lupus—causative drugs include:

- Isoniazid
- Procainamide
- Hydralazine
- Minocycline
- Penicillamine
- Anticonvulsants.

Further information

Keane M, Lynch J Pleuropulmonary manifestations of SLE, Rare diseases 7. *Thorax* 2000; **55**: 159–66

Polymyositis and dermatomyositis

These are two separate disorders:
- Polymyositis is an inflammatory myopathy, causing symmetrical proximal muscle weakness
- Dermatomyositis is an inflammatory myopathy with a characteristic rash

Creatine kinase levels raised up to 50 times normal. Antinuclear and myositis specific antibodies positive (Jo-1). Dermatomyositis is frequently associated with underlying malignancy, including lung, oesophagus, breast, colon, and ovary, so therefore needs thorough investigation. Pulmonary complications are a common and frequent cause of death and occur in both conditions.

Pulmonary fibrosis in 20–30%. Patients present with dyspnoea. Mostly there is basal fibrosis—usually similar to UIP, but can develop a more acute pneumonitis resembling acute interstitial pneumonia (p 272).
- *HRCT* shows patchy consolidation and peripheral reticular pattern
- *Histology* may show features of organizing pneumonia and fibrosing alveolitis, and therefore may have better response to treatment
- Lung involvement frequently associated with antisynthetase antibodies
- May require treatment with steroids or cyclophosphamide

Ventilatory failure due to intercostal and diaphragmatic muscle weakness. Restrictive defect on PFTs.

Organizing pneumonia Poorer prognosis if associated with features of fibrosis.

Pulmonary hypertension secondary to lung disease.

Pulmonary vasculitis causing haemoptysis or, rarely, alveolar haemorrhage.

Aspiration pneumonia in 20%, associated with marked increase in mortality. Caused by dysphagia and pharyngeal muscle weakness and regurgitation.

Criteria for diagnosis of poly/dermatomyositis

- Symmetrical proximal muscle weakness developing over weeks or months
- Elevated serum muscle enzymes, creatine kinase, and aldolase
- Typical EMG findings:
  - Myopathic potentials (low amplitude, short duration, polyphasic)
  - Fibrillation
  - Complex repetitive discharges
  - Typical muscle biopsy findings—endomysial inflammation
- Dermatological features of dermatomyositis:
  - Gottron's papules, involving fingers, elbows, knees, and medial malleoli
  - Heliotrope sign around the eyes
  - Erythematous rash around back, shoulders, upper chest, and face

Systemic sclerosis

This disease affects women more than men (4:1), and often presents in the fifth decade. It is a clinical diagnosis and there are 4 types:

- ***Limited cutaneous*** (formerly known as CREST). Accounts for 60% of systemic sclerosis cases. Patients often have longstanding Raynaud's, and develop non-pitting oedema of the fingers, which become 'sausage-shaped'. Develop thick shiny skin after few weeks–months. Later they can develop skin changes on the hands, face, and neck, microstomia, digital and facial telangectasias, intra- and subcutaneous calcification, and oesophageal dysmotility (74%). Patients can also develop pulmonary fibrosis (26%), pulmonary hypertension (21%), cardiac (9%) and renal disease (8%), but less commonly than in diffuse cutaneous disease
- ***Diffuse cutaneous*** Abrupt onset disease, with widespread symmetrical itchy painful swelling of fingers, arms, feet, legs, and face, and associated constitutional symptoms. There is oedema, which is replaced by tight shiny skin, bound to underlying structures, within a few months. There is cutaneous thickening, as well as hypo- or hyperpigmentation. Raynaud's phenomenon is present, as well as skin sclerosis on the trunk and upper arms, arthropathy, renal disease (18%), pulmonary fibrosis (41%), pulmonary hypertension (17%), and cardiac (12%) and GI disease (68%)
- ***Overlap syndromes***, or mixed connective tissue disease, have features of systemic sclerosis together with those of at least one other autoimmune rheumatic disease, such as SLE, rheumatoid arthritis, polymyositis. Over time other organ involvement may develop and evolve into a more defined disease
- ***Systemic sclerosis sine scleroderma*** Vascular or fibrotic visceral features without skin scleroderma. May or may not have Raynaud's phenomenon. May develop interstitial lung disease, oesophagitis, arrhythmias, malabsorption, pseudo-obstruction, renal failure. Less than 2% of cases.

Systemic sclerosis pulmonary disease is the most common cause of death in patients with systemic sclerosis.

Pulmonary fibrosis is seen at post-mortem in up to 75% of patients. Antinuclear antibody is positive in 60%, of speckled or nucleolar type. Pulmonary involvement is seen particularly if Scl 70 antibody is present. Anticentromere antibodies, however, are associated with reduced risk.

- *Present* with dyspnoea and a history of Raynaud's
- *Examination* Signs of systemic sclerosis, fine bibasal crepitations
- *PFTs* show restrictive defect and reduced kCO. Rapidly falling kCO is a poor prognostic sign. HRCT is performed if PFTs are abnormal. Mostly non-specific interstitial pneumonitis (NSIP) pattern on HRCT, but can be UIP pattern. May need open lung biopsy to confirm diagnosis
- *Treatment* with steroids and cyclophosphamide. A randomized controlled trial of oral cyclophosphamide vs. placebo in patients with active alveolitis and scleroderma-related interstitial lung disease showed a modest but significant effect on FVC, dyspnoea and quality of life (Taskin DP et al. NEJM 2006; 354: 2655–66)

- *Prognosis* Systemic sclerosis associated interstitial lung disease has better prognosis than pure UIP. This may be related to slower disease progression, rather than any greater response to immunosuppressive treatment. 15% of patients have progressive and severe disease. Associated increased risk of lung cancer.

Pulmonary hypertension May be isolated or secondary to interstitial lung disease. Isolated pulmonary hypertension is characteristic of limited cutaneous disease, especially in those with cutaneous telangectasias and anticentromere antibodies. Pathologically similar to primary pulmonary hypertension. Sub-intimal cell proliferation, endothelial hyperplasia, and the obliteration of small intrapulmonary vessels.

- *Present* with dyspnoea, right ventricular hypertrophy, and right heart failure
- *Diagnosis* by echocardiography
- *Treatment* as for PPH (see p 392). May respond to prostacyclin infusions, or may need transplant
- *Prognosis* better than for those with PPH.

Chest wall limitation by skin scleroderma over chest ('hide-bound chest').

Organizing pneumonia See p 270.

Aspiration pneumonia Uncommon and due to oesophageal dysmotility.

Sjögren's syndrome

- Inflammation and destruction of primarily the salivary and lachrymal glands
- Keratoconjunctivitis sicca or xerostomia (dry eyes and dry mouth) is evidence of primary disease, but when associated with connective tissue disease, especially rheumatoid arthritis, is secondary Sjögren's
- Classical Sicca Syndrome includes dry eyes and mouth, and parotid or salivary gland enlargement
- Pulmonary involvement occurs in about 25%.

Pleurisy

Airways inflammation Bronchial hyperresponsiveness, chronic bronchitis, and small airways disease. Mild abnormalities on PFTs, rarely significant.

Dry cough Atrophy of mucus gland in trachea and bronchi and lymphoplasmocytic infiltrate (xerotrachea). Possibly a higher incidence of chest infections. Treatment: nebulized saline, physiotherapy.

Organizing pneumonia Rare.

Diffuse lung disease Often asymptomatic, but may have cough, dyspnoea, and crackles on examination. PFTs show a restrictive defect and lymphocytic interstitial pneumonia (LIP) or UIP pattern on CT.

Lymphoma Unusual, but is 40 times more common in Sjögren's syndrome, especially in patients with high levels of immunoglobulins, autoantibodies, and cryoglobulins. Usually B-cell lymphoma. Can mimic organizing pneumonia.

Ankylosing spondylitis

- Chronic inflammatory disease causing spinal ankylosis with sacroiliac joint involvement
- 90% of Caucasian patients are HLA B27 positive.

Pulmonary fibrosis occurs in 2%, especially those with advanced disease. Typically bilaterally in the upper lobes. May develop cysts/cavities and become colonized with *Aspergillus*, which can require treatment.

Pleural involvement Pleuritis and apical pleural thickening.

Restrictive defect Due to fixed deformity of the thorax, limiting breathing and leading to respiratory failure due to nocturnal hypoventilation. Nocturnal NIV may be indicated.

Behçet's syndrome

- Systemic vasculitis involving arteries and veins of all sizes with recurrent oral ± genital ulceration and chronic relapsing uveitis, which can cause blindness
- Marked geographical distribution, with greatest prevalence in Turkey, Iran, and Japan
- Musculoskeletal, skin, neurological, GI, and major artery and vein involvement.

Pulmonary arterial aneurysms, arterial and venous thrombosis, and pulmonary infarcts in <5%. Recurrent haemoptysis is the main manifestation. This can be massive and fatal. Pulmonary aneurysms are seen as non-cavitating shadows on CXR and confirmed by CT. These are associated with DVT, therefore making anticoagulation difficult due to possible haemoptysis from the aneurysm.

Pleural effusion rare.

Autoantibodies: disease associations

Antinuclear antibody (ANA)	+ve in
SLE	99%
Rheumatoid arthritis	32%
Juvenile rheumatoid arthritis	76%
Chronic active hepatitis	75%
Sjögren's syndrome	68%
Systemic sclerosis	64%
Polymyositis	
Polyarteritis nodosa	
Myasthenia gravis	
Autoimmune thyroid disease	
Extensive burns	
Normal controls	0–2%
Extractable nuclear antigen (ENA)	**(done by lab if ANA positive)**

Anti-double-stranded DNA—SLE

Anti Sm—SLE

Antitopoisomerase 1—diffuse scleroderma

Anticentromere—limited scleroderma

Anti Scl-70—pulmonary fibrosis in scleroderma

Anti Jo-1—myositis

Anti Ro—Sjögren's, SLE, fetal heart block

Anti RNP—SLE, scleroderma, myositis, mixed connective tissue disease, and rheumatoid arthritis

Rheumatoid factor	+ve in
Rheumatoid arthritis	70–80%
Sjögren's syndrome	<100%
Felty's syndrome	<100%
Systemic sclerosis	30%
Still's disease	Rarely positive
Infective endocarditis	<50%
SLE	<40%
Normal controls	5–10%

Also: Neoplasms after radio- or chemotherapy
Hyperglobulinaemic states
Dermatomyositis

Chapter 23

Cor pulmonale

Definition Cor pulmonale is the traditional term for changes in the cardiovascular system resulting from the chronic hypoxia (and usually hypercapnia) of chronic lung disease, mainly pulmonary hypertension and fluid retention. It does not include similar changes seen in some left-sided disorders such as mitral incompetence.

Causes and pathophysiology Cor pulmonale can occur in most situations where there is chronic hypoxia.

- Most often in the setting of hypoxic and hypercapnic COPD
- Hypoventilation syndromes (scoliosis, neuromuscular diseases)
- Much less common when there is no associated rise in $PaCO_2$ (e.g. with interstitial lung diseases).

Cor pulmonale is often also referred to as 'right heart failure', which is misleading as the cardiac output in cor pulmonale is usually normal or high with increased peripheral perfusion (hence, the 'bounding pulse' of type II ventilatory failure). The right ventricle (RV) can cope with much higher pressures than usually occur in cor pulmonale, such as in idiopathic pulmonary arterial hypertension, if allowed time to adapt. In true right heart failure the RV fails to develop an adequate cardiac output, e.g. following right-sided MI, or pulmonary emboli that occlude a large proportion of the pulmonary vascular bed. This also produces a raised JVP, but in contrast there will be a low cardiac output and poor peripheral perfusion.

Cor pulmonale results from the following sequence of events

- Lung disease causes hypoxia with cyanosis and often polycythaemia
- Hypoxia is sensed both within the kidney and via the carotid body, generating increases in sympathetic activity and renal vasoconstriction
- Increased sympathetic activity (and other mechanisms) leads to renal retention of salt and water
- This extra salt and water is mainly held in the capacitance vessels (the large veins) often with a raised JVP
- If vascular permeability rises (particularly when the $PaCO_2$ rises, producing peripheral vasodilatation and an increase in capillary pressure), extra fluid accumulates in dependent tissues, mainly the ankles
- A raised JVP and ankle oedema in this setting are NOT due to impaired right ventricular function, but to fluid overload and increased vascular permeability.

Patients often present with their first episode of ankle swelling during an exacerbation of their COPD, when for the first time the $PaCO_2$ rises and the PaO_2 falls far enough to provoke the above events. Body weight may not actually rise suddenly with the onset of ankle oedema; however, the extra salt and water retained leading up to the exacerbation moves into the subcutaneous tissues, probably from the CO_2-induced vasodilatation raising mean capillary hydrostatic pressure.

The hypoxia also raises the pulmonary artery pressure (PAP), but to modest levels for which the RV can easily compensate, particularly if it builds up slowly. Loss of pulmonary vascular bed from emphysema will also raise PAP. The ECG often shows right ventricular hypertrophy. During an exacerbation, extra hypoxia will produce further rises in PAP with which the RV usually copes, helped by the raised JVP providing a larger pre-load to increase RV filling. Excessive diuresis can lead to a true fall in right-sided output due to inadequate filling of the RV.

Clinical features

- The underlying disease causing the hypoxia, e.g. COPD/bronchiectasis
- Easily visible veins and a raised JVP
- Cyanosis and a suffused conjunctiva (polycythaemia and vessel dilatation from the raised CO_2)
- Peripheral vasodilatation with a full 'bounding' pulse
- Ankle swelling and pitting oedema
- Right ventricular hypertrophy (sternal heave uncommon, masked by hyperinflated lung between heart and chest wall; more often seen with the higher pressures of IPAH)
- Tricuspid incompetence (not usually severe).

Investigations

- CXR—enlarged pulmonary arteries/underlying lung disease
- FBC—may have associated polycythaemia
- Oximetry—cor pulmonale is unlikely if awake SaO_2 over 92%
- Blood gases—cor pulmonale progressively more likely as PaO_2 drops below 8 kPa (equivalent $SaO_2 \approx 91\%$), and $PaCO_2$ rises above 6 kPa
- ECG—may indicate right axis deviation, p pulmonale (right atrial hypertrophy), and right bundle branch block
- Echo—dilated or hypertrophied RV, tricuspid regurgitation, estimate of PAP, and exclude other diagnoses such as a patent ASD
- Overnight oximetry—to reveal unexpected degrees of hypoxia, e.g. from OSA or diaphragm paralysis.

Management Minimal ankle oedema needs no treatment. 'Trimming' the ankles to normal is unnecessary and may reduce RV output by reducing filling. If the oedema is more substantial then the following may help:

- Treat underlying condition to raise PaO_2 and lower $PaCO_2$
- Raise PaO_2 through added oxygen, provide long-term oxygen at home
- In hypoventilation syndromes, home overnight NIV likely to be the correct management
- Promote a limited diuresis with judicious use of diuretics
- Always elevate legs when sitting.

In general, 'cor pulmonale' is over-treated. It is usually a relatively harmless by-product of hypoxia, rather than a problem in its own right. Treating the blood gas disturbance, and making it easier for the patient to get his shoes on, are the main therapeutic aims. The long-term oxygen trials showed that improving the PaO_2 was useful, not that lowering the pulmonary artery pressure was important.

Further information

Stewart AG *et al.* Hormonal, renal, and autonomic nerve factors involved in the excretion of sodium and water during dynamic salt and water loading in hypoxaemic chronic obstructive pulmonary disease. *Thorax* 1995; **50**: 838–45

Chapter 24

Cystic fibrosis

General principles

Definition and pathophysiology

- Multisystem disease due to mutations in the gene encoding for the cystic fibrosis transmembrane conductance regulator (CFTR), a complex chloride channel
- CFTR is essential for regulating salt and water movement across membranes
- Faulty regulation causes viscous secretions
- In the lungs, these secretions result in colonization with pathogenic bacteria, causing a massive inflammatory response, including elastase release. This contributes to lung damage and subsequent development of irreversible bronchiectasis
- In the pancreas, the exocrine ducts become blocked by secretions, leading to pancreatic enzyme insufficiency, pancreatic destruction, and diabetes mellitus.

Genetics

- Autosomal recessive
- Gene found on the long arm of chromosome 7
- Carrier frequency of this gene in Caucasians 1 in 25. 1 in 2500 UK live births have cystic fibrosis
- CF is rare in Afro-Caribbeans, but is seen in patients of Asian origin in the UK and USA
- Heterozygote advantage through resistance to *E. coli* diarrhoea and cholera has probably led to persistence of CFTR mutations, despite the lethal homozygous form
- More than 1500 different mutations in the CFTR gene are recognized to cause clinical disease
- The most common mutation is ΔF508, which accounts for around 67% of CF alleles in the UK and northern Europe. This is a deletion of 3 nucleotides resulting in the omission of a single amino acid, phenylalanine, at the 508 residue
- 13 other mutations have a frequency of greater than 1%, accounting for 85% of CF alleles altogether. These can be effectively screened for. They include G542X (3.4%), G551D (2.4%), W1282X (2.1%), and 3905insT (2.1%)
- Different mutations may be associated with particular clinical subgroups. The phenotype–genotype relationship is closest for pancreatic disease
- Non-CFTR 'modifier' genes (such as TNFα, mannose binding lectin, and α_1-antitrypsin), as well as environmental factors, probably further influence the clinical picture and account for phenotypic variation.

Screening In the UK, neonatal heel-prick for immunoreactive trypsin measurement is now offered routinely as part of a new national screening programme. Prenatal second trimester fetal ultrasound may identify presence of echogenic bowel, which can occur in CF. These babies are then screened at birth. Those with relatives with CF are advised to have preconception CF genotyping, as are the partners of a patient with CF.

Diagnosis Patients are usually diagnosed with CF as neonates or children (genetic screening, family history, failure to thrive, meconium ileus, rectal prolapse, cough, recurrent chest infections). Diagnosis is based on compatible clinical findings, with biochemical or genetic confirmation. The sweat chloride test is an important laboratory test, particularly in children. Some patients are diagnosed with CF in adult life. They usually have different alleles leading to a milder phenotype.

Management The ongoing care of CF patients moves to the adult CF centre around the age of 16–18 (often when the patient leaves school), although a period of transitional care may occur between ages 14–16. A multidisciplinary team approach is recommended, consisting of respiratory physician, specialist nurse, physiotherapist, pharmacist, dietician, and psychologist, with regular additional input from gastroenterology and endocrine teams.

This transition can be a difficult time, as the patient begins to take more responsibility for their care and treatment. Some may have periods of rebelling, not taking medications or performing physiotherapy, despite recognizing the need to do so.

Improved treatment and nutrition of CF patients has led to an increase in median survival, to around 30 years. The predicted lifespan for a baby born with CF now is 42 years.

The main management issues for the adult CF patient are:

- **Lung disease**
  - Maintaining lung function
  - Monitoring lung bacteriology, including screening for multi-resistant and transmissible organisms
  - Consideration of referral for heart–lung or liver transplant, if and when appropriate
- **Nutrition**
  - Nutritional support, weight, enzyme replacement, vitamins
- **GI**
  - Annual screening for biliary cirrhosis and portal hypertension
- **Endocrine**
  - Annual screening for CF-related diabetes (CFRD)
  - Annual screening for osteoporosis
- **Fertility advice**
- **Ensuring psychosocial well-being.**

CF pulmonary sepsis: aetiology

Chronic pulmonary sepsis and its complications cause much of the morbidity and mortality in CF. The airways of a CF patient are chronically colonized by pathogenic bacteria from an early age. Bronchiectasis is usually established by a young age (around 5 years).

- Patients commonly expectorate variable volumes of purulent sputum, even when well
- When organism levels are high, patients may feel generally unwell or more tired, or have anorexia, weight loss, temperature >38°C
- They may have symptoms of dyspnoea, increased volume of more purulent sputum, haemoptysis, wheeze, and chest ache
- Examination and CXR can be unchanged from normal
- FEV_1 levels are a reliable marker of infection and tend to decrease by ≥10%
- With effective antibiotic treatment, FEV_1 levels should rise to the pre-infection normal. If they do not, further antibiotics may be necessary, and other diagnoses or unusual organisms should be considered
- In practice: the FEV_1 is the best marker of disease progression and can be used to assess overall decline, as well as to determine an exacerbation and response to treatment (as PEFR would be used in asthma).

Organisms Airway colonization changes over time, with increasing age and organisms become more resistant to antibiotics. Goals of management should be initially to prevent infection, then to eradicate it, and finally to control the infection. Material for culture should be collected; most commonly sputum, but BAL if necessary. Polymicrobial infection is common.

Typical progression of organism colonization with time is:

- ***Staphylococcus aureus***
- ***Haemophilus influenzae***
- ***Pseudomonas aeruginosa*** worsens lung function and CXR appearance. Most patients with CF are chronically infected with *Pseudomonas* by their early teens. Non-mucoid species colonize initially and these may be asymptomatic or intermittent. These can be eradicated. Mucoid species then follow and permanent eradication is rare. Decreasing the *Pseudomonas* load produces clinical benefit.

Other organisms

- ***Stenotrophomonas maltophilia*** Gram-negative bacteria, often with multiple antibiotic resistance
- ***Burkholderia cepacia complex*** There are at least 10 different strains, or genomovars, of *Burkholderia cepacia*. Some are associated with a worse clinical outcome and some are not. These organisms are resistant to many antibiotics. It is crucial that *Burkholderia cepacia* colonized patients are separated from non-colonized patients, as the organism is highly transmissible. This means separate clinics, separate spirometers, and side rooms on a different ward are necessary. **'Cepacia syndrome'** is the severe worsening of pulmonary infection with septicaemia,

which can be rapidly fatal. This is caused by one strain, genomovar III, or *Burkholderia cenocepacia*. CF patients infected with this strain are usually not accepted for transplant, as studies have shown they do less well.

- **MRSA**
- **NTM**

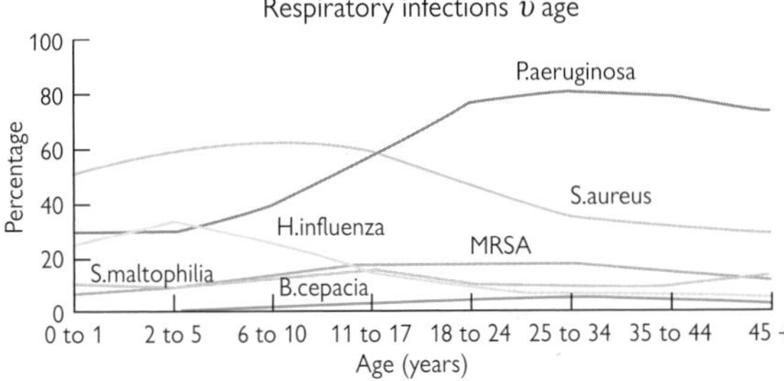

Fig. 24.1 Prevalence of selected respiratory pathogens in patients with CF over time. (From Goss *Thorax* 2007; **62**: 360–7.) Reproduced with the permission of the American Society for Microbiology.

Further information

Goss CH. Exacerbations in cystic fibrosis. *Thorax* 2007; **62**: 360–7

CF pulmonary sepsis antibiotics: 1

Antibiotic courses in patients with CF need to be longer and at higher doses than in non-CF patients. The choice of antibiotics is based on clinical response more than *in vitro* resistance patterns, but recent sputum culture results will also guide therapy. If *Pseudomonas* has previously been isolated, it may need to be covered in the current antibiotic regime.

- In practice, be guided by the last sputum culture result
- It is usually appropriate to give the patient the same regime they had during their last exacerbation, provided there was a good clinical response
- Microbiology advice should be sought if necessary.

Staphylococcus aureus A significant pathogen causing exacerbations. Prevention and eradication are important, even if the patient is asymptomatic. In adults, a minimum of 2 weeks of treatment should be given when *Staphylococcus aureus* is cultured, with flucloxacillin, erythromycin if penicillin-resistant, tetracycline, sodium fusidate, rifampicin, or clindamycin. There is no published evidence that long-term treatment in adults has any additional benefit.

Haemophilus influenzae When isolated (usually in young children) should be treated with amoxicillin, co-amoxiclav, second-generation cephalosporin, tetracycline, or chloramphenicol (toxicity risk), even if the patient is asymptomatic.

Pseudomonas aeruginosa

- **Oral antibiotics** The *Pseudomonas* colonized patient who develops a mild exacerbation should receive 2 weeks of an oral quinolone (such as ciprofloxacin), as well as their usual nebulized colistin. There are problems with resistance, so therefore should not be used more frequently than every 3 months.
- **IV antibiotics** Should be used when oral and nebulized treatments have failed, or patient is unwell. An aminoglycoside plus a β-lactam are given, which have a synergistic effect when used in combination. Treatment should be for a minimum of 10 days. Once or twice a day aminoglycoside dosing is used in many centres (5–7 mg/kg), rather than tds, providing high efficacy and fewer toxic effects (Nicolau DP *et al. Antimicrob Agents Chemother* 1995; **39:** 650–5).

Drug levels should be checked before and 1 h after the third dose, and adjusted if necessary. Bacterial toxicity is achieved by the high peak and safety is ensured by low trough. Renal function should also be checked during the IV course. Local policies may vary on frequency of checking. Some centres, especially in northern Europe, recommend that patients with chronic *Pseudomonas* colonization should receive 2 weeks of IV antibiotic therapy every 3 months routinely. This policy is not widely adopted in the UK, although, as the threshold for starting treatment is low, the number of antibiotic courses is similar using both regimes.

- **Aerosol anti-pseudomonal antibiotics** Once the patient is chronically *Pseudomonas* colonized, twice daily nebulized colistin is used long-term (1–2 mega units bd in 3–4 mL saline after physiotherapy) to try and minimize *Pseudomonas* levels. If colistin causes wheezing, it can either be given in 6 mL saline or reconstituted with 3–4 mL water for injection or salbutamol added. The nebulizer used should have a one-way valve in the exhaust tubing and this tubing should be vented to the outside. If colistin is not tolerated or is ineffective, aminoglycosides designed for IV injection can be tried (e.g. gentamicin 40 or 80 mg bd, made up with saline to 4 ml). Neither gentamicin or tobramycin are licensed for this use. A new preservative-free form of tobramycin (TOBI) has been developed and licensed for nebulization; it has been found in studies to improve pulmonary function and increase weight gain. Although it is expensive, it is becoming established in long-term management of CF patients in the UK. Administer all via nebulizer with exhaust tubing vented to outside as above.

- **First isolate of non-mucoid *Pseudomonas*** should be treated aggressively with 4–6 weeks of oral ciprofloxacin 750 mg bd and concurrent 6 weeks of nebulized colistin 1 mega unit bd. 80% of newly infected patients have *Pseudomonas* eradicated by this regime. If this is not successful, they should have IV therapy with 2 drugs and nebulized colistin.

Satisfactory aminoglycoside levels

- od regime: trough <1 mg/L and repeat in the first week
- tds regimes:
    - gentamicin/tobramycin: pre 1–2 mg/L, post 9–12 mg/L
    - amikacin: pre <10 mg/L, post 28–32 mg/L

Any reports of dizziness or balance problems may suggest early ototoxicity. This must be taken seriously as there is a cumulative dose effect. The aminoglycoside should be stopped and ENT referral made for middle ear testing.

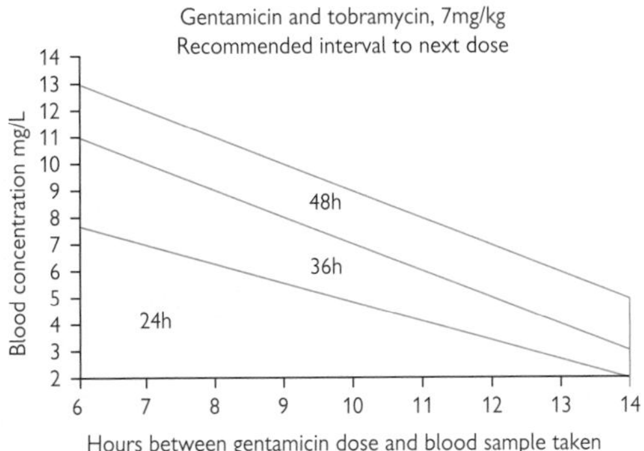

Fig. 24.2 Gentamicin and tobramycin dosing algorithm. Reproduced with the permission of the BMJ (Antimicrodial Agents and Chemotheropy, Mar. 1995, p 626–31).

CF pulmonary sepsis antibiotics: 2

Burkholderia cepacia is characteristically resistant to antibiotics, including colistin and aminoglycosides. Conventional IV therapy may be effective. Should be treated with combination of 2–3 IV antibiotics, such as ceftazidime and an aminoglycoside. Possible synergistic combinations are chloramphenicol and minocycline, chloramphenicol and ceftazidime, or a quinolone with a β-lactam/carbopenem. Co-trimoxazole also used.

MRSA is not more pathogenic than *Staphylococcus aureus*. Nebulized vancomycin can be used for persisting sputum colonization, but IV vancomycin or teicoplanin are required for MRSA exacerbations. Oral rifampicin, sodium fusidate, or linezolid may be beneficial.

Macrolides have additional anti-inflammatory effects, as well as antimicrobial effects. They do not exhibit intrinsic anti-pseudomonal activity, but there is *in vitro* synergy between macrolides and anti-pseudomonal antibiotics. They also seem to improve clinical status compared with placebo or other antibiotics. This is seen with erythromycin, but especially azithromycin, which decreases sputum viscoelasticity and affects the biofilm formed by *Pseudomonas*. It is administered either once daily or three times a week, e.g. at dose of 250 mg/day with LFT monitoring, and has been found to improve FEV_1 and decrease exacerbations when used over 6 months. Larger trials are needed to assess its long-term effects.

Southern KW. Azithromycin for CF. *Eur Respir J* 2004; **24:** 834–8

Further Information

CF Trust. *Antibiotic Treatment for Cystic Fibrosis*, 2nd edn, 2002.

IV antibiotic administration

- If patients are unwell or if they are commencing a new antibiotic, they should be admitted to hospital. Otherwise the majority of IV antibiotic courses can be administered at home, after an initial assessment and with home support from nursing staff. Many patients are relatively well during courses of IV antibiotics and are able to continue attending work or college, although it can take them considerable extra time to administer the antibiotics
- Courses of IV antibiotics are often administered prophylactically before surgery
- Most antibiotic regimes involve two weeks of IV antibiotics. This may require the siting of an intravenous cannula with a microbiological filter (to make it last longer), or preferably a long-line
- Many patients have an indwelling port-a-cath that can be accessed when required
- Review patients after 1 week of treatment to ensure there is adequate clinical progress. If there is no improvement, review microbiological sensitivities and change treatment as appropriate.

Port-a-caths

- Inserted in patients with difficult IV access, or those needing frequent courses of IV antibiotics
- Usually accessed/needled by a trained nurse, patient, or family member. Should be accessed only with a Huber point needle of the appropriate length; do not use standard needles, which may damage the port
- Should be flushed with 5–10 mL of 100 u/mL heparin monthly and with 5 mL of 10 U/mL heparin at the end of each IV dose
- Avoid taking blood from port-a-cath as this increases the risk of blockage and infection. Other complications include venous obstruction, tip dislocation, and leakage
- If port-a-cath blocks: inject 20–50 mL heparinized saline; gently alternating between irrigation and aspiration may clear small occlusions. Urokinase 25 000 units in 3 mL 0.9% saline instilled into port may help a blockage
- Infected or fractured lines need removal by surgeons.

Antibiotic desensitization Antibiotic sensitivity is a major problem in patients with CF as repeated antibiotic courses are associated with the development of allergic reactions, especially to β-lactams. Rashes are common, but anaphylaxis can occur. Document any drug reactions, provide an adrenaline pre-filled syringe, and give first doses of a new antibiotic in hospital. Desensitization regimes can be helpful and are used for specific antibiotics that have previously caused an allergic reaction. Such regimes need to be given at the start of the antibiotic course each time it is used, and during the course if doses are missed for more than one day. Give a dilute antibiotic dose over 20 min, followed by slightly stronger concentration, and repeat for 7 concentration strengths until full antibiotic strength is given. Takes 3–4 h. Stop infusion if any side-effects are noted. Local policy may advise another desensatization regime.

Management of an exacerbation

Diagnose an exacerbation on 2–4 of the following:

- Increase in productive cough or dyspnoea
- Change in appearance or volume of sputum
- New signs on auscultation
- New CXR signs
- Decreased appetite
- Fall in respiratory function
- Fever
- 10% fall from baseline FEV_1.

Most patients with CF will know when they need antibiotics for an exacerbation.

Investigations

- FEV_1
- Oxygen saturation
- Blood gases
- CXR—exclude pneumothorax
- CRP—relatively non-specific, but can be a useful monitoring tool
- Repeat sputum M, C & S, AFBs. Consider *Aspergillus* precipitins.

Treatment with appropriate antibiotics, O_2, physiotherapy, nutrition, NIV, consider ITU/resuscitation status if necessary—liaise with CF consultant.

Other pulmonary interventions

Physiotherapy Dedicated CF physiotherapists aim to teach effective airway clearance. This improves secretion clearance, decreases airflow obstruction, and improves ventilation. Patients should do this themselves twice daily on a long-term basis. Several techniques are used: active cycle of breathing control (tidal volume breathing, then deep inspiration, and passive expiration, followed by forced expiration to mobilize secretions prior to coughing/huffing), autogenic drainage, with percussion if patients are not clearing their chest well, flutter devices, and positive expiratory pressure mask. More intensive physiotherapy is administered during exacerbations, by family and/or physiotherapist. Physiotherapists also have important role in assessment of functional ability with exercise testing and evaluating treatment and encouraging aerobic exercise.

Recombinant DNase (dornase alfa or pulmozyme), a nebulized mucolytic that cleaves DNA from dead neutrophils, decreasing sputum viscosity and aiding its clearance. It is recommended in patients with an FVC >40% predicted, to improve pulmonary function. It is used once daily 2500 U via a specific nebulizer. It is only continued in patients who gain objective benefit, with improved lung function; for example, 10% improvement in spirometry and shuttle walk test. It is expensive and only effective in 30–40%.

Hypertonic saline Use of regular inhaled hypertonic saline has been found to increase mucociliary transport and hence decrease exacerbations and improve lung function. It is re-emerging as a therapeutic aid to expectoration.

Respiratory support Respiratory failure and cor pulmonale can occur with later stage disease. Home oxygen may be required. Nocturnal non-invasive ventilation may be necessary as a bridge to transplant if the patient has chronic respiratory failure. If support is needed for acute deterioration related to infection with a major reversible component, this may be non-invasive initially, but the patient may need intubation and ventilation. Such decisions should be made with the patient, their family, and their CF consultant. These decisions can be difficult and factors, such as being on the transplant list, may be relevant.

Steroids Short oral courses seem to improve lung function, but side-effects, such as growth impairment, osteoporosis, diabetes, and cataracts, are significant. They are used in ABPA, severe unresponsive exacerbations, and occasionally in terminal care to improve the sense of well-being in a patient.

Immunization Annual influenza, as well as pneumococcal vaccination.

Transplant The role of transplantation in patients with CF is well established. Patients should be considered for transplant when their life expectancy is less than 2 years and their quality of life is severely impaired, despite optimal medical therapy.

- FEV_1 ≤30% predicted or FEV_1 >30% with rapid progressive deterioration, e.g. increasing number of admissions, rapid fall in FEV_1, massive haemoptysis
- Hypoxia (PaO_2 <7.3 kPa) and hypercapnia ($PaCO_2$ >6.7 kPa) are associated with <50% survival at 2 years without transplantation, and so are useful guidelines, but patients should be referred for assessment on the basis of FEV_1 criteria even in the absence of severe hypoxia/hypercapnia
- Young female patients with rapid deterioration have a poor prognosis and should be considered for early referral.

Some patients do not want a transplant and full psychosocial assessments are necessary. Whilst on the transplant waiting list, the patient should have optimal nutrition and physical care. Average waits are around 1 year and some patients will inevitably die on the waiting list. Bilateral lung transplant is usually the procedure of choice. Living-donor lobar transplantation is also performed, particularly in children and small adults. Following transplantation, the main immediate problems are infection and acute rejection. Later, 40% of patients go on to develop bronchiolitis obliterans (see p 328). One-year survival following transplant is around 58%.

Other pulmonary disease

Pneumothorax The risk of spontaneous pneumothorax increases with age. It occurs in around 20% of male CF patients and slightly fewer females. It is associated with a poor prognosis. It should be managed according to the standard pneumothorax guidelines (p 381), with initial aspiration if patient is not breathless and chest tube if this fails. The lung may take some time to reinflate, and require prolonged drainage and suction. Continue physiotherapy during this. Persistent air leak may require surgical input, ideally with a limited procedure, such as local abrasion. Pleurodesis should be avoided if possible in those for whom future lung transplant is an option, as this can lead to increased bleeding when the pleura is dissected, but this is not an absolute contraindication. Liaise with the transplant centre, as the transplant surgeon may want to perform the pleurodesis.

Allergic bronchopulmonary aspergillosis (see p 466) Difficult to diagnose in CF as nearly 50% of CF patients have *Aspergillus* hypersensitivity with positive skin prick tests and 25% have positive precipitins. The incidence is around 10%. Screened for annually and advised to avoid compost heaps and hay/stables. ABPA is indicated by:

- Asthma-like symptoms with new CXR changes
- Raised IgE >500 IU/L or IgE RAST
- Eosinophilia >500/mm^3 or
- Hyphae in sputum.

Treatment should be with oral steroids for 2 weeks and, if there is a clinical improvement, these should be continued at decreasing doses for 2–3 months. Intensive physiotherapy is also an important part of the treatment regime. There is some trial evidence that antifungal agents, such as itraconazole 200 mg bd for 4 months, should be used in addition and may have a steroid-sparing role. Itraconazole can cause liver dysfunction, so monitor LFTs.

Non-tuberculous mycobacteria (see p 518) Significance is unclear and treatment may not produce a clinical benefit. Should be screened for annually. If culture positive, repeat twice and consider 12–18-month course of antibiotics.

CF 'asthma' Some CF patients have coexisting asthma and some have asthma-like symptoms of prolonged exhalation, wheeze, and crackles due to underlying lung inflammation. This is difficult to diagnose, as these symptoms and a variable PEFR are found in most CF patients, due to bronchial hyperreactivity. Occurs in 2–37% of patients. Bronchial hyperreactivity is found in at least 40% of patients with CF. There may be bronchodilator responsiveness, also bronchoconstriction after exercise or nebulized hypertonic saline. Treat with the standard asthma stepwise treatment: short-acting bronchodilator, inhaled corticosteroid, long-acting β_2 agonist, theophyllines (which may aid mucociliary clearance), leukotriene receptor antagonist (limited evidence in CF, but may decrease eosinophilic inflammation), oral steroids.

Haemoptysis Small volume haemoptysis is common, especially with concurrent infection and advanced disease. Check clotting and platelets; consider group and save. Stop NSAIDs, give IV antibiotics, vitamin K 10 mg od, and tranexamic acid 15–25 mg/kg/day in 4 divided doses.

Massive haemoptysis (see p 43) >500 mL blood. Usually reflects bronchial artery bleeding and can be fatal. Needs in-patient support and monitoring. Cross-match blood. Sit upright and give ice-cold drink to cause pulmonary vasoconstriction. Nebulized adrenaline (5–10 mL of 1 in 10 000). Bolus dose of octreotide 50 μg over 15 min, then octreotide infusion 400 μg in 20 mL 5% dextrose at 2.5–5 mL per h. May require bronchial artery embolization, bronchial artery ligation, or surgical resection.

Non-pulmonary disease

Nutritional management The maintenance of good nutrition correlates with survival. Nutrition is more problematic as respiratory disease progresses (raised basal metabolic rate, increased work of breathing, ongoing infection, and inflammation). Dietician input is crucial. High calorie, high protein diets are encouraged. Patients may need dietary supplements or, if necessary, supplemental overnight feeding via nasogastric tube or gastrostomy. Perform weight and body mass index measurements at the annual review. Aim for BMI >20.

- ***Pancreatic enzyme supplementation*** to avoid high faecal fat/energy loss. The smallest dose of pancreatin, containing lipase, required to control steatorrhoea should be used. Typical preparations are Creon® (contains lipase, protease, and amylase) 10 000, 25 000, or 40 000, taken pre-meals. Typically patients take 10–20 tablets per day. The dietician can educate patients to adjust the dosage according to the fat and protein content of each meal. Constant re-education is often required to optimize enzyme supplementation. High strength pancreatic enzyme preparations have been found to be associated with the development of colonic strictures, or fibrosing colonopathy; hence maximum levels of lipase of 10 000 units/kg/day have been recommended
- ***Vitamins*** Fat-soluble vitamins are not absorbed well in patients with CF and these need replacement. Vitamins A, D, and E should be started when pancreatic insufficiency is diagnosed and vitamin K if there is evidence of liver disease, with prolonged prothrombin time. Vitamins should be taken at meal times with pancreatin. Vitamin levels should be checked at annual review
- ***Salt tablets*** in hot weather, due to excessive losses in sweat.

Gastrointestinal disease

- ***Distal intestinal obstructive syndrome (DIOS)/abdominal pain*** (meconium ileus equivalent). Bloating, abdominal pain, possible palpable caecal mass, and complete or incomplete intestinal obstruction. Abdominal X-ray shows empty colon and ileal distension with air-fluid levels. Occurs secondary to dehydration, or rapidly increased doses of pancreatic enzymes. Rarely needs surgery. Medical treatment with senna and oral acetylcysteine 200 mg tds and gastrografin® 50–100 mL tds for 5 days is usually adequate. If not, perform gastrografin® enema to determine site of obstruction. This can be therapeutic. Oral intestinal lavage with Kleen Prep® solution and up to 10 L of fluid over 1–2 days can also be given. The treatment is considered to have worked when fluid is passed from the rectum and symptoms have resolved. If not resolving, may need further imaging to rule out intussusception
- ***Reflux*** More common in patients with CF than the general population. Symptoms may occur during physiotherapy, which require changes to positioning/tipping. May require treatment with a proton pump inhibitor to prevent development of Barrett's oesophagus
- ***Pancreatitis*** Can occur in those patients who are pancreas-sufficient. Seen in up to 15% adults with CF. May present as severe acute attack or chronic recurrent abdominal pain. Not usually as unwell as

non-CF patients with pancreatitis. Raised amylase and abnormal USS/CT. Treat with bowel rest, protein pump inhibitor, IV rehydration.

Liver and biliary disease

- ***Liver screening—cirrhosis, portal hypertension*** Reduced bile production and deranged bile acid composition leads to biliary obstruction, portal tract inflammation, and eventual fibrosis and focal biliary cirrhosis. Cirrhosis affects 2–25% of CF patients. Annual screening liver USS is performed, as blood tests can be unhelpful (although ALP most sensitive). Biopsy unhelpful as patchy disease. Established cirrhosis can lead to variceal bleeds, so annual screening endoscopies are performed in those with cirrhosis. Cirrhosis may need treatment with ursodeoxycholic acid, porto-systemic shunts, and sclerotherapy. Liver transplant may be necessary.

Metabolic disease

- ***CF-related diabetes (CFRD)*** is becoming increasingly common as the median age of survival with CF increases. Pancreatic damage in CF (due to fibrosis) causes decreased insulin secretion. Approximately 50% of 30-year-olds will have CFRD. Presents insidiously and non-specifically, with weight loss or fall in lung function, and not with ketoacidosis. Screening glucose tolerance test or random/fasting glucose should be performed annually and more frequently in those on overnight enteral feeds or those with clinical symptoms suggestive of diabetes. Once diabetes is diagnosed, patients should not be managed on a hypoglycaemic diet. Lower doses of insulin are usually required than in IDDM. There is no indication for oral hypoglycaemics. Microvascular complications can occur and annual screening for these should be performed
- ***Osteoporosis*** Several studies have confirmed an increased incidence of low bone mass in CF and increased fracture risk, particularly ribs. Risk factors include malabsorption of vitamin D and calcium, low body mass index, decreased physical activity, delayed puberty, steroid use, diabetes. Treatment is with calcium and vitamin D supplements to maintain vitamin D levels, weight-bearing exercises, hormones for delayed puberty (ethinylestradiol or testosterone), bisphosphonates.

Other organ systems

- ***Arthropathy and CF vasculitis*** Acute or subacute arthritis occurs in around 5% of patients with CF. It often responds to NSAIDs. Sometimes arthritis is associated with skin lesions, such as purpura or erythema nodosum. Up to 40% may be ANCA positive. Purpuric vasculitis is associated with more severe lung disease
- ***Nasal polyps and sinusitis*** Nasal polyps occur in 30% and can cause nasal obstruction. Treatment with topical or systemic steroids and decongestants is usually not helpful and polypectomy may be required, often more than once. Asymptomatic sinusitis is common and can cause mucosal swelling. Consider sinus CT if problematic
- ***Stress incontinence*** occurs in both men and women, caused by coughing. It has been recognized as an increasing problem. Pelvic floor exercises can be taught by physiotherapists.

Other issues

Fertility

Women with CF are usually subfertile. When planning a pregnancy, their physical state should be optimized with antibiotics and nutrition. The outcome of a pregnancy is improved by optimizing and maintaining pulmonary function and weight gain during the pregnancy. Close monitoring throughout is required. Pregnancy does not affect survival when compared with the entire adult female CF population, but impaired pulmonary function with FEV_1<60% predicted is likely to be the main predictor of worse maternal and fetal outcome. Breast-feeding is possible, but intensifies the nutritional strain put on the mother. Most CF antibiotics are safe to use in pregnancy, but avoid ciprofloxacin, chloramphenicol, metronidazole, and IV colistin. Care with aminoglycoside levels.

Men are infertile due to failure of the normal development or blockage of the vas deferens, seminal vesicle, ejaculatory duct, and body and tail of epididymis. Testicular histology is normal and hence one option is surgical sperm retrieval for intracytoplasmic sperm injection (ICSI) into an egg, performed by fertility clinics.

Genetic counselling and screening should be offered to patients with CF and their partners.

Psychosocial support Trained psychologists offer personal and family support regarding education, employment, financial benefits, burden of treatment, and adapting to progressive disease. Pre-transplant psychological assessment is carried out, as well as terminal care and bereavement counselling. Also treat depression, anxiety, and emotional difficulties, with referral to psychiatric services if necessary. Social worker involvement to help with benefit entitlements, travel insurance, disabled car badge.

Care of the dying CF patient When all acknowledge that there are no further treatment options, the focus of care should adjust to being palliative, with an emphasis on symptom relief, at home or in hospital.

Future developments Gene therapy. Replacing CFTR function to prevent progressive airways disease. Work is focusing on finding a suitable vector for delivery, such as nebulizer and airway epithelial implantation. Progress so far has been disappointing, but work is ongoing.

Further information

CF Trust.Standards for the clinical care of children and adults with cystic fibrosis in the UK 2001.
www.cff.org (USA)

www.cftrust.org.uk, www.cysticfibrosis.co.uk (both UK)

CF mutation database: www.genet.sickkids.on.ca

Seeing the patient with CF in clinic

Routine visit

- Fill in paperwork for UK CF database (now called PORT CF)—contains basic data such as height, weight, oxygen saturation, number of hospital admissions, and details of antibiotic use, as well as regular medications
- Check spirometry, weight, oxygen saturation
- Antibiotics if required

At the annual review

- Fill in paperwork for UK CF database (now PORT CF)—contains basic data such as height, weight, number of days off school/work, number of complications, antibiotic use, organisms cultured, supplemental feeding, fertility, glucose level, transplant status, and treatment compliance
- Weight
- Height (until they stop growing)
- Radiology
  - CXR (calculate the Northern score; see CF annual review documentation)
  - Liver and biliary system USS (Doppler if known cirrhosis)
- Bloods
  - FBC and clotting studies
  - U&E, LFTs
  - Fasting glucose tolerance test
  - HbA1c if established diabetes
  - *Aspergillus* species RAST and precipitins
  - IgA, IgG, IgM, and IgE
  - Fat-soluble vitamin levels A, D, E, and K, if available
- Sputum
  - M, C&S including *B. cepacia*, *S. aureus*, *Aspergillus*, and MRSA
  - NTM
- Physiotherapy review
- Exercise testing (6-min walk test or shuttle walk test)
- Respiratory function
  - Spirometry
  - Oximetry and, if <92%, blood gas
  - ± KCO, lung volumes
- Dietician
  - Full assessment and review of dietary intake, enzyme and vitamin use
- CF nurse review
- Psychologist review
- Social worker review
- Doctor review

Chapter 25

Eosinophilic lung disease

Eosinophilic lung disease

Definition Pulmonary eosinophilias are disorders classically associated with CXR infiltrates and a raised blood eosinophil count, although eosinophilic infiltration of the lung can occur *without* blood eosinophilia.

- Eosinophils are phagocytes that are produced in bone marrow and circulate for up to 10 h before localizing in tissues
- Their blood levels are usually tightly regulated
- In health they accumulate in the GI tract mucosa, but they may be attracted to other tissues by chemoattractant mechanisms, including mast cell activation and complement activation
- Eosinophils can survive in the tissues for weeks if appropriate cytokines are present
- Persisting high eosinophil levels cause tissue damage, due to their pro-inflammatory effects
- Eosinophils accumulate in allergic or hypersensitivity disease, parasitic infections, and cancer
- Steroids and severe sepsis both decrease eosinophil levels
- Asthma can cause a raised eosinophil count, especially if there is associated eczema, but an absolute eosinophil count of $>1 \times 10^9$/L is very unusual and raises the possibility of an alternative diagnosis, such as Churg–Strauss syndrome
- Normal eosinophil counts are below 0.4×10^9/L (1–3% of peripheral WCC)
- Counts of 0.4×10^9/L upwards can be seen in pulmonary eosinophilia.

Table 25.1 Causes of CXR infiltrates ± blood eosinophilia

Condition	Characteristic points
Asthma with allergic bronchopulmonary aspergillosis (ABPA)	Known asthma, with worsening symptoms, over weeks to months. Associated systemic symptoms. Raised blood eosinophil count, positive *Aspergillus* skin test, raised IgE, raised *Aspergillus* precipitins
Simple pulmonary eosinophilia (Löffler's syndrome)	Foreign travel. Symptoms for days to weeks. Cough, malaise, anorexia, rhinitis, night sweats, fever, dyspnoea, wheeze. Sputum contains eosinophils and larvae. Low-level blood eosinophilia
Tropical pulmonary eosinophilia	Foreign travel. Symptoms for weeks to months, with remissions and relapses. Cough, wheeze, sputum, dyspnoea, chest pain, fever, weight loss, fatigue. Sputum contains eosinophils. Raised blood eosinophil count, high IgE
Chronic eosinophilic pneumonia	Symptoms for weeks–months, with associated systemic symptoms. Cough, sputum, haemoptysis, dyspnoea, recent onset asthma, fever, weight loss, night sweats. Sputum eosinophilia, but blood levels can be normal
Acute eosinophilic pneumonia	Short duration of symptoms, <5 days. Fever, cough, dyspnoea, and myalgia. Unwell, hypoxic. High BAL eosinophil count, no blood eosinophilia
Hypereosinophilic syndrome	Symptoms for weeks–months. Associated systemic symptoms and other organ involvement. Fever, weight loss, cough, night sweats, pruritus. High blood eosinophil count
Churg–Strauss syndrome	Rhinitis, past history of asthma. Other organ involvement. Associated systemic symptoms. Longer duration of symptoms, weeks–months. Blood eosinophilia and eosinophilic tissue infiltration
Drug-induced pulmonary eosinophilia	Recent new drug. Possible associated skin reaction. Symptoms within hours–days. Spectrum of illness, from mild to severely unwell, with cough, dyspnoea, fever, and hypoxia. Eosinophilic tissue infiltration, but blood eosinophilia not universal

Causes of eosinophilic lung disease 1

Asthma and ABPA (see p 468)

- Fever or worsening asthma symptoms may be caused by type 1 and 2 hypersensitivity reactions to *Aspergillus fumigatus*
- Untreated can cause central bronchiectasis
- ***CXR*** shows fleeting shadows
- ***Blood*** eosinophilia
- ***Aspergillus skin prick test*** is positive and serum aspergillus IgG precipitins are positive. IgE levels are raised
- ***Treatment*** is with steroids and antifungal agents may be necessary.

Simple pulmonary eosinophilia (Löffler's syndrome)

- Caused by parasitic infection, usually *Ascaris lumbricoides*, but also *Strongyloides* and *Ankylostoma*
- Occurs worldwide, especially in SE Asia, Africa, Central and South America
- The eggs of the parasite are found in the soil and are ingested. After 10–14 days, larvae migrate from the intestine via lymph and blood to the liver and lung. From the lung, they pass up the bronchial tree to be swallowed, to develop into roundworms in the gut
- The passage of larvae through the lung causes an allergic reaction. This may be asymptomatic, but may cause cough, malaise, anorexia, rhinitis, night sweats, low-grade fever, occasional wheezing, and dyspnoea. The illness lasts around 2 weeks
- ***CXR*** shows transient bilateral shadows that are discrete and perihilar. They disappear usually between 6 and 12 days, but can take up to 1 month
- ***Sputum*** also contains eosinophils and larvae
- ***Blood*** eosinophilia at a low level
- ***Stool examination*** reveals parasites, but only 2–3 months later when the adult worms are passed
- ***Treatment*** is with an antihelminth agent, such as mebendazole for 3 days or levamisole as a single dose. Steroids may be necessary if the pulmonary manifestations are severe.

Tropical pulmonary eosinophilia

- Hypersensitivity to migrating larvae of filarial worms *Wucheria bancrofti* and *Brugia malayi*, similar to Löffler's syndrome
- Occurs in the Indian subcontinent, SE Asia, and the South Pacific islands
- Insidious onset of cough, wheeze, sputum, dyspnoea, and chest pain, with associated fever, weight loss, and fatigue. Symptoms last for weeks to months, with remissions and relapses
- ***Examination*** reveals crepitations
- ***CXR*** shows bilateral uniform mottling of the lung fields, especially in the middle and lower zones. There may be cavitation and pleural effusion
- ***Sputum and BAL*** contain eosinophils
- ***PFTs*** may be obstructive initially, but can become restrictive in longstanding untreated cases

- ***Histology*** shows eosinophilic bronchopneumonia and eosinophilic abscesses
- ***Blood eosinophil count*** is raised. IgE is raised
- ***Filarial complement test*** is positive
- ***Treatment*** is with a filaricide, diethylcarbamazine, for 3 weeks. This rapidly improves symptoms.

Drug-induced pulmonary eosinophilia

- Pulmonary shadowing develops within hours to days of starting the drug and resolves usually within 1 week of stopping it
- It is due to an allergic reaction in the pulmonary vessel wall caused by the drug and occurs again on drug re-challenge
- There may be an associated skin reaction
- The drug should be avoided in the future and steroids given if necessary
- Severity of illness varies, from mild to severely unwell, with cough, dyspnoea, fever, hypoxia. May occur in those with concomitant asthma
- Tissue eosinophilia, but may not have blood eosinophilia
- Possible drugs include ampicillin, carbamazepine, chlorpropamide, cocaine (inhaled), diclofenac, inorganic chemicals such as nickel, methotrexate, nitrofurantoin, penicillin, phenytoin, sodium aminosalicylate, sulphonamides, tetracycline.

Causes of eosinophilic lung disease 2

Chronic eosinophilic pneumonia

- Unknown cause
- Women:men = 2:1. Occurs in middle age
- Insidious onset over weeks to months, with cough, sputum, possibly haemoptysis, dyspnoea, recent onset asthma, weight loss, night sweats, and high fever. Differential diagnosis includes TB
- **Diagnosis** is usually clinical and radiological, but may need BAL or open lung biopsy
- **CXR** shows peripheral dense opacities with ill-defined margins (photographic negative of pulmonary oedema)
- **CT** shows peripheral air space infiltrates
- **Sputum** eosinophilia
- **BAL** eosinophil count high
- **Blood** eosinophilia may not occur. ESR is raised
- **Treatment** is with steroids, such as prednisolone 30–40 mg/day, and improvement is usually rapid, with the CXR clearing within 2–3 days and normal in 2 weeks. Decrease steroid dose once stable, but continue for 6 months
- Relapses common when steroids stopped and they may need further courses.

Acute eosinophilic pneumonia Unknown cause, occurs in any age or sex. Presents with fever, cough, dyspnoea, and myalgia.

Diagnostic criteria:

- Acute febrile illness of <5 days duration
- Hypoxic respiratory failure
- Interstitial or alveolar CXR infiltrates
- BAL eosinophils >25%
- No parasitic, fungal, or other infection
- Prompt and complete response to steroids
- Failure to relapse after stopping steroids.

May be unwell and hypoxic, requiring ventilatory support. No peripheral blood eosinophilia. High-dose steroids should be given until the respiratory failure resolves and then the dose can be tapered over 2–4 weeks.

Hypereosinophilic syndrome

- Unknown cause. Rare
- Most common in men aged 30–40
- Present with fever, weight loss, night sweats, cough, and pruritus
- **Diagnosis** based on:
    - Marked blood eosinophilia of $>1.5 \times 10^9$/L for 6 months or more
    - Signs and symptoms of eosinophilic tissue infiltration on histology
    - No evidence of another cause of eosinophilia

- Pulmonary involvement with interstitial infiltrates and pleural effusions on CXR. Cardiovascular involvement also occurs, with myocarditis, endocardial fibrosis, restrictive cardiomyopathy, valvular damage, and mural thrombus formation. These may cause considerable morbidity and mortality. Skin may be involved with urticaria and angioedema; CNS involved with encephalopathy, arterial and venous embolism, peripheral neuropathy, or mononeuritis multiplex; GI tract with gastritis, nausea, diarrhoea, alcohol intolerance and hepato- or splenomegaly; joints with effusions and Raynaud's. Kidney and muscles can also be infiltrated by eosinophils. Can be fatal
- **Blood** eosinophil levels may be as high as 70%. IgE levels are high
- **Treatment** is with high-dose steroids (e.g. 60 mg prednisolone), which improves about 50% of cases. May need to use other immunosuppressants, such as cyclophosphamide, hydroxyurea, azathioprine, or interferon alpha. Treatment should be tapered according to falling eosinophil counts and end-organ improvement.

Churg–Strauss syndrome (see p 660)

- Severe asthma, blood eosinophilia, and pulmonary infiltrates occur as part of a small and medium vessel vasculitis
- There may be eosinophilic tissue infiltration
- ANCA usually, but not always positive
- Treatment with steroids and immunosuppression.

Chapter 26

Extreme environments: flying, altitude, diving

Lung disease and flying

Problems Flying presents problems for three reasons:
- Extra hypoxia
- Volume changes in gas compartments
- Closed environment and disease transmission

Extra hypoxia Some aeroplanes may be pressurized to the equivalent of about 5000 ft (1500 m). This gives an atmospheric pressure of about 85 kPa and an FiO_2 of about 18 kPa, compared with 21 kPa at sea level. In normal subjects this causes inconsequential falls in PaO_2 and SaO_2.

However, some companies pressurize to the minimum allowed, 8000 ft (2400 m, same as some of the lower ski resorts in Colorado), FiO_2 16 kPa (equivalent to breathing 15% O_2 at sea level), and even in normal subjects the SaO_2 may fall to 90% or so. The new Airbus 380 is pressurized to only 8000 ft, but the new Boeing 787, built from largely carbon fibre, will apparently allow greater pressurization and humidity levels.

Patients with lung disease and a degree of hypoxia will be nearer the steep part of the haemoglobin dissociation curve, and will experience bigger proportional falls in oxygen carriage by the blood. The estimated PaO_2 at 8000 ft (the lowest cabin pressurization likely to be encountered) is estimated by the formula:

$$\text{Estimated } PaO_2 \text{ at 8000 ft} = (0.24 \times PaO_2 \text{ at sea level}) + (2.7 \times FEV_1/VC) + 3$$

e.g. sea level PaO_2 = 8 kPa, FEV_1/VC = 0.40, estimated PaO_2 = 6 kPa.

This is a rough approximation, and will vary considerably from patient to patient, particularly due to differences in hypoxic drive. An alternative is to give the patient a hypoxic mixture to breathe for 15 min minimum and measure the PaO_2/SaO_2. This is most easily achieved by feeding a 40% Venturi mask with 100% nitrogen, which simulates a little under 8000 ft (equivalent to 16% O_2). Even this will not necessarily predict that a patient will or will not run into trouble. Empirically, oxygen is often prescribed if the in-flight PaO_2 at 8000 ft, estimated from the above equation or by experimentation, is less than 7 kPa or 86% SaO_2. This is not evidence-based, so a simple recommendation based on sea level oximetry measurements is likely to be as valid.

Simple recommendations for oxygen when flying

Sea level SaO_2	
SaO_2 >92%	No oxygen required
SaO_2 90–92%	Perform challenge test
SaO_2 <90%	Recommend oxygen

These are not quite the same as the BTS guidelines, which are more complex and consider comorbidities. 2 L/min via nasal cannulae, or 28% Venturi mask, is usually sufficient to raise the SaO_2 to sea level equivalent. Airlines vary as to whether they charge for this and at least a month should be allowed to arrange it. A MEDIF form or equivalent will require completion by the GP or specialist. Occasionally patients are allowed to bring their own oxygen on board as hand luggage. Some airlines prohibit using oxygen during take-off and landing.

Volume changes in gas compartments Ascent to the equivalent of 5000 ft will increase gas in trapped compartments by 20%, and ascent to 8000 ft by nearly 40%. A pneumothorax or non-communicating bullae will therefore increase by this amount. Therefore, it is advised that patients with current pneumothoraces should not fly. In addition, it used to be advised not to fly within 6 weeks of a pneumothorax because of the slightly higher chance of a recurrence and the lack of adequate emergency medical treatment on board. This has recently been changed to 1 week after full radiographic resolution or 2 weeks in the case of traumatic pneumothorax. The same arguments are applied to patients having had recent thoracic surgery (for whatever reason) who are now advised not to fly for 2 weeks after surgery. None of this is really evidence-based and the risks of ignoring these guidelines are not known. It is probable that the risk of a second pneumothorax within this period is only high enough to worry about in patients with pre-existing lung disease.

Closed environment Patients with infectious diseases such as TB should not fly. There seems to be a significant risk of infecting others.

Further information

Cottrell JJ Aircraft cabin pressures. *Chest* 1988; **98**: 81

British Thoracic Society guidelines, www.brit-thoracic.org.uk/page246.html

British Lung Foundation/BTS patient leaflet on flying with a lung condition, www.brit-thoracic.org.uk/c2/uploads/air_20patient_20info.pdf

BLF advice, www.britishlungfoundation.org/air-travel.asp

Altitude sickness

Definitions of acute mountain or high altitude sickness are not precise, but include several symptoms provoked by the hypoxia.

Pathophysiology Some of the pathophysiology is well understood and explains some of the symptoms and signs. These largely fall into two categories, minor and major.

Minor, due to hyperventilation provoked by the hypoxia, and include:

- Light-headedness/fatigue
- Numbness/tingling of extremities
- Nausea/vomiting and anorexia
- Headache
- Insomnia/sleep disturbance
- Periodic ventilation during sleep.

These symptoms are common, develop over 6–12 h after arrival, and affect at least a quarter of those flying to Colorado for a skiing holiday (altitude 2400–3400 m, ~10 000 ft, barometric pressure 70 kPa, inspired oxygen tension 14.5 kPa, average SaO_2 on arrival 89–90%). Most of the symptoms are due to a respiratory hypocapnic alkalosis and resolve as the kidney retains $[H^+]$ and excretes $[HCO_3^-]$, returning pH towards normal. This allows further hyperventilation and the rise in SaO_2 helps resolve any of the symptoms due to the hypoxia itself. This scenario tends to be common in those with a higher hypoxic drive (measured at sea level, as it encourages greater hypocapnia and alkalosis). Confusingly, these symptoms may also indicate the early development of the more major category.

Major, those due to the hypoxia itself. These are more serious, can develop rapidly, and tend to occur more in those with a lower hypoxic drive. There is also a genetic component influencing susceptibility, related to the ACE gene. In ***high altitude pulmonary oedema (HAPE)*** the hypoxia provokes a *non-uniform* pulmonary vasoconstriction, raising pulmonary artery pressure (PAP); hence some pulmonary capillaries are unprotected and receive the full rise in PAP. Fluid leakage into alveoli, pulmonary oedema, and capillary damage (with pulmonary haemorrhage) produce clinically apparent disease. The dominant symptoms/signs are:

- Extra breathlessness/cough
- Cyanosis
- Blood tinged frothy sputum
- Crackles on auscultation/raised JVP.

In ***high altitude cerebral oedema (HACE)*** hypoxia also causes increased cerebral blood flow, cerebral oedema, retinal haemorrhages, cerebral thrombosis, and petechial haemorrhages. The dominant symptoms are:

- Ataxia (may be the first sign)
- Confusion/disorientation/hallucinations/behavioural change
- Severe headache/reduced conscious level
- Papilloedema.

Both HAPE and HACE are potentially fatal.

Management Risk factors are mainly the rate and degree of altitude attained. Keep ascent to ≤300 m/day and rest every third day. The minor form of altitude sickness is likely to resolve spontaneously over a few days with simple symptomatic treatment, analgesics, and plenty of hydration. However, prophylaxis, or early treatment on symptom appearance, with acetazolamide, is very effective, as are limiting further ascent and encouraging descent. ***Acetazolamide*** provokes a mild metabolic acidosis (by reducing $[H^+]$ availability for excretion in the distal tubule) and 'pre-acclimatizes' the subject to allow greater hyperventilation in response to hypoxia without the usual alkalosis. It is recommended when rapid ascent to altitudes ≥2500 m is unavoidable (such as a package ski trip to Aspen). 500 mg per day (slow release) for the 2 days prior to ascent is probably adequate for most subjects (or as treatment after symptoms develop). The commonest side-effect is a harmless and reversible tingling of the extremities. ***Temazepam*** has been shown to reduce the periodic breathing at night (by reducing the arousals that help maintain the periodicity) and does not appear to worsen the hypoxia or reduce vigilance levels the following day.

The best predictor of severe altitude sickness is a prior episode. It may be possible to predict likely problems based on sea level estimates of a poor hypoxic response, but this has not been fully validated.

The management of the more severe forms of altitude sickness that tend to occur with rapid ascent to over 4000 m, pulmonary and cerebral oedema, is urgent.

Management of severe altitude sickness

- Increase inspired oxygen tension by rapid descent, extra inspired oxygen, or a local pressurized environment (e.g. a portable hyperbaric chamber such as the Gamow bag)

HAPE

- Sit upright and keep warm
- Nifedipine (20 mg bd up to qds + loading dose, 10 mg sublingually) to reduce PAP
- Acetazolamide may help by also reducing PAP, as well as increasing the effective ventilatory response to altitude hypoxia

HACE

- Dexamethasone (4 mg qds + loading dose, 8 mg) to reduce cerebral oedema.

Improvement is usually rapid once the inspiratory oxygen tension is raised. Prophylaxis for this more severe form of altitude sickness is more controversial, but graded ascent is important, acetazolamide probably helps, and nifedipine is used by some, particularly if there is a history of a previous episode.

Further information

Information for patients. www.thebmc.co.uk/world/mm/mm1.htm

Information for patients. www.familydoctor.org/247.xml

Information for patients and doctors. www.high-altitude-medicine.com

Diving

Problems Increased recreational diving has raised the awareness of respiratory problems at depth. These can essentially be divided into five:

- Barotrauma, e.g. ruptured bullae and pneumothorax
- Worsening of pre-existing disorder whilst at depth, e.g. asthma
- Nitrogen gas evolved from solution in body fluids
- Breath-hold diving and ascent hypoxia
- Pulmonary oedema.

Pathophysiology

Barotrauma *(second commonest cause of death in SCUBA divers after drowning)* During descent, any air-containing cavity in the body will be compressed by the rise in external pressure. If there is any communication with the airways (e.g. middle ear, lung bullae) then gas will slowly move into the air space. On ascent the airspace will expand and, if air cannot escape quickly enough, may lead to rupture, of the eardrum or the bullae, for example. *A tension pneumothorax can be rapidly fatal in this situation.* Obstructive lung diseases in general can predispose to ruptured alveoli. In addition to pneumothoraces, the escaped air can produce a pneumomediastinum, causing chest pain, and a radiolucent band (air in the pericardium) along the cardiac border on CXR. Breathing 100% O_2 will clear the air more quickly. Air emboli can also occur and produce a wide range of symptoms; hyperbaric oxygen may be required.

Pre-existing lung disease The onset of asthma during a dive can be disastrous and may be provoked by the dry gases breathed from SCUBA gear (self-contained underwater breathing apparatus). See *BSAC recommendations on asthma and diving* (opposite). Many lung diseases, such as cystic fibrosis, COPD (FEV_1 <80% predicted), fibrotic lung disease, previous pneumothorax (with no pleurodesis), and lung bullae are considered contraindications to diving. However, recently, BSAC has adopted the pragmatic approach of accepting that in individuals with a history of spontaneous pneumothorax, who have had no pneumothorax for 5 years, the risk of pulmonary barotrauma is small and not significantly greater than for many in the general population, e.g. smokers. Such individuals may dive provided that a CT scan of the chest and lung function tests (including flow–volume loops) show no reason to suggest that there is significant residual lung disease.

The bends or caisson disease (caisson are underwater air chambers in which people work). During periods of high pressure, extra nitrogen dissolves into the blood and other tissue fluids. This takes many minutes. On ascent this nitrogen literally bubbles off. If the amount coming out of solution is too great, nitrogen bubbles act as emboli and limit blood flow. This produces micro-infarction with activation of inflammatory and clotting cascades and damage to several organs, e.g. joints, spinal cord, brain. Limited diving times and slow ascents reduce this problem, as do breathing mixtures containing helium, rather than nitrogen. Severe cases require treatment in hyperbaric chambers.

Breath-hold diving During breath-hold diving, increased pressure on the chest elevates alveolar and arterial PO_2. This extends breath-hold time, particularly with prior hyperventilation to reduce $PaCO_2$. During the dive,

O_2 is used and PO_2 falls. On ascent, with rarefaction of the thoracic gas, PO_2 falls quickly with possible loss of consciousness and drowning.

Pulmonary oedema has been reported whilst SCUBA diving in cold water, but the mechanism is not clear.

British Sub Aqua Club (BSAC) recommendations re asthma

- Asthma may predispose to air-trapping leading to pulmonary barotrauma and air embolism, which may be fatal. An acute asthma attack can also cause severe dyspnoea that may be hazardous or fatal during diving
- These theoretical risks should be explained fully to the asthmatic diver. There is little, if any, evidence that the mild controlled, asthmatic that follows the guidelines below is at more risk
- Asthmatics may dive if they have allergic asthma, but not if they have cold-, exercise-, or emotion-induced asthma
- All asthmatics should be managed in accordance with British Thoracic Society Guidelines
- Only well-controlled asthmatics may dive
- Asthmatics should not dive if needed a *therapeutic* bronchodilator in the last 48 h, or have had any other chest symptoms.

Control of asthma

- The asthmatic should not need more than occasional bronchodilators, i.e. daily usage would be a disqualifying factor, but inhaled steroids/cromoglicate/nedocromil are permissible
- During the diving season he/she should take bd peak flows. A deviation of 10% from best values should exclude diving until within 10% of best values for at least 48 h before diving
- The medical examiner should perform an exercise test such as the 18 in (43 cm) step test for 3 min, or running outside (not a bicycle ergometer) to increase the heart rate to 80% (210 minus age). A decrease in PEFR of 15% at 3 min post-exercise should be taken as evidence of exercise-induced bronchoconstriction and, hence, disbars. The patient should be off all bronchodilators for 24 h before the test
- A β_2 agonist may be taken pre-diving as a *preventative*, but not to relieve bronchospasm at the time.

Further information

Aberdeen emergency number for hyperbaric chambers, 07831 151523. www.hyperchamber.com

British Thoracic Society guidelines, www.brit-thoracic.org.uk/bts_diving_guidelines_html

Diving and medical conditions, www.bsac.org/page/42/medical-matters.htm

Diving and pneumothorax, www.bsac.org/page/192/pneumothorax-and-diving.htm

Diving, medical forms and certificates, www.bsac.org/page/100/uk-sdm-forms.htm

Plymouth Diving Disease Research Centre, *www.ddrc.org/docs/contact.htm* (24 h help line and register of hyperbaric chambers) 01752 209999. email enquiries@ddrc.org

Cochard G *et al.* Pulmonary oedema in scuba divers. *Undersea Hyperb Med* 2005; **32:** 39–44

Chapter 27

Gastrointestinal disease and the lung

Hepatic hydrothorax and hepatopulmonary syndrome

Hepatic hydrothorax Predominantly right-sided pleural effusion occurring in patients with liver disease and no cardiorespiratory disease, often with minimal ascities. The ascitic fluid accumulates in the chest as a result of diaphragmatic defects. Occurs in 5–12% of patients with cirrhosis and portal hypertension. Spontaneous bacterial empyema can occur and is associated with mortality of 20%. Diuretics are rarely effective. The definitive treatment is liver transplantation.

Hepatopulmonary syndrome (HPS) is the triad of:
- Chronic liver disease and portal hypertension
- Abnormal intrapulmonary peripheral vascular vasodilatation with decreased pulmonary vascular resistance (right to left shunt) and subsequent ventilation–perfusion abnormalities
- Arterial hypoxia.

It occurs in 4–29% of patients with chronic liver disease. The mechanism is thought to be related to the release of vasoactive mediators from portal hypertension causing altered bowel perfusion, which in turn leads to pulmonary vascular dilatation, with the formation of vascular spider naevi on the pleura. Patients with cirrhosis who develop hepatopulmonary syndrome have a worse prognosis.

Presentation is with progressive dyspnoea and cyanosis. Examination reveals clubbing and telangiectasia, with associated stigmata of chronic liver disease.

Diagnosis
- ***Hypoxia*** on blood gases <8.6 kPa on air, at rest and upright. Platypnoea and orthodeoxia are present, that is, breathlessness and desaturation on sitting upright, caused by preferential perfusion of basal pulmonary vasculature. Lying flat relieves this. These changes may be seen in other lung diseases, but in the presence of liver disease is suggestive of HPS. Hypoxia is poorly reversed with 100% oxygen, due to the pulmonary shunting
- ***Contrast-enhanced echocardiogram*** is positive. Contrast/saline bubbles are injected peripherally, and are normally seen only in the right heart and are then filtered by the pulmonary bed. In the presence of intrapulmonary shunts, these are seen in the left ventricle. (False-positive results occur if right-to-left cardiac shunt present, which can be excluded during echocardiogram)
- ***Pulmonary technetium-99 perfusion scan*** assesses the shunt fraction. Normally, the radiolabelled albumin is trapped in the pulmonary capillary bed. In the presence of intrapulmonary or cardiac shunts, there is significant uptake of radiolabelled albumin in the brain or spleen. A shunt index fraction of >20% indicates severe hepatopulmonary syndrome
- ***CT chest*** is performed to rule out other pulmonary comorbid disease

Treatment

- Oxygen if PaO_2 <8 kPa
- Avoid vasodilators. There is minimal evidence for pharmacological intervention
- Mainstay of treatment is liver transplantation, which reverses the condition. Hypoxia may take months to improve. Severe hypoxia (PaO_2 <6 kPa) is associated with increased mortality post-transplant, as there is increased risk of hepatic ischaemia
- Transjugular intrahepatic portosystemic shunt (TIPS) is ineffective
- Coil embolization can be tried in selected cases with AV communications.

Prognosis is poor, with a mortality of 40% in 2.5 years.

Portopulmonary hypertension

Portopulmonary hypertension (POPH) is pulmonary artery hypertension occurring in association with portal hypertension. It occurs in an estimated 2–5% of patients with cirrhosis and is present in around 16% of those referred for liver transplant. The mechanism is unclear, but probably relates to a hyperdynamic circulation, high cardiac output, cytokine release, and possible pulmonary emboli.

Defined as:

- Elevated pulmonary artery pressure (>25 mmHg at rest, >30 mmHg during exercise)
- Increased pulmonary vascular resistance due to pulmonary vasoconstriction and obliterative vascular remodelling (>120 dyn/s/cm^5)
- Abnormal left ventricular end diastolic/wedge pressure (<15 mmHg)
- In the setting of portal hypertension (portal pressure >10 mmHg).

Presentation Dyspnoea on exertion, possibly syncope, chest pain, fatigue, palpitations, haemoptysis, and orthopnoea. There may be signs of volume overload with raised JVP and pedal oedema. P2 may be loud, with pulmonary and tricuspid regurgitation, as well as stigmata of chronic liver disease. It is usually diagnosed 4–7 years after the diagnosis of portal hypertension.

Diagnosis

- ***Hypoxia*** on blood gases, but less so than in hepatopulmonary syndrome
- ***CXR*** may be normal or show prominent pulmonary arteries and enlarged right heart
- ***ECG*** shows RVH, RBBB, RAD, and sinus tachycardia
- ***kCO*** may be decreased
- ***Echocardiography*** is the main screening test and is diagnostic if the right ventricular pressure is >50 mmHg
- Exclude other causes of pulmonary hypertension
- ***Right heart catheterization*** with vasodilator studies is performed
- The changes in the vessels in POPH are the same histologically as those seen in IPAH (see p 388).

Treatment Options are the same as for patients with IPAH, with vasodilators, prostacyclin, and endothelin antagonists (see p 394). Avoid β-blockers, so manage varices with banding. Anticoagulation is not advised due to the risk of variceal bleeding. LTOT if PaO_2 <8 kPa. Liver transplantation may reverse mild to moderate POPH, although symptoms may take weeks to months to resolve. Severe POPH is not reversed and is associated with significant intra- and post-operative morbidity and mortality. A few cases of heart–lung–liver transplants have been reported.

Prognosis is poor in severe POPH, with a median survival after diagnosis of 6 months, without transplant.

Further information

Hoeper M *et al.* Portopulmonary hypertension and hepatopulmonary syndrome. *Lancet* 2004; **363**: 1461–8

Budhiraja R, Hassoun P. Portopulmonary hypertension. A tale of two circulations. *Chest* 2003; **123**: 562–76

Inflammatory bowel disease, coeliac disease, and pancreatitis

Inflammatory bowel disease (IBD) Pulmonary involvement tends to occur after the onset of the IBD, but can predate it. Pulmonary involvement is found in up to a quarter of patients, but this is usually subclinical. Patients can develop a variety of clinical syndromes, including airway inflammation, subglottic stenosis, chronic bronchitis, bronchiectasis, and chronic bronchiolitis. Bronchoscopy may reveal inflammatory tissue within the large airway walls, which on biopsy shows mucosal ulceration, basal cell hyperplasia, basement membrane thickening, and submucosal inflammatory cell infiltration. IBD is also associated with the development of interstitial lung disease, such as cryptogenic organizing pneumonia (COP), pulmonary infiltrates with eosinophilia, or neutrophilic necrotic parenchymal nodules. Pulmonary involvement tends to be steroid-responsive. Inhaled steroids can be tried for chronic bronchitis, but oral or intravenous steroids may be required for worsening lung involvement. Note that drugs used in the treatment of IBD may also cause lung disease, such as sulfasalazine (alveolitis), mesalazine, or infliximab (both: pulmonary infiltrates and eosinophilia; infliximab: reactivation of latent TB).

Ulcerative colitis Pulmonary involvement is usually asymptomatic or may be associated with dry cough. Minimal interstitial change may be suggested by abnormal pulmonary function tests. Restrictive, obstructive, or reduced kCO defects may be seen. Usually normal CXR and CT. No specific treatment indicated.

Crohn's disease Pulmonary involvement less common than in ulcerative colitis, but similar changes found.

Coeliac disease May be associated with idiopathic lung fibrosis, causing restrictive defect. Also may be at increased risk of asthma, bird fancier's lung, and haemosiderosis. Increased risk of lymphoma and malignancy in GI tract.

Pancreatitis Acute pancreatitis is frequently associated with exudative pleural effusion. Raised amylase in the pleural fluid is suggestive (see p 55). Adult respiratory distress syndrome (ARDS) may develop, which requires supportive care and mechanical ventilation (see p 101).

Further information

Mahadeva *et al.* Clinical and radiological characteristics of lung disease in inflammatory bowel disease. *Eur Respir J* 2000; **15**: 41–8

Chapter 28

Hypersensitivity pneumonitis

Causes

Definition Group of lung diseases caused by inhalation of organic antigen to which the individual has been previously sensitized. Hypersensitivity pneumonitis (HP; previously termed extrinsic allergic alveolitis) is often divided into 'acute' and 'chronic' forms based on the time-course of presentation. Acute HP often follows a short period of exposure to a high concentration of antigen, and is usually reversible. Chronic HP typically follows a period of chronic exposure to a low antigen dose and is less reversible. These two presentations may overlap and 'subacute' forms of the disease are recognized.

Epidemiology Exact prevalence unknown. At least 8% of budgerigar and pigeon keepers and up to 5% of farmers may develop HP. Hypersensitivity pneumonitis is thought to be more common in non-smokers (mechanism unclear; may reflect inhibition of alveolar macrophage function by smoke).

Causes Many different antigens have been reported to cause HP, ranging from the relatively common (bird-fancier's lung and farmer's lung in the UK; summer-house HP in Japan) to the more unusual and exotic (shell lung—proteins on mollusc shells; pituitary snuff-taker's disease; sericulturist's lung—silk worm larvae proteins; sax lung—yeast on saxophone mouthpieces). Important examples are listed in Table 28.1.

Table 28.1 Causes of hypersensitivity pneumonitis—examples

Antigen	Sources	Diseases
Organisms		
Thermophilic actinomycetes *(Micropolyspora faeni, Thermoactinomyces vulgaris), Aspergillus* spp	Mouldy hay; sugarcane; compost; mushrooms; contaminated water in humidifiers and air conditioners	Farmer's lung; bagassosis; compost lung; mushroom worker's lung; humidifier lung
Aspergillus clavatus	Mouldy barley	Malt worker's lung
Trichosporon cutaneum	House dust	Summer-house HP (Japan)
Cladosporium spp	Ceiling mould	Hot tub lung
Animal protein		
Bird proteins	Bloom on bird feathers and droppings	Bird fancier's lung
Rat proteins	Rat droppings	Rat lung
Chemical		
Toluene diisocyanate	Paints	Isocyanate HP

Pathophysiology Pathogenesis of HP is not fully understood, and may involve T-cell mediated immunity and granuloma formation (type IV hypersensitivity) and/or antibody–antigen immune complex formation (type III hypersensitivity). It is not an atopic disease, and is not characterized by a rise in tissue eosinophils or IgE (type I hypersensitivity); this may, in part, be due to the small particle size of offending antigens, which tend to be deposited more distally in the air-spaces than the larger particles associated with asthma. Lung histology specimens typically reveal an interstitial inflammatory infiltrate, often with accompanying bronchiolitis and organizing pneumonia. Non-caseating granulomata are often present, and typically are ill-defined and single (cf. sarcoidosis, where granulomata are well-defined and are grouped subpleurally or near bronchi). Chronic HP is characterized by fibrosis, and often the absence of granulomata and airways involvement, particularly if antigen exposure has ceased.

Diagnosis

Clinical features

Acute HP

- Breathlessness, dry cough, and systemic symptoms (fever, chills, arthralgia, myalgia, headache) occur 4–8 h after exposure to antigen
- Examination: crackles and squeaks on auscultation, fever
- In the absence of ongoing exposure, symptoms settle spontaneously within 1–3 days. Episodes may be recurrent.

Chronic HP

- Progressive exertional breathlessness, dry cough, sometimes systemic symptoms (weight loss) over the course of months–years. May be history of acute episodes
- Examination: crackles and squeaks on auscultation, clubbing rare, may be features of cor pulmonale.

Investigations

- ***Imaging: acute HP***
    - *CXR* Diffuse small (1–3 mm) nodules or infiltrates, sometimes ground glass change, apical sparing. Normal in up to 20% of cases
    - *HRCT* Patchy ground-glass change and poorly defined nodules. Areas of increased lucency (enhanced on expiratory HRCT) occur due to air trapping from bronchiolar involvement
    - Both CXR and HRCT appearances may quickly normalize following removal from antigen exposure
- ***Imaging: chronic HP***
    - *CXR* Typically upper- and mid-zone reticulation
    - *HRCT* Diffuse well-defined centrilobular nodules, ground-glass change, increased lucency from air trapping. May mimic IPF
- ***PFTs*** Typically restrictive pattern with reduced gas transfer and lung volumes; mild obstruction is also sometimes observed. Hypoxia may occur
- ***Bloods*** Acute hypersensitivity pneumonitis associated with neutrophilia but not eosinophilia. Inflammatory markers often increased
- ***Serum antibody (IgG) precipitin*** results are presented either as an ELISA or as a number of precipitin lines, referring to the number of different epitopes an individual responds to. Precipitins to organic antigens are found in 90% of patients, but are also present in up to 10% of asymptomatic farmers and 50% of pigeon breeders. Precipitin levels often fall in the absence of ongoing antigen exposure
- ***BAL*** lymphocytosis (>40% of cells) is a typical finding, but not in itself diagnostic
- ***Transbronchial or surgical lung biopsy*** may be required in cases of diagnostic uncertainty. TBB may provide insufficient tissue for adequate histological analysis
- ***Inhalation antigen challenge*** may be unpleasant, and is not recommended routinely

Diagnosis is based on the combination of history of antigen exposure and typical clinical and HRCT features. The most diagnostically useful clinical features are an onset of symptoms 4–8 h after exposure, a history of recurrent episodes of symptoms, the presence of weight loss, and the finding of crackles on examination. An absence of serum precipitins is very unusual but described. Atypical presentations require further investigation to support the diagnosis, such as BAL lymphocytosis or characteristic histological features on lung biopsy.

Differential diagnosis

- Atypical pneumonia
- Idiopathic interstitial pneumonias (particularly IPF and COP)
- Sarcoidosis
- Vasculitis
- Occupational asthma (e.g. from isocyanates)
- Drug-induced lung disease (including pesticides)
- Organic dust toxic syndrome (follows very high levels of exposure to agricultural dusts, symptoms transient, benign course)
- Silo-filler's disease (variable respiratory manifestations following exposure to nitrogen dioxide in silos; ranges from mild bronchitis to fatal bronchospasm)

Management

Management centres on antigen avoidance, which is frequently difficult. If complete removal from antigen is unrealistic (e.g. farmers), measures to reduce exposure may be of benefit (such as respiratory protection with high performance, positive pressure masks; avoidance of particularly heavy exposure; improved ventilation and use of air filters; drying of hay prior to storage).

In acute HP, symptoms typically resolve following cessation of antigen exposure and treatment is usually not required. Removal from exposure may also result in symptomatic and physiological improvement in chronic HP, although this is less certain and established pulmonary fibrosis is often irreversible.

When treatment is required, corticosteroids are frequently used although there is a lack of randomized controlled evidence to support this. Steroids may hasten the resolution of impaired pulmonary function in acute HP, although their effect on long-term outcome is unclear. A typical regimen is prednisolone 40–60 mg daily for up to a month, and then slowly reduce dose over several months. Inhaled steroids have not been studied in detail, although may be of some benefit.

Prognosis Highly variable. Prognosis is usually excellent following removal from antigen exposure in acute HP, although progression to respiratory failure and death may very rarely occur after short-term exposures of very high intensity. Recurrent episodes of acute HP do not necessarily progress to chronic HP and fibrosis, and chronic HP may develop in the absence of previous acute HP episodes. Development of chronic HP with ongoing exposure may eventually lead to cor pulmonale and death, although again this is variable and many patients do not exhibit disease progression despite chronic exposure. Persistent low-dose exposure (e.g. budgerigar in the house) may be more likely to progress to the chronic fibrotic form of HP than intermittent high-dose exposure (e.g. pigeon fanciers), which predisposes more to episodes of acute HP.

Further information

Schuyler M. Hypersensitivity pneumonitis, Lesson 6, Volume 14 in PCCU Education Series online at www.chestnet

Chapter 29

Hyperventilation syndrome

Definition Poorly defined, and the term is falling into disfavour, dysfunctional breathing being the alternative. Most respiratory physicians still use hyperventilation syndrome to describe breathlessness and over-breathing associated with fear, stress, and anxiety, in the absence of any demonstrable physiological abnormality.

Usually part of a spectrum of physical symptoms (e.g. chest pain, palpitations/tachycardia, fatigue, dizziness, parasthesiae, headache, diarrhoea, inappropriate sweating, etc.) from an anxiety or panic disorder. Other specialties may have been consulted due to the mixed symptomatology.

Pathophysiology Hyperventilation syndrome can occur *de novo*, or follow a respiratory disorder that has resolved—such as an attack of mild asthma. It appears to be based on a heightened awareness of breathing, and concerns as to what the shortness of breath signifies. The $PaCO_2$ is intermittently low, with a respiratory alkalosis. Recordings of breathing pattern often show a rather chaotic pattern.

Clinical features

- Intermittent episodes of breathlessness largely unrelated to exercise, although can be worsened by exercise
- May be associated with symptoms of respiratory alkalosis, such as numbness, tingling of the extremities, feelings of impending doom, and light-headedness, occasionally to the point of losing consciousness (cerebral vasoconstriction due to the hypocapnia)
- Sensation of not being able to take a satisfactory breath
- No history suggestive of an alternative current respiratory disorder, although there may have been one previously
- History of some stressful situation in the patient's life
- Previous episodes.

Diagnosis is essentially one of exclusion, but with additional confirmatory findings.

- No evidence of a cardiac cause for the breathlessness
- No evidence of a respiratory cause, i.e. normal lung function, normal CXR, and normal SaO_2 at rest and on exercise to the point of breathlessness (SaO_2 may even rise on exercise)
- Irregular breathing pattern at rest and on exercise
- No evidence of pulmonary hypertension
- No evidence to support pulmonary emboli
- No evidence of hyperthyroidism
- Low $PaCO_2$, raised pH, on blood gases (and a normal A–a gradient)
- No metabolic acidosis on blood gases (e.g. ketoacidosis, lactacidosis)
- Unresolved psychological issues, or social phobia/agoraphobia.

Differential diagnosis Important pathological causes to exclude are:

- Subtle interstitial lung disease with a normal CXR: consider HRCT
- Mild asthma with normal basic PFTs: consider PEFR monitoring, exercise provocation, or bronchial reactivity testing
- Pulmonary hypertension/thromboembolic disease: consider cardiac echo or CTPA
- Hyperthyroidism
- Unexpected acidosis: e.g. renal failure, lactacidosis, ketoacidosis.

Management It is important not to dismiss the patient's symptoms, implying it is 'all in the mind'. The patient has a real symptom, which requires a real explanation. There are no controlled trials of management, but most clinicians will offer an explanation based on an 'over-awareness' of respiratory sensations, heightened by anxiety. It is important to explain that the associated symptoms of tingling and light-headedness are well recognized and harmless.

Old recommendations to rebreathe into a paper bag have not stood the test of time and are rather impractical in the middle of a supermarket. Because cold peripheries often accompany an episode (vasoconstriction), placing the cold palms on to the cheeks can help suppress the desire to breathe, thought to be related to the diving reflex: again, this is an untested remedy.

Careful explanation may be enough. A short period on an anxiolytic (e.g. diazepam 2–5 mg bd) may be helpful, to demonstrate that the symptoms can be controlled. Management of the psychological problem may be possible. Some experienced respiratory physiotherapists can help patients control their symptoms and divert the anxiety away from breathing.

Failure to respond should always prompt a reconsideration of whether an underlying disorder is gradually progressing to the point where an investigation becomes abnormal. On the other hand, repeated investigations will confirm the patient's concern that 'the doctors think there is something wrong.'

Prognosis Some patients improve quickly with explanation. Some tend to relapse at times of stress. Some prove resistant to any treatment and probably should be seen in the clinic regularly, but infrequently, to reduce their likelihood of involving other medical services with another pointless round of investigations.

Nijmegen hyperventilation score (Table 29.1) Filled in by a patient; a score of 22 or over is highly suggestive of hyperventilation syndrome.

Table 29.1 Example of Nijmeqen hyperventilation score

Before treatment	Never 0	Rare 1	Sometimes 2	Often 3	Very often 4
Chest pain			✓		
Feeling tense				✓	
Blurred vision		✓			
Dizzy spells			✓		
Feeling confused			✓		
Faster/deeper breathing					✓
Shortness of breath				✓	
Tight feeling in the chest					✓
Bloated feeling in the stomach			✓		
Tingling fingers	✓				
Unable to breath deeply				✓	
Stiff fingers or arms			✓		
Tight feeling around mouth	✓				
Cold hands or feet	✓				
Heart racing (palpitations)				✓	
Feeling anxious				✓	
Total score	34				

Chapter 30

Idiopathic interstitial pneumonias

Overview

Definition The IIPs comprise a group of diffuse lung diseases of unknown aetiology that primarily involve the pulmonary interstitium—the area between the alveolar epithelium and capillary endothelium, as well as the septal and bronchovascular tissues that make up the fibrous framework of the lung. These primarily interstitial processes, however, also frequently involve the airways, vasculature, and alveolar airspaces. The underlying pathological process is one of varying degrees of inflammation and fibrosis.

The terminology used to describe the IIPs may be confusing; these conditions have been subject to much reclassification, reflecting the lack of understanding of their underlying aetiology and pathogenesis. Idiopathic pulmonary fibrosis (IPF; previously termed cryptogenic fibrosing alveolitis) is the commonest IIP and is characterized by the histological pattern of usual interstitial pneumonia (UIP). The other IIPs are distinct disease entities and are all rare. They all represent a subgroup of interstitial (or diffuse parenchymal) lung diseases.

Diagnosis Made from a combination of clinical, HRCT, and histological features—distinguish from other causes of diffuse lung disease (see Chapter 6). Histological patterns are the most specific and form the basis for the current classification of IIPs. Surgical lung biopsy is recommended for most cases of suspected IIP with the exception of patients exhibiting typical clinical and HRCT features of IPF. Transbronchial biopsies have a very limited role due to the generally patchy distribution of the IIPs, although they may be useful in the diagnosis of acute interstitial pneumonitis (AIP) and cryptogenic organizing pneumonia (COP), as well as the exclusion of other causes of diffuse lung disease (e.g. sarcoidosis).

Treatment The optimal treatment of many of the IIPs is poorly established, and there is a lack of supportive data from randomized controlled trials. Steroids and immunosuppression are the mainstay of treatment, but these are often ineffective and have significant side-effects. Treatment may alter both the HRCT and histological pictures, and if possible should be delayed until a diagnosis has been made.

The conditions currently included within the classification of idiopathic interstitial pneumonias, together with their key clinical, imaging, and histological features and prognosis, are presented in Table 30.1 opposite and discussed in detail in the remainder of this chapter. They are listed in order of frequency.

Further information

ATS/ERS. International Multidisciplinary Consensus Classification of the Idiopathic Interstitial Pneumonias. *Am J Resp Crit Care Med* 2002; **165**: 277–304

Table 30.1. Idiopathic interstitial pneumonias: summary of key features

Idiopathic pulmonary fibrosis (IPF) [previously cryptogenic fibrosing alveolitis (CFA)]	Idiopathic *Onset* over years *HRCT* fibrosis, honeycombing, minimal ground glass, subpleural, and basal distribution *Histology* usual interstitial pneumonia (UIP): areas of interstitial fibrosis (made up of foci of proliferating fibroblasts) interspersed with normal lung (temporal and spatial heterogeneity), minimal inflammation *Prognosis* poor
Non-specific interstitial pneumonia (NSIP)	Idiopathic or disease-associated *Onset* over months–years *HRCT* diffuse ground glass, fine reticulation, minimal honeycombing *Histology* varying degrees of inflammation and fibrosis, more uniform appearance than UIP *Prognosis* variable, can be good
Cryptogenic organizing pneumonia (COP) [previously idiopathic bronchiolitis obliterans organizing pneumonia, BOOP]	Idiopathic or disease-associated *Onset* over months *HRCT* areas of consolidation, basal, subpleural, and peribronchial predominance *Histology* alveolar spaces 'plugged' with granulation tissue, ± extension into bronchioles *Prognosis* generally good
Acute interstitial pneumonia (AIP)	Idiopathic Many similarities to ARDS *Onset* over days *HRCT* diffuse ground glass and patchy consolidation *Histology* diffuse alveolar damage: interstitial oedema, intra-alveolar hyaline membranes, followed by fibroblast proliferation and interstitial fibrosis *Prognosis* poor
Respiratory bronchiolitis associated interstitial lung disease (RB-ILD)	Idiopathic, occurs in smokers *Onset* over years Symptoms usually mild *HRCT* centrilobular nodules, ground glass, thick-walled airways *Histology* pigmented macrophages in bronchioles *Prognosis* good
Desquamative interstitial pneumonia (DIP)	Idiopathic, occurs in smokers *Onset* over weeks–months *HRCT* ground glass *Histology* pigmented macrophages in alveolar air spaces (perhaps a more extensive form of RB-ILD), temporally uniform appearance *Prognosis* good
Lymphoid interstitial pneumonia (LIP)	Idiopathic or disease-associated *Onset* over years *HRCT* ground glass, often reticulation *Histology* diffuse interstitial lymphoid infiltrates *Prognosis* variable

Idiopathic pulmonary fibrosis (IPF): diagnosis

Definition Chronic interstitial pneumonia of unknown cause characterized histologically by temporal and spatial heterogeneity, with areas of fibrosis and architectural distortion interspersed with areas of normal lung. This occurs as different areas of lung are in varying stages of evolution of the pathological process. The histological appearance of idiopathic pulmonary fibrosis (previously known as cryptogenic fibrosing alveolitis) is usual interstitial pneumonia (UIP).

Epidemiology Prevalence figures vary from 6 to 14/100 000, although prevalence may be 175/100 000 in patients >75 years old. Slightly more common in males. Mean age at presentation 67. Familial form well described, but very rare.

Causes and pathophysiology The development of fibrosis was previously thought to reflect a response to chronic inflammation resulting from an unknown initial injury. This key role of inflammation in the pathogenesis of IPF has been questioned, however, based partly on the observations that inflammation is not a major feature of pathological specimens, and that responses to 'anti-inflammatory' treatment with steroids are often poor. An alternative theory is that repeated alveolar epithelial injury leads directly to wound healing and fibrosis, and this concept of 'fibrosis without inflammation' has been demonstrated both in animal models and other human diseases. The nature of the lung injury remains obscure: postulated triggers include inhalation of metal dust and wood dust, smoking, or exposure to the Epstein–Barr virus. Cytokine production (e.g. plasminogen activator inhibitors, matrix metalloproteinases, transforming growth factor β) by alveolar epithelial cells may play an important role in the development of fibrosis. Host genetic factors are also likely to be important in modifying the wound-healing response.

Clinical features

- Typically presents with gradual onset exertional breathlessness and cough; average of 9 months of symptoms prior to presentation
- 5% of patients are said to be asymptomatic, although this is likely to be an underestimate
- Arthralgia occurs in about 20%
- Fine basal late inspiratory crackles
- Clubbing in up to 50%
- Cyanosis and cor pulmonale in severe disease.

Investigations

- ***Blood tests*** Raised ESR and CRP and mild anaemia may occur; positive rheumatoid factor and/or ANA may occur at low titres in the absence of associated connective tissue disease
- ***PFTs*** Typically restrictive pattern with reduced vital capacity and transfer factor; smokers may exhibit coexisting obstructive defect. Oxygen saturations are frequently reduced, particularly on exertion; ABGs may demonstrate type I respiratory failure

- ***CXR*** Peripheral and basal reticular shadowing, may extend to other zones, sometimes with honeycombing; rarely may be normal
- ***HRCT*** features include bilateral, peripheral, and subpleural reticulation, with honeycombing, traction bronchiectasis, architectural distortion, and minimal or no ground-glass change. Predominantly basal initially, more extensive later in disease course. Extent of disease on CT correlates with physiological impairment. Predominant ground-glass appearance suggests an IIP other than IPF—consider lung biopsy
- ***BAL*** is not routinely required and is rarely helpful. Typically shows neutrophilia, sometimes mild eosinophilia. Marked eosinophilia (>20%) or lymphocytosis (>50%) should raise possibility of alternative diagnosis
- ***Lung biopsy*** (via VATS or thoracotomy) if there is diagnostic doubt
- ***Gallium and DTPA*** scanning are seldom of use in clinical practice.

Histology Usual interstitial pneumonia, a fibrosing pattern characterized by temporal and spatial heterogeneity: patches of active fibroblastic foci (reflecting acute injury) are interspersed with honeycombing/architectural distortion (reflecting chronic scarring) and areas of normal lung, reflecting varying stages of evolution of the disease process in different areas of lung. Interstitial inflammation is minimal. Significant inter-observer disagreement between expert pathologists regarding the presence of a UIP pattern on lung biopsy has been reported, however, and an overall diagnosis taking into account clinical, radiological and histological features is recommended.

Diagnosis can be confidently made in most cases on the basis of clinical and HRCT findings. Lung biopsy is not generally required in patients with typical clinical and HRCT features of IPF, but should be considered in the presence of unusual features (e.g. predominant ground glass/nodules/consolidation/upper lobe involvement on HRCT, or young patient). When required, biopsies should be obtained at VATS or thoracotomy; transbronchial biopsies provide smaller samples, which rarely give diagnostic information due to the patchy distribution of disease.

Differential diagnosis

- Left ventricular failure (a common clinical misdiagnosis in IPF, and patients are often prescribed inappropriate diuretics)
- Asbestosis (may mimic clinically and radiologically; occupational history and presence of pleural plaques may suggest this diagnosis)
- Connective tissue disease (may mimic clinically and radiologically, and precede extrapulmonary manifestations of disease)
- Chronic hypersensitivity pneumonitis (suggested by typically upper/mid-zone predominance, micronodules, ground glass, areas of reduced attenuation)
- Drug-induced lung disease.

IPF: management 1

Treatment choices are hindered by a lack of large well-conducted placebo-controlled trials. There is currently no evidence that any drug treatment improves survival or quality of life. Drugs should not be used routinely, but may be considered in a closely observed trial of therapy. They may be of benefit in patients with other IIPs misdiagnosed as IPF. Drug treatments include:

- ***Oral corticosteroids*** Prior to the reclassification of IIPs, studies suggested that corticosteroids may improve lung function (in around 20–30% of patients) and symptoms (in around 50%). However, these studies probably included patients with conditions other than IPF that are associated with a better treatment response and prognosis (e.g. NSIP). Significant side-effects may affect at least a quarter of patients (e.g. hyperglycaemia necessitating insulin, osteoporosis, myopathy, peptic ulcer disease, cataracts, raised intraocular pressure, psychosis). Consider routine septrin prophylaxis (960 mg 3 times/week) against PCP
- ***Azathioprine*** in combination with prednisolone may improve survival compared with prednisolone alone; again this may reflect studies undertaken on individuals with IIPs other than IPF. Side-effects appear to be uncommon. Use of azathioprine alone has not been investigated
- ***Cyclophosphamide*** does not appear to improve survival and side-effects are common
- ***Colchicine*** appears to have a comparable effect to prednisolone and may be better tolerated
- Penicillamine and ciclosporin have not been studied in detail.

Management protocol The following recommendations are adapted from the BTS guidelines. In all cases they should be considered in the context of the individual patient's clinical condition, comorbidity, and wishes, particularly in view of the often unpredictable disease course, unknown efficacy of treatment, and high frequency of serious side-effects.

Initial assessment and decision to treat On presentation, all patients should have full clinical assessment, pulmonary function tests, and HRCT chest. In general, decisions regarding treatment are based on severity and rate of progression of symptoms, changes in pulmonary function, and HRCT appearance. Predominant ground-glass appearance on HRCT suggests an IIP other than IPF, and may be associated with steroid responsiveness—consider lung biopsy prior to starting treatment. Predominantly reticular patterns are usually less steroid-responsive.

Indications for trial of treatment

- Severe or rapidly progressive symptoms
- Predominantly ground-glass appearance on HRCT (consider biopsy)
- Consider in the context of a reticular pattern on HRCT if lung function significantly impaired or patient requests treatment.

If mild/moderate symptoms or a long history, and without predominant ground glass on HRCT (i.e. a reticular/mixed pattern), consider withholding treatment and follow-up within 3 months. If stable on follow-up, review 3-monthly for at least 1 year and regularly thereafter; consider trial of treatment if lung function deteriorates or symptoms worsen.

Monitoring Disease progression and response to treatment are best assessed by serial measurements of VC and TLCO; document them at each clinic attendance. Changes in VC or TLCO of 10–15% or more are considered significant in terms of assessing treatment response or disease progression. Changes in symptoms such as exercise tolerance and cough frequency/severity may also be useful.

Recommended treatment Oral prednisolone (0.5 mg/kg) is the mainstay of treatment. Consider IV methylprednisolone in very ill patients. Reassess lung function after 1 month (some recommend treating for a longer period before response to therapy is formerly assessed, e.g. 3–6 months):

- Improvement (increase in VC or TLCO by 10–15% or more) or stable: slowly reduce prednisolone dose (e.g. reduce by 5 mg weekly to 20 mg and review—if no worse, reduce by 5 mg a month to maintenance dose of 10 mg and continue at 10 mg for 1 year, and consider further reduction after this). Consider combination treatment with azathioprine (regimens vary; an example is initial daily dose of 50 mg for 4 weeks, then increase by 50 mg each week to maximum of 2–3 mg/kg, although do not exceed 150 mg daily; check WCC weekly until established on maximum dose for 2 weeks, then check WCC and LFTs every 6–8 weeks). Azathioprine is used less frequently in patients with a predominantly ground-glass HRCT appearance, who may be treated with prednisolone alone
- Deterioration (decrease in VC or TLCO by 10–15% or more): quickly reduce prednisolone dose (e.g. reduce by 10 mg weekly to 10 mg daily, and more slowly after this). Supportive treatment (see below). Consider lung transplant referral.

Patients who are unable to tolerate treatment

- Consider trial of azathioprine alone if prednisolone is not tolerated
- Colchicine may be tried as an alternative to prednisolone alone.

Further information

British Thoracic Society. BTS guidelines on the diagnosis, assessment and treatment of diffuse parenchymal lung disease in adults. *Thorax* 1999; **54** (suppl. 1): S1–30

IPF: management 2

Supportive treatment Consider use of home oxygen if very limited by breathlessness and in respiratory failure. Use of oxygen during exercise may improve exercise tolerance. Encourage pulmonary rehabilitation programme, if no contraindications. Cough may be troublesome; consider oral codeine. Opioids are frequently required for palliation of severe breathlessness.

Lung transplantation Patients with IPF are often referred for consideration of transplantation too late and most die whilst on the waiting list (which is around 12 months in the UK). Single lung transplant in IPF leads to an 80% survival at 1 year and 55% at 3 years. Guidelines recommend referral of all suitable patients with histological or radiographic evidence of UIP, irrespective of vital capacity and without delaying for trials of treatment. These are not widely applied in the UK, and, in practice, referral is often considered following failure of first-line treatment in symptomatic patients aged <65 years, with TLCO <40% predicted, fall in FVC ≥10% over 6 months, oxygen desaturation <88% on 6-min walk, and/or honeycombing on HRCT.

Causes of acute deterioration in patients with previously stable IPF

- Accelerated decline of IPF—an important cause of death in even mild–moderate, apparently stable IPF; mechanism poorly understood; biopsy often shows diffuse alveolar damage
- Pneumothorax—collapsed lung is often relatively resistant to re-expansion, making treatment difficult
- Infection (especially if immunocompromised), e.g. PCP
- Pulmonary embolism
- Acute deterioration may also occur post-operatively following major surgery, e.g. cardiac or orthopaedic—the reasons behind this are unclear.

Prognosis is variable: some decline rapidly, others remain stable or decline slowly over years. Several studies have demonstrated a median survival of 2.5–3.5 years, although prognosis is difficult to predict for individual patients. One study has shown oxygen desaturation <88% during 6-min walk, whilst breathing air is associated with 35% 4-year survival (compared with 69% in patients who do not desaturate below this level). More extensive fibroblastic foci on lung biopsy have also been shown to correlate with shorter survival. Death is commonly due to respiratory failure and/or infection. Risk of developing lung cancer is increased.

Future developments Therapeutic agents currently under evaluation include:

- ***Pirfenidone*** (antifibrotic, inhibits collagen synthesis and reduces fibroblast proliferation). No improvement in primary end-point (desaturation during 6-min walk) compared with placebo, although possible benefit in secondary end-points (vital capacity and prevention of acute exacerbation of IPF).

- ***Interferon γ-1b*** (antifibrotic, inhibits fibroblast proliferation and down-regulates transforming growth factor β). A large study of IPF patients unresponsive to corticosteroids showed no difference from placebo in disease progression or functional deterioration, and a trend towards improved survival with interferon γ-1b (particularly in the mild-to-moderate disease group with FVC>62% predicted). A further larger study (INSPIRE) is ongoing.
- ***Anticoagulation*** A placebo-controlled study suggested a possible survival benefit from anticoagulation in addition to prednisolone, particularly following acute exacerbations of IPF, but the study was small, open label, and with differential drop-out between groups; further studies needed
- Oral ***co-trimoxazole*** as a disease-modifying agent; pilot studies have been promising
- Oral ***N-acetylcysteine*** (an antioxidant, increases lung glutathione levels) at a high dose (600 mg tds) in combination with prednisolone and azathioprine appears to confer a small improvement in lung function when compared with prednisolone and azathioprine alone (no effect on mortality). The combination of prednisolone and azathioprine has not in itself been compared with placebo, however-they may be more toxic, and so this 'triple combination' cannot be recommended at present
- ***Bosentan*** (endothelin receptor 1 antagonist). Studies are ongoing
- ***Etanercept*** (TNF-α blockade). Studies are ongoing
- ***Imatinib*** (PDGF receptor antagonist and c-Abl tyrosine kinase inhibitor). Studies are ongoing
- ***Sirolimus*** (or rapamycin, a macrolide and immunosuppressant). Studies are ongoing.

Non-specific interstitial pneumonia (NSIP)

Definition The term NSIP is a description of a histological pattern rather than a specific clinical entity. This form of IIP is poorly understood, and may be subject to further reclassification in the near future. Patients with NSIP on lung biopsy have a generally better prognosis and greater response to steroids when compared with patients with IPF. NSIP may be idiopathic or occur in association with other systemic conditions, most notably connective tissue diseases.

Epidemiology Typically affects younger patients than IPF, with age of onset 40–50 years. May rarely affect children.

Causes/associations

- Idiopathic
- Connective tissue disease (NSIP may be the first manifestation of disease)
- Hypersensitivity pneumonitis
- Drugs
- Infection
- Immunodeficiency (including HIV, post bone marrow transplant, chemotherapy)

Clinical features There are few specific clinical features that help distinguish NSIP from other IIPs. Described features include:

- Breathlessness, cough
- Weight loss is common
- Onset gradual or subacute, typical symptom duration before diagnosis varies 0.5–3 years
- Crackles at lung bases, later more extensive
- Clubbing in a small proportion of patients

Investigations

- ***HRCT*** frequently shows diffuse symmetrical ground-glass change, with or without reticulation and traction bronchiectasis. The confluent and homogeneous appearance contrasts with the patchy heterogeneous distribution seen in IPF. Honeycombing is rare
- ***PFTs*** typically restrictive pattern, but impaired gas transfer in only 50%. Desaturation on exertion is common
- ***BAL*** lymphocytosis common
- ***Lung biopsy***
- Investigations to exclude underlying disease (see above)

Histology Variable, ranging from a predominantly 'cellular' pattern (mild–moderate interstitial inflammation, no fibrosis) to a 'fibrotic' pattern (interstitial fibrosis, more homogeneous appearance than in UIP and lack of fibroblastic foci or honeycombing, lung architecture may be relatively preserved). NSIP may be subclassified based on the relative proportions of inflammation and fibrosis: NSIP 1 (primarily inflammation), NSIP 2 (inflammation and fibrosis), and NSIP 3 (primarily fibrosis). Features of both NSIP and UIP are sometimes seen on biopsies from the same individual—in such cases, the diagnosis is considered to be IPF (indicating a poor prognosis).

Diagnosis Clinical and HRCT features are non-specific and surgical lung biopsy is required for diagnosis. Consider the presence of associated diseases (see list above).

Management Treatment is with corticosteroids (see p 265 for example of protocol). Additional immunosuppressive treatments may be considered in patients who fail to respond to corticosteroids alone (see p 265).

Prognosis Variable. Most patients improve or remain stable on treatment. 'Cellular' pattern on biopsy is associated with a good prognosis. Disease progression to death occurs, but is unusual.

Cryptogenic organizing pneumonia (COP)

(formerly bronchiolitis obliterans organizing pneumonia, BOOP)

Definition Cryptogenic organizing pneumonia (COP) is a disease of unknown cause characterized by 'plugging' of alveolar spaces with granulation tissue that may also extend up into the bronchioles. In addition to the 'cryptogenic' form, organizing pneumonia may also occur in the context of other diseases (see below). Use of the name BOOP is no longer recommended, as it erroneously suggests a primarily airways disease and is easily confused with bronchiolitis obliterans, a distinct disease entity.

Epidemiology More common in non-smokers. Mean age of onset 55 years, although can affect any age. Males = females.

Causes of organizing pneumonia

- Cryptogenic (COP)
- Organizing pneumonia secondary to:
  - Infection (including pneumonia, lung abscess, bronchiectasis)
  - Drug reaction or radiotherapy
  - Connective tissue disease (particularly myositis, rheumatoid arthritis, Sjögren's)
  - Diffuse alveolar damage
  - Hypersensitivity pneumonitis
  - Eosinophilic pneumonia
  - Inflammatory bowel disease
  - Post bone marrow transplant
  - Lung malignancy or airways obstruction
  - Pulmonary infarction.

Clinical features

- Typically short (<3 months) history of breathlessness and dry cough, often with malaise, fevers, weight loss, and myalgia. Often presents as a 'slow to resolve chest infection', frequently after several courses of antibiotics
- Breathlessness is usually mild, although a minority of patients experience severe breathlessness, and rapid onset of respiratory failure and sometimes death
- Examination may be normal or reveal crackles. Clubbing is absent.

Investigations

- ***Blood tests*** Raised CRP and ESR, neutrophilia
- ***PFTs*** Mild–moderate restrictive pattern is typical, although mild airways obstruction may also be seen in smokers. Mild hypoxaemia is common
- ***CXR*** classically shows patchy consolidation, sometimes with nodular shadowing. May present as a solitary mass on CXR

- ***HRCT*** Areas of consolidation with air bronchograms, sometimes with associated ground glass or small nodules. Often basal, subpleural, and peribronchial. May migrate spontaneously. Reticulation may suggest poor response to treatment. Less common appearance is as a solitary mass that may cavitate and that is often mistaken radiologically for a lung cancer. Septal thickening may occur
- ***TBB*** often confirms diagnosis, but there is concern that the relatively small samples may not effectively exclude associated diseases. Usually adequate in patients with typical clinical and HRCT features who are subsequently followed up closely. Surgical lung biopsy (at VATS) is otherwise required
- ***BAL*** if performed, shows lymphocytosis, neutrophilia, and eosinophilia.

Histology Alveolar spaces 'plugged' with granulation tissue (fibrin, collagen-containing fibroblasts, often with inflammatory cells), sometimes with extension up into the bronchiolar lumen. Patchy. Lack of architectural distortion. Examine for evidence of underlying cause, e.g. infection, vasculitis.

Diagnosis Usually made on the basis of clinical and HRCT features and transbronchial biopsy. Surgical lung biopsy may be required in atypical cases or if an underlying disease is suspected. Remember that the histological finding of 'organizing pneumonia' is non-specific, and search for secondary causes (see list above). Lung cancers may be surrounded by patches of organizing pneumonia, and biopsy of these areas in patients with a solitary lung mass may give misleading results.

Differential diagnosis

- Infective consolidation
- Connective tissue disease, vasculitis
- Lymphoma, alveolar cell carcinoma
- Lung cancer (when COP presents as lung mass).

Management Steroids are the mainstay of treatment. Optimal dose and duration unknown. Typical initial dose of oral prednisolone is 0.75 mg/kg daily. Slowly taper the dose over a period of several months (see p 264, for example). Additional treatment with azathioprine or cyclophosphamide may be considered in patients with minimal response to steroids; intravenous pulses of cyclophosphamide may be tried in addition to steroid treatment in critically ill patients.

Prognosis Generally good. Most patients respond to steroids, and improve within a week of starting treatment. Consider alternative diagnosis (e.g. lymphoma) if no improvement on steroid doses >25 mg/day. Relapse is common on reduction of steroid dose, and treatment courses of 6–12 months are usually required. A minority improve spontaneously. Lack of steroid response and progressive respiratory failure and death are rare, but well-documented.

Further information

Cordier J-F Organising pneumonia. *Thorax* 2000; **55**: 318–28

Acute interstitial pneumonia (AIP)

Definition Rapidly progressive form of interstitial pneumonia characterized histologically by diffuse alveolar damage. May be considered as an idiopathic form of ARDS. Formerly known as Hamman–Rich syndrome.

Epidemiology Poorly described. Mean age of onset is 50, but may occur at any age. Patients often previously healthy.

Clinical features

- Often preceded by 'viral'-type illness, with systemic symptoms, e.g. fevers, tiredness, myalgia, arthralgia
- Rapid onset (over days) of breathlessness; usually presents <3 weeks after symptom onset
- Widespread crackles on examination.

Investigations

- ***CXR*** Bilateral diffuse airspace shadowing with air bronchograms, progressing to widespread reticulation and ground glass; often spares costophrenic angles, heart borders, and hila
- ***HRCT*** Bilateral diffuse ground glass and patchy airspace consolidation in early stages; later traction bronchiectasis, cystic change, reticulation
- ***PFTs*** Restrictive, reduced gas transfer. Often profound hypoxia and respiratory failure
- ***BAL*** Increased total cells, red blood cells, and haemosiderin. Non-diagnostic, but may be useful in excluding infection
- ***Lung biopsy*** required for diagnosis. Transbronchial biopsy may be diagnostic; the risk of pneumothorax is higher in mechanically ventilated patients (about 10%), although serious complications are rare. Surgical lung biopsy is otherwise required.

Histology Diffuse alveolar damage: hyaline membranes, oedema, interstitial inflammation, and alveolar septal thickening, progressing to organizing fibrosis and sometimes honeycombing.

Diagnosis based on lung biopsy and exclusion of causes of ARDS.

Differential diagnosis

- ARDS (ARDS is of known cause, whereas AIP is idiopathic; often otherwise indistinguishable on clinical and histological grounds)
- Accelerated decline of IPF (with diffuse alveolar damage on biopsy)
- Connective tissue disease (causing diffuse alveolar damage)
- Diffuse infection (community-acquired pneumonia, PCP, CMV)
- Drug-induced pneumonitis
- Acute hypersensitivity pneumonitis
- Acute eosinophilic pneumonia
- Cardiogenic pulmonary oedema
- Pulmonary haemorrhage/vasculitis.

Management No treatment demonstrated to be of benefit. In practice, treat infection (including consideration of unusual organisms) and consider steroids (often given at high dose, e.g. intravenous methylprednisolone). High flow oxygen. ITU admission and mechanical ventilatory support usually required.

Prognosis Overall mortality at least 50%, although difficult to predict in individuals. Survivors may stabilize, develop chronic progressive interstitial lung disease, or experience recurrent exacerbations.

Respiratory bronchiolitis-associated interstitial lung disease (RB-ILD)

Definition 'Respiratory bronchiolitis' is a pathological term referring to the accumulation of bronchiolar pigmented macrophages in cigarette smokers, and is asymptomatic in nearly all cases. A minority of smokers with respiratory bronchiolitis, however, develop a form of interstitial lung disease known as respiratory bronchiolitis-associated interstitial lung disease (RB-ILD). The exact relationship between RB-ILD and DIP is unclear—they may be considered as different forms of the same underlying disease, with DIP associated with a more extensive accumulation of macrophages throughout alveolar spaces.

Epidemiology Invariably occurs in current or previous smokers, typically >30 pack years. Male:female 2:1. Usual age of onset 30–40 years.

Clinical features

- Usually mild breathlessness and cough
- Small proportion have severe dyspnoea and respiratory failure
- Often crackles on examination.

Investigations

- ***PFTs*** often show restrictive or combined obstructive and restrictive picture, with mildly impaired gas transfer
- ***CXR*** Thick-walled bronchi, reticular or ground-glass change, may be normal
- ***HRCT*** Centrilobular nodules, ground-glass change, thick-walled airways, often with associated centrilobular emphysema
- ***BAL*** typically reveals pigmented alveolar macrophages.

Histology Accumulation of pigmented brown macrophages in terminal bronchioles. Patchy bronchiolocentric distribution. These findings are frequently incidental in smokers, and so the diagnosis of RB-ILD requires consideration of clinical and imaging features in conjunction with histology.

Management Smoking cessation is the mainstay of treatment. Corticosteroids are occasionally used, with uncertain benefit.

Prognosis Available data are limited; prolonged survival is common, although improvements in symptoms or physiology appear to occur in only a minority of patients.

Desquamative interstitial pneumonia (DIP)

Definition Interstitial lung disease that occurs in smokers and is associated with the pathological finding of abundant pigmented macrophages located diffusely throughout alveolar air spaces. It may represent a more extensive form of RB-ILD, in which macrophages are restricted to peribronchiolar regions. The term DIP is misleading, as desquamation of epithelial cells is not responsible for the histological findings as previously thought; a more accurate term is 'alveolar macrophage pneumonia', although this is not in widespread use.

Epidemiology Very rare. Majority of patients are smokers, although may also occur following inhalation of inorganic dusts, including passive inhalation of cigarette smoke. Typically occurs aged 30–50.

Clinical features Onset of breathlessness and cough over weeks–months is typical. Clubbing is common.

Investigations

- *PFTs* Mild restrictive pattern common, sometimes with reduced gas transfer
- *CXR* may be normal, or may demonstrate reticular or ground-glass pattern particularly affecting lower zones
- *HRCT* Ground glass seen in all cases, typically lower zone or peripheral predominance. Reticulation and honeycombing may be present, although tend to be mild
- *BAL* Increase in pigmented macrophages.

Histology Diffuse accumulation of pigmented macrophages in alveolar air spaces. Changes are uniform.

Diagnosis Clinical and HRCT features are non-specific and surgical lung biopsy is required for diagnosis.

Management Smoking cessation. Corticosteroids are often used, although their efficacy has not been studied.

Prognosis Usually good prognosis. Improvement in ground glass on HRCT may correlate with response to treatment. Survival 70% after 10 years. Fluctuating course with remissions and relapses may occur.

Lymphoid interstitial pneumonia (LIP)

Definition Interstitial pneumonia characterized by diffuse lymphoid infiltrates and often lymphoid hyperplasia. Previously considered to be a precursor to pulmonary lymphoma, and difficult to distinguish from lymphoma histologically, it is now considered a distinct entity and is thought to only rarely undergo neoplastic transformation.

Epidemiology Very rare. Commoner in women. May occur at any age.

Causes/associations

- Idiopathic
- Connective tissue disease—particularly Sjögren's syndrome, also rheumatoid arthritis, SLE
- Immunodeficiency, e.g. HIV
- Infection, e.g. PCP, hepatitis B
- Autoimmune disease, e.g. haemolytic anaemia, Hashimoto's thyroiditis, pernicious anaemia, chronic active hepatitis, primary biliary cirrhosis, myasthenia gravis
- Drugs.

Clinical features Gradual onset breathlessness and cough over several years. Fever, weight loss may occur. Crackles may be heard on examination.

Investigations

- ***Blood tests*** Mild anaemia may occur; poly- or monoclonal increase in serum immunoglobulins is common
- ***CXR*** Lower zone alveolar shadowing or diffuse honeycombing
- ***HRCT*** Predominant ground-glass change, often with reticulation and sometimes honeycombing and nodules
- ***BAL*** Non-clonal lymphocytosis
- Investigations to identify underlying cause (see above).

Histology Diffuse interstitial lymphoid infiltrates, predominantly involving alveolar septa, sometimes with lymphoid hyperplasia or honeycombing. Cellular NSIP, follicular bronchiolitis, and lymphoma may give similar appearances.

Management Steroids are frequently used and often appear to improve symptoms.

Prognosis Progression to extensive fibrosis occurs in around one-third of patients.

Chapter 31

Lung cancer

Epidemiology and types

Epidemiology

- Nearly 38, 000 new cases diagnosed per annum in the UK
- Commonest cause of cancer death in men and women in the UK
- 2:1 male:female, but numbers decreasing in men, increasing in women, because of increasing smoking
- More women die from lung cancer than from any other cancer, including breast
- 90% smoking-related
- Stopping smoking decreases the risk, but the risk remains higher than in non-smokers
- Risk of lung cancer may be increased by asbestos exposure, arsenic and heavy metal exposure, and coexistent idiopathic pulmonary fibrosis (IPF).

Types of lung cancer In practical terms, lung cancer is divided into two groups, which influence management and treatment decisions.

Non-small cell lung cancer (NSCLC)

- Accounts for 75–80% of all lung cancers
- *Squamous cell carcinoma* is the commonest histological type. Usually presents as a mass on CXR, but may cavitate and look radiologically like a lung abscess. Rarely, there may be multiple cavitating lesions. Patients with hypercalcaemia are most likely to have squamous cell carcinoma
- *Adenocarcinoma* may not necessarily be smoking-related. Can occur in scar tissue or sites of fibrosis. Can be a lung primary or a secondary from adenocarcinomas at other sites, especially if causing pleural infiltration and subsequent pleural effusion
- *Alveolar cell carcinoma* is rare. It can rarely cause copious sputum production (bronchorrhoea). Typically causes fluffy air space shadowing on CXR.

Small cell lung cancer (SCLC)

- Accounts for 20–25% of all lung cancers
- Most aggressive of lung cancer subtypes
- Usually disseminated by the time of diagnosis (haematogenous spread)
- Frequently *metastasizes* to liver, bones, bone marrow, brain, adrenals, or elsewhere
- Syndrome of inappropriate secretion of antidiuretic hormone (SIADH) with hyponatraemia is common in small cell lung cancer
- Surgery usually not appropriate
- Chemo- and radiosensitive
- Untreated extensive stage small cell lung cancer is rapidly progressive and has a median survival of 6 weeks.

WHO histological classification of lung tumours, 2004

- Squamous cell carcinoma
- Small cell carcinoma
- Adenocarcinoma
- Large cell carcinoma
- Adenosquamous carcinoma
- Sarcomatoid carcinoma
- Carcinoid tumours
- Salivary gland tumours
- Pre-invasive lesions.

Clinical features

Smokers and ex-smokers with chest symptoms, especially those aged over 50, need investigation.

Symptoms and signs

These may be due to local tumour effects, metastatic tumour effects, or paraneoplastic manifestations. Many patients have no specific signs. In some, the lung cancer may be an incidental finding on CXR performed for another reason.

Local tumour effects

- Persistent cough, or change in usual cough
- Haemoptysis
- Chest pain (suggests chest wall or pleural involvement)
- Unresolving pneumonia or lobar collapse
- Unexplained dyspnoea (due to bronchial narrowing or obstruction)
- Wheeze or stridor
- Shoulder pain (due to diaphragm involvement)
- Pleural effusion (due to direct tumour extension or pleural metastases)
- Hoarse voice (tumour invasion of the left recurrent laryngeal nerve)
- Dysphagia
- Raised hemi-diaphragm (phrenic nerve paralysis)
- SVCO (see p 300)
- Horner's syndrome (meiosis, ptosis, enopthalmos, anhidrosis) due to apical or Pancoast's tumour
- Pancoast's tumours can directly invade the sympathetic chain, brachial plexus, and rib. Cause weakness of small muscles of the hand—C5/6, T1 motor loss, and shoulder pain

Metastatic tumour effects

- Cervical/supraclavicular lymphadenopathy (common, present in 30%, and may be an easy site for diagnostic biopsy)
- Palpable liver edge
- Bone pain/pathological fracture due to bone metastases
- Neurological sequelae secondary to cerebral metastases (median survival of NSCLC with brain metastases is 2 months)
- Hypercalcaemic effects (due to bony metastases or direct tumour production of parathyroid-hormone-related peptide or parathyroid hormone) see p 304
- Dysphagia (compression from large mediastinal nodes)

Paraneoplastic syndromes

Endocrine syndromes are due to the ectopic production of hormones or hormonally active peptides. Neurological syndromes are due to antibody mediated CNS damage.

- Cachexia and wasting
- Clubbing (up to 29% of patients; any cell type, more common in squamous and adenocarcinoma)
- Gynaecomastia
- SIADH (mainly SCLC) in up to 15% of patients see p 306

- Ectopic ACTH (Cushing's syndrome, but due to rapid development; biochemical changes predominate, mainly SCLC) in 2–5% of patients
- Hypertrophic pulmonary osteo-arthropathy (HPOA, often in association with clubbing, any cell type; more common in squamous and adenocarcinoma)
- Lambert–Eaton myasthenic syndrome (or LEMS)—with SCLC. Affects proximal limbs and trunk, with autonomic involvement (dry mouth, constipation, erectile failure) and hyporeflexia (although reflexes return on exercising the affected muscle group), and only a slight response to edrophonium. Symptoms may predate lung cancer by up to 4 years. Caused by auto-antibodies against P/Q-type voltage-gated calcium channels. Decreased acetylcholine release at motor nerve terminals leads to the proximal weakness. Diagnosis made by auto-antibody detection on radio-immunoprecipitation assay. EMG shows increased amplitude of muscle action with high frequency stimulation and repeated muscle contraction may lead to increasing strength and reflexes. Treatment of underlying SCLC causes neurological improvement. If weakness is severe, IV immunoglobulin or plasmapheresis may give short-term benefits. 3,4-Diaminopyridine may increase muscle strength in 85% of patients. Prednisolone alone or with azathioprine or ciclosporin can increase muscle strength and provide long-term control in non-responders
- Cerebellar syndrome (usually SCLC)
- Limbic encephalitis (SCLC, also breast, testicular, other cancers. Occurs within 4 years of diagnosis of cancer. Personality change, seizures, depression, sub-acute onset confusion and short-term memory loss. Diagnosed by pathological or radiological involvement of limbic system. Anti-Hu antibodies positive in 50% if associated with lung cancer.)
- Glomerulonephritis.

Lymphangitis carcinomatosa Infiltration of pulmonary lymphatics by tumour. May be due to lung cancer or breast, prostate, stomach, or pancreatic malignancies. Causes shortness of breath, cough, and is often associated with systemic signs of advanced malignancy. May be visible on CXR as fine linear shadowing throughout both lung fields. Septal lines present. May look like pulmonary oedema. Easily diagnosed on CT. Oral steroid treatment and diuretics can give symptomatic relief, but it is usually a short-lived response. Often part of a rapid decline.

Further information

Maddison P, Newsom-Davies J. Treatment for Lambert–Eaton myasthenic syndrome. *Cochrane Database Syst. Rev* 2005: CD003279

Investigations

Patients should be referred under the '2-week cancer wait' scheme and should be seen within 14 days of referral. The aim of the investigations is to reach a histological diagnosis and tumour stage, in order to determine the most appropriate treatment. Current government guidelines recommend patients should receive treatment without undue delay: within 31 days of the decision to treat and within 62 days of their urgent referral.

In out-patients

- ***History and examination,*** including smoking and occupational histories
- ***Spirometry*** pre-biopsy or surgery
- ***CXR*** (PA and possibly lateral)—location of lesion, pleural involvement, pleural effusion, rib destruction, intrathoracic metastases, mediastinal lymphadenopathy. CXR can be normal
- ***Blood tests,*** including sodium, calcium, and liver function tests. Check clotting if biopsy planned
- ***Sputum cytology*** only indicated in patients who are unfit for bronchoscopy or biopsy
- ***Diagnostic pleural tap,*** if effusion present
- ***Fine-needle aspiration*** of enlarged supraclavicular or cervical lymph nodes.

Radiology

- ***CT chest, liver, adrenals (contrast-enhanced) to assess tumour site and size*** Lung cancers frequently metastasize to the mediastinal lymph nodes, liver, and adrenals. CT can locate lesions amenable to biopsy (either the primary tumour or a metastasis). Assesses size of local and regional lymph nodes. Poor at assessing whether enlarged nodes are reactive (inflammatory) or represent metastatic spread (79% sensitive, 78% specific). Can assess tumour invasion to mediastinum and chest wall
- ***Ultrasound scan*** of neck or liver may provide information about enlarged lymph nodes or metastases suitable for biopsy
- ***MRI*** Used to answer specific questions relating to tumour invasion/borders. Good for assessing brachial plexus involvement. No role in nodule assessment
- ***Bone scan*** Indicated if any suggestion of metastatic disease, such as bony pain, pathological fracture, hypercalcaemia, raised alkaline phosphatase. Highly suggestive of bony metastases if multiple areas of increased uptake. Solitary lesion may require further evaluation
- ***CT head*** Only indicated if any neurological evidence of metastatic disease, such as persistent vomiting, fit, focal neurological signs, headache, unexplained confusion, or personality change, especially if aggressive local treatment is considered for primary tumour
- ***Positron emission tomography (PET scanning)*** Imaging technique, where metabolically active tissues such as tumours take up more of a radiolabelled 18-fluorodeoxyglucose (FDG) molecule. They then show as a 'hot-spot'. Improves the rate of detection of local and distant metastases in patients with NSCLC. Useful for assessing regional and mediastinal lymph nodes (88% sensitive, 93% specific). This is increased

if abnormal nodes are identified on CT. Becoming more widely used and should be interpreted with the CT. Perform in:

- All patients considered for radical therapy to look for involved lymph nodes and distant metastases
- Patients with N2–3 disease on CT of uncertain significance, who are otherwise surgical candidates
- Candidates for radical radiotherapy
- Limited stage SCLC staged by standard staging methods to identify metastases, as SCLC avidly takes up FDG

PET positive nodes that would exclude a patient from surgery should be confirmed as malignant with a biopsy, unless the pre-test probability of malignancy is high. PET may reveal a distant abnormality other than the primary lung cancer, which could be a solitary metastasis or a second cancer. It is important therefore to biopsy isolated PET abnormalities before determining that a patient's cancer is not resectable

False negatives occur in tumours with a low metabolic activity (such as bronchoalveolar cell, carcinoid), small nodules, and hyperglycaemic patients. ***False positives*** occur in patients with benign pulmonary nodules with a high metabolic rate, such as infective granulomata.

Patients fast 4 h before the test and if they have diabetes, glucose should be within the normal range

Multidisciplinary team (MDT)

Should include a chest physician, radiologist, thoracic surgeon, oncologist, pathologist, lung cancer nurse, and palliative care specialist, who meet regularly in order to discuss patients and plan the most appropriate course of management.

The Department of Health in the UK has produced guidelines for performance in lung cancer care. These encourage access to the MDT in decision making for the treatment and investigation of all patients with lung cancer.

Further information

NICE lung cancer guidelines 2005. www.nice.org.uk

Giving information to lung cancer patients. BTS Lung Cancer and mesothelioma Specialist Advisory Group. April 2008. www.brit-thoracic.org.uk/Portals/0/Clinical%20Information/Lung%20Cancer/WTSTPBTSfinds210408.pdf

Diagnostic procedures

Investigations are performed to obtain a tissue diagnosis and to stage cancer in order to determine the most appropriate treatment. Aim to achieve diagnosis and staging with as few procedures as possible. Establishing diagnosis and presence of metastatic spread at a single test is desirable if possible. Aspects of further investigation may be inappropriate if the patient has advanced disease, is frail with comorbid conditions, or does not want to pursue diagnosis. This should be documented in their notes, to aid audit and cancer service evaluation.

Bronchoscopy Method of obtaining histological and cytological specimens. Suitable for central tumours. Tumours can be washed, brushed, and biopsied. Bronchoscopic samples are more likely to be histologically positive if there is:

- An ill-defined lesion on the CXR
- An endobronchial component to the tumour
- Tumour less than 4 cm from the origin of the nearest lobar bronchus
- A segmental or larger airway leading to the mass.

Greater diagnostic yield if performed after CT scan, as radiologically abnormal areas can be targeted. Tumour position bronchoscopically may contribute to operative decisions: tumour confined to a lobar bronchus may be resectable with lobectomy, tumour <2 cm from the main carina requires pneumonectomy, left vocal cord paralysis indicates inoperability due to tumour infiltration of the left recurrent laryngeal nerve, and a splayed carina occurs secondary to enlarged mediastinal nodes.

Transbronchial needle aspiration of lymph nodes can be performed to aid staging at the time of bronchoscopy. Also EUS-FNA (endoscopic ultrasound guided fine-needle aspirate) or endoscopic bronchial ultrasound (EBUS)—all may reduce need for mediastinoscopy/otomy and are less invasive (see p 754).

CT/USS-guided biopsy of tumour or of an enlarged lymph node, especially in the neck, or of a metastasis (see box opposite). 85–90% sensitivity in lesions >2 cm. Biopsy of a metastasis gives valuable staging information as well as also diagnosing the primary.

Mediastinoscopy Biopsy of enlarged mediastinal lymph nodes to determine whether they are inflammatory or have malignant invasion. Suprasternal notch incision under general anaesthetic, blunt dissection, palpation, and endoscopic visualization and biopsy of nodes: paratracheal, prevascular, tracheobronchial, and anterior subcarinal. 93% sensitivity, 96% specificity. Technically more difficult if SVCO. Bleeding in <0.3%, left recurrent laryngeal nerve injury in 1%, pneumothorax, mediastinal emphysema, infection, oesophageal perforation (all rare). Repeat mediastinoscopies have lower positive yield and higher complication rate.

Mediastinotomy Biopsy of aorto-pulmonary, sub-aortic, phrenic, or hilar nodes. Metastatic involvement of these nodes does not necessarily preclude curative surgical resection with a pneumonectomy. Also can assess direct tumour invasion of central pulmonary artery or thoracic aorta, which would preclude curative surgery. Right or left parasternal incision, blunt dissection, palpation, and endoscopic visualization and biopsy of nodes.

Thoracoscopy may be required to determine whether a pleural effusion contains malignant cells or is inflammatory, for example, due to pneumonia caused by an obstructing lesion. Malignant effusions are evidence of T4 disease and hence are a contraindication to surgery.

Operative It is sometimes difficult to obtain definitive cytology or histology pre-operatively. If there is a high suspicion of malignancy, surgery can be performed regardless. Patients undergoing surgery are given a pathological stage, which is sometimes different to the clinical stage. This is because resection margins, lymph nodes, and the pleura can be sampled histologically.

Radiologically guided lung biopsy

Indications

- New or enlarging mass, not amenable to bronchoscopy
- Multiple chest nodules in patient not known to have malignancy
- Persistent undiagnosed single or multiple focal infiltrates
- Hilar mass.

Pre-biopsy preparation

- Discuss with MDT
- Recent spirometry, with FEV_1 >35% predicted
- Check APTT and PT ratios <1.4 and platelets >100 000/mL. If not, discuss with haematologist to determine whether it is safe to proceed
- Recent imaging available
- High risk patients should have overnight admission following biopsy
- Written information for patient, with informed signed consent.

Biopsy preparation

- Perform without sedation if possible
- Use USS if possible
- Local anaesthetic to skin and subcutaneous tissue
- Perform at least two passes, may use FNA or cutting needle. FNA high diagnostic yield for malignant lesions (95%), but less for benign (10–50%). Cutting needles as good for malignancy and better for benign diagnoses. Operator decision.

Post-biopsy

- Observation by staff for 1 h in case of complications
- Erect CXR 1 h after biopsy and reviewed by doctor
- Manage any pneumothorax according to BTS guidelines (p 373). Small pneumothoraces often resolve spontaneously, but may need in-patient admission if there are concerns.

Complications

- 20% chance of pneumothorax, 3% require chest drain
- Haemoptysis 5%, death 0.15%.

Manhire A *et al.* Guidelines for radiologically guided lung biopsy. *Thorax* 2003: **58**: 920–34

Staging

Clinical and radiological tools categorize tumour size, location, regional and distant spread, and aid determination of most appropriate treatment. They can also therefore give prognostic information.

- **Small cell lung cancer** is staged as:
  - ***Limited*** confined to ipsilateral hemi-thorax and supraclavicular lymph nodes. Median survival with treatment 12 months, without treatment 12 weeks
  - ***Extensive*** everything else. Median survival with treatment 8 months, without treatment 6 weeks
- **Non-small cell lung cancer** is commonly classified using TNM staging system (see box opposite). Frequency of patient stage at diagnosis:
  - I and II—20%
  - III—35%
  - IV—45%.

Table 31.1 Lung cancer clinical staging and survival

Stage	TNM subset	After treatment survival (%)	
		1 year	5 years
0	Tis	?	?
IA	T1 N0 M0	91	61
IB	T2 N0 M0	72	38
IIA	T1 N1 M0	79	34
IIB	T2 N1 M0	61	24
	T3 N0 M0	55	22
IIIA	T1 N2 M0	50	13
	T2 N2 M0	50	13
	T3 N1–2 M0	56	9
IIIB	T4 N0–2 M0	37	7
	T1–4 N3 M0	32	3
IV	Any T, Any N, M1	20	1

TNM Staging of Lung Cancer (American Joint Committee on Cancer and the Union Internationale Contre le Cancer)

Extent of primary tumour (T)

- Tx Primary tumour cannot be assessed, or tumour proven by presence of malignant cells in sputum or bronchial washings but not visualized by imaging or bronchoscopy
- T0 No evidence of primary tumour
- Tis Carcinoma *in situ*
- T1 Tumour <3 cm surrounded by lung or visceral pleura, without bronchoscopic evidence of invasion more proximal than the lobar bronchus
- T2 Tumour >3 cm, or in main bronchus, >2 cm distal to carina or invading visceral pleura, or associated with atelectasis or obstructive pneumonitis that extends to the hilar region, but does not involve whole lung
- T3 Tumour of any size which invades chest wall, diaphragm, parietal pericardium, mediastinal pleura, or tumour in main bronchus <2 cm distal to carina, or associated atelectasis or obstructive pneumonitis of the entire lung
- T4 Tumour of any size invading: mediastinum, heart, great vessels, trachea, oesophagus, carina, vertebral body, or separate nodules in the ipsilateral lobe as primary tumour, or malignant pleural or pericardial effusion

Regional lymph nodes (N)

- Nx Cannot be assessed
- N0 No regional lymph node metastasis
- N1 Ipsilateral peribronchial and/or ipsilateral hilar nodes and intrapulmonary nodes involved by direct extension of tumour
- N2 Ipsilateral mediastinal and/or subcarinal nodes
- N3 Contralateral mediastinal, hilar nodes, or any scalene or supraclavicular nodes

Distant metastasis (M)

- Mx Cannot be assessed
- M0 No distant metastasis
- M1 Distant metastasis present, including separate nodules in different lobes

Further information

Mountain CF. Revisions in the International System for staging lung cancer. *Chest* 1997; **111**: 1710–17

Mountain CF, Dresler CM. Regional Lymph Node Classification for Lung Cancer Staging. *Chest* 1997; **111**: 1718–23

Non-small cell lung cancer (NSCLC): surgery

Much of the investigation of lung cancer is to determine whether a patient has disease that is potentially curable by surgery. Other treatment options include chemotherapy, radiotherapy, and best supportive care, i.e. symptom-based conservative management. The MDT decides the most appropriate choice of treatment which is then discussed with the patient.

Surgery

The aims of surgery for lung cancer are to completely excise the tumour and local lymphatics, with minimal removal of normal functioning lung parenchyma.

- Stages I and II non-small cell lung cancers are usually amenable to surgery if the patient is fit enough (see below). This has a high chance of cure in stage I (70% in IA), and a reasonable chance in stage II. 10–20% of NSCLC patients undergo resection
- In stage IIIA tumours, surgery alone is unlikely to be curative, but adjuvant chemotherapy and radiotherapy can improve survival rates. These patients should be recruited to clinical trials
- Stages IIIB and IV are inoperable
- Stages 0/tumour *in situ* often will have no defined primary lesion amenable to resection. The natural progression of these tumours is still unknown; they may progress or regress with time.

Resectability of a tumour implies likelihood of complete removal by surgery; this is different from patient operability, which is determined by the patient's fitness for surgery.

Fitness for surgery

- *Age* is not a contraindication, but increasing age is associated with an increased peri-operative morbidity. Higher mortality risk if over 80 and if pneumonectomy, rather than lobectomy (14% mortality vs 7%, respectively). Right pneumonectomy has higher mortality than left pneumonectomy (more lung removed). 2-year post-operative survival similar to that of other age groups
- *Lung function* FEV_1 >1.5 L post-bronchodilator for lobectomy, >2 L post-bronchodilator for pneumonectomy or more than 60% of predicted. Borderline cases may require further lung function assessment (arterial saturations, full PFTs including TLCO, isotope perfusion scan, exercise testing) in order to calculate whether predicted post-operative FEV_1 >40% in association with TLCO >40%
- *Cardiovascular* Postpone surgery if patient has had MI within 6 weeks. Cardiology opinion if patient has had MI within 6 months. Echo if they have heart murmur. Pre-operative ECG for all
- *CNS* If any history of TIAs, strokes, or carotid bruits: need carotid Doppler studies and vascular surgeon opinion if necessary
- *Nutritional* Requirements should be optimized, with advice from a dietician if necessary. Patients presenting with a pre-operative weight loss of 10% or more ± performance status ≥2 are more likely to have advanced disease or comorbidities. Therefore require careful staging and search for evidence of comorbidity.

EGFR inhibitors EGFR (epidermal growth factor receptor) is an important mediator of cell growth, differentiation, and survival. It is over-expressed in 40–80% of NSCLC patients. New EGFR inhibitors include:

- ***Gefitinib (Iressa)*** Oral preparation used vs. placebo in patients refractory or intolerant of their latest chemotherapy. No significant difference in median survival time between the two groups
- ***Erlotinib (Tarceva)*** Shown to significantly improve survival in patients with previously treated stage IIIB or IV NSCLC vs. placebo (6.7 vs. 4.7 months, $p = 0.001$). No benefit shown in combination with chemotherapy as a first-line treatment. Used as second- or third-line therapy in NSCLC, but funding issues in UK.

Response evaluation criteria in solid tumours (RECIST)—method of measuring response of a tumour to treatment (particularly in chemotherapy trials)

Target lesion = all measurable lesions up to a maximum of 5 lesions per organ and 10 lesions in total, representative of all involved organs. Record and measure sum of their longest diameter.

Non-target lesions = all other sites of disease, which are recorded at baseline. Measurements of these lesions are not required, but presence or absence of each is noted during follow-up.

Evaluation of target lesions

- ***Complete response (CR)***—disappearance of all target lesions
- ***Partial response (PR)***—at least a 30% decrease in the sum of the longest diameter of target lesions
- ***Progressive disease (PD)***—at least a 20% increase in the sum of the longest diameter of target lesions
- ***Stable disease (SD)***—neither sufficient shrinkage to qualify for PR, nor sufficient increase to qualify for PD.

Evaluation of non-target lesions

- ***Complete response (CR)***—disappearance of all non-target lesions and normalization of tumour marker level
- ***Incomplete response/stable disease (SD)***—persistence of one or more non-target lesion(s) and/or maintenance of tumour marker level above the normal limits
- ***Progressive disease (PD)***—appearance of one or more new lesions and/or unequivocal progression of existing non-target lesions.

Further information

Burdett S *et al.* Chemotherapy and surgery vs. surgery alone in NSCLC. *Cochrane Database Syst Rev* 2007; **3**: CD006157

Gilligan D *et al.* Pre-operative chemotherapy in patients with resectable NSCLC. *Lancet* 2007; **369**: 1929–37

The International Adjuvant Lung Cancer Trial Collaborative Group. Cisplatin-based adjuvant chemotherapy in patients with completely resected NSCLC. *NEJM* 2004; **350**: 351–60

NSCLC Collaborative Group. Chemotherapy in NSCLC: a meta-analysis using updated data on individual patients from 52 randomised clinical trials. *BMJ* 1995; **311**: 899–909

NSCLC: radiotherapy

May be given for:

- Curative intent (high dose)
- Palliative control (high dose)
- Symptom relief (low dose).

Radiotherapy has no benefit following complete primary tumour surgical resection.

CHART (continuous hyperfractionated accelerated radiotherapy) is high-dose radiotherapy given with curative intent.

- Recommended for patients with localized chest disease <5 cm, stage I–II with performance status 0–1, who are resectable, but unfit for surgery or do not want surgery
- Small radiation doses tds for 12 days (54 Gy in 36 fractions over 12 days)
- Patients are often in-patients for the duration of their therapy to facilitate their frequent radiotherapy sessions
- Less morbidity than conventional radical radiotherapy
- A large randomized control trial has shown an improvement in 2-year survival from 20% with conventional radical radiotherapy to 29% with CHART. The largest benefits were in patients with squamous cell carcinoma. Overall 75% 1 year survival, 55% 2 year survival, 18% 5 year survival.
- Severe dysphagia more likely with CHART in the first 3 months than with conventional radiotherapy
- Need PFTs including lung volume and TLCO before CHART. FEV_1 should be ≥1.5l
- Not performed in all UK centres; lack of radiographers may limit availability.

High-dose palliative radiotherapy is given to patients with symptomatic disease, good performance status, no evidence of metastases, and who will be able to tolerate a high-dose regime. An example of such a regime would be 36–39 Gy in 12–13 fractions over 6 weeks. Improves median survival by 2 months.

Low-dose radiotherapy is given for symptom relief in patients who would be unable to tolerate high-dose palliative radiotherapy or those with evidence of metastases. Symptoms palliated include pain, haemoptysis, breathlessness, or cough.

Urgent radiotherapy is used in combination with oral steroids for relief of superior vena cava obstruction by tumour, although stenting performed via CT angiography is now the treatment of choice, where possible. Radiotherapy takes approximately 10 days to be effective.

Chemoradiotherapy is used to improve tumour radiosensitization for localized disease. There may be some additional advantages with treatment of potential distant micrometastases. Some early survival benefits have been shown, and further studies are ongoing.

Further information

Saunders M *et al.* CHART vs. conventional radiotherapy. *Lancet* 1997; **350**: 161–5

WHO/ECOG performance status

0 = Fully active, able to carry on all pre-disease performance without restriction
1 = Restricted in physically strenuous activity, but ambulatory and able to carry out work of a light or sedentary nature, e.g. light house work, office work
2 = Ambulatory and capable of all self-care but unable to carry out any work activities. Up and about more than 50% of waking hours
3 = Capable of only limited self-care, confined to bed or chair more than 50% of waking hours
4 = Completely disabled. Cannot carry on any self-care. Totally confined to bed or chair

Oken MM *et al.* Toxicity and response criteria of the Eastern Cooperative Oncology Group. *Am J Clin Oncol* 1982; **5:** 649–55

Small cell lung cancer: treatment

Surgery Limited stage small cell lung cancer may be appropriate for surgical resection if there is no evidence of metastases. This is rare. It requires further assessment with brain and bone scanning ± bone marrow biopsy if there is an unexplained abnormal FBC. The patient should also be considered for post-operative combination chemotherapy for treatment of micro-metastases, especially if histology was only determined at operation.

Chemotherapy

Combination chemotherapy is used for limited and extensive SCLC.

- Etoposide with either cisplatin or carboplatin is the standard regime
- Given 3 weekly, commonly for 6 cycles
- Different regimes are selected according to performance status
- Patients with performance status 3 may benefit from less intensive out-patient chemotherapy on a 3 weekly basis
- Patients are carefully assessed and, if there is no sign of a response to treatment based on CXR or CT scan, they are switched to second-line agents, such as single agent topotecan or combination cyclophosphamide, doxorubicin and vincristine
- 80–90% response if limited disease; 60–80% if extensive disease
- Chemotherapy may increase median survival to 12 months in limited disease.

Radiotherapy

- Patients with limited stage disease who are reasonably well should have consolidation radiotherapy to the chest disease, either with the first or second cycle of chemotherapy or after completion if they have a response or partial response
- Prophylactic cranial radiotherapy is advised at completion of chemotherapy for those with limited disease or those with extensive disease and good prognostic factors. This improves survival by 5.4%
- In patients with extensive disease, including cerebral metastases, or poorer performance status, chemotherapy is given first. If there is a good response, palliative thoracic radiotherapy may be given
- Of benefit to symptomatic bone metastases, cord compression, SVCO.

Further information

Jackman DM, Johnson BE. Small cell lung cancer. *Lancet* 2005; **366**: 1385–96

Lung cancer: emerging areas

Radio-frequency ablation (RFA) applied via a probe inserted into a nodule/tumour under CT guidance with sedation. Barbs/tines extrude from needle once in the tumour and cause tissue death by thermal necrosis. Lesions initially increase in size and density, and may cavitate, but then become fibrotic scar tissue. May become a tool to treat patients with primary lung cancer unsuitable for curative surgery/radiotherapy due to comorbid disease, used with radiotherapy. The size of the cancer that can be treated is limited (maximum 5 cm, best results with <3 cm). Peripheral lesions are easier to access. Side-effects of therapy: pleuritic chest pain, pneumothorax, haemoptysis, haemorrhage, low grade fever. FEV_1 should ideally be >1 L. Tumour follow-up with contrast-enhanced imaging as ablated tissue does not enhance. Used currently mainly in pulmonary metastases from gastrointestinal or renal cell cancers, or sarcomas, which are not suitable for surgical resection, but also some data for primary NSCLC. In 153 patients with primary or metastatic medically inoperable lung cancer, 78% 1-year survival rate, 57% 2-year, 27% 5-year (Simon CJ *et al. Radiology* 2007; **243:** 268–75). No long-term RCT reported.

Biological therapies such as oral thalidomide acting as an angiogenesis inhibitor are being tried. These may offer medium-term survival benefits in both SCLC and NSCLC.

Targeted molecular therapy Lung cancer is said to be at the leading edge of targeted molecular therapy, which may become more effective than using traditional cytotoxic agents. The presence or absence of these molecular target molecules seems to determine response to traditional treatments. The cellular targets under investigation include epidermal growth factor receptor (EGFR), protein kinase C, vascular endothelial growth factor, cyclo-oxygenase 2, plus expression of various genes, including excision repair cross complementation protein gene, which has a role in DNA repair. Gene expression profiling may be used to determine the prognosis and response to therapy and to identify the mechanisms of tumour biology. In the future, lung cancer staging may also address the molecular biology of a tumour.

Further information

Dy GK, Adjei AA. Novel targets for lung cancer therapy. *J Clin Oncol* 2002; **20**: 2881–94

BTS Recommendations to respiratory physicians for organising the care of patients with lung cancer. *Thorax* 1998: **53** (suppl. 1): S1–8

www.bacup.org.uk

www.cancerguide.org

www.cancerresearchuk.org

www.lungcanceronline.org

www.nice.org.uk/CG024NICEguideline

www.roycastle.org, patient network, telephone 0800 358 7200

Superior vena caval obstruction (SVCO): aetiology and clinical assessment

Obstruction of the flow of blood in the superior vena cava results in the symptoms and signs of SVCO. It is caused by two different mechanisms (which may coexist): *external compression or invasion* of the superior vena cava by tumour extending from the right lung (four times more common than the left lung), lymph nodes, or other mediastinal structure; or due to *thrombosis* within the vein.

Aetiology The commonest cause is malignancy. Lung cancer and lymphoma together cause 94% of SVCO.

Malignant causes

- *Lung cancer* Up to 4% of lung cancer patients will develop SVCO at some point during their disease. Up to 10% of small cell lung cancers present with SVCO
- *Lymphoma* Up to 4% of lymphoma patients will develop SVCO, most commonly in non-Hodgkin's lymphoma. This usually occurs due to extrinsic compression of the SVC by enlarged lymph nodes
- *Other malignant causes* Thymoma, mediastinal germ cell tumours, tumours with mediastinal metastases (commonest is breast cancer).

Benign causes include granulomatous disease, intrathoracic goitre, and central venous lines, port-a-caths, and pacemaker wires (causing thrombosis). In the past SVCO was commonly due to untreated infection, e.g. syphilitic thoracic aortic aneurysm or fibrosing mediastinitis (due to actinomycosis, tuberculosis, blastomycosis, or *Aspergillus*). These are all now rare.

Clinical features

- Facial and upper body oedema with facial plethora, often with increased neck circumference, and a cyanotic appearance
- Venous distension of the face and upper body. SVCO due to malignancy usually develops over days to weeks, so an adequate collateral circulation does not have time to develop. Pemberton's sign—facial plethora, distress, and sometimes stridor after lifting the arms above the head for a few minutes—may suggest the diagnosis
- Breathlessness
- Headache—worse on bending forwards or lying down
- Cough/haemoptysis or other signs of an underlying lung malignancy
- Hoarse voice
- Dysphagia
- Syncope/dizziness (reduced venous return)
- Confusion.

Diagnosis is usually made clinically from the signs of facial and upper body swelling, with distension of superficial veins across the chest wall, neck, and upper arms.

Investigations The investigation and treatment of SVCO was previously considered a medical emergency. SVCO is now not considered to be immediately life-threatening, making treatment less urgent and allowing a definitive diagnosis to be made prior to treatment. The exception to this rule is the patient who presents with stridor or laryngeal oedema, which is a medical emergency.

- ***CXR*** Up to 85% have an abnormal CXR (as lung malignancy is the commonest underlying disorder). Mediastinal widening is common
- ***CT chest with contrast*** can stage the underlying malignancy and image the venous circulation and collateral blood supply
- ***Tissue diagnosis*** Usual practice is to obtain a tissue diagnosis of the underlying disease before starting treatment, as the underlying diagnosis can alter treatment markedly. Symptomatic obstruction will have been developing for some weeks prior to presentation and, in the clinically stable patient, a delay of 24–48 h whilst the correct underlying diagnosis is obtained is warranted. Radiotherapy prior to biopsy can lead to problems making a subsequent histological diagnosis, and, similarly, high-dose steroids can make the diagnosis of lymphoma difficult
- ***Cytological diagnosis*** may be obtained from:
  - Pleural fluid
  - Ultrasound guided biopsy of an extrathoracic lymph node (e.g. supraclavicular or cervical nodes—low risk)
  - Bronchoscopy, or mediastinoscopy if no endobronchial disease, may be needed, depending on CT features. There may be increased risk of bleeding post-biopsy because of venous congestion, and anaesthesia is theoretically more risky because of possible associated tracheal obstruction or pericardial effusion (potentially leading to haemodynamic compromise due to cardiac tamponade), though these can be anticipated from the CT scan
  - Sputum

►► SVCO: management

This is usually in two phases.

- Initial general treatment: oxygen, analgesia, sitting the patient up (to reduce venous pressure), and steroids (in some)
- Followed by treatment of the underlying disease causing the SVCO, dependent on the tissue diagnosis. The major differential in terms of treatment is small cell carcinoma (initial chemotherapy), non-small cell carcinoma (initial radiotherapy), and lymphoma (chemotherapy). The presence of SVCO usually means that surgical resection of a NSCLC is not possible.

►► SVCO: management (*cont.*)

Steroids Limited trial data to support the use of steroids in SVCO, prior to definitive treatment, but most would start them fairly promptly (e.g. dexamethasone 8 mg bd, avoid in the evening as affects sleep). They may reduce oedema and improve symptoms. Ideally a tissue diagnosis should be obtained before commencing steroids, but may not always be possible. The problem arises where the underlying diagnosis is lymphoma, where steroids may alter the histology, making a definitive diagnosis more difficult. In an older smoker, with an obvious CXR mass (in whom the diagnosis is likely to be lung cancer), steroids can probably be started without risk to the underlying histology.

Radiotherapy 90% of patients are oedema-free by 3–4 weeks. In those with a poor response to radiotherapy, only 25% survive 1 year.

Intraluminal stents are used for malignant SVCO, and may be a first-line treatment whilst radiotherapy is planned. Successful in 90% of cases, with relief of symptoms in most patients within 48 h. They do not preclude subsequent radiotherapy or chemotherapy. In SCLC, however, chemotherapy will improve SVCO rapidly, so stent insertion may not be necessary. It is not clear whether post-procedure anticoagulation is required. Some centres advocate the use of low-dose warfarin anticoagulation (i.e. 1 mg/day), aiming for an INR of <1.6. Thrombosis in the SVC is not a contraindication to the procedure, as clot can be dispersed mechanically or with thrombolysis at the time of the procedure.
Stent complications Stent migration is the major complication, but most patients do not live long enough for this to be a major problem.

Anticoagulation Some recommend prophylactic anticoagulation in the presence of SVCO. Small increased risk of intracerebral bleeding, but the benefits of SVCO treatment may be limited by subsequent SVC thrombus if anticoagulation is not started. This is controversial.

SVCO due to thrombosis is usually in association with central venous lines or pacemaker wires. If the clot is less than 5 days old (as judged by symptoms) thrombolysis is warranted. Subsequent oral anticoagulation may reduce recurrence.

Prognosis depends on the underlying disease, and is unrelated to the duration of SVCO at presentation. The majority of SVCO is due to mediastinal spread of carcinoma of the lung, so the overall prognosis is generally poor, but depends on the patient's performance status, stage and extent of disease, and the cell type.

Further information

Rowell NP, Gleeson FV. Steroids, radiotherapy, chemotherapy and stents for SVCO in carcinoma of the bronchus: a systematic review. *Clin Oncol (R Coll Radiol)* 2002; **14**: 338–51

Hypercalcaemia

Definition and aetiology A serum calcium level over 2.75 mmol/L is considered abnormal; borderline values need repeating. In malignancy, a raised calcium is due to increased osteoclast activity, either from bony metastases or the production of parathyroid-hormone-related protein. A serum level over 3.25 mmol/L is rare outside malignancy, although can occur in sarcoidosis.

Clinical features Values over 3 mmol/L are usually symptomatic. Common symptoms are confusion, weakness, nausea, reduced fluid intake, and constipation. There may be a short QT interval on ECG and renal failure.

Investigations Exclude other causes of hypercalcaemia and identify the tumour, although in most patients with malignant hypercalcaemia the diagnosis of malignancy will already be known. The parathyroid hormone (PTH) will be suppressed in malignant hypercalcaemia, but raised in hyperparathyroidism. The phosphate will tend to be low in hyperparathyroidism and hypercalcaemia due to ectopic PTH, and low/normal in sarcoidosis, metastatic bone disease, and with excess vitamin D. Check for renal failure.

►► Management of hypercalcaemia

- Isotonic saline infusion (250 ml/h initially, to reverse dehydration, but avoid fluid overload, reducing to 150 ml/h) with furosemide to increase calcium excretion
- Steroids help, but less so than in sarcoid-associated hypercalcaemia, partly through reduced intestinal absorption.

In addition to this initial management:

- Reduce bone reabsorption with bisphosphonates (takes a few days for maximum effect). The bisphosphonates can also reduce the pain of secondary bony deposits and may reduce pathological fracture rate.
  - *Intravenous preparations* Disodium pamidronate, 10 mL vial of 3 mg/mL, or 10 mL vial of 6 mg/mL infused over 2 h. Works for several weeks. Sodium clodronate, 300 mg (1 x 5 mL vial of 60 mg/mL) daily for 7 days or 1.5 g single dose (5 x 5 mL vials of 60 mg/mL). Zoledronic acid, 4 mg vial reconstituted in water and given over 2 h, repeated monthly if required
  - *Oral preparations* Sodium clodronate, one 800 mg tablet bd.

Syndrome of inappropriate secretion of ADH (SIADH)

Definition and aetiology Excessive retention of water relative to electrolytes due to inappropriate production of ADH. Hence there is hyponatraemia (<135 meq/L), hypo-osmolality, a urine osmolality >100 mosmol/kg, a urine sodium concentration usually above 40 meq/L, normal acid–base (and potassium), and usually a low plasma urea concentration. Diuretic-induced hyponatraemia will be accompanied by evidence of dehydration, e.g. raised urea. Causes of SIADH include:

- Drugs, e.g. carbamazepine, fluoxetine, high-dose cyclophosphamide
- Post major surgery
- Pneumonia
- HIV infection
- CNS disorders, e.g. stroke, infection, psychosis
- Small cell lung cancer, either ectopic ADH production or stimulation of normal ADH production (poor prognostic factor).

Clinical features Lethargy and confusion often when sodium levels fall below 130 meq/L and nearly always when below 120 meq/L.

Investigations A low sodium in the presence of a low urea and an appropriate clinical setting may be adequate to make a diagnosis. If sodium depletion/water overload are a possible alternative cause of hyponatraemia, they should be accompanied by a urine osmolarity <100 mosmol/kg (or a specific gravity <1.003 or a urine sodium <40 meq/L). Therefore, values increasingly above this are suggestive of SIADH (unless the patient is on loop diuretics when, of course, the urinary sodium concentration will be higher).

►► Management of inappropriate ADH secretion

- Fluid restriction (0.5–1.0 L/day) will help, but is often unpleasant for the patient
- Demeclocycline (450 mg bd, tetracycline derivative) blocks ADH action at the distal renal tubules and can be used long term
- Salt tablets/extra-dietary salt
- May resolve over a few weeks following chemotherapy
- Hypertonic saline is rarely indicated and can provoke brainstem damage (demyelination) through rapid changes in osmolality.

Future developments

New drugs specifically blocking the ADH receptor in the distal tubule are under investigation.

Spinal cord compression

This is a medical emergency requiring prompt treatment within 24 h to prevent irreversible paraplegia and loss of bowel and bladder function.

Definition and aetiology Spinal cord compression occurs commonly in patients with metastatic cancer (in about 5% of all cancer patients, particularly breast, lung, and prostate cancer). It may be the first presentation of cancer, but often occurs in patients with a known primary tumour. Cord compression is commonly caused by direct spread from a vertebral metastasis into the extradural space or, less commonly, from pressure on the cord from a primary tumour in the posterior mediastinum or the retroperitoneum, or by pressure from a mass of retroperitoneal nodes. It is unusual to have a metastasis within the cord itself, although meningeal spread can occur. Spinal cord compression causes interruption of the arterial supply to the cord and subsequent infarction.

Clinical features Patients frequently experience back pain initially, due to associated vertebral collapse. This precedes any neurological signs. Pain is not, however, universal. Neurological signs may be non-specific: weak legs, constipation, urinary incontinence. Leg weakness develops over hours–days, with associated sensory loss. Loss of bladder and bowel sensation is a late sign and usually heralds irreversible paraplegia within hours or a few days. Examination reveals bilateral upper motor neuron signs in the legs, with increased tone, weakness, brisk reflexes, and extensor plantars. There may be sensory loss in the legs, particularly with a loss of proprioception and a sensory level on the trunk. Sensory loss in the saddle area, with decreased rectal tone, suggests a cauda equina lesion. The bladder may be palpable.

Investigations

Have a low threshold for investigating a patient with known cancer with back pain

- ***MRI*** of the spine is the investigation of choice to demonstrate the level of the cord compression
- ***CT*** is less reliable, but can also be helpful, if MRI is not available
- ***Plain spine XR*** may show vertebral metastases, but this is usually unhelpful, as there is no imaging of the spinal cord. Time should not be wasted in obtaining a plain XR
- ***Bone scan*** shows vertebral metastases, but again does not image the spinal cord. Earlier scans showing bony metastases may alert the physician to the possibility of future cord compression
- If patient is not known to have underlying malignant disease, a search for a primary tumour should be performed, but must not delay treatment of the spinal cord compression. Take full history (weight loss, anorexia, specific symptoms) and perform full examination, CXR, blood tests, PSA, and myeloma screen.

▶▶ Management of spinal cord compression

This depends on tumour type and overall prognosis. Discuss with oncologist and/or neurosurgeon to determine which definitive treatment(s) are the most appropriate for the patient.

- High-dose steroids (dexamethasone IV 4 mg/6 h). These should be started whilst waiting for MRI scan, if the clinical picture suggests cord compression
- Radiotherapy to the metastasis or tumour causing cord compression, particularly if there are multiple sites of cord compression or if surgery is not advised
- Surgical decompression of the cord, reconstruction, and stabilizing the spinal column
- Catheter if in urinary retention
- Care for pressure areas
- DVT prophylaxis
- Consider chemotherapy, if appropriate, for underlying cancer causing the spinal cord compression, once the initial treatment has taken place
- Rehabilitation, ideally in unit with spinal cord expertise.

Early referral to physiotherapists and occupational therapists with oncology expertise.

A recent Dutch study showed 66% of patients with metastatic cord compression (from all cancers) admitted to rehabilitation centres were discharged and the average survival post-discharge was 808 days. 52% were alive at 1 year.

Prognosis Patients who are mobile at presentation have the best prognosis and are likely to have preserved neurological function following treatment. If there is some preserved motor function, 25% will be able to walk post-treatment. If paraplegia is present pre-treatment, less than 10% will be able to walk afterwards. Loss of bladder function for more than 24–48 h cannot be reversed.

Further information

Conway R *et al.* What happens to people after malignant cord compression? Survival, function, quality of life, emotional well-being and place of care 1 month after diagnosis. *Clin Oncol* 2007; **19**: 56–62

Eriks IE *et al.* Epidural metastatic spinal cord compression: functional outcome and survival after in-patient rehabilitation. *Spinal Cord* 2004; **42**: 235–9

Pulmonary carcinoid tumours

These are uncommon primary lung tumours, comprising 1–2% of all lung tumours. Equal male/female incidence; typical age at presentation is 40–50 years. They are a form of neuroendocrine tumour and can have similar histological appearances to small cell lung cancer.

Pathophysiology Although typically slow growing benign tumours, more aggressive subtypes exist, with metastatic potential. Commonly they are located endobronchially, but can also be located peripherally in the lung parenchyma.

Clinical features

- Endobronchial carcinoids can cause isolated wheeze, dyspnoea, infection, haemoptysis, or persistent lobar collapse
- Parenchymal carcinoids are often asymptomatic, being detected on routine CXR
- Carcinoid syndrome, with flushing, tachycardia, sweats, diarrhoea, wheeze, and hypotension, occurs in 1% of pulmonary carcinoid tumours
- Carcinoid tumours can also be associated with Cushing's syndrome, due to ectopic tumour ACTH production.

Investigations

- ***CXR*** may reveal a well-defined tumour, which should be further characterized on CT. *Tumourlets* is the description given to multiple endobronchial or parenchymal carcinoid tumours. PET has decreased sensitivity for detecting carcinoid tumours compared with NSCLC (75% in one study)
- ***Bronchoscopy*** is performed for accessible endobronchial carcinoid tumours. They typically appear to be intraluminal, cherry red, and covered with intact epithelium. Bronchial brushings may be adequate for a histological diagnosis. Bronchial biopsy can be associated with brisk or torrential bleeding, so care should be taken. Some avoid biopsy altogether and proceed to surgical resection based on a clinical diagnosis. CT-guided biopsy may be preferred for peripheral tumours
- ***Histological diagnosis*** can be difficult as the appearances can be similar to those of small cell lung cancer. Special stains and immunohistochemistry are used to help differentiate between the two. Clinically, however, these tend to be quite different conditions and clinical details can aid pathological diagnosis. Carcinoid tumours are characterized as being *typical* or *atypical*. They each have a characteristic pattern:
    - *Typical carcinoids* have no necrosis, occasional nuclear pleomorphism, and absent or late mitoses. Distant metastases are rare and metastasis to lymph nodes occurs in 5–15% of cases. The 5-year survival is 100% and 10-year survival is 87%
    - *Atypical carcinoids* may show focal necrosis and often have nuclear pleomorphism. There is increased mitotic activity. They have distant metastases in 20% and metastasize to the lymph nodes in up to 48% of cases. The 5-year survival is 69% and 10-year survival is 52%

Management

- Patients with isolated pulmonary carcinoid tumours should be considered for surgical resection. Resection is ideally limited, removing minimal amounts of normal lung parenchyma. Tumour resection is associated with resolution of any features of the carcinoid syndrome
- If the tumour is atypical or close to the resection margin, patients should be followed up with repeat CXR on an annual basis. Radiotherapy is not performed
- Tumour size does not relate to the presence of lymph node metastases and therefore local lymph nodes should be sampled peri-operatively
- In the 1% with carcinoid syndrome, serotonin antagonists, such as octreotide, can be used for treatment. Isolated liver metastases can be treated with arterial embolization. Metastatic aggressive carcinoid tumours can be treated with chemotherapy, such as etoposide, cisplatin, 5-fluorouracil, and streptozotocin.

Further information

Hage R *et al.* Update in pulmonary carcinoid tumours: a review article. *Ann Surg Oncol.* 2003; **10**: 697–704

Pulmonary nodules 1

Definition These are focal, round, or oval areas of increased opacity in the lung, measuring less than 3 cm in diameter. They are detected on CXR or CT. Greater use of CT and thinner slice spiral CT scanning has led to increased detection rates. CT allows the precise localization of a nodule and reliable determination of its features. It has a high sensitivity of detecting nodules of >5 mm in diameter. Volumetric analysis using CT-aided software means that a 3D nodule can be simulated, to aid nodule characterization and assess whether its volume has increased over time.

Table 31.1 Causes of pulmonary nodules

Benign	Malignant
Infectious granulomata	Lung cancer
Non-infectious granulomata	Solitary metastasis
Bronchial adenoma	
Benign hamartoma (developmental abnormality, containing cartilage, epithelium, and fat. Can contain smooth muscle. Slow growing. Can be seen at any age, especially 40+; often calcify.)	

- The majority of pulmonary nodules are benign, although exact numbers depend on the characteristics of the population screened
- 20–30% of patients with lung cancer may present with a solitary pulmonary nodule
- Of the nodules detected on CT in smokers with a normal CXR, between 1% and 2.5% will be malignant
- The Early Lung Cancer Action Project screening programme in the USA used CT scans in over-60-year-olds, with at least a 10-pack year history of smoking, and found non-calcified nodules in 23%, which were seen on CXR in 7%. 11% of these nodules were malignant on biopsy
- Early detection of these malignant nodules might alter the management of the patient, with surgical resection of a stage 1 cancer.

Management options for patients with pulmonary nodules

Observation Baseline CT scan showing nodule ≥ 4 mm, then repeat after an arbitrary time interval, such as 3 and 12 months, or 3, 6, and 12 months. If the nodule has increased in size or shows features of malignancy, consider biopsy or proceed straight to surgical resection. PET scan may be helpful in combination with CT if the nodule is indeterminate or increasing in size, but cannot be biopsied.

CT-PET scan useful in lesions >7 mm

Biopsy Difficult on small nodules <7 mm, and those behind a rib or scapula.

Resection If nodule has features of malignancy and biopsy not possible. Local practice varies.

Chemotherapy or radiotherapy If nodule proven to be malignant, but surgical treatment is not indicated due to performance status.

Combined modality treatment

Pulmonary nodules 2

Factors that suggest a pulmonary nodule is malignant

- Size >1 cm
- Smokers, older age
- Increasing volumetrically determined growth rates over time
- Increased enhancement with contrast, suggesting increased vascularity (>15 Hounsfield units)
- Increased FDG uptake with PET compared with normal tissue. Estimated sensitivity of PET is 97% for identifying a malignant process
- Occult extrathoracic disease identified on PET scanning
- Irregular or spiculated margin, with distortion of adjacent vessels—the 'corona radiata' sign
- Associated ground-glass shadowing
- Cavitation with thick irregular walls
- Pseudocavitation within nodule—bronchoalveolar cell carcinoma.

Factors that suggest a pulmonary nodule is benign

- Stable or decreasing size for 2 years
- Nodule resolves during follow-up
- Non-smoker
- Lack of enhancement with contrast
- Smooth, well-defined margins (although 21% of smooth nodules may be malignant)
- Benign pattern of calcification: central, diffuse solid, laminated, or 'popcorn like'—related to prior infections or calcification in a hamartoma
- Intranodular fat—likely hamartoma
- Cavitation with thin smooth walls
- Younger age
- Resident in histoplasmosis endemic areas, such as North America.

Pulmonary nodule with extrathoracic malignancy

In a patient with pre-existing malignancy, a pulmonary nodule could be a metastasis, new lung cancer, or benign disease. The histology of the extra-pulmonary neoplasm and the patient's smoking history influence this. These cases need discussion within the cancer MDT to determine whether nodule biopsy or treatment of the underlying primary cancer would be the most appropriate management.

One study determined the likelihood of a pulmonary nodule being a new primary or metastasis based on the site of the original cancer:

- ***New lung primary more likely*** if the primary tumour is head and neck, bladder, breast, bile ducts, oesophagus, ovary, prostate, stomach
- ***Metastasis more likely*** if the primary tumour is melanoma, sarcoma, testes
- ***Either new primary or metastasis possible*** if the primary tumour is salivary gland, adrenal, colon, parotid, kidney, thyroid, thymus, uterus.

Further information

Ost D *et al.* The solitary pulmonary nodule. *NEJM* 2003; **348**: 2535–42

Erasmus J *et al.* Solitary pulmonary nodules. *Radiographics* 2000; **20**: 43–66

Quint L *et al.* Solitary pulmonary nodule with extra pulmonary neoplasms. *Radiology* 2000;

217: 257–61

Henschke CI *et al.* Early lung cancer action project: overall design and findings from baseline screening. *Lancet* 1999; **354**: 99–105

Lung cancer screening

This is an area that is currently under investigation. Screening programmes are based on the premise that the early detection of lung cancer and any subsequent intervention will improve the patient's survival. There is no evidence yet of reduction in lung cancer mortality from screening studies. To be detectable on CXR, a lung cancer needs to be 1 cm diameter, and 3–4 mm diameter to be detectable on CT.

Screening studies

- Four previous CXR screening studies in the 1970s were negative, of which the ***Mayo Lung Project*** has been the most studied. This compared 4-monthly CXR and sputum cytology for 6 years in smokers 45 years old or older of 20+ per day, with infrequent or no screening in a control group. 206 cancers were found in the study group and 160 in the control group, but all-cause mortality was not affected by screening, even at 20 years
- More recent studies have used low-dose spiral CT scanning. The ***Early Lung Cancer Action Project (ELCAP)*** in New York recruited 1000 symptom-free volunteers aged 60+ with a 10 pack-year history of smoking, who would be fit for a thoracotomy. There was no control group. Baseline CXR and CT were performed. Non-calcified nodules were present in 23% of patients at baseline on CT. Repeat CT was performed for nodules <5 mm; nodules >6 mm were biopsied and nodules >11 mm received standard care. 2.7% of all the patients entered had malignant nodules with stage 1 disease in 2.3%. All but one patient had their cancer surgically resected
- ***International ELCAP*** screened 31 567 asymptomatic over-40-year-olds at risk for lung cancer between 1993 and 2005. The median age was 61. 13% had a positive result requiring follow-up at baseline CT and 5% at annual CT. Lung cancer was diagnosed in 1.5% of people (85% stage 1), with 411 having resection and 57 having radiotherapy ± chemotherapy. There was no non-treatment randomized control group, so it is still difficult to interpret whether the earlier diagnosis and intervention led to longer survival. (Henschke CI *et al. NEJM* 2006;355:1763-71)
- Further research is needed to demonstrate a clear detection survival benefit, before national screening programmes are instituted.
- Large randomized studies of CT vs. CXR are ongoing and the results are awaited. The role of PET in screening also needs to be evaluated.

Further information

Ellis JRC *et al.* Lung cancer screening. *Br J Radiol* 2001; **74**: 478–85

Marcus PM. Lung cancer screening: an update. *J Clin Oncol* 2001; **19**: 83s–6s

Kawahara M. Screening for lung cancer. *Curr Opin Oncol* 2004; **16**: 141–5

Chapter 32

Lung transplantation

Patient selection

Lung transplantation was first performed successfully in the early 1980s, and since then the number of candidates for transplantation has increased significantly. However, there is a significant shortage of donor organs, and so an increasing number of patients (up to 10–15%) die on the waiting list. There are five transplant centres in the UK: Harefield, Papworth, Birmingham, Manchester, and Newcastle. Approximately 100 lung transplants and 50 heart–lung transplants are carried out in the UK annually. Average waiting times in the UK are around 12 months for lung transplantation and 16 months for heart–lung transplantation. Matching is carried out according to size and major blood groups; HLA matching is not carried out.

Underlying conditions Most common diagnoses, in order:
- COPD (including α_1-antitrypsin deficiency)
- Cystic fibrosis
- Idiopathic pulmonary fibrosis
- Idiopathic pulmonary arterial hypertension
- Pulmonary hypertension secondary to congenital cardiac disease (Eisenmenger's syndrome)
- Others, including sarcoidosis, lymphangioleiomyomatosis, Langerhans' cell histiocytosis, collagen vascular disease-related lung disease, bronchoalveolar cell carcinoma (successful transplantation has been carried out, although tumour recurrence in the donor lung is common).

Indications Referral for transplant assessment should be considered in patients with chronic end-stage lung disease despite maximal medical therapy, whose life expectancy is 2–3 years or less (so that transplantation would be expected to prolong their survival). Candidates should be functionally disabled but still able to walk, with no significant cardiac, renal, or hepatic impairment. Suggested age limits are 55 years for heart–lung, 60 years for bilateral lung, and 65 years for single lung transplant.

General referral criteria for lung transplantation

- Normal renal function, with creatinine clearance >50 mL/min
- Normal left ventricular function and normal coronary arteries
- Preserved liver synthetic function
- No osteoporosis
- No systemic sepsis
- BMI >17
- No psychiatric disorder
- No history of malignancy within 5 years.

Contraindications

Absolute

- Severe extrapulmonary organ dysfunction (including renal, hepatic, and cardiac disease)
- Active cancer or recent history (within 2 years) of cancer with substantial likelihood of recurrence; a 5-year disease-free interval is recommended (excluding cutaneous squamous or basal cell carcinomas)
- Severe psychiatric illness or non-compliance with treatment/follow-up
- Incurable chronic extrapulmonary infection (including HIV, active hepatitis B and C)
- Active or recent (6 months) substance addiction (cigarette smoking, alcohol, narcotics)
- Significant chest wall/spinal deformity

Relative

- Age >65 years
- Chronic medical conditions that are poorly controlled or associated with target-organ damage (hypertension, diabetes, coronary artery disease)
- Severe or symptomatic osteoporosis (risk of post-transplant fractures and poor quality of life; start treatment prior to transplant)
- Daily requirement for >20 mg prednisolone
- Severe obesity (BMI >30) or malnutrition (BMI <17)
- Inability to walk, with poor rehabilitation potential
- Mechanical ventilation (excluding NIV) or acute critical illness
- Extensive pleural thickening (from infection or prior surgery, e.g. pleurodesis)—procedure is technically more difficult
- Active collagen vascular disease
- Pre-operative colonization of the airway with pan-resistant bacteria, fungi, or mycobacterium in cystic fibrosis: there are no clear data to support exclusion of pan-resistant *Pseudomonas*, although it remains a relative contraindication in some centres. *B. cepacia* colonization (particularly with genomovar III), however, is high risk and an absolute contraindication in many centres

Contentious

- Non-tuberculous mycobacterium, especially *M. chelonae*
- Aspergilloma (ABPA is not generally a contraindication, though patients would not be transplanted during an exacerbation, and would be treated with prophylactic voriconazole)
- Portal hypertension (prophylactic variceal sclerotherapy may be offered).

Further information

Orens JB *et al.*, International guidelines for the selection of lung transplant candidates: 2006 update. *J Heart Lung Transplant* 2006; **25**: 745–55

Glanville AR, Estenne M. Indications, patient selection and timing of referral for lung transplantation. *Eur Resp J*. 2003; **22**: 845–52

Specific conditions

Timing of referral This can be difficult; life expectancy should be <2–3 years, but patients must be fit for the procedure during a waiting time of up to 16 months. The decision should not be based on a single factor; instead, a combination of clinical, laboratory, and functional assessments should be considered. Patients with CF and IPF have particularly high waiting list mortalities, suggesting inappropriately late referral for these conditions. Disease-specific guidelines for referral:

Chronic obstructive pulmonary disease

- BODE index (incorporating BMI, FEV_1, degree of dyspnoea, and 6-min walk; p 169) >5
- History of hospitalization for exacerbation associated with acute hypercapnia ($PaCO_2$ >6.7kPa; 49% 2-year survival)
- Pulmonary hypertension or cor pulmonale, despite oxygen therapy
- FEV_1 <20% predicted and either TLCO <20% or homogeneous distribution of emphysema (median survival 3 years with medical therapy)
- Patients should be on maximal medical therapy, have completed pulmonary rehabilitation, have stopped smoking for at least 6 months (if in doubt, check urinary cotinine levels), and ideally <60 years old

Cystic fibrosis

- Defining referral criteria is especially difficult for patients with CF, due to considerable inter-individual variation in course and prognosis
- FEV_1 ≤30% predicted or FEV_1 >30% with rapid progressive deterioration, e.g. increasing frequency of exacerbations, rapid fall in FEV_1
- History of ITU admission for pulmonary exacerbation
- Oxygen-dependent respiratory failure, hypercapnia, or pulmonary hypertension
- Severe recurrent haemoptysis despite embolization
- Refractory and/or recurrent pneumothorax
- Young (<20 years) female patients with rapid deterioration have a poor prognosis and should be considered for early referral
- Invasive ventilation is a contraindication in most centres

Idiopathic pulmonary fibrosis

- Given the poor prognosis and high waiting-list mortality associated with IPF, guidelines recommend referral of all suitable patients with histological or radiographic evidence of UIP, irrespective of vital capacity and without delaying for trials of treatment; these are not widely applied in the UK
- TLCO <40% predicted, fall in FVC ≥ 10% over 6 months, oxygen desaturation <88% on 6-min walk, honeycombing on HRCT (each associated with high mortality)

Idiopathic pulmonary arterial hypertension

- New York Heart Association (NYHA) functional class III or IV, rapidly progressive disease/failing medical therapy, low (<350 m) or declining 6-min walk test, mean right atrial pressure >15 mmHg, cardiac index <2 L/min/m^2.

Investigations and surgical approaches

Investigations prior to referral Consult transplant referral centre for details and avoid repetition of investigations. Important investigations include full PFTs, tests of exercise performance (e.g. 6-min walk), sputum microbiology, ECG, echo, HRCT chest, LFTs, viral serology (e.g. HIV, CMV, hepatitis B and C), 24-h creatinine clearance, stress echo, and/or coronary angiography. If on waiting list, inform transplant centre of changes in clinical condition. Remember that the referring physician remains responsible for continuing regular medical care of the patient, to ensure they remain optimally treated during the waiting period, with particular attention to:

- Maintenance of nutrition (may require PEG feeding)
- Avoidance of obesity
- Maintenance of mobility, continuing exercise and rehabilitation
- Monitoring comorbid disease: heart, kidney, liver, bones. Optimize treatment of diabetes, systemic hypertension, osteoporosis, peptic ulcer disease, gastro-oesophageal reflux and sinus disease
- Early NIV if indicated
- Avoiding intubation, if possible.

Surgical approaches for transplant

Single lung (50% of procedures)

- Technically easier, allows two recipients from one donor
- Used successfully in all patients except CF and bronchiectasis
- Over-distension of the compliant native lung in emphysema is uncommon, but may be problematic

Bilateral sequential (25%)

- Sequential right and left single lung transplants at one time
- Selective lung ventilation may render cardiopulmonary bypass unnecessary

Heart–lung (25%)

- Indicated in Eisenmenger's syndrome, or advanced lung disease with concurrent LV dysfunction or coronary disease
- Cor pulmonale is not in itself an indication, as right ventricular hypertrophy resolves rapidly following lung transplantation alone
- Certain patients without cardiac disease may undergo a 'domino' procedure, where they receive a combined heart–lung transplant, because this is technically easier, and their healthy heart is then used for a patient needing a heart transplant

Living lobar transplantation

- Bilateral grafting of lower lobes from two living adult donors to replace lungs of child or small adult
- Appears to be safe for the donor, with lung volume reductions of about 15%, but potential for 300% overall mortality (2 donors and one recipient)
- Not widely performed in the UK

Follow-up

Patients are usually discharged about one month after transplant, following post-transplant bronchoscopy with BAL and biopsy. They will be followed up closely by their transplant centre, but may also attend general respiratory clinics intermittently between transplant centre visits. Be alert to possible complications (pp 326–9). Spirometric values are generally very stable from 3 months after transplantation, and sustained falls ≥10–15% warrant further investigation. Remember drug interactions (particularly ciclosporin and tacrolimus) if new medications are added. Check immunosuppressant drug blood levels and perform routine blood tests according to the local transplant centre policy.

Outcomes

Survival

- Survival rates: 85% 1-year, 63% 3-year, 50% 5-year. Median survival is 4.5 years
- Compared with patients on the waiting list, lung transplant conveys a survival benefit to patients with CF and IPF, but not emphysema
- Rate of death is highest in first year (infection, primary graft failure)
- Risk factors for early death are pre-existing pulmonary hypertension, ventilator dependence, recipient age >50, donor age >50
- No survival difference between single- and double-lung transplant.

Functional

- Lung function usually normalizes after bilateral transplant and markedly improves following single-lung transplant. In COPD, FEV_1 increases to 50–60% of predicted value after single-lung transplant
- Arterial oxygenation rapidly normalizes
- 6-min walk distance typically doubles; most patients resume active lifestyle although fewer than 40% of patients return to work
- Limited data on quality of life: initial improvement suggested, but effects after 1 year are unclear.

Routine surgery after lung transplant

Routine surgery >3 months after transplant can be carried out locally, but inform the transplant centre. Routine antibiotic prophylaxis is adequate; there is no increased risk of SBE. The morning dose of calcineurin inhibitor (ciclosporin, tacrolimus) should be omitted, as there is a risk of nephrotoxicity with hypovolaemia.

Future developments are likely to address both the shortage of donor organs (e.g. living lobar transplantation, the 'non-heart beating donor', xenotransplantation, and further research in lung preservation) and the development of more effective treatments for chronic rejection (new immunosuppressive drugs, induction of immune tolerance).

Complications 1

Early graft dysfunction

- Characterized by pulmonary infiltrates, hypoxaemia, and diffuse alveolar damage or organizing pneumonia on biopsy; not uncommon during first few days after transplant. Clinical severity ranges from very mild acute lung injury to acute respiratory distress syndrome
- Presumably related to preservation and ischaemia–reperfusion injury
- Exclude other causes, e.g. volume overload, pneumonia, rejection, occlusion of venous anastomosis, aspiration
- Treatment is supportive (mechanical ventilation)
- High mortality (40–60%).

Airway complications

- Anastomotic stenosis most common and typically occurs weeks–months after transplant; suggested clinically by localized wheeze, recurrent pneumonia, or suboptimal lung function. Treat with stent placement via bronchoscopy
- Complete dehiscence of bronchial anastomosis now rare, and requires immediate surgery or retransplantation
- Partial dehiscence is managed conservatively: drain pneumothorax, reduce steroid dose.

Infection

Bacteria

- May occur early (first month after transplant) or late (associated with bronchiolitis obliterans syndrome)
- Most commonly due to Gram-negative organisms, particularly *Pseudomonas aeruginosa*
- Recipients with cystic fibrosis are not at greater risk than other patients; an exception is *B. cepacia* colonization, which is associated with a high risk of often lethal postoperative infections.

CMV

- CMV-seronegative recipients from seropositive donors are at particular risk of severe infection, including pneumonitis; this is usually treated successfully with ganciclovir
- Increases risk of bacterial or fungal superinfection
- Ganciclovir prophylaxis probably results in later, less severe infection.
- CMV infection may be a risk factor for development of bronchiolitis obliterans syndrome.

Aspergillus

- *Aspergillus* frequently colonizes the airways after lung transplant, but clinically apparent infection develops in only a minority of patients
- Peak disease incidence at 2 months after transplant
- Sites of disease include airways (may lead to mucosal oedema, ulceration, and pseudomembranes; usually responds to itraconazole, voriconazole, or amphotericin B), fresh bronchial anastomosis, lung parenchyma, and disseminated aspergillosis (associated with high mortality).

Drug-related Immunosuppressive drugs must be taken lifelong following transplantation. Agents used include ciclosporin or tacrolimus, azathioprine or mycophenolate mofetil, and prednisolone. They are associated with many drug interactions and side-effects, particularly nephrotoxicity and osteoporosis. Ciclosporin and tacrolimus blood levels need to be closely monitored.

Further information

Kotloff A Medical complications of lung transplantation. *Eur Resp J*, 2004; **23**: 334–42

Knoop *et al.* Immunosuppressive therapy after human lung transplantation. *Eur Resp J* 2004; **23**: 159–71

Complications 2

Acute rejection

- Very common, particularly within 3 months of transplant. Rare after 12 months
- Asymptomatic, or may be associated with malaise, fever, dyspnoea, cough, hypoxia. May present similarly to pneumonia or COP
- **CXR** may be normal or show non-specific infiltrates
- Common finding is fall in **spirometry** >10%, although this does not distinguish from other complications, particularly infection
- Refer back to the transplant centre if these problems develop within 3 months of the transplant
- Ideally confirm histologically: transbronchial biopsies are safe and typically show perivascular lymphocytic infiltrates. Routine surveillance transbronchial biopsies are increasingly used to detect acute rejection prior to falls in lung function.
- **Treatment** IV methylprednisolone pulses. The majority of patients respond quickly; consider switch in immunosuppressive agent from cyclosporin A to tacrolimus if ongoing or recurrent acute rejection
- Acute rejection is the main risk factor for the development of chronic rejection
- Acute rejection is an uncommon cause of breathlessness after 3 months and other common causes of SOB should be considered.

Chronic rejection

- A significant problem, accounting for poor long-term prognosis following lung transplant
- Uncommon in first 6 months, but prevalence subsequently increases steadily, affecting 50–60% of patients at 5 years
- **Pathogenesis** incompletely understood, likely involves immune-mediated injury to epithelial and endothelial cells, possibly with an environmental trigger; risk factors for development include previous episodes of acute rejection, CMV pneumonitis, presence of anti-HLA antibodies pre-transplant, and perhaps gastro-oesophageal reflux, community respiratory virus infection, and medical non-compliance
- **Clinically** Insidious onset of breathlessness and cough, and progressive airflow obstruction on spirometry
- Manifest histologically as ***bronchiolitis obliterans***, a fibroproliferative process affecting small airways. Histological confirmation is difficult: transbronchial biopsies have a low sensitivity, so a clinical diagnosis of 'bronchiolitis obliterans syndrome (BOS)' is defined as an unexplained and sustained (≥3 weeks) fall in FEV_1 to <80% of peak value post-transplant. 'Potential BOS' is defined as FEV_1 81–90% of baseline and/or forced mid-expiratory flow ($FEV_{25-75\%}$) to ≤75% of baseline, and indicates the need for close monitoring/further investigation
- **CXR** unhelpful; **HRCT** may show expiratory air trapping and peripheral bronchiectasis
- *P. aeruginosa* colonization is common, with recurrent purulent tracheobronchitis

- **Treatment** is challenging, and involves either modified or increased immunosuppression (e.g. switch ciclosporin to tacrolimus; high-dose steroid pulses and antilymphocyte antibodies; inhaled cyclosporin may have a role), and if effective this acts only to reduce the rate of disease progression. Infection is investigated and treated aggressively, sometimes with reductions in immunosuppression. Azithromycin is often used for deteriorating BOS. Gastro-oesophageal reflux is treated, sometimes with surgery. Total lymphoid irradiation is sometimes recommended when other immunomodulatory treatments have failed
- **Prognosis** is poor: mortality is 40% within 2 years of diagnosis; the rate of decline is very variable between individuals
- Retransplantation is the only definitive treatment and is controversial.

Recurrence of primary disease Documented in sarcoidosis, lymphangioleiomyomatosis, giant cell interstitial pneumonitis, diffuse pan-bronchiolitis, and bronchoalveolar cell carcinoma.

Malignancy Increased risk of certain malignancies, e.g. lymphoma (and other EBV-related post-transplant lymphoproliferative diseases), skin, lip, vulval, and perineal carcinomas, *in situ* cervical cancer, and Kaposi's sarcoma.

- Most lymphomas appear within the first year, and the lung allograft is the most common site of involvement, with pulmonary nodule(s) ± mediastinal lymphadenopathy. Lymphocyte aggregates from acute rejection may mimic the appearance of post-transplant lymphoproliferative disease on small transbronchial biopsy specimens. Lymphomas presenting after the first year are more commonly disseminated or intra-abdominal (e.g. presenting with tonsillar enlargement, peripheral lymphadenopathy, skin nodules, or bowel complications such as intussusception). Patients should be referred back to the transplant centre for treatment, rather than the local haematologist. The usual treatment is a reduction in immunosuppression or rituximab (monoclonal antibody against CD20 on B cells)
- Lung cancer occurs in patients with COPD and IPF. Unclear if transplantation itself increases the risk of lung cancer. May progress unusually rapidly, mimicking infection.

Differential diagnosis of CXR nodules following lung transplant

- Post-transplant lymphoproliferative disease
- Infection (*Pseudomonas*, *Nocardia*, aspergilloma, TB)
- Disease recurrence
- Primary lung cancer.

Further information

Boehler, E. Post-transplant bronchiolitis obliterans. *Eur Resp J* 2003; **22**: 1007–18

Chapter 33

Mediastinal abnormalities

The mediastinum is the area within the centre of the chest containing the heart, great vessels, nerves, lymph nodes, trachea, oesophagus, and thymus. Two-thirds of mediastinal masses are benign. Age 20–40, presence of symptoms and anterior location of a mass are all associated with an increased likelihood of malignancy. Common symptoms of mediastinal disease include cough, chest pain, and dyspnoea, as well as symptoms relating to any structure being compressed, such as dysphagia, stridor, or SVCO. Mediastinal disorders can also be asymptomatic. They may be found incidentally following a CXR.

Anatomy

Anterior mediastinum The area behind the body of the sternum and in front of the fibrous pericardium. Contains the thymus, which also extends superiorly.

Posterior mediastinum The area in front of the vertebral bodies and behind the fibrous pericardium. Contains the spinal nerve roots, the descending aorta and oesophagus, the azygos and hemiazygos veins, the thoracic duct, and vagus and splanchnic nerves.

Superior mediastinum The area located between the thoracic inlet superiorly, the manubrium of the sternum anteriorly, by the superior 4 thoracic vertebrae posteriorly and inferiorly where a horizontal plane would cross through the sternal angle. It contains the aortic arch and its large branches and the upper half of SVC. It also contains the trachea, the oesophagus, the thoracic duct, and the phrenic, vagus, cardiac, and left recurrent laryngeal nerves.

Middle mediastinum The area containing the heart and pericardium, the ascending aorta, the lower half of the SVC, part of the azygos vein, the pulmonary arteries and veins, the tracheal bifurcation, phrenic nerves, and the IVC.

These areas are easily seen on a lateral CXR.

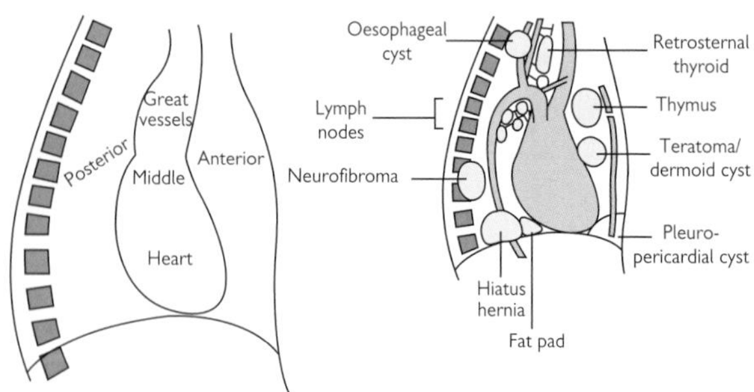

Fig. 33.1. Anterior, posterior, superior, and middle mediastinum

Likely nature of mediastinal mass according to anatomical site

Anterior mediastinal mass

- Thymoma (superior)
- Thyroid (superior)
- Germ-cell tumour
- Lymphoma
- Ascending aortic aneurysm
- Pleuropericardial cyst
- Pericardial fat pad
- Morgagni anterior diaphragmatic hernia (p 343)

Superior mediastinal mass

- Bronchogenic cyst

Posterior mediastinal mass

- Neural tumour
- Foregut duplication or cyst
- Lipoma
- Descending aortic aneurysm
- Bochdalek posterior diaphragmatic hernia (p 343).

Approach to the patient with a mediastinal mass

- Full history
- Examination, including skin, lymphadenopathy (neck, axillae, groins) and testes
- Look for fatiguability: ptosis, opthalmoplegia, inability to maintain upward gaze
- Look for signs of SVCO or stridor
- Blood tests, including AFP, βHCG, anti-acetyl choline receptor antibody
- CXR and lateral CXR (if not already done)
- Arrange CT scan of chest
- Try and locate old CXRs.

Mediastinal abnormalities 1

Neural tumours mostly occur in the posterior mediastinum. 75% are benign in adults.

- ***Schwannomas and neurofibromas*** are benign peripheral nerve sheath tumours. They may be multiple. Usually asymptomatic, although can cause segmental pain. Slowly enlarge and, rarely, can cause cord compression, with dumb-bell shaped tumours straddling the intervertebral foramen. Can be surgically excised
- ***Malignant peripheral nerve sheath tumours or neurosarcomas*** include new malignant growths and benign neurofibromas that have undergone malignant change. They may cause systemic features of malignancy and can invade locally and metastasize
- ***Autonomic nervous system tumours*** including neuroblastomas and ganglioneuromas, range from benign to malignant. Surgical removal is the treatment of choice, with radiotherapy and chemotherapy if the tumour is malignant.

Thymoma Tumour of epithelial origin arising in the thymus. May contain functioning thymic tissue. M = F. Rare below age 20. Myasthenia gravis is present in 30–40% of patients with a thymoma; this is often unimproved after thymectomy and may even develop after the thymoma is removed. 20% of patients presenting with myasthenia gravis are found to have a thymoma, particularly if patients are over 50 and male. This group is likely to have positive acetylcholine receptor (AChR) autoantibodies, which bind to AChRs at the postsynaptic motor endplate, decreasing available acetylcholine binding sites, causing nerve fatigability.

Patients with thymomas are usually symptomatic with pain, dyspnoea, dysphagia, or myasthenia gravis symptoms. Thymomas contained within the thymic capsule tend to be benign, although they do have malignant potential; those that have extended outside the capsule are malignant, and may involve local structures or metastasize. Diagnose with CT and treat with surgical excision of the thymus, avoiding prior FNA or biopsy as this may cause tumour seeding outside the capsule. Consider post-operative radiotherapy and chemotherapy for invasive tumours, especially those not completely excised. Thymectomy is indicated in patients with myasthenia gravis even without thymoma, as it may lead to symptomatic improvement. This gives best results in those with detectable AChR antibody levels and younger patients early in the disease course, particularly those with severe disease.

Thymic cyst may be congenital or acquired secondary to inflammation. Asymptomatic unless large and causing symptoms of compression. Benign, but usually treated with surgical excision, as diagnostic certainty may be difficult.

Thymic carcinoid Not associated with myasthenia gravis and behaves aggressively, with local recurrence and metastasis. May be associated with Cushing's syndrome. Treatment with surgery, chemotherapy, or octreotide.

Also: thymic carcinoma, thymic lipoma, and thymic hyperplasia.

Germ cell tumours Arise from immature germ cells, which fail to migrate during development. Tend to be in an anterior and mid-line location.

- ***Mature cystic teratomas*** represent 80% of germ cell tumours. These are benign and occur in young adults. M = F. Often asymptomatic, but can erode surrounding structures and cause symptoms. CXR shows well-defined mass, which may contain flecks of calcification. Treatment is by surgical excision
- ***Seminoma*** occurs in men age 20–40 years. Mediastinal seminomas are malignant and almost always arise within the thymus and are histologically indistinguishable from those occurring in the testes. Can be primary mediastinal tumour or metastasis from testicular tumour; therefore always examine testes. Patients frequently present with chest pain. CXR shows non-calcified lobulated anterior mediastinal mass, confirmed with CT. Serum AFP is normal and this aids diagnosis. Diagnose with surgical biopsy. Surgical excision is not recommended as is usually incomplete. Treatment is with cisplatin-based chemotherapy initially, which can cause infertility and therefore patients may wish to consider sperm banking before treatment. Tumours are radiosensitive, so radiotherapy used if they are bulky. Long-term survival expected in 80%. Better prognosis than non-seminomatous germ cell tumours
- ***Non-seminomatous germ cell tumours*** (including choriocarcinoma, teratocarcinoma, and yolk sac tumours) are all malignant and occur in men in their 30s. They are symptomatic due to local invasion and they metastasize. CXR shows mediastinal mass and diagnosis is with surgical biopsy. βHCG and AFP are raised. Treatment is with cisplatin-based chemotherapy. βHCG and AFP are markers of disease and fall with tumour response.

Thyroid Retrosternal goitre occurs, especially in older women. Usually asymptomatic unless large and compressing the trachea, causing dyspnoea and stridor. May be seen on plain CXR. CT and radioactive iodine isotope scans are helpful in diagnosis. Flow–volume loops are abnormal if there is tracheal compression. Surgery is recommended if there is airway compromise, but can lead to tracheomalacia afterwards.

Also: parathyroid adenoma

Mediastinal abnormalities 2

Lymphoma The mediastinum is frequently involved in patients with Hodgkin's lymphoma. CT scan is necessary to assess the extent of this and to assess response to treatment. To establish the histological diagnosis of lymphoma, an adequate tissue sample is required; this should be from a biopsy, rather than a fine-needle aspirate. This may be best achieved surgically, via mediastinoscopy. Examine patient for peripheral lymph nodes, as these may be easier to biopsy. Treatment is with chemotherapy initially.

Enlarged lymph nodes

- ***Metastases*** from breast, lung, and oesophageal cancer
- ***Castleman's disease*** Giant lymph node hyperplasia. Rare. Two forms:
  - *Angio-follicular hyperplasia* causing mediastinal or hilar lymph node mass. Often asymptomatic or may cause cough or wheeze due to localized compression. Non-progressive. May have fever and raised ESR. Nodal biopsy shows follicles of pericapillary lymphocytes and proliferation of the plump and eosinophilic capillary endothelial cells. Removal of nodes may improve symptoms. Can also occur on pleura
  - *Multicentric Castleman's disease* is a more aggressive disease that may occur in association with HIV infection. Lymphoproliferative disorder with prominent systemic symptoms, as well as generalized lymph node enlargement, hepatosplenomegaly, paraproteinaemia, and skin rash. Biopsy shows prominent plasma cell infiltration. Related to IL-6 over-production and human herpes virus-8 infection. Treatment is with steroids ± chemotherapy (doxorubicin, vincristine, and cyclophosphamide), but prognosis is poor. Can progress to non-Hodgkin's lymphoma. Rapidly fatal without treatment

Also: lymphangioma

Cysts

- ***Foregut duplications or bronchogenic cysts*** can be related to the oesophagus or the airways, especially near the carina. Lined by respiratory epithelium. Often diagnosed in childhood, as they cause dyspnoea, stridor, or cough due to limited space to expand. Seen on CXR and CT and treated with surgical excision
- ***Pleuropericardial cysts*** mostly occur at the cardiophrenic angles and can measure up to 25 cm diameter. M = F. Usually asymptomatic, but may cause chest pain. CXR shows smooth round shadow abutting the heart. Excision can be carried out at thoracoscopy, but conservative management is favoured. Also known as springwater cysts.

Inflammation

- ***Mediastinitis*** occurs after oesophageal perforation or rupture, due to malignancy, instrumentation, or vomiting (Boerhaave's syndrome). Patients are ill, with pain and fever. CXR may show widened mediastinum or air in the mediastinum. Pneumothorax or pleural effusion may also be seen. Treatment includes repairing the defect, parenteral feeding, and antibiotics. High morbidity and mortality
- ***Mediastinal fibrosis*** Rare idiopathic condition that occurs in middle age. Symptoms depend on which aspects of the mediastinum are involved, but may include dyspnoea, wheeze, haemoptysis, hoarse voice, dysphagia, pulmonary hypertension, SVCO. CXR shows a widened mediastinum. Diagnosis made on biopsy, particularly to exclude malignancy. Treatment is supportive; steroids and surgical debulking ineffective. Prognosis variable, depending on sites involved. May be associated with retroperitoneal fibrosis, radiotherapy, methysergide, auto-immune disease, or infection with TB, histoplasmosis, *Aspergillus*, or *Nocardia*.

Mediastinal emphysema or pneumomediastinum. Can be caused by sneezing, straining, Valsalva manoeuvres, vomiting, substance abuse, parturition, positive pressure ventilation, instrumentation, or trans-bronchial biopsy. Usually symptomless, but occasional pain. Hamman's sign may be present (click with each heart beat on auscultation over lung). Treat with high-flow oxygen. Resolves spontaneously.

Vascular Aortic aneurysms are usually asymptomatic, but symptoms relate to compression of adjacent structures. May diagnose on CXR as a widened mediastinum. This is best imaged via CT or MRI. Surgery should be considered to prevent death from rupture.

Further information

Duwe BV *et al.* Tumors of the mediastinum. *Chest* 2005; **128**: 2893–909

Chapter 34

Paediatric lung disorders pertinent to adult patients

This chapter concentrates on pulmonary conditions that occur in childhood and may become increasingly relevant to adult practice.

Chronic lung disease of prematurity

Chronic lung disease of prematurity (CLD), formerly known as bronchopulmonary dysplasia (BPD). Advances in neonatal medicine have led to the improved survival of premature babies with immature lungs and respiratory disease. Babies born at lower gestational ages are surviving into adulthood, due to therapy with antenatal steroids to prevent respiratory distress syndrome and the use of artificial surfactant to decrease the surface tension of the neonatal alveolar membrane. There have also been improvements in ventilatory techniques. CLD usually occurs in babies who have been mechanically ventilated.

Usually caused by barotrauma from prolonged ventilation, high-pressure ventilation, and/or ventilation with high oxygen concentrations.

Typical presentation is a premature baby who remains oxygen-dependent after 36 weeks post-conceptional age. It is now infrequent in those born at 30+ weeks and weighing more than 1200 g. Mortality of 25–30% with severe CLD. May require prolonged home oxygen therapy, up to 1 year or beyond. 50% of infants with CLD will need hospital re-admission during their first year with respiratory infection. Some may have significant pulmonary sequelae during childhood and adolescence, with chronic hypoxia and pulmonary hypertension, but the majority of children with CLD do not have significant ongoing respiratory symptoms. Children may have disabilities associated with prematurity, such as cerebral palsy or learning difficulties.

Pathology Cytokine-mediated scarring and repair. *Early inflammatory phase:* bronchial necrosis, alveolar destruction, capillary permeability, and associated obliterative bronchiolitis. *Subacute fibroproliferative phase:* type II pneumocyte hyperplasia, bronchial and bronchial smooth muscle hypertrophy, and interstitial and peri-alveolar fibrosis. *Chronic fibro-proliferative phase* airway remodelling for up to 1 year. Prior to surfactant use, these changes were more severe.

PFTs Functional respiratory abnormalities persist with increased airway resistance and airway hyperresponsiveness. RV and RV/TLC are raised, indicative of air trapping. Air trapping improves over 3–4 years as lung growth occurs; however, small airway abnormalities persist, at least until the age of 10.

Chest radiology Persisting mild to moderate abnormalities, with multi-focal areas of reduced lung attenuation and perfusion, bronchial wall thickening, and decreased bronchus:pulmonary artery diameter ratios on CT. These radiological abnormalities correlate with physiological evidence of air trapping.

Adulthood There are few longitudinal studies beyond childhood and it is unclear what the significance of CLD of prematurity is to adult lung disease.

Viral wheeze and asthma

A controversial area. Wheezing is common in infants and toddlers, and is often due to viral respiratory tract infections, causing a viral-induced wheeze. This has been found to be associated with passive cigarette smoke exposure, contact with other children, and not being breast-fed. This transient early wheezing is distinct from childhood asthma. The children are not atopic and have no family history of such. The wheeze has resolved usually by the age of 3, although they may persist in having airway hyperactivity for many years. Children with asthma tend to have a family history of eczema with concomitant atopic dermatitis and develop their symptoms at any age, but usually slightly later (by the age of 5). Half of them have mild symptoms, which regress by puberty. Those with more severe disease, requiring regular inhaled steroids, often have disease that persists into adult life. Treatment for young children is based on persistent symptoms and atopy. Drugs which may be effective include inhaled corticosteroids and leukotriene receptor antagonists.

Congenital abnormalities

Tracheomalacia Floppy trachea, usually associated with oesophageal atresia. Rarely will require intubation or tracheostomy.

Congenital lobar emphysema Over-inflation of a lobe due to localized bronchomalacia or bronchial obstruction. May cause wheeze or produce chest deformity. Often resolves spontaneously.

Diaphragmatic hernia A diaphragmatic defect, causing bowel to be present in the chest. This may cause respiratory distress soon after birth and may have been detected during the antenatal period by USS, or it may be completely asymptomatic and found incidentally on CXR, with bowel seen in the chest. There are two types. ***Bochdalek hernia*** is the congenital absence of posterolateral part of diaphragm, with associated hypoplastic lung due to bowel limiting growth. Treatment is with surgical repair of the diaphragmatic defect, but survival rate is only 50% due to underlying lung problems. ***Morgagni hernia*** is anteromedial herniation through the foramen of Morgagni, which is more commonly found in adulthood. It may be asymptomatic or cause symptoms of fullness, tightness, or pain in the anterior chest; it does not cause intestinal obstruction. CXR shows a cardiophrenic angle density. Surgical repair is difficult and is usually not necessary.

Cystic adenomatoid lung Excessive overgrowth of bronchioles with multiple cysts occurring in a section of lung. Commonly affects left lower lobe. Can be diagnosed antenatally. Can present in the same way as congenital lobar emphysema. May be mistaken for diaphragmatic hernia. Treatment is by resection of the affected lobe, but there may be space-occupying effects of the abnormal lobe that can cause morbidity and mortality, e.g. due to vena cava obstruction.

Pulmonary sequestration/sequestrated segment Segment of lung parenchyma with no bronchial connection that is unventilated. May be supplied by aberrant artery from the aorta and have anomalous pulmonary drainage to the right atrium. Can be intralobar, sharing pleura with the rest of the lung, or extralobar, which is separated from the lung by a lining of pleural tissue. Mostly left-sided; 75% are situated between the diaphragm and left lower lobe. Associated with other congenital abnormalities in 60% of cases. Can be a chance finding on CXR at any age, when cystic change may be seen in this area. Contrast CT or MRI may aid diagnosis. Surgical resection may be necessary if there is repeated infection in this segment.

MacLeod's syndrome Focal hyperlucency of lung or lobe, due to parenchymal and vascular maldevelopment, following a childhood bronchitis or bronchiolitis. Usually asymptomatic, and is diagnosed on CXR, which shows a hypertranslucent lung with reduced vascular markings and a small pulmonary artery.

Chapter 35

Pleural effusion

Clinical features and imaging

A pleural effusion results from the accumulation of abnormal volumes (>10–20 ml) of fluid in the pleural space. Pleural effusions are common and are associated with many different diseases; see Chapter 8 for a step-by-step approach to the diagnosis of a patient with a pleural effusion, differential diagnosis of transudates and exudates, and details of pleural fluid analysis.

Clinical features

- May be asymptomatic, or associated with breathlessness, dry cough, pleuritic chest pain (suggesting pleural inflammation), chest 'heaviness', and sometimes pain referred to the shoulder or abdomen
- Signs on examination include reduced chest expansion, reduced tactile vocal fremitus, a stony dull percussion note, quiet breath sounds, and sometimes a patch of bronchial breathing above the fluid level. A friction rub may be heard with pleural inflammation.

Imaging

CXR

- Sequential blunting of posterior, lateral, and then anterior costophrenic angles are seen on radiographs as effusions increase in size
- PA CXR will usually detect effusion volumes of 200 mL or more; lateral CXR is more sensitive and may detect as little as 50 mL pleural fluid
- Classical CXR appearance is of basal opacity obscuring hemidiaphragm, with concave upper border. Massive effusion may result in a 'white-out' of the hemithorax, with mediastinal displacement away from the effusion; lack of mediastinal shift in such cases raises the possibility of associated volume loss due to bronchial obstruction from a primary lung cancer
- Other CXR appearances include rounded or lentiform shadowing in loculated interlobar effusions, and diffuse shadowing throughout the hemithorax on supine films
- CXR appearance may suggest the underlying diagnosis, e.g. bilateral effusions with cardiomegaly in cardiac failure; massive effusions are most commonly due to malignancy.

Ultrasound is extremely sensitive at detecting fluid volumes of 100 mL or more, and is useful for distinguishing pleural fluid from pleural masses or thickening, and for demonstrating loculation.

CT chest with pleural contrast is useful in distinguishing benign and malignant pleural disease: nodular, mediastinal, or circumferential pleural thickening are all highly specific for malignant disease. CT may also reveal evidence of extrapleural disease, e.g. lymphadenopathy or parenchymal change, which may suggest a diagnosis such as cancer or tuberculosis.

Role of ***MRI*** is unclear; it may have increasing role in distinguishing benign from malignant pleural disease.

Pleural thickening

- Pleural fibrosis and thickening may follow previous episodes of pleural inflammation. Causes include previous empyema, tuberculous pleuritis, rheumatoid pleuritis, haemothorax, thoracotomy, and asbestos exposure (diffuse pleural thickening, p 111)
- May be asymptomatic or cause breathlessness
- CXR features include blunting of the costophrenic angle or apices, sometimes with associated calcification
- Ultrasound or CT may be required to distinguish from a pleural effusion
- Treatment is difficult and usually unnecessary; decortication may be considered.

Malignant pleural effusion: causes and investigations

Epidemiology Commonest cause of exudative pleural effusion in patients older than 60 years. About 40 000 cases of malignant effusion each year in the UK.

Causes Most malignant effusions are metastatic, with lung and breast the most common primary sites (Table 35.1).

Table 35.1 Primary sites and frequency

Primary site	Approximate frequency (%)
Lung	37
Breast	16
Lymphoma	10
Mesothelioma	10
Genitourinary tract	9
Gastrointestinal tract	7
Unknown primary	10

Other, rarer tumours include sarcoma, melanoma, leukaemia, and myeloma; almost any malignant tumour may spread to the pleural cavity. ***Mesothelioma*** is an important cause of malignant effusions and is discussed on p 114.

Clinical features Breathlessness is the main symptom; chest pain, cough, weight loss, and anorexia may also be present. A small proportion of patients are asymptomatic. Effusions may be unilateral or bilateral, and are frequently large volume.

Differential diagnosis Consider other potential causes of pleural effusion in patients known to have cancer, e.g. due to pneumonia, pulmonary embolism, radiotherapy, pericardial disease, or drugs.

Investigations A strategy for investigating the patient with an undiagnosed pleural effusion is detailed on p 48. Key investigations in patients suspected to have a malignant effusion are:

1. ***Pleural fluid cytology*** Sensitivity for malignancy is about 60%; yield is increased by analysis of a second, but not a third sample. Immunostaining of malignant cells may provide clues as to the likely primary site. Visualization of monoclonal cells in fluid on flow cytometry may support a diagnosis of lymphoma.
2. ***CT chest with pleural contrast*** Nodular, mediastinal, or circumferential pleural thickening on CT are highly specific for malignant disease. May also demonstrate extrapleural disease, e.g. lymphadenopathy.

3. ***Pleural biopsy histology*** Required in cytology-negative cases. Options:

- *CT-guided* cutting needle biopsy has been demonstrated to be a more effective diagnostic test for malignant pleural disease than Abrams' pleural biopsy (sensitivity 87% in CT-guided biopsy group vs. 47% in Abrams' group)
- *Ultrasound-guided* needle biopsies are also effective and relatively straightforward to perform
- *Thoracoscopy* is an extremely useful investigation allowing direct visualization of the pleural space with a high sensitivity (90%) for biopsies. Therapeutic talc poudrage (talc is 'puffed' directly on to the pleural surfaces) may be performed at same time, with a pleurodesis success rate >80%. Can be performed under general anaesthesia, although well tolerated with sedation and local anaesthesia. Complications (such as empyema) are rare.

Serum tumour markers (CEA, CA19–9, CA15–3, CA125, PSA) may be helpful in the investigation of patients with malignant effusion of unknown primary, although their diagnostic and prognostic value are limited.

Prognosis Median survival 3–12 months from diagnosis; shortest in lung cancer, longest in mesothelioma and ovarian cancer. Pleural fluid pH <7.3 tends to be associated with shorter survival (median survival 2.1 months) and decreased success of pleurodesis.

Further information

Antunes G *et al.* BTS guidelines for the management of malignant pleural effusions. *Thorax* 2003; **58** (suppl. II): ii 29–38

Maskell NA *et al.* Standard pleural biopsy vs CT-guided cutting-needle biopsy for diagnosis of malignant disease in pleural effusions: a randomised controlled trial. *Lancet* 2003; **361**: 1326–31

Malignant pleural effusion: management

Key points influencing the management of malignant effusions are:

- Symptoms, performance status, and wishes of the patient
- Sensitivity of the primary tumour to chemotherapy, e.g. small cell lung carcinoma, lymphoma, ovarian and breast carcinoma may respond to chemotherapy, although in some cases pleural effusions remain problematic and require additional treatment
- Extent of lung re-expansion following effusion drainage.

Treatment options

Observation and follow-up if asymptomatic.

Therapeutic pleural aspiration of 1–1.5 L pleural fluid to improve breathlessness. Can be performed at the bedside as a day-case procedure, avoiding hospital admission. Useful in the palliation of breathlessness in patients with a poor prognosis and in rare cases where effusion reaccumulates very slowly. Most effusions recur within 1 month of aspiration, and these patients should be considered for pleurodesis; repeated aspiration may be inconvenient and uncomfortable for the patient, and carries a risk of complications such as empyema, pneumothorax, and tumour seeding (in mesothelioma).

If the breathlessness does not improve following fluid aspiration, then there is little to be gained by repeated aspiration and other causes of breathlessness should be considered, e.g. lymphangitis carcinomatosa, pulmonary embolism.

Intercostal chest drainage and pleurodesis The aim of pleurodesis is to seal the visceral pleura to the parietal pleura with adhesions to prevent pleural fluid accumulating. The success of pleurodesis depends on the degree of apposition of the visceral and parietal pleura, which depends on the degree of lung re-expansion following drainage of the effusion. 'Trapped lung' occurs when tumour encases the visceral pleura and prevents lung expansion. Lung expansion may also be inhibited by a proximal airway obstruction or by a persistent air leak (e.g. after tearing of a friable tumour-infiltrated lung on re-expansion). Trapped lung may also be caused by non-malignant, fibrotic processes, e.g. rheumatoid pleuritis, haemothorax, tuberculosis.

The patient should be admitted and the effusion drained with an intercostal tube. If lung fully re-expands on CXR, proceed to pleurodesis (see p 775). If lung fails to re-expand fully (trapped lung; CXR shows a pneumothorax or hydropneumothorax), consider chest drain suction, which may encourage lung expansion and allow pleurodesis.

Treatment options for trapped lung or failed pleurodesis

- *Pleurodesis* may be successful despite only partial lung re-expansion and should still be considered. It may be repeated if unsuccessful initially
- *Repeated therapeutic pleural aspiration*
- *Intrapleural fibrinolytics* (e.g. streptokinase 250 000 IU) may be of benefit in the management of multiloculated effusions resistant to drainage and pleurodesis, encouraging free fluid drainage and in some cases enabling successful pleurodesis. Haemorrhage is a theoretical complication, although it appears to be uncommon
- *Thoracoscopy* enables the disruption of pleural adhesions and may have a role in facilitating pleurodesis in select patients with trapped lung
- *Long-term in-dwelling pleural catheter* may be beneficial in patients with trapped lung and frequent accumulation of symptomatic effusions, and avoids the need for recurrent pleural aspiration. The most frequent complications are tumour seeding around the drain site and pleural space infection. Can be inserted as a day-case procedure. Needs additional out-patient support (e.g. trained district nurse or respiratory specialist nurse), although most patients perform the drainage themselves after education
- *Pleuroperitoneal shunts* are effective in patients with trapped lung or failed pleurodesis, in the absence of multiple loculations. Shunting of fluid may occur spontaneously, at high pressures, or may require manipulation of a percutaneous pump chamber, inserted at thoracoscopy or mini-thoracotomy. Main problem is shunt occlusion, which occurs in at least 10% of cases and necessitates shunt removal. Malignant spread may also occur
- *Surgical parietal pleurectomy* may be performed as VATS (video-assisted thoracoscopic surgery). The procedure is effective in the management of refractory malignant effusions. May be useful in a minority of patients with good performance status and prognosis. Not suitable for patients with heavily diseased visceral pleura and trapped lung; consider in patients who have failed pleurodesis
- *Palliative care team* involvement should also be considered.

Parapneumonic effusion and empyema: definition and clinical features

Definition and pathophysiology Pleural effusions occur in up to 40% of patients with pneumonia. An initial sterile exudate (simple parapneumonic effusion) may in some cases progress to a complicated parapneumonic effusion and eventually empyema (Fig. 35.1).

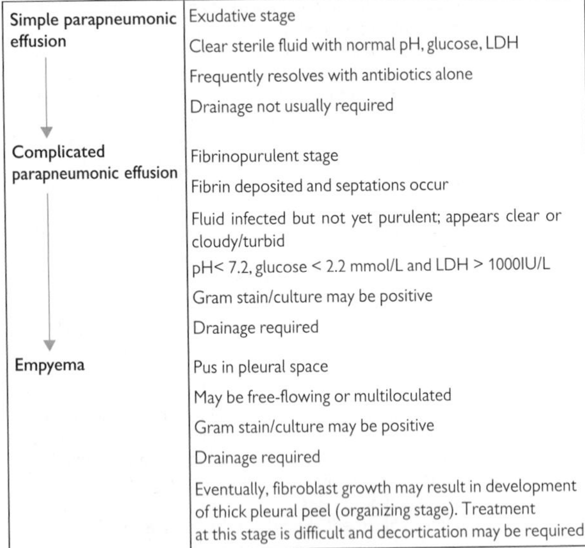

Simple parapneumonic effusion ↓	Exudative stage Clear sterile fluid with normal pH, glucose, LDH Frequently resolves with antibiotics alone Drainage not usually required
Complicated parapneumonic effusion ↓	Fibrinopurulent stage Fibrin deposited and septations occur Fluid infected but not yet purulent; appears clear or cloudy/turbid pH< 7.2, glucose < 2.2 mmol/L and LDH > 1000IU/L Gram stain/culture may be positive Drainage required
Empyema	Pus in pleural space May be free-flowing or multiloculated Gram stain/culture may be positive Drainage required Eventually, fibroblast growth may result in development of thick pleural peel (organizing stage). Treatment at this stage is difficult and decortication may be required

Fig. 35.1 Parapneumonic effusion and empyema: definition and clinical features.

Pleural infection may also occur in the absence of a preceding pneumonic illness ('primary empyema')

Clinical features

Common

- Consider the diagnosis particularly in cases of 'slow to respond' pneumonia, pleural effusion with fever, or high-risk groups with non-specific symptoms such as weight loss
- Similar to clinical presentation of pneumonia: fever, sputum production, chest pain, breathlessness
- Anaerobic empyema may present less acutely, often with weight loss and without fever.

Rare

- Infected pleural fluid may spontaneously drain through the chest wall *(empyema necessitatis)* or into the lung, leading to a bronchopleural fistula and severe pneumonia
- History of atypical chest pain, vomiting, or oesophageal instrumentation suggests possible underlying oesophageal rupture (measure pleural fluid amylase)
- History of a recent sore throat may suggest Lemierre's syndrome (acute oropharyngeal infection with *Fusobacterium* species leads to septic thrombophlebitis of the internal jugular vein and subsequent metastatic infection and abscess formation, commonly in the lungs and pleura; consider ultrasound of internal jugular vein if suspected); see p 446.

Risk factors for developing empyema include diabetes, alcohol abuse, gastro-oesophageal reflux, and intravenous drug abuse. Anaerobic infection is associated particularly with aspiration or poor dental hygiene. Empyema may rarely occur following bronchial obstruction from a tumour or foreign body. Many patients, however, have no apparent risk factors.

Differential diagnosis includes malignancy, tuberculosis (when the pleural fluid is usually lymphocytic), and rheumatoid pleuritis.

Parapneumonic effusion and empyema: bacteriology and investigations

Bacteriology

- ***Community-acquired*** infection (% of cases):
  - *S. milleri* (28%)
  - *Anaerobes* (19%)
  - *S. pneumoniae* (14%)
  - Staphylococci (12%)
  - Other less common organisms include other streptococci, enterobacteria, *H. influenza*, *Pseudomonas*, TB, and *Nocardia*. *Legionella* may very rarely cause empyema
- ***Hospital-acquired*** infection (% of cases):
  - MRSA (27%)
  - Staphylococci (22%)
  - Enterobacteria (20%)
  - Enterococci (12%)
  - Others include streptococci, *Pseudomonas*, and anaerobes.

Gram-negative organisms may occur in mixed growths with other Gram-negatives or with anaerobes.

Investigations

- ***Diagnostic pleural tap*** is essential if pleural infection is suspected. Frankly purulent or turbid/cloudy pleural fluid, organisms on pleural fluid Gram stain or culture, or pleural fluid pH <7.2 are all indications for chest tube drainage. 40% of pleural infections are culture-negative. Identification of anaerobes is improved following inoculation of blood culture bottles with pleural fluid
- ***Ultrasound*** typically shows echogenic effusion that may be septated, and is useful in guiding pleural tap in patients with small or loculated effusions or following an unsuccessful 'blind' tap. Very small effusions (<10 mm maximal thickness on ultrasound) probably do not require tapping and can be observed
- ***Contrast-enhanced CT*** may be useful both in supporting the diagnosis and visualizing the distribution of fluid. Empyema is associated with pleural enhancement and increased attenuation of extrapleural subcostal fat. The displacement of adjacent lung by empyema may help to distinguish from a parenchymal lung abscess. Empyemas frequently appear lenticular and may exhibit the 'split pleura' sign of enhancing separated visceral and parietal pleura. Absence of pleural thickening on CT is unusual in empyema. CT may also sometimes identify a proximal endobronchial obstructing lesion
- ***Blood cultures*** positive in only 13% of cases, but in these cases they are often the only positive microbiology
- ***Bronchoscopy*** is only indicated if a bronchial obstructing lesion is suspected

Parapneumonic effusion and empyema: management and outcome

Management

*1. **Antibiotics*** All patients with pleural infection should be treated with antibiotics; refer to local hospital prescribing guidelines. Typical choices:
- *Community-acquired* empyema—second-generation cephalosporin (e.g. cefuroxime) plus metronidazole as anaerobic cover. Ciprofloxacin and clindamycin together may be appropriate. Add macrolide if *Legionella* is suspected
- *Hospital-acquired* empyema—cover Gram-positive and Gram-negative organisms and anaerobes. MRSA infection is common. Consult with microbiology team. One option is meropenem and vancomycin.

Rationalize with culture and sensitivity results (although note that anaerobes are frequently difficult to culture and may coexist with other organisms). Avoid aminoglycosides, which penetrate the pleural space poorly.

Switch to oral antibiotics when apyrexial and improving clinically. Co-amoxiclav is a useful single agent with anaerobic cover (not if penicillin allergic). Optimal duration of antibiotic treatment unclear, although likely to be at least 3 weeks.

*2. **Chest tube drainage***

Indications for chest tube drainage

- Frankly purulent or turbid/cloudy pleural fluid
- Organisms on pleural fluid Gram stain or culture
- Pleural fluid pH <7.2

Consider earlier chest tube drainage in the elderly and patients with comorbidity, and loculated effusions, as these are associated with a worse outcome.

Drain insertion should ideally be carried out under ultrasound or CT guidance, as effusions are frequently loculated. Ideal chest tube size remains subject to debate. Small (10–14 French) flexible tubes are more comfortable and have been demonstrated to be as effective as large drains in the management of empyema. Usually apply suction (–20 cm water) and flush regularly (e.g. 30 ml normal saline every 6 h) to prevent occlusion. Consider drain removal when clinical improvement occurs. If there is no indication for drainage, give antibiotics and monitor closely. If slow to improve or deteriorate, re-sample the effusion and consider chest drain.

*3. **Intrapleural fibrinolytics*** Current evidence suggests that intrapleural streptokinase has no effect on mortality, need for surgery, or hospital stay, and the routine use of fibrinolytics is therefore not recommended.

4. ***Nutritional support*** Dietician review, consider supplementary nasogastric feeding. Intravenous feeding may be required.

5. ***Surgery*** Consult with thoracic surgeon if there are ongoing features of sepsis and residual pleural collection after 7 days despite tube drainage and treatment with antibiotics. Surgical techniques include:

- *Video-assisted thoracoscopic surgery* (VATS) allows the breakdown of adhesions and drainage of residual collection, but it is frequently unsuccessful in chronic empyema with very thickened visceral pleura
- *Thoracotomy and decortication* Removal of fibrinous and infected tissue from the pleural space: a major surgical procedure
- *Open thoracic drainage* Resection of segments of several ribs adjacent to the empyema and insertion of large-bore drains into the cavity: a more minor procedure that can be performed under local anaesthesia, but results in open chest wound for long period (typically around 5 months).

Difficulties in management

Chest drainage ceases despite residual pleural collection

- Attempt to flush drain with normal saline
- Ensure that drain is not kinked at skin insertion site or lying subcutaneously
- Consider CT to assess extent of residual collection and drain position
- Remove drain if persistently blocked
- Consider further image-guided chest drain(s), surgery

Failure to clinically improve despite antibiotics and chest drain

- Review microbiology results and ensure appropriate antibiotics
- CT to assess extent of residual collection and drain position
- Surgical referral
- Options if unfit for surgery:
    - Further image-guided small-bore drains into loculated effusions
    - Large-bore drain
    - Surgical rib resection and open drainage under local anaesthesia

Outcome About 15% of patients require surgery. Empyema 1-year mortality is about 15%. Increased age, renal impairment, low serum albumin, hypotension, and hospital-acquired infection are associated with a poor outcome. CXR may remain abnormal despite successful treatment of empyema, with evidence of calcification or pleural scarring or thickening.

Further information

Davies CWH *et al.* BTS Guidelines for the management of pleural infection. *Thorax* 2003; **58** (suppl. II): ii 18–28

Maskell NA *et al.* UK controlled trial of intrapleural streptokinase for pleural infection. *NEJM* 2005; **352**: 865–74

Tuberculous pleural effusion

Definition and epidemiology Tuberculous pleural effusion usually develops from a delayed hypersensitivity reaction to mycobacteria released into the pleural space. It is a common manifestation of primary tuberculosis in regions with a high prevalence, affecting children and young adults; it may also be associated with reactivation of tuberculosis in older individuals. May occur more commonly in the setting of HIV co-infection.

Rarely, tuberculosis may present as pseudochylothorax or tuberculous empyema.

Clinical features

- Clinical features are similar to those of pulmonary tuberculosis, i.e. fever, sweats, weight loss, and dyspnoea, although it may present acutely with pleuritic chest pain and fever, mimicking pneumonia
- Effusions are typically small–moderate in volume, although can be massive

Investigations

- Associated parenchymal infiltrate on ***CXR*** in less than one-third of cases
- ***Tuberculin skin tests*** positive in two-thirds of cases
- ***Pleural fluid*** lymphocytosis, exudative effusion, pH and glucose moderately depressed, mesothelial cells rare. Pleural fluid acid-fast bacilli (AFB) smears are positive in around 5–10% of cases; pleural fluid cultures are positive in 25% of cases and take 2–6 weeks
- Blind ***Abrams' pleural biopsy*** alone has a sensitivity of 75%, but this increases to nearly 90% when histology and culture of both the fluid and biopsy are analysed
- ***Thoracoscopic biopsies*** have a sensitivity of nearly 100%
- Measurement of ***adenosine deaminase*** (an enzyme released by macrophages after phagocytosis of mycobacterium) in pleural fluid may be of benefit in regions where tuberculosis is highly prevalent; a raised value is very sensitive for pleural tuberculosis, but is non-specific and may also occur in empyema and malignancy
- ***PCR*** for mycobacterial DNA in the pleural fluid may be useful diagnostically, but is not widely available
- ***Induced sputum*** for acid-fast bacilli may have a diagnostic role in high-risk patients with lymphocytic effusions, even in the absence of parenchymal disease on CXR

Treatment and outcome

- Tuberculous pleural effusions resolve spontaneously in the majority of cases, but two-thirds of untreated patients go on to develop pulmonary tuberculosis within 5 years and so treatment is recommended
- Treatment is the same as for pulmonary tuberculosis (p 494)
- Pleural fluid volumes may increase during effective treatment and therapeutic thoracentesis is often required
- Steroids may reduce fluid volumes, but do not affect long-term outcome
- Pleural thickening and calcification are common long-term consequences of tuberculous pleural effusion.

Other causes

Pleural effusion due to pulmonary embolism

- Fourth commonest cause of pleural effusion in the USA
- Consider in all patients with undiagnosed pleural effusion, particularly if there is a history of pleuritic chest pain or of breathlessness/hypoxia out of proportion to the size of the effusion
- Frequently complicates other disease processes, e.g. occurs in one-fifth of patients with cardiac failure and pleural effusions
- Effusions are usually small (<one-third of hemithorax) and unilateral, although may be bilateral
- Pleural fluid analysis is non-diagnostic; appearance varies from clear to bloody, 80% are exudates and 20% transudates. Bloodstained pleural fluid is not a contraindication to anticoagulation
- Imaging investigations, such as CTPA of the chest, are required to make the diagnosis; these should be performed prior to thoracentesis if pulmonary embolism is strongly suspected.

Rheumatoid arthritis-associated pleural effusion

- Pulmonary changes may be the first manifestation of rheumatoid arthritis
- Rheumatoid pleurisy is more common in men (70% are in men)
- Pleural fluid may be yellow-green, serous, turbid, or bloody
- May be unilateral or bilateral
- Pleural fluid glucose level is frequently low (<1.6 mmol/L), and progressively falls in chronic effusions
- Pleural fluid pH is commonly reduced (<7.3)
- Low pleural fluid complement levels (C4 <0.04 g/L) may also favour the diagnosis
- Elevated pleural fluid rheumatoid factor titre is found, but it is not more diagnostically helpful than serum rheumatoid factor
- Typically persist for months to years, although duration may be several weeks
- Some cases may respond to treatment with steroids

Haemothorax

- Haemothorax is defined as a pleural effusion with a haematocrit >50% of peripheral blood haematocrit
- Causes include trauma, iatrogenic, malignancy, pulmonary infarction, benign asbestos-related pleural effusion, pneumonia, post-cardiac injury syndrome, pneumothorax, thoracic endometriosis, and aortic rupture
- Massive haemothorax defined as >1500 cm^3 of blood in hemithorax, and is most commonly due to trauma. Traumatic haemothorax is said to require a chest drain and sometimes thoracotomy; all cases should be discussed immediately with the cardiothoracic surgical team
- Large volumes of residual blood in the pleural space will clot and may lead to pleural thickening, empyema, or trapped lung. Tube drainage is difficult and thoracoscopy or thoracotomy with decortication are often needed. However, undrained cases can resolve without intervention

Pleural effusion after coronary artery bypass grafting

- Small, typically left-sided pleural effusions occur in the majority of patients post-CABG, and most resolve spontaneously
- Larger (>25% of hemithorax) effusions can be subdivided:
  - Pleural effusions occurring ***within 30 days*** of surgery. Classically bloody and eosinophilic exudate, with high LDH; probably related to post-operative bleeding into pleural space
  - Pleural effusions ***more than 30 days*** after surgery. Typically clear and lymphocytic exudate; cause unknown, perhaps immunological or a form of post-cardiac injury syndrome
- Main symptom in each case is breathlessness; chest pain and fever are unusual
- Management consists of repeated therapeutic thoracentesis to alleviate breathlessness. Recurrent effusions after 1 year are rare and may be difficult to treat; NSAIDs, prednisolone, or thoracoscopy and pleurodesis may be considered
- Differential diagnosis of pleural effusion post-CABG includes pulmonary embolus, cardiac failure, pleural infection, post-cardiac injury syndrome, chylothorax.

Pleural effusion following asbestos exposure

The main differential diagnosis is between benign asbestos pleural effusion (p 110) and mesothelioma (p 114).

Further information

Light RW. Pleural effusions after coronary artery bypass graft surgery. *Curr Opin Pulm Med* 2002; **8**: 308–11

Chapter 36
Pneumoconioses

Overview and causative mineral dusts

- Pneumoconioses are non-neoplastic pulmonary diseases caused by the reaction of the lung to the inhalation of mainly mineral, but also organic, dusts
- Inhaled particles of dust size <5 μm reach the terminal airways and alveoli and settle on the epithelial lining. From here they are slowly cleared by macrophages or alveolar cells. They may pass into the lymphatic system, be cleared via the airway, or remain in the alveolus
- The dust particles can lead to an inflammatory reaction within the lung, depending on their physical and chemical properties
- The inflammation causes characteristic alterations in pulmonary structure and radiological abnormalities
- Of the diseases caused by inhalation of mineral dusts, many are becoming less common in the UK, due to improved protection of workers from dusts and decreasing levels of mining. Newer industrial nations may see increasing numbers of cases of pneumoconiosis
- Organic dusts causing hypersensitivity pneumonitis and extrinsic asthma are discussed on p 249 and 142. Asbestos-related diseases are discussed separately on p 107.

Table 36.1 Causative mineral dusts

Mineral dust	Disease	Examples of exposure
Coal dust	Simple pneumoconiosis Progressive massive fibrosis Caplan's syndrome	Coal mining, especially hard coal
Silica	Silicosis Caplan's syndrome	Foundry work, sandblasting, stone cutting, hard rock mining
Asbestos	Asbestosis Benign asbestos-related pleural disease Mesothelioma Lung cancer	Mining, milling, and fabrication Installation and removal of insulation
Beryllium	Acute berylliosis Beryllium granulomatosis	Mining, fabrication of electrical and electronic equipment, workers in nuclear and aerospace industry
Iron oxide	Siderosis	Welding
Barium sulphate	Baritosis	Mining
Tin oxide	Stannosis	Mining
Aluminium	Like silicosis (bauxite worker's lung, Shaver's disease)	Mining, firework, painting, and armament manufacture

Types of mineral dust exposure

Non-fibrous mineral dusts

- Silica
- Coal dust
- Mixed mineral dusts containing quartz: slate, kaolin, talc, non-fibrous clays.

Fibrous mineral dusts

- Asbestos
- Other mineral fibres.

Metal dusts and fumes

- Iron, aluminium, beryllium, cobalt.

Chest disease in coal miners It was recognized many years ago that coal miners had higher levels of respiratory disease than the general population. Coal miners can get any or all of:

- Chronic bronchitis
- COPD
- Pneumoconiosis.

They may be eligible for compensation for all of these. It has been difficult to establish the independent effects of coal dust due to high smoking rates amongst miners. However, it is now thought that coal dust contributes to the COPD and bronchitis caused by smoking, because:

- Miners have an increased prevalence of cough, sputum, and decreased FEV_1 when compared with non-miners. The risk of cough increases with increasing dust exposure
- FEV_1 declines in proportion to the amount of dust exposure
- In smokers the response to dust is probably different to that of non-smokers, with worse disease at a given level of exposure.

In the past, tuberculosis has also been a major problem amongst miners and their families, relating to their socio-economic conditions.

SWORD is the Surveillance of Work-related and Occupational Respiratory Disease scheme run in the UK to monitor the numbers of patients with occupational lung diseases. Patients with a clinical diagnosis of an occupational lung disease are confidentially reported by respiratory or occupational health physicians.

Further information

www.dti.gov.uk/coalhealth

Coal-worker's pneumoconiosis

This is the condition caused by the deposition of coal dust within the lung and its associated inflammatory reaction.

There are two types:

- Simple pneumoconiosis, which can progress to
- Complicated pneumoconiosis, also known as progressive massive fibrosis (PMF).

These are common diseases amongst coal miners who work in poorly ventilated conditions. The risk of pneumoconiosis varies with different compositions of coal from different geographical areas, but the larger the amount of dust to which the miner is exposed, the greater the risk of developing pneumoconiosis. It is now rare for miners under the age of 50 to be diagnosed with pneumoconiosis in the UK.

Pathology

Simple pneumoconiosis Coal dust is inhaled into the alveolus and is engulfed by macrophages, forming a black stellate lesion, the coal macule. This causes cytokine release and subsequent inflammatory cell recruitment, leading to fibroblast activation. These coal macules are found throughout the lung, especially in the upper zones of the upper and lower lobes, and often associated with surrounding bronchiolar dilatation. They are not palpable. Regional lymph nodes also become blackened. In time, larger nodules develop, containing reticulin and collagen between the macrophages, and associated bronchiolar dilatation leading to focal emphysema is seen.

Progressive massive fibrosis occurs on this background, but with aggregation of the fibrotic nodules to form larger lesions, 2–10 cm diameter. Macroscopically, these look like large black scars, extending from the lung parenchyma to the chest wall. The central area of these nodules may be necrotic and the outer rim is firm and collagenous. It is not understood what causes the progression of small nodules to PMF, although continued exposure to coal dust in the presence of simple pneumoconiosis makes this development more likely.

Clinical features

Simple pneumoconiosis is usually asymptomatic with no associated clinical signs. This is a relatively benign disease.

Progressive massive fibrosis is usually associated with cough, productive of mucoid or blackened sputum, and breathlessness, particularly on exertion, and may in time lead to the development of cor pulmonale. Examination is unremarkable, with no clubbing and no crepitations audible (the presence of crepitations suggests a different diagnosis).

Investigations

- ***CXR*** In *simple pneumoconiosis* there is nodular shadowing, with nodules of varying size, up to 10 mm, particularly in the upper and middle zones. Pneumoconiosis can be graded according to the number of different sized nodules, p = <1.5 mm, q = 1.5–3 mm, and r = 3–10 mm. Nodule numbers increase with increasing dust inhalation and usually stop forming when the miner has left the work environment. *PMF* is diagnosed when one or more opacities of >1 cm diameter are present, on the background of simple pneumoconiosis. These lesions are often located in the upper lobes and enlarge, becoming increasingly radiodense and clearly demarcated with time. They may distort the adjacent lung and cause emphysema. The lesions continue to progress out of the work environment
- ***HRCT*** of *simple pneumoconiosis* shows parenchymal nodules 1–10 mm in size, with upper zone predominance. In *PMF*, nodules of >1 cm are seen, with irregular borders and associated parenchymal distortion and emphysema. Larger lesions may have cavitation and necrosis. They may also have areas of calcification
- ***PFTs*** *Simple pneumoconiosis*: FEV_1 and FVC are normal, although TLCO may be slightly decreased. *PMF*: signs of airway obstruction due to emphysema, and restriction due to loss of lung volumes. TLCO is reduced.

Management Minimization of dust exposure with improved mine ventilation, respirator provision, and monitoring of dust levels. Miners have CXR every 4 years and are moved to less dusty work if they show signs of pneumoconiosis, to prevent the development of PMF. Miners with signs of coal worker's pneumoconiosis are entitled to industrial injury benefits from British Coal. No increased risk of lung cancer with pneumoconiosis or PMF.

Caplan's syndrome Miners with seropositive rheumatoid arthritis or positive serum rheumatoid factor can develop large well-defined nodules. These occur on a background of simple pneumoconiosis and in those with a relatively low coal dust exposure. They may be multiple and may cavitate. They cause no significant functional impairment and have no malignant potential.

Silicosis

This is a chronic nodular densely fibrosing pneumoconiosis, caused by the prolonged inhalation of silica particles.

- Long lag time of decades between exposure and clinical disease
- Insidious onset, progressive
- Larger radiological opacities than those seen in coal-worker's pneumoconiosis and more rapid progression
- The pattern of disease depends on the level and duration of the silicone dust exposure.

Silica is present mostly as crystalline quartz, which is mined and quarried, and used in industries such as ceramics, brick-making, and stone masonry. It is becoming less prevalent in Western societies, due to changes in silica working conditions.

Pathology Quartz and cristobalite forms of crystalline silica cause silicosis. When they accumulate within the airways, lymphocytes and alveolar macrophages engulf the particles and are removed into the lymphatic system. Any remaining silica dust causes focal aggregations of macrophages, which are, in time, converted into fibrosing nodules. Silica dust can cause surfactant secretion from the alveolus due to local irritation. This leads to further macrophage recruitment. Large nodules are formed by the aggregation of smaller nodules.

Different types of silicosis There are four types, and the distinction is often not clear.

- ***Acute silicosis*** is caused by intense exposure to fine dusts, such as those produced by sand blasting. It may become apparent in workers within a few months to a year of starting work. Rapid deterioration over 1–2 years, with treatment being ineffective. Rare now, due to regulation of silica levels in the workplace
  - *Clinically* dry cough, shortness of breath, and a feeling of tightness on breathing deeply. Rapid deterioration over a few weeks. Fine crepitations are heard over the lower zones bilaterally. Respiratory failure
  - *CXR* Patchy bilateral lower air space consolidation, which may look like pulmonary oedema
  - *Pathology* Irregular fibrosis adjacent to alveolar spaces filled with a lipoproteinaceous exudate, similar to that found in alveolar proteinosis.
- ***Subacute silicosis*** This is the classic picture of silicosis, which is now quite rare. Dry cough, gradual onset of shortness of breath
  - *CXR* Upper and mid-zone nodules are present, measuring between 3 and 5 mm diameter. Initially indistinct, but become clearer with time. Nodules coalesce and calcify and can progress to progressive massive fibrosis (PMF). Associated calcified hilar lymphadenopathy (egg shell calcification) and possible pleural thickening. Nodules continue to develop with continued exposure, but due to long lag time will also develop when patient stops being exposed. In some cases with heavy exposure to silica, patients may develop progressive upper zone fibrosis with sparse nodularity

  - *PFTs* Slow decline, including TLCO, with mild restrictive pattern, unless the silicosis has caused emphysema, when obstructive or mixed picture is seen
  - *Pathology* Dust particles within the alveoli are phagocytosed by macrophages. They are removed to the lymphatics, where they lodge and cause diffuse inflammatory change. Layers of collagen are deposited around the dust particle. Nodules are found within the secondary pulmonary lobule, where they cause fibrosis
- ***Chronic silicosis*** occurs with lower dust concentrations than those seen in active silicosis
  - *CXR* A few upper and mid-zone nodules occur, which become calcified after 10 years or so. There is no associated parenchymal distortion. There may be associated hilar lymphadenopathy.

If there is further silica exposure, this disease may progress, with coalescence of nodules.

- ***Silicotuberculosis*** Increased likelihood of active TB infection in people with silicosis, most likely due to the reactivation of quiescent lesions. Silica within the lung is thought to affect the efficacy of the macrophage at clearing *Mycobacterium tuberculosis*. TB can be difficult to diagnose, due to multiple pre-existing CXR nodules. Cavitation may occur, which does not occur with silicosis alone. Haemoptysis, fever, and new soft CXR opacities should prompt sputum examination and BAL. Confirmed TB should be treated with the usual 3 or 4 drug regime. Non-tuberculous mycobacterial infection is also more common.

Management Prevention of silicosis by monitoring and minimizing dust levels with adequate ventilation. Masks can be useful for short-term use, if the high levels of dust are transiently unavoidable. Disability benefits available from the Department for Work and Pensions. Small increased risk of lung cancer with silicosis and associated PMF.

Berylliosis

Beryllium is a light, strong industrial metal. It is mined and often used as an alloy in the manufacture of fluorescent tubes for lighting and televisions, radiological equipment, in atomic reactors, and in heat-resistant ceramics. Cases of berylliosis are now rare, as beryllium levels have been tightly regulated to avoid sensitization. However, due to the long latent period between exposure and granuloma formation, as well as accidental beryllium exposure, cases are still occurring. There are two types of disease.

- ***Acute beryllium disease*** is an acute alveolitis due to the direct effects of high-dose inhaled beryllium fumes. There is subsequent widespread airway oedema and pulmonary oedema, which causes dyspnoea, cyanosis, and widespread inspiratory crepitations. CXR shows pulmonary oedema. It may be self-limiting if mild, but if severe is usually fatal. Corticosteroids may prevent progression, but the patient is often left with residual pulmonary impairment
- ***Subacute and chronic berylliosis*** is a hypersensitivity-type skin or pulmonary disease that occurs a long time after beryllium exposure in a minority of individuals. It can be clinically indistinguishable from sarcoidosis. It has also been seen in the wives of beryllium workers and those who live near beryllium refineries. Inhalation of beryllium or the exposure of beryllium to a skin abrasion causes initial sensitization in 2–19% of exposed individuals. Only low levels of exposure are required for this. There is a cell-mediated immune response, with the production of numerous inflammatory cytokines, which cause granulomatous inflammation. Following a long latent period, which may be months to 10 years plus after exposure, non-caseating granulomatous tissue reactions occur in the lungs or on the skin. Similar to sarcoidosis. There is a genetic predisposition to the response to beryllium exposure and it is HLA-mediated (HLA-DPB1(Glu69)). HLA status could be used to identify workers at high risk of berylliosis (but is not routinely used at present).

Clinical features of chronic berylliosis

- ***Symptoms*** Cough, dyspnoea. Macular skin lesions, which do not spontaneously resolve
- ***Signs*** No clubbing or crepitations in early disease, but both occur with established fibrosis. Hepato/splenomegaly and macular skin lesions. Do not get uveitis or erythema nodosum.

Investigations

- ***CXR*** Fine reticulonodular appearance throughout both lungs. Finer nodules than those seen in sarcoidosis. Progression to irregular interstitial fibrosis, with irregular linear opacities seen in the lung bases. Hilar lymphadenopathy can occur, but always in association with interstitial lung disease
- ***HRCT*** Subpleural micronodular change, thickened interlobular septae, traction bronchiectasis, and honeycombing. There may be ground-glass shadowing
- ***BAL*** High levels of T-lymphocytes
- ***PFTs*** Restrictive defect, with decreased KCO

- ***Pathology*** Non-caseating granuloma. May be indistinguishable from sarcoidosis. May develop irregular fibrosis with bulla and cyst formation

No single test to distinguish berylliosis from sarcoidosis.

Management Corticosteroids to try and prevent disease progression. Continue indefinitely as few patients gain complete resolution of symptoms, CXR or PFTs. Annual screening of beryllium-exposed workers with CXR. If they develop breathlessness or skin rashes, this may be an indication to start oral steroids to delay progression to interstitial fibrosis.

Prognosis Progressive disease, although those with very low exposure who develop CXR changes may find they resolve. Associated delayed skin sensitivity (anergy) to tuberculin. Granulomata do not spontaneously resolve, although can be excised if causing problems, such as troublesome lesions on the skin. Interstitial fibrosis occurs in the lungs, which is progressive and leads to cyanosis and death. Other complications include pneumothorax, hypercalcaemia, hypercalciuria, and nephrocalcinosis.

Differential diagnosis

- Sarcoidosis
- Tuberculosis.

In clinic

- Ask patients with suspected sarcoidosis about possible exposure to beryllium
- Monitor PFTs and CXR to assess disease response or progression.

Chapter 37

Pneumothorax

Clinical features and investigations

Definition A pneumothorax is air in the pleural space. May occur with apparently normal lungs (primary pneumothorax) or in the presence of underlying lung disease (secondary pneumothorax). May occur spontaneously or following trauma.

Epidemiology

- Annual incidence of primary pneumothorax is around 9 per 100 000
- Primary pneumothoraces occur most commonly in tall thin men aged between 20 and 40. They are less common in women (male : female 5: 1)—consider the possibility of underlying lung disease (e.g. lymphangioleiomyomatosis, catamenial pneumothorax)
- Cigarette smoking is a major risk factor for pneumothorax, increasing the risk by a factor of 22 in men and 9 in women. The mechanism is unclear; a smoking-induced influx of inflammatory cells may both break down elastic lung fibres (causing bulla formation) and cause small airways obstruction (increasing alveolar pressure and the likelihood of interstitial air leak)
- May rarely be familial.

Causes and pathophysiology

Primary

Pathogenesis is poorly understood; they are presumed to occur following an air leak from apical bullae, although small airway inflammation is often also present and may contribute by increasing airways resistance.

Secondary

- Underlying diseases include: COPD (60% of cases), asthma, interstitial lung disease, necrotizing pneumonia, tuberculosis, PCP, cystic fibrosis, Langerhans cell histiocytosis, lymphangioleiomyomatosis, Marfan's syndrome, oesophageal rupture, lung cancer, catamenial pneumothorax, and pulmonary infarction
- Pneumothorax may be the first presentation of the underlying disease.

Clinical features

- Classically presents with acute onset of pleuritic chest pain and/or breathlessness. Breathlessness is often minimal in young patients and is more severe in secondary pneumothorax
- Signs of pneumothorax include tachycardia, reduced expansion, hyper-resonant percussion note, and quiet breath sounds on the pneumothorax side. These are frequently absent in small pneumothoraces. Hamman's sign refers to a 'click' on auscultation in time with the heart sounds, due to movement of pleural surfaces with a left-sided pneumothorax
- May feel 'bubbles' and 'crackles' under the skin of the torso and neck if there is subcutaneous emphysema
- Presents in ventilated patients with acute clinical deterioration and hypoxia or increasing inflation pressures.

Investigations

- ***CXR*** is the diagnostic test in most cases, revealing a visible lung edge and absent lung markings peripherally. Blunting of the ipsilateral costophrenic angle due to bleeding into the pleural space is common. Pneumothoraces are difficult to visualize on supine films: look for a sharply delineated heart border, hemidiaphragm depression, and increased lucency on the affected side
    - Width of the rim of air surrounding the lung on CXR may be used to classify pneumothoraces into small (rim of air <2 cm) and large (≥2 cm). A 2-cm rim of air approximately equates to a 50% pneumothorax in volume
    - Tiny pneumothoraces that are not apparent on PA CXR may be visible on lateral chest or lateral decubitus radiographs
    - CXR appearance may also show features of underlying lung disease, although this can be difficult to assess in the presence of a large pneumothorax
- ***CT chest*** may be required to differentiate pneumothorax from bullous disease, and is useful in diagnosing unsuspected pneumothorax following trauma and in looking for evidence of underlying lung disease
- ***ABGs*** frequently show hypoxia and sometimes hypercapnia in secondary pneumothorax

Prognosis

- Average of 30% (range 16–54% in studies) of primary pneumothoraces recur, most within 2 years. Continued smoking increases the risk of recurrence. Risk of recurrence increases with each subsequent pneumothorax: risk of recurrence is around 30% after a first pneumothorax, about 40% after a second, and >50% after a third
- Mortality of secondary pneumothorax 10%
- Recurrence of secondary pneumothorax occurs in 39–47%, and is associated with age, pulmonary fibrosis, and emphysema. Recurrence rates may be as high as 80% in patients with Langerhans cell histiocytosis or lymphangioleiomyomatosis.

Further information

Sahn SA, Heffner JE. Spontaneous pneumothorax. *NEJM* 2000, **342**: 868–74

Initial management

There is considerable variation amongst clinicians regarding optimal pneumothorax management. The treatment algorithms presented on pp 380–1 follow the BTS guidelines.

General management points

- Management is determined by the degree of breathlessness and hypoxia, evidence of haemodynamic compromise, the presence and severity of any underlying lung disease, and to some extent the pneumothorax size
- Severe breathlessness out of proportion to pneumothorax size may be a feature of impending tension pneumothorax
- Secondary pneumothorax has a significant mortality (10%), and should be managed more aggressively. Treat also the underlying disease.

Aspiration

- Procedure described on p 779
- Halt the procedure if painful, or if the patient coughs excessively; do not aspirate >2.5 L of air, as this suggests a large air leak and aspiration is likely to fail
- Ideal timing of repeat CXR following aspiration is unknown; it may be advisable to wait several hours before performing the CXR, in order to detect slow air leaks
- Aspiration is successful if the lung is fully or nearly re-expanded on CXR
- If initial aspiration of a primary pneumothorax fails, repeat aspiration should be considered (unless ≥ 2.5 L has already been aspirated). At least one-third of patients will respond to second aspiration, although the optimal timing of repeat aspiration is unclear.

Chest drainage

- Procedure described on p 757
- Associated with significant morbidity and even mortality, and not required in the majority of patients with primary spontaneous pneumothorax
- Small (10–14F) drains are sufficient in most cases; consider large-bore (24–28F) drain in secondary pneumothorax with large air leak, severe subcutaneous emphysema, or in mechanically ventilated patients
- Never clamp a bubbling chest drain (risk of tension pneumothorax)
- When air leak appears to have ceased, clamping of the drain for several hours followed by repeat CXR may detect very slow or intermittent air leaks, thereby avoiding inappropriate drain removal; this is controversial, however, and should only be considered on a specialist ward with experienced nursing staff. Addition of washing-up liquid to water in underwater seal bottle aids visualization of bubbling in very slow air leaks.

- If drain water level does not swing with respiration, the drain is kinked (check underneath dressing, as tube enters skin), blocked, clamped, or incorrectly positioned (drainage holes not in pleural space; check CXR)
- Heimlich flutter valves (or thoracic vents) are an alternative to underwater bottle drainage, and are being used increasingly in some centres. They allow greater patient mobilization, and sometimes out-patient management of pneumothorax.

Oxygen

All hospitalized patients should receive high flow (10 L/min) inspired oxygen (unless CO_2 retention is a problem). This reduces the partial pressure of nitrogen in blood, encouraging removal of air from the pleural space and speeding up resolution of the pneumothorax.

Persistent air leak

- Defined as continued bubbling of chest drain 48 h after insertion
- Consider drain suction (–10 to –20 cmH_2O), insertion of large-bore drain, and/or thoracic surgical referral
- Check that persistent bubbling is not the result of 'outside' air being sucked down the drain, e.g. following drain displacement such that a hole lies outside the pleural cavity, or, if enlargement of the drain track occurs, allowing outside air to enter and then be released down the drain.

Discharge

Prior to discharge, discuss flying and diving (see p 378), and advise to return to hospital immediately if breathlessness worsens. Document this in medical notes.

Further management

Out-patient follow-up

- Repeat CXR to ensure resolution of pneumothorax and normal appearance of underlying lungs
- Discuss risk of recurrence and emphasize smoking cessation, if appropriate
- Ascent to altitude with a pneumothorax is potentially hazardous. Guidelines recommend that patients should not fly for at least one week from the resolution of spontaneous pneumothorax on CXR. This time interval is arbitrary, however, and patients should understand that there is a high initial risk of recurrence that falls with time, and they may wish to avoid flying for a longer period, e.g. 1 year
- Advise never to dive in the future, unless patient has undergone a definitive surgical procedure.

Surgical management

Indications for cardiothoracic surgical referral

- Second ipsilateral pneumothorax
- First contralateral pneumothorax
- Bilateral spontaneous pneumothorax
- Persistent air leak (>5–7 days of drainage)
- Spontaneous haemothorax
- Professions at risk (e.g. pilots, divers) after first pneumothorax.

Note that these are guidelines only, and patient choice will also influence the decision for surgical intervention.

Surgical treatments aim to repair the apical hole or bleb, and close the pleural space. Options:

- *Video-assisted thoracoscopic surgery (VATS)* Recurrence rates are higher than for open thoracotomy (4% vs. 1.5%), although less invasive procedure and probably shorter hospital stay. Pleural abrasion (rather than talc poudrage) is usually favoured for closure of the pleural space. Often the procedure of choice in young patients with primary pneumothorax
- *Open thoracotomy* Apical bleb resected, pleural space closed by pleural abrasion or parietal pleurectomy. Effective procedure with a recurrence rate <1%, but probably prolonged recovery rates compared with VATS
- *Transaxillary minithoracotomy* uses a relatively small axillary incision and may be a less invasive alternative to open thoracotomy.

Chemical pleurodesis

- Talc or tetracycline most commonly used; procedure described on p 775
- Can be performed via intercostal drain or at VATS
- Failure rates around 10–20%, and some concern about the long-term safety of intrapleural talc; therefore not recommended in younger patients
- Consider pleurodesis via intercostal drain only as a last resort in older patients with recurrent pneumothorax in whom surgery would be high risk (e.g. patients with severe COPD)
- Likelihood of successful pleurodesis in the setting of an incompletely re-expanded lung with a persistent air leak remains uncertain, although it may be attempted if surgery is not an option.

Treatment algorithm for primary pneumothorax

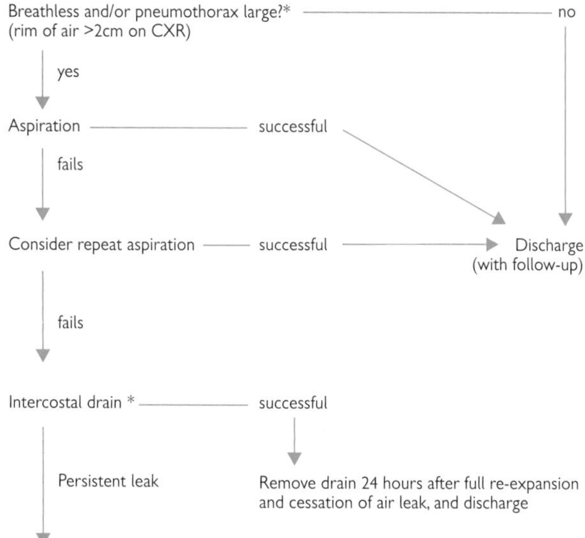

Fig. 37.1 Treatment algorithm for primary pneumothorax.

*Some disagreement exists regarding this point: in the setting of a relatively asymptomatic patient with a large pneumothorax, the risk of intervention may outweigh the risk of the pneumothorax, and conservative management may be considered.

Treatment algorithm for secondary pneumothorax

Consider in-patient observation without aspiration in relatively asymptomatic patients with tiny (<1 cm) pneumothoraces.

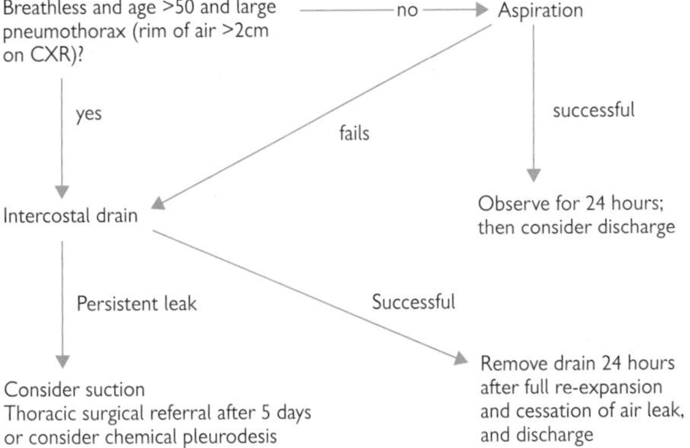

Fig. 37.2 Treatment algorithm for secondary pneumothorax.

Further information

Henry M *et al.* BTS Guidelines for the management of spontaneous pneumothorax. *Thorax* 2003; **58** (suppl. II): ii39–52

Specific situations

Tension pneumothorax

- Pneumothorax acts as a one-way valve, with air entering the pleural space on each inspiration and unable to escape on expiration. The progressive increase in pleural pressure compresses both lungs and mediastinum and inhibits venous return to the heart, leading to hypotension and potentially cardiac arrest
- Occurrence is not related to pneumothorax size, and tension can occur with very small pneumothoraces in the context of air trapping in the lung from obstructive lung disease
- Typically presents with acute respiratory distress, agitation, hypotension, raised jugular venous pressure, and tracheal deviation away from the pneumothorax side. Reduced air entry on affected side
- May present with cardiac arrest (pulseless electrical activity), or with acute deterioration in ventilated patients.

►► Management of a tension pneumothorax

- If strong clinical suspicion, give high-flow oxygen and insert large-bore cannula into second intercostal space in mid-clavicular line on side of pneumothorax
- Do not wait for a CXR if patient seriously compromised or cardiac arrest has occurred
- Do not wait for a CXR if the diagnosis is clinically certain
- Hiss of escaping air confirms diagnosis
- Aspirate air until the patient is less distressed and then insert chest drain in mid-axillary line, leaving cannula in place until finished and the underwater seal is bubbling satisfactorily.

Iatrogenic pneumothorax

- Causes include transbronchial biopsy, transthoracic needle lung biopsy, subclavian line insertion, mechanical ventilation, pleural aspiration, pleural biopsy, external cardiac massage, and percutaneous liver biopsy
- Presentation may be delayed, even several days after procedure
- Most cases do not require intervention and improve with observation, although aspiration is sometimes required
- Drainage is seldom needed, although is more commonly required in patients with COPD. The exception is mechanically ventilated patients, who will require an intercostal drain in the majority of cases.

Traumatic pneumothorax

- Up to half may not be clinically apparent or visible on CXR; chest CT is required for diagnosis
- Majority of patients require intercostal drain. Ensure adequate analgesia; intercostal nerve block may be required
- Consider VATS early if persistent air leak.

Subcutaneous (or 'surgical') emphysema

- Occurs as air tracks below skin under pressure from the pleural space
- May result from large air-leaks, particularly in the presence of underlying lung disease, such as COPD. Also may occur if chest drain is blocked or displaced so that holes lie subcutaneously
- Harmless in majority of cases, although rarely may result in significant respiratory compromise from upper airway compression
- Treat with high-flow (10 L/min) inspired oxygen (unless CO_2 retention a problem). Check that the drain is patent (swinging, bubbling)
- Management if unwell: oxygen, large-bore chest drain on suction. If the airway is compromised, consider anaesthetizing and incising areas of affected skin, and 'milking' out subcutaneous air; subcutaneous drains are sometimes used, and in rare cases tracheostomy is required.

Pneumothorax in HIV

- Most commonly occurs as a result of PCP. Empirical treatment of PCP is advised (see p 478)
- Use of nebulized pentamidine may increase the risk of pneumothorax
- Consider early intercostal drainage and surgical referral.

Pneumothorax in cystic fibrosis

- Associated with severe underlying lung disease
- Subsequent ipsilateral and contralateral pneumothorax common
- Manage as for secondary pneumothorax, although intercostal drainage frequently required
- Give course of intravenous antibiotics
- In cases of persistent air leak despite suction, discuss management with cardiothoracic surgical team at local transplant centre. Partial pleurectomy is effective in preventing recurrence. Pleurodesis renders later transplant technically more difficult, but it is not an absolute contraindication to transplantation.

Catamenial pneumothorax

- Pneumothorax occurring at the same time as menstruation
- Usually recurrent
- Pathogenesis is unknown; possibilities include pleural endometriosis or transfer of air into pleural spaces through a diaphragmatic defect from the peritoneal cavity at menstruation
- Treatment options: VATS, pleurodesis, ovulation-suppressing drugs.

Re-expansion pulmonary oedema

- Occurs in up to 14% of cases following treatment, and causes breathlessness and cough with evidence of oedema in the re-expanded lung (and sometimes both lungs) on CXR
- More common in young patients with large primary pneumothoraces, and may be associated with late presentations to hospital
- May be precipitated by early use of suction (<48 h)
- Self-resolving in most cases, although may rarely be fatal.

Chapter 38

Pulmonary hypertension

Classification

Definition Pulmonary hypertension is a mean pulmonary artery pressure (PAP) >25 mmHg with a pulmonary capillary or left atrial pressure <15 mmHg.

A rise in pulmonary artery pressure can be due to:

- Increased pulmonary blood flow, e.g. atrial septal defect with left to right shunting
- Increased resistance in the pulmonary vascular bed, e.g. vascular remodelling in pulmonary arterial hypertension
- Elevated pulmonary venous pressure, e.g. left ventricular failure.

WHO classification of pulmonary hypertension, 2003

1. Pulmonary arterial hypertension
- Idiopathic pulmonary arterial hypertension (IPAH, previously known as primary pulmonary hypertension)
- Familial pulmonary arterial hypertension (FPAH)
- Related to:
  - Collagen vascular disease
  - Congenital systemic to pulmonary shunts
  - Portal hypertension
  - HIV infection
  - Drugs/toxins: anorectic agents (fenfluramine, dexfenfluramine), rape seed oil, others
  - Very likely causes: amphetamine, L-tryptophan
  - Possible: methamphetamine, cocaine, chemotherapy agents
  - Other (glycogen storage diseases, haemoglobinopathies, myeloproliferative disorders, hereditary haemorrhagic telangiectasia, splenectomy)
- Associated with significant venous or capillary involvement
  - Pulmonary veno-occlusive disease
  - Pulmonary capillary haemangiomatosis
  - Sickle cell disease

2. Pulmonary venous hypertension
- Left-sided atrial or ventricular heart disease
- Left-sided valvular heart disease

3. Pulmonary hypertension associated with hypoxaemia
- Chronic obstructive pulmonary disease
- Interstitial lung disease
- Sleep disordered breathing
- Alveolar hypoventilation disorders
- Chronic high-altitude exposure

4. Pulmonary hypertension due to chronic thrombotic and/or embolic disease
- Thromboembolic obstruction of proximal pulmonary arteries
- Obstruction of distal pulmonary arteries
  - Pulmonary embolism (thrombus, tumour, ova, parasites, foreign material)

5. Pulmonary hypertension associated with miscellaneous disorders
- Inflammatory
  - Langerhans cell histiocytosis
  - Sarcoidosis
  - Other
- Extrinsic compression of the central pulmonary veins
  - Fibrosing mediastinitis
  - Lymphadenopathy/tumours

Idiopathic pulmonary arterial hypertension (IPAH)

Definition Idiopathic pulmonary arterial hypertension (IPAH), previously called primary pulmonary hypertension (PPH), is a rare disease of uncertain aetiology. It is defined as a mean pulmonary artery pressure >25 mmHg at rest (or >30 mmHg on exercise) with a pulmonary capillary or left atrial pressure <15 mmHg. By definition there is no demonstrable cause. The presence of resting pulmonary hypertension is significant, as more than 70% of the vascular bed must be lost for the pulmonary arterial pressure to rise.

Epidemiology The incidence of IPAH in Europe and the USA is 1–2 cases per million population per year. The mean age at diagnosis is 36, with a female preponderance of about 2:1. Although rare, it is important to diagnose, as it affects a young age group and has an extremely poor outcome without treatment.

Pathophysiology Vasoconstriction and secondary thickening of peripheral 'resistance' blood vessels in association with smooth muscle cell and endothelial cell proliferation and thrombosis lead to raised pulmonary vascular resistance. The mechanism for this is poorly understood, but the identification of a mutation in BMPR2, which is present in 70% of familial cases of PAH, has improved understanding. BMPR2, bone morphogenetic protein receptor type II, is a receptor in the transforming growth factor beta (TGFB) receptor superfamily and is an important regulator of apoptosis and proliferation. It is hypothesized that defective signalling via this pathway may result in abnormal endothelial proliferation and cell growth in response to various insults, with an inability to terminate the proliferative response to injury. Due to incomplete disease penetrance in the presence of a mutation in BMPR2 (15–20%), it is thought that the genetic abnormality may have to be accompanied by some additional environmental factor, e.g. hypoxia to cause PAH. Allelic variations in the serotonin transporter have also been identified.

An imbalance between prostacyclin (a potent vasodilator and platelet inhibitor) and thromboxane A2 (a potent vasoconstrictor and platelet agonist) has been identified in PAH. Unfavourable imbalances between other regulators of vascular tone and smooth muscle cell growth, including endothelin-1, nitric oxide, and serotonin have also been implicated in the disease.

Acute hypoxia causes reversible changes in vascular tone, with chronic hypoxia inducing structural vascular remodelling, which can add significantly to morbidity in certain lung diseases.

Aetiology

- *Idiopathic IPAH* This is a disease for which, strictly speaking, no cause is found, although a number of risk factors have been identified, and BMPR2 mutations may be present in up to 25%. The identified risk factors for IPAH have in common an ability to damage the pulmonary endothelium, which may provoke an excessive proliferative response, progressing to IPAH.
- *Familial IPAH* A familial predisposition is seen in 6–10% of IPAH cases, where the disease is transmitted in an autosomal dominant fashion. Incomplete penetrance and anticipation are seen, with presentation at a younger age in successive generations. The responsible gene has been localized to chromosome 2 (locus 2q 31–32). Abnormal cardiovascular responses to exercise have been demonstrated in asymptomatic carriers of BMPR2.
- *Associations*
  - *Anorexigens* are associated with the development of PAH, with an increased incidence with longer duration of use. A raised PAP can occur after only 4 weeks of drug use.
  - *CNS stimulants* Cocaine and methamphetamine are associated with the development of PAH.
  - *Scleroderma* Post mortem studies show histological changes consistent with PAH in up to 80% of patients with scleroderma spectrum disease, including SLE, mixed connective tissue disease, and RA. The reported lifetime incidence of PAH in scleroderma varies, but may be about 15%. In all of these diseases there is a strong association between PAH and Raynaud's phenomenon, suggesting pathological similarities between these two conditions.
  - *HIV* PAH is found in HIV infected individuals, regardless of the route of infection. The incidence is about 0.5%, 6–12 times higher than the general population. The development of PAH is independent of CD4 cell count, but is associated with duration of infection. The mechanism is unclear.
  - *Portal hypertension* PAH is seen in up to 5% of patients with portal hypertension, increasing with duration of liver disease. The mechanism is uncertain, but it appears that cirrhosis without portal hypertension is insufficient for the development of PAH.
  - *Hereditary haemorrhagic telangiectasia* PAH occurs in around 15% of patients with HHT, an autosomal dominant vascular dysplasia. Mutations in the ALK-1 receptor (also in the TGFB receptor superfamily) are implicated.

Prognosis is variable, depending on haemodynamic compromise with cardiac index, right atrial pressure, and mean pulmonary artery pressure at presentation being linked to prognosis. The median survival in NYHA functional class 3 (symptomatic on mild exertion) is 2.8 years and 6 months in NYHA class IV (symptomatic at rest) without treatment.

IPAH: clinical features

The symptoms of idiopathic pulmonary arterial hypertension are non-specific, leading to an average delay in diagnosis of 3 years from first symptoms.

Presenting features

- Exertional breathlessness, due to the inability to increase cardiac output with exercise
- Chest pain (right heart angina)
- Syncope, due to a fall in systemic blood pressure on exercise
- Palpitations
- Oedema, or other signs of right-sided fluid overload.

Examination Signs consistent with right heart fluid overload and right ventricular hypertrophy are associated with advanced disease and include:

- Raised JVP, with giant V waves
- Right ventricular heave
- Wide splitting of S2 with loud P2
- Murmur of tricuspid regurgitation
- Hepatomegaly
- Ascites
- Peripheral oedema
- Cyanosis.

Investigations These are aimed at making a diagnosis of idiopathic pulmonary arterial hypertension by excluding possible underlying causes for the pulmonary hypertension. In 85% of patients presenting with symptoms caused by established pulmonary hypertension, a CXR and ECG will be abnormal.

- ***CXR*** may show enlarged pulmonary arteries and an enlarged cardiac silhouette, with pruning of peripheral vessels
- ***ECG*** Right atrial hypertrophy, right axis deviation, and RVH
- ***Arterial blood gas*** Hypoxia and hypocapnia (correlating with disease severity), with a fall in oxygen saturation on exercise
- ***Pulmonary function tests*** The lung volumes may be normal, or show a mild restrictive or obstructive defect with a reduced TLCO (late in the disease course)
- ***HRCT chest*** to exclude underlying lung disease
- ***Ventilation–perfusion scanning/CTPA*** to exclude chronic thromboembolic disease as a cause. V/Q is more sensitive than CTPA
- ***Echocardiography*** The most useful diagnostic test in pulmonary hypertension. Typically shows enlargement of right-sided cardiac chambers with paradoxical interventricular septum movement, and tricuspid regurgitation. The systolic pulmonary artery pressure can be estimated from the velocity of the tricuspid regurgitant jet, using Doppler techniques, and the estimated right atrial pressure from the IVC calibre. Pericardial effusions may be present and represent a poor prognosis

- ***Right heart catheterization*** to confirm the pulmonary artery pressure, pulmonary capillary wedge pressure and cardiac output (with a Swann–Ganz catheter, by thermodilution or Fick). Vasodilator testing (usually with inhaled nitric oxide) should be performed to identify patients who will respond to calcium-channel blockers. Also needed to exclude a left to right intracardiac shunt.
- ***Selective pulmonary angiography*** is rarely required as CTPA and V/Q can detect nearly all cases of thromboembolic disease
- ***Blood tests*** Routine tests, including autoantibodies (anti-centromere antibody, anti SCL-70, and RNP) if connective tissue disease suspected as a cause, HIV, TSH, thrombophilia screen, serum ACE.

IPAH: general management

The diagnosis of idiopathic pulmonary arterial hypertension is made when all other causes have been excluded. The management in this section applies to IPAH.

General management

- ***Anticoagulation*** All patients with pulmonary hypertension are at risk of venous thromboembolism and *in situ* pulmonary arterial thrombosis, and therefore should be on life-long warfarin. A small thrombus can have catastrophic effects in a patient who is already severely compromised. Studies show an increased survival with warfarin in IPAH, which may reflect reversal of an underlying pro-thrombotic state, as well as the prevention of *in situ* thrombus formation. Additional beneficial effects are seen when combined with a vasodilator. There is no published data on the use of warfarin in other causes/associations of pulmonary hypertension
- ***Long-term oxygen*** Hypoxaemia is due to reduced cardiac output, ventilation/perfusion mismatching, and right–left shunting through a patent foramen ovale. Added oxygen may reduce any further rise in PAP resulting from additional hypoxic pulmonary vasoconstriction
- ***Diuretics and digoxin*** Diuretics may be useful for the treatment of oedema, but excess preload reduction may limit their usefulness. Digoxin has been shown to improve cardiac output acutely in IPAH, though its longer-term effects are not known
- ***Immunization*** Annual influenza and one-off pneumococcal vaccination
- ***Contraception*** may be required, as pregnancy is poorly tolerated in IPAH with a 30–50% mortality.

A **National Pulmonary Hypertension Service** was set up in the UK in 2001 to coordinate diagnosis and treatment in five regional centres, recognizing the need to provide best care (with complex interventions) and optimize funding for expensive treatments. The five UK centres are:

- London—Hammersmith Hospital (general)
  - Royal Brompton Hospital (adult congenital heart disease)
  - Royal Free Hospital (connective tissue disease)
  - Great Ormond Street Hospital for Children (children)
- Cambridge—Papworth Hospital
- Sheffield—Royal Hallamshire Hospital
- Newcastle—Freeman Hospital
- Glasgow—Western Infirmary

Recent guidelines suggest referral to a specialist centre after CXR, ECG, simple spirometry, and echocardiogram (but not cardiac catheterization, as this should be done in parallel with a vasodilator study in a specialist centre).

Recommendations on the management of pulmonary hypertension in clinical practice. *Heart* 2001; **86**: S1

IPAH: disease-targeted therapy

In IPAH there is impaired production of the vasodilators nitric oxide and prostacyclin, and over-production of the vasoconstrictor endothelin by the pulmonary endothelium. Imbalance of these factors also leads to vascular remodelling. ***Vasodilator responsiveness*** is measured during right heart catheterization with incremental doses of a short-acting vasodilator, such as inhaled nitric oxide, or intravenous epoprostenol or adenosine. A positive vasodilator response is defined as a drop in mean pulmonary arterial pressure by more than 10 mmHg to less than 40 mmHg with an unchanged or increased cardiac output. Only about 5-10% of patients are responders. Vasoresponders should be considered for first-line therapy with calcium-channel blockers. Non-responders should receive prostacyclin analogues, endothelin receptor antagonists, and/or phosphodiesterase inhibitors.

Calcium-channel blockers (CCBs)

- High-dose nifedipine (30–240 mg daily) and diltiazem (120–900 mg daily) are recommended in patients with a positive acute vasodilator response. They should then be followed to determine if they are long-term CCB responders (about 2/3). This group has an excellent prognosis (>90% 10-year survival). CCBs should not be used in those with a negative vasodilator challenge, as they may increase mortality.
- Side-effects include hypotension and oedema, which may limit use
- Amlodipine has more selective vasodilating properties, and at doses of 2.5–5 mg daily may be useful in those intolerant of the other agents, or if right ventricular function is impaired
- Calcium antagonists should be started in hospital and titrated with careful monitoring
- Verapamil is not used, because of its negative inotropic effects.

Prostacyclin analogues Prostacylin is a potent vasodilator. It inhibits platelet aggregation, and has antiproliferative and cytoprotective properties. Side-effects include jaw pain, diarrhoea, and arthralgias.

- *Epoprostenol* This potent vasodilator acts via increasing intracellular cAMP. It is a prostacyclin analogue (PGI_2). It is the only drug shown to improve survival in a randomized controlled trial. It probably has its effects as a selective pulmonary vasodilator, and potentially through vascular remodelling and platelet adhesion. It also improves exercise capacity and haemodynamics. It is inactive within the circulation after 5 min and therefore needs to be given by continuous intravenous infusion via a portable pump and Hickman line. Pump failure can be life-threatening. Side-effects include jaw pain, diarrhoea, headache, flushing, and nausea and are usually dose related
- *Treprostinil* is a prostacyclin analogue that can be given as a continuous subcutaneous infusion, as it has greater *in vivo* stability than epoprostenol. It improves symptoms, exercise capacity, and pulmonary haemodynamics. Pain at the infusion site is the major side-effect
- *Beraprost* is the first orally active prostaglandin analogue, with a half-life of about 40 min. A qds dose has been shown to increase 6-min walk distance, without improvement in pulmonary haemodynamics, but initial improvements have not been maintained at 9 and 12 months, and it is not used in the UK

- *Iloprost* is a prostacyclin analogue and is more potent than epoprostenol. It has a half-life of 25 min and can be given by continuous intravenous infusion or nebulizer (6–9 times a day)
- Even though patients may be vasodilator non-responders, they may benefit from long-term treatment with disease-targeted therapy
- Prostaglandin treatment doubles the time on the lung transplantation waiting list, and improves transplantation outcomes. Improved haemodynamics may lead to some patients coming off transplant waiting lists
- Failure to show improved exercise capacity following one month's treatment with prostaglandin therapy is often considered an indication for lung transplantation
- Tolerance develops to intravenous prostaglandin therapy, with increasing dose requirements over time. The mechanism for this is unclear.

Endothelin receptor antagonists Endothelin is a powerful vasoconstrictor and pro-inflammatory mediator, and causes smooth muscle cell proliferation. Plasma levels raised in some forms of pulmonary hypertension.

- *Bosentan* is an oral endothelin receptor A and B antagonist that has been shown to improve exercise capacity, haemodynamics, and time to clinical worsening. It is the first oral therapy approved for the treatment of IPAH and PAH related to connective tissue disease. Side-effects include liver enzyme abnormalities. Three-year survival for a cohort of mainly WHO functional class III patients starting on bosentan is greater than 85%. The major side-effect is reversible liver transaminitis, causing discontinuation in approximately 3%
- *Sitaxentan* is a selective endothelin type A receptor antagonist. The type B receptor on the endothelium clears endothelin from the circulation, but also contributes to vasoconstriction on the smooth muscle cell. There is no clear evidence for superiority over the dual blockade of bosentan, although liver side-effects may be lower
- *Ambisentan* is another selective type A blocker, with a different structure from sitaxentan and bosentan, giving it a better liver safety profile. It has not yet received a UK licence.

Phosphodiesterase inhibitors e.g. sildenafil augment the vasodilatory effects of nitric oxide and improve exercise capacity and haemodynamics in IPAH in patients in functional classes II and III.

Current practice Start patients with a negative vasodilator response on one of the above three classes of drug. Unwell patients in NYHA functional class IV will usually start on an infusion of epoprostenol, but if unable to cope with the practicalities of a continuous infusion, will be considered for other treatment modalities. Functional class III patients usually start on an endothelin-receptor antagonist, given the long-term data available for these agents. Functional class II patients may be considered for sildenafil or endothelin receptor antagonists. As in many other diseases, such as asthma or systemic hypertension, when patients are failing on monotherapy, other therapies may be added. Data for various combinations are available from case series and some randomized studies, but larger studies are needed to show unequivocal benefit.

IPAH: surgical treatments, end of life care, and future developments

Surgical treatments

Atrial septostomy Creation of a right–left shunt by balloon atrial septostomy aims to increase systemic blood flow by bypassing the pulmonary circulation, particularly in patients with syncope or severe right heart failure. It is a palliative procedure and can be used for symptom control prior to transplantation, with the defect being closed at the time of transplant. Arterial desaturation occurs following the procedure, but is normally offset by the increased cardiac output seen with increased oxygen delivery. It is not indicated in severe left heart failure or in patients with impaired left ventricular function.

Transplantation Improves survival and quality of life in patients with pulmonary hypertension. In those with preserved left ventricular function, lung transplant is the procedure of choice. Return of normal right ventricular function is found after transplantation.

- As for all diseases needing transplantation, timing of referral and operation is crucial, as organ availability is limited
- The incidence of obliterative bronchiolitis appears to be higher post-transplantation for IPAH than in transplantation for other diseases, although the reason for this is uncertain.

End of life care Palliative care may be warranted to improve symptoms such as fatigue, breathlessness, abdominal bloating, nausea, and pain (see p 713).

Future developments Combination therapies are likely to be used more frequently in the future. A number of agents are currently being investigated, including vasoactive intestinal peptide (VIP) and drugs with anti-proliferative effects such as simvastatin, imatinib, and rapamycin.

Non-idiopathic pulmonary hypertension: causes

The majority of patients with pulmonary hypertension seen by a respiratory specialist will have PHT due to chronic hypoxic lung disease, such as COPD. In this case, the pulmonary hypertension is often an incidental finding in a patient with a chronic respiratory disease.

Chronic hypoxia causes pulmonary vasoconstriction and in the longer term vascular remodelling.

- A significant proportion of COPD patients will develop PHT, possibly up to 25%. The level of PAP in these patients is much lower than that seen in patients with IPAH
- COPD with pulmonary hypertension has a much poorer prognosis than COPD without pulmonary hypertension. In patients with a PAP <25 mmHg, the 5-year survival is >90%. In those with a PAP >45 mmHg, the 5-year survival is <10%. Whether this is due to the pulmonary hypertension itself, or whether the pulmonary hypertension is a marker of worse hypoxia and disease severity is unclear
- PHT in COPD was thought to be due to hypoxia and emphysematous destruction of the vascular bed, but neither of these factors correlates well with PAP. Cigarette smoke may have a direct effect on the intrapulmonary vessels, with the up-regulation of mediators leading to aberrant vascular structural remodelling and physiological changes in vascular function

Alveolar hypoventilation, e.g. due to neuromuscular disease. Both alveolar hypoxia and hypercapnia produce pulmonary vasoconstriction, thereby increasing pulmonary artery pressures.

Chronic thromboembolic pulmonary hypertension (CTEPH) is a frequent cause of pulmonary hypertension. Recent data suggest that CTEPH occurs in up to 4% of cases of acute non-fatal pulmonary embolism, higher than previously thought. Pathogenesis is uncertain, with no consistent defect in fibrinolytic activity demonstrated. Natural history of pulmonary thromboemboli is resolution or near total resolution of clot, with restoration of normal pulmonary haemodynamics within 30 days in 90% of patients. Right-sided pressures return to normal in most patients by 2 weeks. In CTEPH, thromboemboli do not resolve, forming endothelialized fibrotic obstructions of the pulmonary vascular bed. *In situ* thrombosis and vascular remodelling of small distal pulmonary arteries also contribute. Peripheral IPAH-like vasculopathic changes are also seen, which has led some to suggest that IPAH and CTEPH are a continuum of disease; *in situ* thrombosis in IPAH can be extensive, and it is possible that *in situ*, rather than embolic, thrombus may be more important in CTEPH. Neovascularization from bronchial and intercostal arteries develops through residual adhesions between the chest wall and visceral pleura. The clinical deterioration parallels the loss of right ventricular functional capacity. Risk factors for CTEPH include increasing age, idiopathic PE, and a larger perfusion defect. Splenectomy is associated, possibly by inducing a pro-thrombotic state due to loss of filtering function of the spleen. Antiphospholipid antibodies are present in 10–20% of patients. The diagnosis is not usually made until advanced pulmonary hypertension is present. Progressive pulmonary hypertension seems to result from changes in the small peripheral resistance vessels in the vascular bed, as opposed to being due to progressive pulmonary events. Secondary hypertensive changes, probably induced by high pulmonary artery pressures, lead to incremental increases in right ventricular afterload, with increasing pulmonary hypertension, ultimately leading to right ventricular failure.

Collagen vascular disease PAH develops in about 15% of patients with scleroderma, and is most frequently seen as an isolated phenomenon in patients with limited cutaneous disease. Also occurs secondary to interstitial lung disease with a very poor prognosis. Life expectancy is <1 year in patients with collagen vascular disease, isolated pulmonary hypertension, and a gas transfer of <25% of normal. Obliteration of the alveolar capillaries and arteriolar narrowing is induced by both the primary vascular disease and any interstitial fibrosis. Other connective tissue diseases, including rheumatoid arthritis and SLE, can also lead to secondary pulmonary hypertension. There is an association with Raynaud's phenomenon and a female predominance is seen.

Drugs and toxins Damage to the pulmonary artery endothelium can be caused by drugs, e.g. anorectic agents such as fenfluramine, dexfenfluramine, cocaine, and amphetamines. The clinical syndrome can be indistinguishable from IPAH. A careful history must therefore be taken. The absolute risk for pulmonary hypertension with anorectic agents is 28 cases per million person-years of exposure. Pulmonary hypertension can develop within weeks of starting the drug.

Pulmonary arteritis PHT secondary to Behçet's or Takayashu's arteritis is associated with systemic arteritis in the supra-aortic trunk. Typical lesions are seen at pulmonary angiography, with *in situ* thrombosis and false aneurysms.

HIV infection Pulmonary hypertension is seen in up to 1 in 200 people who are HIV positive, in the absence of AIDS. It is hypothesized that HIV-infected macrophages release vasoactive cytokines that lead to endothelial damage and proliferation. Antiretroviral drugs may have a beneficial effect on pulmonary haemodynamics.

Congenital heart disease and shunts Pressure overload caused by systemic to pulmonary shunts, e.g. ventricular septal defect and patent ductus arteriosus, lead to PAH. The role of atrial septal defects in the development of PAH is uncertain, with some suggesting they may be bystanders in IPAH.

Portal hypertension Porto-pulmonary hypertension, seen in patients with portal hypertension (of whatever cause), is probably due to the failure of the liver to remove vasoactive substances from the portal circulation, with their resultant accumulation and presentation to the pulmonary arterial endothelium.

Hyperthyroidism is also recognized as a cause.

Non-idiopathic pulmonary hypertension: management

In this group of patients the diagnosis is usually made from echocardiography, and the treatment is optimal management of the underlying lung disease, with the addition of oxygen and diuretics. Recent guidelines on the management of pulmonary hypertension suggest that the management protocol for patients with idiopathic pulmonary arterial hypertension (see p 392) may also be suitable for patients with secondary hypertension, but there is no evidence for most of these treatments in this context. In particular, evidence for treating pulmonary hypertension in hypoxic COPD, other than with long-term oxygen therapy, does not exist. Current studies will establish if agents such as bosentan or sildenafil are of benefit in patients with secondary causes of pulmonary hypertension.

Disease-specific management

- **Chronic thromboembolic pulmonary hypertension** Patients with chronic thromboembolic pulmonary hypertension have a 5-year survival of <10%, if the PAP >50 mmHg. Pulmonary thromboendarterectomy is the treatment of choice for proximal obstructive disease. This is the surgical removal of organized thrombotic material, and aims to strip away the pulmonary arterial endothelium, starting proximally and extending out to remove all clot in the subsegmental levels. It is done on cardiopulmonary bypass with circulatory arrest. The PAP usually falls within 48 h of surgery. Operative mortality is <10% in experienced hands
- ***Scleroderma*** Very few patients with scleroderma-associated PAH have a positive vasodilator response and the significance of it, when present, is uncertain. These patients are treated similar to vasodilator non-responder IPAH algorithms. Patients with systemic sclerosis should be screened annually for pulmonary hypertension, even if no symptoms are present
- ***Pulmonary hypertension associated with left heart disease*** should not be treated with pulmonary vasodilators as these will increase flow to an already overloaded left heart. Treatment should be aimed at the left-sided cardiac abnormality.

Further information

Recommendations on the management of pulmonary hypertension in clinical practice. *Heart* 2001; **86** (S1): i1–i13

Peacock A. Primary pulmonary hypertension. *Thorax* 1999; **54**: 1107

Diagnosis and management of pulmonary arterial hypertension: ACCP evidence-based clinical practice guidelines. *Chest* 2004; **126**: suppl.

Pulmonary arterial hypertension. *N Engl J Med* 2004; **351**: 1655–65

Treatment of pulmonary arterial hypertension. *N Engl J Med* 2004; **351**: 1425–36

Patient group, www.pha-uk.com

Chapter 39

Pulmonary thromboembolic disease

Epidemiology and pathophysiology

Definition A pulmonary embolism (PE) is a clinically significant obstruction of part or all of the pulmonary vascular tree, usually caused by thrombus from a distant site.

Epidemiology

- The overall annual incidence is 60–70/100 000, with a UK annual death rate of 100/million. The estimated overall population incidence of DVT is 0.5 per 1000 person years
- PE may account for up to 15% of all post-operative deaths. It is the commonest cause of death following elective surgery, and the commonest cause of maternal death
- Post mortem studies have consistently shown a frequency of 7–9%, and large in-patient studies have shown a frequency of around 1%, with a mortality of 0.2%. The mortality is much higher in patients with serious underlying comorbid disease
- The incidence is likely to be stable, but improved diagnostic methods mean that it is probably reported more frequently.

Pathophysiology

- 75% of thrombi are generated in the deep venous system of the lower limbs and pelvis, probably initiated by platelet aggregation around venous valve sinuses. Activation of the clotting cascade leads to thrombus formation, with Virchow's triad (venous stasis, injury to the vessel wall, and increased blood coaguability) predisposing to thrombus formation. Venous stasis is increased by immobility and dehydration, and leads to local accumulation of platelets and clotting factors. In addition, coagulation factors may be altered in various disease states, e.g. in the acute phase response, malignancy, and autoimmune disease
- 20% of leg thrombi embolize, with a higher incidence in above than below knee clots. Large clots may lodge at the bifurcation of the main pulmonary arteries, causing haemodynamic compromise. Smaller clots will travel more distally, infarcting the lung and causing pleuritic pain. These are more commonly multiple and bilateral, and are found most often in the lower lobes, where blood flow is greatest
- Thrombi can also develop in the right heart following myocardial infarction
- Septic emboli are found in endocarditis, in association with intraventricular septal defects (paradoxical emboli), AV shunts, or central venous access.

Haemodynamic effects of PE depend on the size of the clot and which area of the pulmonary vascular tree it subsequently obstructs, as well as the pre-existing state of the myocardium and pulmonary parenchyma.

- As the pulmonary vasculature in a healthy lung has a large capacitance, the mean pulmonary artery pressure (PAP) does not rise until at least 50% of the vascular bed has been occluded
- As the PAP rises, right ventricular afterload increases, with a resulting increase in right ventricular end-diastolic pressure.

- The right ventricle will start to fail acutely as the PAP reaches over 40 mmHg
- This causes a reduction in pulmonary blood flow, leading to reduced left ventricular filling and a reduction in systemic blood pressure
- Adequate blood volume for right-sided heart filling is vital. The secondary effects are much worse if right-sided filling cannot be maintained, e.g. if the patient is dehydrated, hypovolaemic, or erect
- Hypoxia results from reduced cardiac output, low mixed venous PaO_2 and higher perfusion to the remaining alveoli, leading to ventilation/perfusion mismatching in the unaffected lung
- Hypoxia will be worse if there is a larger premorbid V/Q spread, e.g. in the elderly and in those with pre-existing lung disease. It is therefore possible for a young healthy person to have a normal PaO_2 and A–a gradient following a PE
- A patient with a PAP of ≥40 mmHg cannot have *acute* PE as this pressure cannot be achieved acutely. In this setting, the raised PAP raises the possibility of *chronic* thromboembolic disease, pulmonary hypertension, or another cause.

Aetiology

Risk factors can be divided into major and minor factors. This division is important for an assessment of clinical probability.

Risk factors for venous thromboembolism (VTE)

Major risk factors (relative risk x 5–20)	
Surgery	Major abdominal/pelvic surgery
	Orthopaedic surgery (especially lower limb)
	Post-operative intensive care
Obstetrics	Late pregnancy (higher incidence with multiple births)
	Caesarean section
	Pre-eclampsia
Malignancy	Pelvic/abdominal
	Metastatic/advanced
Lower limb problems	Fracture, varicose veins
Reduced mobility	Hospitalization
	Institutional care
Previous proven VTE	
Minor risk factors (relative risk x 2–4)	
Cardiovascular	Congenital heart disease
	Congestive cardiac failure
	Hypertension
	Central venous access
	Superficial venous thrombosis
Oestrogens	Oral contraceptive pill (especially third-generation higher oestrogen containing)
	Hormone replacement therapy
Miscellaneous	Occult malignancy
	Neurological disability
	Thrombotic disorders
	Obesity
	Inflammatory bowel disease
	Nephrotic syndrome
	Dialysis
	Myeloproliferative disorders
	Behçet's disease

Risk of malignancy Occult cancer will be present in 7–12% of patients presenting with idiopathic venous thromboembolism (VTE). Malignancy may be detected by careful clinical assessment, routine blood tests, and chest radiography. Screening for malignancy in these patients is not recommended, unless suspected clinically. These patients are more likely to have a poor prognosis, because of regional spread or distant metastases at diagnosis.

Inherited thrombophilias

- 25–50% of patients with VTE have an identifiable inherited thrombophilia, e.g. antiphospholipid syndrome, deficiency of antithrombin III, a prothrombin gene defect, protein C or protein S deficiency
- These usually need to interact with an additional acquired risk factor to cause VTE
- Factor V Leiden deficiency is present in 5% of the population and 20% of patients presenting with thrombosis
- Current recommendations do not advocate routine screening for inheritable thrombophilias, unless in specific circumstances (see below), as the number needed to test to prevent an episode of VTE would be very high. In addition, detecting a heritable thrombophilia does not predict a significantly higher rate or earlier occurrence of VTE in the absence of a secondary risk factor

Thrombophilia testing is recommended in:

- Patients with recurrent venous thrombosis
- Patients <40 with venous thrombosis with no obvious risk factors
- First venous thromboembolism with a clear family history in first-degree relatives
- Thrombosis secondary to pregnancy, oral contraceptive pill, hormone replacement therapy
- Thrombosis at an unusual site—cerebral, mesenteric, portal, or hepatic veins

All but factor V Leiden deficiency and the prothrombin gene mutation need to be tested for when the patient is off anticoagulants.

'Economy class syndrome' refers to thromboembolic disease association with long distance sedentary travel, with an increasing incidence of disease with increasing distance travelled. A 2001 study of 135.29 million passengers showed an incidence of PE of 1.5 cases/million for travel over 5000 km, compared with 0.01 cases/million for travel under 5000 km. For travel over 10 000 km, the incidence increased to 4.8 cases/million.

Clinical features

Acute PE typically presents in four main ways.

- ***Pulmonary infarction and haemoptysis*** (in 60%) ± pleuritic pain. Arterial blood gases may be normal, and ECG changes uncommon. Localizing signs may be present, e.g. pleural rub
- ***Isolated dyspnoea*** (in 25%) Defined as acute breathlessness in the absence of haemorrhage or circulatory collapse. The thrombus is more likely to be central, with hypoxia on blood gases. The patient may have sudden onset and unexplained breathlessness, in the presence of risk factors for VTE
- ***Collapse, poor reserve*** (in 10%) May be due to a small PE, often in an elderly patient with limited cardiorespiratory reserve. These patients can rapidly decompensate with even a relatively small PE. The clinical findings may be non-specific and reflect the underlying disease process, rather than the PE itself
- ***Circulatory collapse in a previously well patient*** Hypotension ± loss of consciousness in 1%. Usually due to extensive pulmonary artery occlusion from massive PE causing marked hypoxia and hypocapnia (due to hyperventilation) and acute right heart failure, with chest pain due to right heart angina, raised JVP, and fainting on sitting up. ECG may be normal, show sinus tachycardia or right heart strain. Echocardiogram shows pulmonary hypertension and right ventricular failure. These patients have the highest mortality, up to 30%.

Chronic thromboembolic disease This typically presents with more insidious onset breathlessness over the course of weeks–months due to increasing load of recurrent small volume clot. See p 398.

Dyspnoea and tachypnoea (a respiratory rate >20) are the commonest presenting features and are absent in only 10% of patients.

Consider PE in the differential diagnosis of:

- Unexplained shortness of breath
- Collapse
- New onset atrial fibrillation
- Signs consistent with right heart failure
- Pleural effusion

Examination of a patient with PE

- May be normal
- Tachycardia and tachypnoea are common
- Atrial fibrillation
- Reduced chest movement (due to pain)
- Pleural rub
- Classically loud P2 and splitting of the second heart sound, with a gallop rhythm (acute right heart strain)
- Hypoxia (with hypocapnia due to hyperventilation, and an increased alveolar–arterial gradient), *but* PaO_2 may be in the normal range in young healthy individuals
- Low-grade fever
- Signs of DVT (common, in around 25%)
- Right heart failure—low cardiac output and raised JVP with reduced BP and perfusion pressure

Diagnosis of acute PE

The diagnosis of a pulmonary embolism can be difficult and involves a clinical assessment of probability. This takes risk factors, clinical presentation, and clinical signs into account. Investigations are then performed, that may add weight to the clinical decision, rather than being stand-alone diagnostic tests. Therefore the estimation of the pre-test clinical probability of PE is of vital importance in interpreting the results of the tests performed.

Pre-test clinical probability scoring systems One example is the BTS pre-test clinical probability scoring system, shown in the box below.

A standard assessment of **pre-test clinical probability** might include:

- (a) Patient has clinical features compatible with PE:
  - raised respiratory rate
  - ± haemoptysis
  - ± pleuritic chest pain
- Plus 2 other factors:
  - 1. Absence of another reasonable clinical explanation
  - 2. Presence of a major risk factor (see box, p 426)
- (a) plus 1 and 2: **HIGH** pre-test clinical probability
- (a) plus 1 or 2: **INTERMEDIATE** pre-test clinical probability
- (a) alone: **LOW** pre-test clinical probability

The Wells and Geneva pre-test probability scores are similar to the above, but include separate scores for clinical features such as heart rate, haemoptysis, and blood gas estimates (Geneva). Local scoring systems may be in place. ***These scoring systems should always be used with the D-dimer result.***

D-dimer has an important role in diagnosing and excluding PE, and should only be used with a pre-test clinical probability assessment following careful clinical evaluation by an experienced clinician. D-dimers are sensitive for thromboembolism, but not specific. They are rarely in the normal range in cases of acute thromboembolism, but are not a valid screening test for PE alone. D-dimers are generated as a result of fibrinolysis, which occurs in many clinical situations, including sepsis, post surgery, pneumonia, neoplasia, inflammatory disease, pregnancy, and advanced age.

- Only a normal result (which excludes PE) is of clinical value
- An abnormal result (however high) does not necessarily imply a significantly increased probability of PE
- The sensitivity ranges from 87% to 99%, depending on the assay used (ELISA (Vidas) or red cell agglutination (SimpliRED)). Specificity is poorer, around 60–70% (so a large number of false positives)
- The different assays have different performance characteristics and these should be known before incorporating them into diagnostic algorithms

- D-dimer testing for excluding PE has been validated as an out-patient test, but not in in-patient groups
- A low or intermediate pre-test clinical probability score, combined with a negative D-dimer has a 92% sensitivity at excluding PE

Modified Geneva score

Age >65 years	1 point
Previous DVT or PE	3 points
Surgery or fracture within 1 month	2 points
Active malignancy	2 points
Unilateral lower limb pain	3 points
Haemoptysis	2 points
Heart rate 75–94 bpm	3 points
Heart rate >95 bpm	5 points
Pain on limb palpation & unilateral oedema	4 points
Low probability	0–3 points
Intermediate probability	4–10 points
High probability	≥11 points

D-dimer test interpretation

- A negative D-dimer test reliably excludes PE in patients with a low (SimpliRED) or intermediate pre-test clinical probability (Vidas). These patients do not need further imaging
- A negative test is unhelpful in those with a high clinical probability and therefore should not be done in this situation
- A positive result needs further investigation, but does not necessarily imply PE
- The D-dimer becomes less useful the longer the period spent in hospital (i.e. increasing false positives), due to clot formation at venepuncture sites, venous stasis due to bed rest, etc.

Assessment and documentation of pre-test clinical probability in PE is paramount. This enables accurate clinical assessment, and may obviate the need for imaging.

An alternative explanation should be sought when PE is excluded.

Investigations

- ***ECG*** Non-specific changes are frequent. Most commonly sinus tachycardia. Atrial fibrillation, right bundle branch block, anterior T-wave inversion (indicating R ventricular strain) are common. The S1Q3T3 pattern is uncommon
- ***CXR*** A good quality departmental CXR is required. No specific features are characteristic in PE, but it may reveal another pathology. Small effusions are present in 40% (80% are exudates, 20% transudates). Focal infiltrates, segmental collapse, and a raised hemi-diaphragm can also occur
- ***Arterial blood gas*** may be normal, especially in the young and healthy. Hypoxia and hypocapnia, due to hyperventilation, with an increased A–a gradient are more common
- ***D-dimer*** (see p 408)
- ***Troponin*** and natriuretic peptides are sensitive markers of right ventricular dysfunction and early data suggest a raised troponin predicts poorer prognosis
- ***CTPA*** is the gold standard investigation, and is now recommended as the initial imaging technique in suspected non-massive PE. It has a sensitivity of >95%, and may enable an alternative diagnosis to be made if PE is excluded. Advances in imaging mean that a 16-slice multi-detector row scanner can image the entire chest with resolution approaching 1 mm, requiring a breath-hold of less than 10 s. Emboli can be detected in sixth-order pulmonary vessels, which are so small that their clinical relevance is uncertain. CTPA should be performed within 1 h in suspected massive PE, and within 24 h of suspected non-massive PE. The sensitivity and specificity of CTPA depends on the location of the emboli, with lower sensitivity for clot confined to the segmental or sub-segmental pulmonary vessels compared with more central clot. CTPA needs specialist reporting.

In those with a high clinical probability but negative CTPA the options are:

- PE has been excluded, stop anticoagulation, or
- Perform further imaging (leg ultrasound, conventional pulmonary angiogram, venous phase CT to include the legs)

In one large prospective multicentre study, with all patients investigated with CTPA and leg ultrasound, those with negative tests and low or intermediate clinical probability were not anticoagulated. Only 0.2% had a definite PE after 3 months of follow-up. Those with negative tests but high clinical probability were investigated further, and PE was identified in 5% (Musset D *et al. Lancet* 2002; **360:** 1914).

A volume of 100–150 ml contrast media is required for CTPA, which poses a substantial risk of nephropathy (in patients with renal insufficiency and diabetes) and sometimes fluid overload (patients with impaired left ventricular function). In these patients, leg ultrasound and/or isotope lung scanning might be safer first line investigations.

- ***Isotope lung scanning*** (ventilation/perfusion or V/Q scan)—mostly now superseded by CTPA. Some units may just perform the Q (perfusion) part of the scan. May be useful as a first-line imaging investigation in patients with a normal CXR and with no concurrent cardiopulmonary disease, in whom a negative scan can reliably exclude a PE. Scans are reported as low, intermediate, or high probability, and the report's meaning must be interpreted in light of the pre-test clinical probability score. Further imaging is necessary for those in whom:
  - The scan is indeterminate
  - There is a discordant scan result and clinical probability.

The clinical significance of the V/Q scan report is:

- Normal = no PE
- Low or intermediate pre-test clinical probability *plus* low probability scan = PE excluded
- High pre-test clinical probability *plus* high probability scan = PE diagnosed
- Any other = need further imaging.

Other imaging techniques

- ***Leg ultrasound***—around 70% of patients with a proven PE have a proximal DVT; hence leg imaging can be used as an alternative to lung imaging in those with clinical DVT. A single examination is not adequate to exclude subclinical DVT (venography is more sensitive). It is safe to withhold anticoagulation in patients with suspected DVT and a single negative leg ultrasound, but these data cannot yet be extrapolated to those presenting with suspected PE. If a leg ultrasound is positive in a patient with clinical features of PE, this excludes the need for further imaging. Up to 50% of patients with a clinically obvious DVT will have a high-probability V/Q scan
- ***Conventional pulmonary angiogram*** is available in a few specialist centres only, where catheter fragmentation of large clots may be of therapeutic benefit. Now mostly superseded by CTPA
- ***CT venography*** is an emerging area. It can be combined with CTPA to image the pelvic leg veins simultaneously
- ***Echocardiogram*** is diagnostic in sub-massive and massive PE. The transoesophageal route is more sensitive, enabling visualization of intrapulmonary and intracardiac clot. May give prognostic information
- ***Transthoracic ultrasound*** is used uncommonly. May show peripheral infarcts with peripheral pulmonary emboli.

►► Management of acute massive PE

Acute massive PE has a mortality of 20%.

1. Oxygen—100%, via non-rebreathe mask
2. IV access. Send baseline bloods, including clotting. Perform ECG
3. Analgesia if required; consider opiates
4. Management of cardiogenic shock—fluids and inotropes may be required in sub-massive or massive PE to maintain right ventricular filling
5. Start IV heparin unless active GI bleeding or intracerebral haemorrhage:
   - Bolus dose 5000–10 000 units or 80 IU/kg
   - Maintenance infusion of 1300 IU/h or 18 units/kg/h
   - Adjust infusion rate until APTT is 1.5–2.5× control. Check APTT4–6 h after initial bolus and 6–10 h after any dose change. When APTT is in the therapeutic range, check it daily
6. Investigation to confirm PE depends on the clinical state of patient. Ideally perform urgent echocardiogram and if this is non-diagnostic, perform a CTPA, but not delaying for more than 1 h. It may, however, be unwise to move a sick patient to the radiology department for a CTPA. If there is circulatory collapse and the patient is peri-arrest and PE is the most likely cause, confirmation of the diagnosis should not be sought, but treatment prioritized. Remember aortic dissection, cardiac tamponade, and acute MI can mimic PE
7. Thrombolysis if collapsed or hypotensive, if no active GI bleeding or intracerebral haemorrhage:
   - Alteplase 100 mg over 2 h given peripherally
   - Or streptokinase 250 000 units in 30 min with 100 000 units/h for 24 h (plus hydrocortisone to prevent further circulatory instability)
   - Or urokinase 4400 IU/kg in 10 min and 4400 IU/kg/h for 12 h
   - Stop the heparin during thrombolysis and restart afterwards
   - In cardiac arrest due to suspected massive PE, 50 mg IV alteplase immediately may be life-saving
8. Consider liaising with cardiothoracic centre to consider embolectomy, particularly if thrombolysis is contraindicated.

Low molecular weight heparin (LMWH) is as effective as standard unfractionated intravenous heparin, and should be given to patients with intermediate or a high pre-test clinical probability prior to imaging.
Unfractionated heparin should be considered in massive PE (faster onset of action) as a first dose bolus prior to commencement of LMWH.
Oral anticoagulation should only be commenced once PE is proven, after initial heparin treatment. Target INR 2.0–3.0 (when achieved, heparin can be stopped). Some centres now advocate out-patient anticoagulation for PE, as well as DVT. Recent data suggest that this is as safe as in-patient anticoagulation, in a carefully selected population, in centres with a well-established out-patient DVT service.

Length of warfarin anticoagulation

- Temporary risk factor: 4–6 weeks. This is an area of some debate
- First episode of idiopathic PE: 3 months is currently recommended, though some still advocate 6 months warfarin treatment

- Recurrent idiopathic PE: no guidelines exist; length of treatment depends on individual circumstances, with risk of bleeding balanced with risk of recurrent event, and often long-term anticoagulation
- Persisting risk factors: lifelong anticoagulation may be recommended

Side-effects
- The risk of bleeding increases with age and concurrent illness
- Higher bleeding rate with concomitant aspirin use, and previous gastrointestinal bleed
- Risk of bleeding relates to duration and intensity of anticoagulation.

Thrombolysis There is emerging evidence to support the use of thrombolysis in certain subgroups of patients with PE; however, this is a controversial area, and the risk/benefit analysis of this treatment must always be carefully considered.

Massive PE causing circulatory collapse. Current BTS guidelines (2003) support the use of early thrombolysis in massive PE. In practice, thrombolysis is usually given to the acutely unwell/peri-arrest patient, when the history and physical findings are suggestive of massive PE, in the absence of another reasonable explanation. There is rarely time for imaging or investigations in this situation.

Non-massive PE is more controversial. Some evidence now supports the use of intravenous alteplase in addition to IV heparin in the treatment of haemodynamically stable submassive PE, in association with pulmonary hypertension or right ventricular dysfunction. Current BTS guidelines recommend thrombolysis only for patients with clinically massive PE. Increasing evidence suggests that individuals with a large clot volume, in the absence of haemodynamic compromise, have better clinical outcomes with thrombolysis. This is due to the prevention of chronic thromboembolic disease, as larger clot volume is a risk factor for this. More data is required.

Contraindications None absolute; rarely a consideration in the life-threatening situation. Risk of major haemorrhage is 3–4 times that of heparin, with a higher incidence of bleeding in the elderly. Active bleeding or recent intracerebral bleed are contraindications.

Embolectomy Rarely done, and only in life-threatening massive PE. Options include surgical embolectomy (few regional centres only) and mechanical clot fragmentation via right heart catheterization.

IVC filter placement There is little evidence to show improved survival or reduction in recurrent PE rate with IVC filters, and changing to low molecular weight heparin may be as effective. IVC filters may, however, be indicated in:
- Acute VTE in patients with an absolute contraindication to anticoagulation
- Patients with massive PE who survive (a second PE may be fatal)
- Recurrent VTE despite adequate anticoagulation
- Post-pulmonary thromboendarterectomy in pulmonary hypertension.

Further information

Konstantinides S *et al.* Heparin plus alteplase compared with heparin alone in patients with submassisve pulmonary embolism. *NEJM* 2002; **347**: 1143–50

Special circumstances

Pregnancy and thromboembolic disease

- The incidence of DVT ± PE in pregnancy is 1 in 1000, rising to 2 in 1000 in the puerperium. The risk of PE in pregnancy is greater with increasing maternal age and with increasing gestational age. More PEs occur during pregnancy than after delivery. There is a 20–30 times increased risk with Caesarean section, compared with normal vaginal delivery. PE is one of commonest causes of maternal death in pregnancy (1/100 000 pregnancies)
- D-dimers are raised in the normal pregnancy and so are usually unhelpful in the investigation of thromboembolic disease
- The CTPA whole-body radiation dose is 2–4 mGy, with an absorbed dose to the fetus of 0.01 mSv. This equates to a risk of fatal cancer to age 15 of <1 in 1 million. The absorbed dose to the breast is 10 mSv (higher in pregnancy). CTPA increases the lifetime breast cancer risk in premenopausal women from 10% to 11.4%, with an even higher risk in pregnancy
- The V/Q scan whole-body radiation dose is 1.5–2 mGy, with an absorbed dose to the fetus of 0.12 mSv. This equates to a risk of fatal cancer to age 15 of 1 in 280,000. The absorbed dose to the breast is 0.28 mSv
- The overall radiation risk depends on the gestation of the fetus and the metabolic activity of the pregnant breast tissue. There is considerable debate as to which imaging technique is best in pregnancy, in terms of radiation risk to both the mother (including breast tissue) and the fetus. The lowest overall risk favours a Q scan as the first-line investigation, especially as this young healthy population are likely to have normal lungs. Some experts suggest a leg ultrasound first (see p 64)
- In those with antenatal thromboembolic disease, low molecular weight heparin (LMWH) is used. Close to delivery, this is changed to unfractionated heparin, as it is easier to monitor and to reverse its effects. It is unclear whether heparin should be stopped or the dose reduced at the time of delivery. LMWH levels can be monitored with anti-Xa levels
- There are case reports of successful thrombolysis, catheter-directed thrombolysis, and embolectomy in massive PE, but no relevant trials
- Warfarin is teratogenic and is contraindicated in pregnancy, although it is safe in breast-feeding
- Anticoagulation should be continued for 6 weeks after delivery or 3 months following initial episode, whichever is longer.

Thromboembolic disease and the oral contraceptive pill/HRT

- The OCP, pregnancy, and hormone replacement therapy (HRT) increase the risk of PE, but the incidence of fatal PE is low—estimated at 1/100 000 OCP users, with a median age of 29
- Risk of fatal PE is twice as high amongst those taking third-generation pills
- Previous history of DVT or PE is a contraindication to the OCP
- Meta-analyses show a relative risk of VTE of 2.1 in HRT users, which is highest in the first year of use.

Flight prophylaxis for thromboembolic disease

- For patients with high risk of a PE, i.e. previous VTE, within 6 weeks of surgery, or current malignancy, the 1997 BTS Guidelines recommend low-dose aspirin, low molecular weight heparin, or formal anticoagulation (INR 2–3) prior to flying
- For those with moderate or low risk, graduated or compression stockings with or without pre-flight aspirin is suggested.

Future developments

Thrombolysis Further research is ongoing regarding the use of thrombolysis in non-massive PE and more data are likely in the next few years.

Low-intensity warfarin therapy A reduced target INR of 1.5–2.0 may be used. A study of a cohort of patients treated for up to 4.3 years, following 6 months of standard warfarin therapy for idiopathic venous thromboembolism, led to a 48% reduction in recurrent VTE, major haemorrhage, or death compared with placebo (Ridker PM *et al*, *NEJM* 2003; **348:** 1425).

Further information

BTS guidelines for the management of suspected acute pulmonary embolism. *Thorax* 2003; **58**: 470–84

Goldhaber SZ. Seminar: pulmonary embolism. *Lancet* 2004; **363**: 1295–1305

Rare causes

Air embolism Air is found within the arterial or venous circulation. Small amounts of air can be tolerated, but large amounts can lodge in the pulmonary vasculature and cause mechanical obstruction and death. This is rare.

Causes Neck vein cannulation, intrauterine manipulations (such as criminal abortion, where a frothy liquid is passed under pressure into the uterus), bronchial trauma, or barotrauma causing air to enter the pulmonary vein and left heart. Air in the left ventricle causes impairment to venous filling and subsequent poor coronary perfusion as air enters the coronary arteries.

Diagnosis *Arterial* air emboli may cause dizziness, loss of consciousness, and convulsions. Air may be seen in the retinal arteries or from transected vessels. *Venous* air emboli may cause raised venous pressure, cyanosis, hypotension, tachycardia, syncope, and a 'mill-wheel' murmur over the praecordium.

Treatment Patients should lie on their right side, with head down and feet up, to allow air to collect and stay at the cardiac apex. From here it can be aspirated via thoracotomy.

Amniotic fluid embolism is estimated to occur in 1 in 25 000–80 000 live births. It is the third commonest cause of maternal death, and the most common cause of death in the immediate post-partum period. Usually catastrophic, 80% of women die, 20–50% of these in the first hour. An anaphylactic-type response to amniotic fluid entering the circulation is seen. Amniotic fluid enters the circulation because of torn fetal membranes, which can occur in Caesarean section, uterine or cervical trauma, or uterine rupture. It has a thromboplastic effect, causing disseminated intravascular coagulation and thrombi to form in pulmonary vessels. Not all women react in this way to amniotic fluid. It is more common in older multiparous mothers, who have had short tumultuous labour, often involving uterine stimulants.

Clinically presents with sudden onset respiratory distress, hypoxia, bronchospasm, cyanosis, cardiovascular collapse, pulmonary oedema, convulsions, coma, and cardiac arrest. Coagulopathy with intractable uterine bleeding and uterine atony is seen.

Diagnosis is clinical. Fetal debris/cells can be identified in blood sampled from the maternal pulmonary artery, but this is not pathognomonic.

Treatment is supportive, whilst the thrombi clear from the maternal lungs. Maintain the circulation with fluids and inotropes. Respiratory support with oxygen and ventilation may be needed. Correct coagulopathy with fresh frozen plasma and packed cells. Control placental bleeding.

Fat embolism Common pathological finding following long bone fractures. Occurs especially with lower limb fractures—pelvis and femur. Commoner in fractures that have not been immobilized. Can also occur after prosthetic joint replacement, cardiac massage, liver trauma, burns, bone marrow transplant, rapid high-altitude decompression, and liposuction. Generally occurs in the young and previously healthy. Presents 24–72 h post-fracture. Marrow fat enters the circulation and lodges in the lungs, causing mechanical obstruction.

Classically presents with hypoxia, coagulopathy, with a transient petechial rash on the neck, axillae, and skinfolds, and neurological disturbance, such as confusion, disorientation, or sometimes coma. Stable patients may deteriorate with low-grade fever, petechial rash, hypoxia, and confusion. Jaundice and renal dysfunction are possible.

Diagnosis is usually made clinically in a patient with a lower limb fracture presenting with tachypnoea and hypoxia. Fat globules can be identified in the urine. CXR shows bilateral alveolar infiltrates. ARDS can develop.

Treatment is with early immobilization of fracture, fluid replacement, oxygen, and supportive care.

Septic, hydatid, and tumour emboli are also causes. Uterine leiomyosarcoma has vascular tropism and can invade the inferior vena cava and obstruct the pulmonary arteries. Teratomas can invade the IVC and pulmonary arteries.

Chapter 40

Respiratory infection: bacterial

Community-acquired pneumonia (CAP)

Community-acquired pneumonia is a common disease, associated with significant morbidity and mortality.

Definition A syndrome of infection that is usually bacterial with symptoms and signs of consolidation of part(s) of the lung parenchyma. This is different to bronchitis (see p 647).

Epidemiology

- CAP is the commonest infectious cause of death and the 6th leading cause of death in the UK and USA (with age-adjusted death rates of between 1 and 24/100 000)
- Up to 40% of UK adults with CAP require hospital admission. Hospital mortality varies between 5% and 12%
- A BTS multicentre UK study showed that 5–10% of patients with CAP require ICU admission
- Mortality is up to 50% in those admitted to ICU
- CAP managed in the community has a mortality of 1%.

Pathophysiology The lung and tracheobronchial tree are usually sterile below the level of the larynx, so an infecting agent must reach this site via a breach in host defences. This may be by micro-aspiration (which occurs in around 45% of healthy individuals overnight), haematogenous spread, direct spread from an adjacent structure, inhalation, or activation of previously dormant infection.

Aetiology Broadly similar pathogens are seen in patients managed in the community and in hospital. A single pathogen is identified in 85% of cases. The proportion of cases with more than one pathogen is unknown.

Risk factors for CAP

- ***Aspiration*** Typically caused by anaerobes and Gram-negative organisms
- ***Alcoholism and diabetes*** Typically associated with bacteraemic pneumococcal pneumonia. Anaerobes and mixed infections are more common in alcoholics
- ***Oral steroids/immunosuppression*** *Legionella* infection may be more common
- ***Cigarette smoking*** is the strongest independent risk factor for invasive pneumococcal disease in immunocompetent patients
- ***COPD*** *Haemophilus influenzae* and *Moraxella catarrhalis* are more common, and COPD is more common in those with bacterial pneumonia
- ***Nursing home residents*** have an increased frequency of CAP, with aspiration, Gram-negative organisms, and anaerobes more common than in age-matched elderly people. *Haemophilus influenzae* is the most common causative organism. *Mycoplasma pneumoniae* and *Legionella* are less common.

Organisms causing community-acquired pneumonia

- *Streptococcus pneumoniae* (the pneumococcus) —the most frequently identified organism, commonest in winter, accounting for two-thirds of all cases of bacteraemic pneumonia. Previous epidemics in the UK have been associated with overcrowding, e.g. in prisons—these are now very rare.
- *Legionella pneumophilia*—most common in the autumn. 52% are travel-related. Epidemics occur related to water-containing systems in buildings, typically in the Mediterranean
- *Staphylococcus aureus*—commonest in winter months. Coincident influenza infection in 39% of those requiring hospital admission and 50% of those admitted to ICU
- *Influenza*—annual epidemics in the winter months, complicated by pneumonia in 3% of community cases. 10% of those admitted to hospital have coincident *Staphylococcus aureus* infection
- *Mycoplasma pneumoniae*—epidemics occur every 4 or 5 years in the UK
- *Chlamydia pneumoniae*—epidemics in the community; whether it has a direct pathogenic role, or is an associated infectious agent, is not clear
- *Chlamydia psittaci*—infection acquired from birds and animals, with 20% of cases having a history of bird contact. Human-to-human spread may occur. Uncommon
- *Coxiella burnetii (Q fever)*—epidemics in relation to animal sources (usually sheep), but occupational exposure only present in 8%. Uncommon.

See p 463 for zoonotic causes of community-acquired pneumonia

CAP: clinical features

- Fever
- Cough
- Sputum
- Shortness of breath
- Pleuritic chest pain
- Non-specific features in the elderly. May present 'off legs' or with confusion, in the absence of fever.

Examination

- Raised respiratory rate (may be the only sign in the elderly)
- Tachycardia
- Localizing signs on chest examination. Reduced chest expansion on the affected side, with signs consistent with consolidation (reduced air entry, with bronchial breathing, reduced percussion note, increased vocal resonance) and crackles. A normal chest examination makes the diagnosis unlikely.

Diagnosis of CAP is made on the basis of:

- Symptoms and signs of an acute lower respiratory tract infection
- New focal chest signs
- New radiographic shadowing, for which there is no other explanation
- At least one systemic feature (e.g. sweating, fevers, aches, and pains)
- No other explanation for the illness.

Most helpful in diagnosis

- Fever, pleuritic pain, dyspnoea, and tachypnoea
- Signs on chest examination.

Specific clinical features of pathogens The aetiological agent cannot be accurately predicted from the clinical features alone, although some features are more statistically likely with one pathogen than another. The exception to this is the presence of chest pain or fever (>39°C) in those admitted to ICU, which predicts a higher likelihood of streptococcal pneumonia.

- *Streptococcus pneumoniae* Increasing age, comorbidity (especially cardiovascular), acute onset, high fever, and pleuritic chest pain
- *Bacteraemic Streptococcus pneumoniae* Alcohol, diabetes, COPD, dry or no cough, female
- *Legionella* Younger patients, smokers, absence of comorbidity, more severe infection, neurological symptoms, evidence of multisystem disease (e.g. abnormal liver enzymes and raised creatine kinase)
- *Mycoplasma pneumoniae* Younger patients, prior antibiotics, less multisystem involvement, but extrapulmonary involvement including haemolysis, cold agglutinins, hepatitis, skin and joint problems
- *Staphylococcus aureus* Recent influenza-like illness
- *Chlamydia psittaci* Longer duration of symptoms prior to admission, headache.

- *Coxiella burnetii (Q fever)* Dry cough, high fever, headache, male. animal exposure e.g. sheep and goats
- *Klebsiella pneumoniae* Low platelet count and leucopenia, male.

Rare causes

- *Acinetobacter* Older patients, history of alcoholism, high mortality
- *Streptococcus milleri* Dental or abdominal source of infection
- *Streptococcus viridans* Aspiration is a risk factor.

CAP: severity assessment

- CAP has a wide range of severity. An assessment of severity enables the most appropriate care to be delivered in the most appropriate clinical setting
- Early identification of patients at high risk of death allows early decisions about hospital admission and possible need for assisted ventilation to be made
- Assessment of disease severity depends on the experience of the clinician; a number of predictive assessment models have been trialled. These severity models should be regarded as adjuncts to clinical assessment, and regular reassessment of the disease is needed.

Poor prognostic factors Those with two or more adverse prognostic factors are at high risk of death and should be managed as for severe CAP.

- ***Age*** (≥65)
- ***Coexisting disease***—including cardiac disease, diabetes, COPD, stroke
- ***Respiratory rate*** ≥30/min—this is one of the most reliable predictors of disease severity
- ***Confusion***—abbreviated mental test score ≤8
- ***Blood pressure***—systolic ≤90 mmHg and/or diastolic ≤60 mmHg
- ***Hypoxaemia***—respiratory failure with PaO_2 <8 kPa and the need for assisted ventilation predicts mortality
- ***Urea*** ≥7 mmol/L
- ***Albumin*** <35 g/L
- ***White cell count***—a WCC >20 or <4 x 10^9/L are both predictive
- ***Radiology***—bilateral or multilobe involvement. In patients admitted to ICU, progression of CXR changes is a poor prognostic marker
- ***Microbiology***—positive blood culture, whatever the pathogen isolated.

A commonly used severity assessment score is ***CURB or CURB-65***, which aims to predict morbidity and mortality in CAP. The Pneumonia Severity Index (PSI) is an alternative, which may be more sensitive, but is much more complicated, and includes information on comorbid disease and laboratory tests before stratifying patients into 5 risk classes. Ewig's score is another severity assessment score.

CURB-65 score core factors

- Confusion—new mental confusion defined (AMTS ≤ 8)
- Urea—≥7 mmol/L. Some scores omit this
- Respiratory rate raised ≥30/min
- Blood pressure—systolic BP ≤90 and/or diastolic BP ≤60
- *65* age ≥65

The presence of the 4 'core' CURB factors correlates with mortality:

- 4 factors present gives a mortality of 83%, 3 factors 33%, 2 factors 23%, 8% with one, and 2.4% in the presence of no core factors

- Low risk of death: age <50, no coexisting disease, CURB score zero patients may be suitable for home treatment
- Pneumonia severity scores aim to contribute to, rather than supersede, a clinical judgement; they include a potential over-emphasis on age.

Abbreviated mental test score

(1 point per question, max = 10)
Age
Date of birth
Time (to nearest hour)
Year
Hospital name
Recognition of 2 people (e.g. nurse, doctor)
Recall address
Date of First World War
Name of monarch
Count backwards 20 to 1

CAP: investigations

General investigations are aimed at confirming the diagnosis, assessing disease severity, guiding appropriate treatment, assessing the presence of underlying disease, enabling identification of complications, and monitoring progress.

- ***Oxygenation assessment*** Those with an oxygen saturation of <92% on admission or with features of severe pneumonia should have arterial blood gases measured. The inspired oxygen concentration must be documented
- *CXR*
    - Consolidation, most commonly in the lower lobes. Also interstitial infiltrates and cavitation
    - Multilobe involvement, more common in bacteraemic pneumococcal infection
    - Pleural effusion, more common in bacteraemic pneumococcal infection
    - Lymphadenopathy, uncommon, but most likely with mycoplasma infection
    - Multilobe involvement, cavitation, or spontaneous pneumothorax suggest *Staphylococcus aureus* infection
    - Upper lobe preponderance suggests *Klebsiella*
- ***CT chest*** Unlikely to add additional information. May be useful if the diagnosis is in doubt or the patient is severely ill and failing to respond to treatment in order to exclude abscess formation, empyema, underlying malignancy, or other interstitial disease process.
- ***Blood tests***
    - FBC—a white cell count (WCC) >15 x 10^9 suggests bacterial (particularly pneumococcal) infection. Counts of >20 or <4 indicate severe infection
    - Deranged renal and liver function tests can be indicative of severe infection, or point to the presence of underlying disease. LFTs may be abnormal, particularly with right lower lobe pneumonia. A raised urea is a marker of more severe pneumonia
    - Metabolic acidosis is associated with severe illness
    - C-reactive protein may be useful in management, with high levels being a more sensitive marker of infection than the white cell count or temperature. Serial measures may be useful in assessing response to treatment.

Microbiological investigations The microbiological cause for CAP is not found in 25–60% of patients and therefore often does not contribute to patient management. Microbiological investigations can help to aid selection of optimal antibiotics, hence limiting antibiotic resistance and the possible problems of *Clostridium difficile* associated diarrhoea. They also inform public health or infection control teams, aiding in the monitoring of pathogen trends causing CAP over time.

- ***Blood cultures*** Recommended for all patients with CAP, ideally before antibiotics are started. About 10% of patients with CAP will have positive blood cultures. The early availability of blood culture results (within 24 h of admission) improves outcome.
- ***Sputum culture and sensitivity*** Useful for those patients who have failed to improve with empirical antibiotic treatment, and in those with non-severe pneumonia admitted to hospital who are expectorating purulent samples and have not received prior antibiotics. Also useful in severe pneumonia. Not routinely recommended for those treated in the community. Sputum examination is recommended for possible tuberculosis in those with weight loss, a persistent cough, night sweats, and risk factors for TB, e.g. ethnic origin, social deprivation
- ***Pleural fluid*** (if present) for M, C, & S and pH to exclude empyema (see p 354)
- ***Viral and atypical pathogens*** In severe CAP only
- ***Serological testing*** Paired samples (from within 7 days of the onset of the illness, repeated 7–10 days later) should be tested together, in those with severe CAP, and in those unresponsive to β-lactam antibiotics. They are unlikely to guide initial treatment though.

Specific serological tests

- ***Pneumococcal pneumonia***
  - Urinary antigen (SpUA) has a sensitivity of 100% and specificity of 60–90% for invasive pneumococcal disease, and should be tested in all patients with severe CAP
- ***Legionnaires' disease*** A number of immunological tests exist to aid in the prompt and accurate diagnosis of *Legionella pneumophilia*:
  - Urinary antigen detection is about 70% sensitive and about 90% specific for serogroup A, and rapid results can be obtained early. A positive urinary antigen test correlates with subsequent ITU admission
  - Direct immunofluorescence tests (DIF)—*Legionella pneumophilia* can be detected on bronchial aspirates
  - Culture is 100% specific (sputum, endotracheal aspirate, BAL, pleural fluid, lung)
  - Serology—antibody levels and PCR are also available
- ***Mycoplasma pneumonia***
  - The complement fixation test (CFT) is the commonest serological assay and is regarded as the gold standard. Culture of *Mycoplasma pneumoniae* is not generally available
- ***Chlamydia***
  - Chlamydial antigen can be detected by DIF in respiratory samples or by CFT
- ***Others***
  - Influenza A and B, adenovirus, respiratory syncytial virus. *Coxiella burnetii* indirect immunofluorescence antibody test

CAP: management

General management

- ***Oxygen*** Hypoxia is due to V/Q mismatching, as blood flows through unventilated lung. Aim for oxygen saturation >92%. If there is severe concomitant COPD, controlled oxygen therapy and close monitoring of blood gases are mandatory. A rising CO_2 in a patient without prior respiratory disease may indicate they are tiring, and need respiratory support—discuss with ITU early
- ***Non-invasive ventilatory support*** **A number of studies demonstrate beneficial effects of NIV in severe CAP. However, following initial improvement in physiological parameters, >50% of patients subsequently deteriorate, requiring intubation. A higher initial respiratory rate (>30) is associated with failure of non-invasive ventilatory support (CPAP or bi-level ventilation). NIV may have a place in the management of severe CAP, but should only be used in a high dependency setting, with very close observation**
- ***Fluids*** Assessment of volume status by JVP (with or without central venous access) and blood pressure is paramount. Encourage oral fluids. Intravenous fluids may be needed if volume depleted and severely unwell. Monitor urine output
- ***Analgesia*** Paracetamol or NSAIDs initially if required. Paracetamol also has an antipyretic role
- ***Nutrition*** Nutritional status is important to the outcome, and nutritional supplements may be of benefit in prolonged illness. Poor nutritional status may increase the risk of acquiring pneumonia
- ***Physiotherapy*** is of no proven benefit in acute pneumonia.

Additional treatments

Bronchoscopy May be helpful, especially after intubation on ITU, to suction retained secretions, particularly if these are causing lobar collapse, to obtain further samples for culture, and to exclude an endobronchial abnormality.

Steroids There is some evidence that these are of benefit in severe bacterial pneumonia.

Monitoring Temperature, respiratory rate, heart rate, blood pressure, mental status, oxygen saturation, and inspired oxygen concentration should be monitored twice daily, and more often in the severely ill.

ICU admission Those fulfilling criteria for severe CAP on admission, or who fail to respond rapidly to treatment, should be considered for transfer for close monitoring, either to a high dependency unit or to ICU. Persisting hypoxia ($PaO_2 \leq 8$ kPa), acidosis, hypercapnia, hypotension, or depressed conscious level, despite maximal therapy, are indications for assisted ventilation. CPAP may be of benefit whilst awaiting for the arrival of the anaesthetist (although this may just be a more effective way of delivering 100% oxygen).

When to discuss patient with CAP with ITU

- Always sooner rather than later
- Respiratory failure (PaO_2 <8 kPa) despite high flow oxygen
- Tiring patient, with a rising CO_2
- Worsening metabolic acidosis, despite antibiotics and optimum fluid management
- Hypotension despite adequate fluid resuscitation.

CAP: antibiotics

- Most antibiotics are used empirically at diagnosis of CAP in the absence of microbiological information. The clinical scenario also guides antibiotic choice, such as the addition of anaerobic cover in an alcoholic who has a high chance of aspiration
- Severity assessment guides antibiotic therapy and the method of antibiotic administration
- Local protocols and antibiotic resistance patterns may also guide choice. Liaise closely with microbiologist.

General points

- Early administration of antibiotics is associated with an improved outcome
- Antibiotics given before admission can influence the results of subsequent microbiological investigations, but this should not delay antibiotic administration in the community if the patient is unwell
- It is vital that there is no delay in the administration of the first antibiotic dose in patients admitted to hospital. The admitting doctor should oversee its administration.

  IV antibiotics will be needed in 30–50% of patients admitted to hospital. Consider IV antibiotics if:
  - Severe pneumonia
  - Loss of swallow reflex
  - Impaired absorption
  - Impaired conscious level

  Oral antibiotics should be used in those with community-managed pneumonia, or those with non-severe hospital-managed pneumonia, with no other contraindications.
- ***Add anaerobic antibiotic cover,*** e.g. metronidazole if possible aspiration pneumonia in an unconscious patient, or if suspicion of a lung abscess on CXR/CT
- Switch from IV to oral antibiotics as soon as possible, usually when a patient has shown clear response to treatment, with a normal temperature for 24 h
- A switch to oral co-amoxiclav, and not an oral cephalosporin is recommended after treatment with IV cephalosporin
- For those treated with benzylpenicillin plus levofloxacin, a switch to oral levofloxacin ± oral amoxicillin is recommended

Length of treatment

There is no evidence to guide treatment length, but consensus suggests

- 5–7 days—non-severe, uncomplicated pneumonia
- 10 days—severe microbiologically undefined pneumonia
- 14–21 days—if Legionella, staphylococcal disease, Gram-negative suspected
- Consult local antibiotic guidelines; concern regarding increasing rates of *Clostridium difficile* has lead to reduced antibiotic course length and alternative empirical antibiotic choice in some centres. There is no evidence that any specific antibiotic (other than clindamycin) is more likely to cause *C. difficile* than any other

Table 40.1 Suggested initial antibiotics for CAP treatment

	Preferred treatment	Alternative (if intolerant of or allergic to preferred treatment)
Community treatment	Amoxicillin 500 mg–1 g tds PO	Erythromycin 500 mg qds PO or clarithromycin 500 mg bd PO
Hospital treatment: not severe pneumonia		
Oral	Amoxicillin 500 mg–1 g tds PO ± erythromycin 500 mg qds PO or clarithromycin 500 mg bd PO	Erythromycin 500 mg qds PO or clarithromycin 500 mg bd PO or levofloxacin 500 mg od PO or moxifloxacin 400 mg OD
If intravenous treatment needed	Ampicillin 500 mg qds IV or benzylpenicillin 1.2 g qds IV *plus* erythromycin 500 mg qds IV or clarithromycin 500 mg bd IV	Levofloxacin 500 mg od IV
Hospital treatment: severe pneumonia	Co-amoxiclav 1.2 g tds IV or cefuroxime 1.5 g tds IV or cefotaxime 1 g tds IV or ceftriaxone 2 g od IV *plus* erythromycin 500 mg qds IV (or clarithromycin 500 mg bd IV)	Levofloxacin 500 mg bd IV *plus* benzylpenicillin 1.2 g qds IV

New fluoroquinolones Moxifloxacin is licensed in the UK for the treatment of non-severe CAP. It is not available for IV use. It has equivalence to the other oral antibiotics used in CAP, but is not recommended for first-line treatment for CAP for community use, given the current low level of pneumococcal resistance in the UK. Levofloxacin is available in oral and IV preparations, and is licensed for severe CAP. In the future, other fluoroquinolones, e.g. gemafloxacin and gatifloxacin, are likely to extend the choice of oral antibiotics for CAP when they are licensed in the UK. The ketolides (e.g. telithromycin) are novel macrolides, with efficacy against penicillin- and erythromycin-resistant pathogens.

Antibiotic resistance Surveillance studies suggest that the UK prevalence of penicillin resistant *S. pnemoniae* is now about 20%. Macrolide resistant organisms may be as high as 25–30%. Worldwide prevalence of pneumococcal resistance to fluoroquinolones is low, at <2%, though this has increased substantially in some countries (e.g. Hong Kong) in recent years (because of the spread of a fluoroquinolone resistant clone).

CAP: treatment failure

A CRP that does not fall by >50% at 4 days suggests either treatment failure, or the development of a complication such as a lung abscess or empyema.

Causes of failure to improve

- Slow clinical response, particularly in the elderly patient
- Incorrect initial diagnosis
  - Pulmonary thromboembolic disease
  - Pulmonary oedema
  - Bronchial carcinoma
  - Bronchiectasis
  - Also consider eosinophilic pneumonia, foreign body aspiration, alveolar haemorrhage, cryptogenic organizing pneumonia, vasculitis or connective tissue disease, drug-induced lung disease
  - Review the history, examination, and radiology
  - Consider repeat imaging, e.g. CT chest
- Secondary complication
  - Pulmonary, e.g. parapneumonic effusion (occurs in 36–57%, most resolve spontaneously, thoracentesis is recommended), empyema, abscess formation, ARDS
  - Extrapulmonary, e.g. septicaemia, metastatic infection (e.g. meningitis, endocarditis, septic arthritis), sequelae of initial insult, e.g. renal failure, myocardial infarction
- Inappropriate antibiotics or unexpected pathogen
  - Review dose, compliance, and route of administration. Send further microbiological specimens
  - Review microbiological data, exclude less common pathogens, e.g. *Legionella, Mycoplasma,* staphylococcal disease
  - Pathogen may be resistant to common antibiotics; 10% of CAP will have a mixed infection
  - Consider tuberculosis, fungal infection
- Impaired immunity
  - Systemic, e.g. hypogammaglobulinaemia, HIV infection, myeloma
  - Local, e.g. bronchiectasis, aspiration, underlying bronchial carcinoma
  - Overwhelming infection

Table 40.2 Recommended antibiotic treatment of specific causative organisms

Pathogen	Preferred antibiotic	Alternative antibiotic
Streptococcus pneumoniae	Amoxicillin 500 mg–1 g tds PO or benzylpenicillin 1.2 g qds IV	Erythromycin 500 mg qds PO or clarithromycin 500 mg bd PO or cefuroxime 0.75–1.5 g tds IV or cefotaxime 1–2 g tds IV or ceftriaxone 2 g od IV
Mycoplasma pneumoniae and *Chlamydia pneumoniae*	Erythromycin 500 mg qds PO/IV or clarithromycin 500 mg bd PO or IV	Tetracycline 250–500 mg qds PO, or fluoroquinolone PO or IV
Chlamydia psittaci and *coxiella burnetii*	Tetracycline 250–500 mg qds PO or 500 mg bd IV	Erythromycin 500 mg qds or clarithromycin 500 mg bd, both PO or IV
Legionella sp.	Clarithromycin 500 mg bd PO, or IV rifampicin 600 mg od or bd, PO or IV	Fluoroquinolone PO or IV
Haemophilus influenzae	***Non-lactamase producing*** amoxicillin 500 mg tds PO or ampicillin 500 mg qds IV ***Lactamase producing*** co-amoxiclav 625 mg tds PO or 1.2 g tds IV	Cefuroxime 750 mg–1.5 g tds IV or cefotaxime 1–2 g tds IV or ceftriaxone 2 g od IV or fluoroquinolone PO or IV
Gram-negative enteric bacilli	Cefuroxime 1.5 g tds or cefotaxime 1–2 g tds IV or ceftriaxone 1–2 g od IV	Fluoroquinolone IV or imipenem 500 mg qds IV or meropenem 0.5–1.0 g tds IV
Pseudomonas aeruginosa	Ciprofloxacin 500–750 mg bd PO ceftazidime 2 g tds IV *plus* gentamicin or tobramycin (NB therapeutic drug monitoring)	Ciprofloxacin 400 mg bd IV or piperacillin 4 g tds *plus* gentamicin or tobramycin (NB therapeutic drug monitoring)
Staphylococcus aureus	***Non-MRSA*** flucloxacillin 1–2 g qds IV ± rifampicin 600 mg od/bd, PO, or IV ***MRSA*** vancomycin 1 g bd (NB therapeutic drug monitoring)	Teicoplanin 400 mg bd IV ± rifampicin 600 mg od or bd PO/IV linezolid 600 mg bd PO/IV

CAP: follow-up

CXR resolution Radiographic improvement lags behind clinical improvement. There is no need to repeat a CXR before hospital discharge in those who have made a satisfactory clinical recovery.

- In one study of CAP, complete radiographic resolution occurred after 6 weeks in 74% of patients, but only in 51% at 2 weeks
- Radiographic resolution is slower in the elderly, those with multilobe involvement at presentation, smokers, and hospital in-patients
- Legionella and pneumococcal pneumonia are slower to resolve (may take 12 weeks or more).

CXR follow-up is recommended around 6 weeks after CAP:

- In all patients with persisting symptoms or clinical signs
- In all patients at higher risk of underlying lung malignancy, i.e. smokers and those over the age of 50.

This is to exclude an underlying condition that may have led to CAP, such as lung cancer. Further investigations, such as bronchoscopy, should be considered at this time in patients with persisting symptoms and/or a persistently abnormal CXR.

- One study showed lung cancer is diagnosed on follow-up in 17% of smokers aged over 60 treated for CAP in the community
- Other studies have shown a prevalence of lung cancer of 11% in current and ex-smokers aged over 50, who are in-patients with CAP and who undergo bronchoscopy prior to discharge.

Vaccination

Influenza vaccination This reduces hospital deaths from pneumonia and influenza by about 65% and respiratory deaths by 45%. It also leads to fewer hospital admissions.

Recommended for 'high-risk' individuals

- Chronic lung disease
- Cardiac, renal, and liver disease
- Diabetes
- Immunosuppression due to disease or treatment
- Those aged over 65
- Long-stay residential care
- Health care workers
- Contraindicated in people with hen egg hypersensitivity (the virus is cultured in chick embryos).

The vaccination contains both A and B subtype viruses and provides partial protection against influenza illnesses. It is modified annually, based on recent viral strains. The protection rate from influenza by vaccination is over 75% for influenza A and 51–97% for influenza B. Antibody levels appear to reduce about 6 years after vaccination.

Pneumococcal vaccination

Recommended for:

- Asplenic individuals (including coeliac disease and sickle cell disease)
- Chronic renal, cardiac, and liver disease
- Diabetes
- Immunodeficiency or immunosuppression (due to disease, including HIV infection, or drugs).

It should not be given during acute infection or in pregnancy. Re-immunization is contraindicated within 3 years.

Further information

British Thoracic Society Guidelines for the management of community acquired pneumonia in Adults. *Thorax* 2001; **56**(S): VI

An updated version of the 2001 guidelines is on the BTS website: http://www.brit-thoracic.org.uk/c2/uploads/MACAPrevisedApr04.pdf

Thomas MF. Community acquired pneumonia. *Lancet* 2003; **362**: 1991–2001

Hospital-acquired pneumonia: clinical features

Definition New radiographic infiltrate in the presence of evidence of infection (fever, purulent sputum, leucocytosis) with onset at least 72 h after hospital admission. It represents around 15% of hospital-acquired infections. Most occur outside the ICU, but those at highest risk are mechanically ventilated patients. Hospital-acquired pneumonia is expensive and prolongs the hospital stay. It requires different antibiotic treatment to community-acquired pneumonia, and is the leading cause of death from hospital-acquired infection. It is also known as nosocomial pneumonia.

Pathophysiology Hospital-acquired pneumonia occurs from haematogenous spread of organisms, aspiration of infected upper airway secretions, or from the inhalation of bacteria from contaminated equipment.

Aspiration is thought to be the most important cause. Around 45% of normal people aspirate during sleep, and this is increased in hospital in-patients (who may be more frail) and in those with chronic disease. These patients' upper airways become colonized with Gram-negative bacteria (in up to 75% within 48 h of admission) and this proportion is even higher in those who have received broad-spectrum antibiotics. In addition, the severely ill may have impaired host defences, making them more susceptible to hospital-acquired pneumonia. Alteration in the gastric pH with illness, and various drugs, means that the gastrointestinal tract is no longer sterile, thereby providing a potential source of bacterial infection. A cerebrovascular event and reduced conscious level are the major risk factors for aspiration.

Risk factors for nosocomial pneumonia

- Age >70
- Chronic lung disease and/or other comorbidity (especially diabetes)
- Reduced conscious level/cerebrovascular accident
- Chest/abdominal surgery
- Mechanical ventilation
- Nasogastric feeding
- Previous antibiotic exposure
- Poor dental hygiene
- Steroids and cytotoxic drugs.

Risk factors for specific organisms

Streptococcus pneumoniae and Haemophilus influenza Increased risk in trauma.
Staphylococcus aureus Increased risk in ventilated neurosurgical patients (especially closed head injury), blunt trauma, and coma.
Pseudomonas aeruginosa Increased risk with intubation >8 days, COPD, prolonged antibiotics.
Acinetobacter spp. Increased risk with prolonged ventilation and previous broad spectrum antibiotics.
Anaerobic bacteria Increased with recent abdominal surgery, aspiration.

Clinical features It presents typically with:

- Fever
- Productive cough
- Raised inflammatory parameters
- New CXR infiltrate
- Deterioration in gas exchange.

Diagnosis is often a clinical one, and identification of the infecting agent can be difficult, especially if the patient has already received broad spectrum antibiotics.

Investigations

- *CXR* usually shows a non-specific infiltrate
- *Blood, sputum, and pleural fluid* should be cultured
- *Arterial blood gas* to determine severity
- *Renal and liver function tests* to assess other organ dysfunction
- *Serological tests* are of little use in nosocomial pneumonia.

Hospital-acquired pneumonia: management

Severity assessment The CURB or CURB-65 pneumonia severity score (see p 180) for community-acquired pneumonia has not been validated in hospital-acquired pneumonia, but may be useful in guiding the treatment needed.

Microbiology

- About 50% are mixed infections
- 30% are due to aerobic bacteria alone (most commonly Gram-negative bacilli and *Pseudomonas*)
- Anaerobes alone are found in about 25%
- *Pseudomonas aeruginosa* and *Staphylococcus aureus* are common causes
- *Peptostreptococcus, Fusobacteroides,* and *Bacteroides* species are commonly isolated, as well as *Enterobacter* spp., *Escherichia coli, Serratia marcescens, Klebsiella,* and *Proteus* spp.
- *Acinetobacter* is a new emerging pathogen
- *MRSA* is increasing in prevalence
- *Viruses* are recognized as causes.

Management

- Patients developing pneumonia within 48 h of arrival in hospital can be treated with standard community-acquired pneumonia antibiotics (see p 430), as the pneumonia is likely to be due to bacteria acquired in the community
- Patients developing pneumonia more than 48 h after hospital admission need antibiotics to cover different organisms
- Intravenous, prolonged treatment is usually needed, with cover for Gram-negative anaerobic bacteria. This is best done by using a second-generation cephalosporin, e.g. cefuroxime 750 mg–1.5 g tds, with an aminoglycoside, e.g. gentamicin 7 mg/kg od (unless renal impairment), with levels at 8–12 h, to determine dose interval
- Supportive treatment is also required, with oxygen, fluids, and ventilation if necessary
- In penicillin-allergic patients clindamycin or ciprofloxacin can be used (as long as *Streptococcus pneumoniae* is not thought to be the infecting agent). Levofloxacin has better pneumococcal cover
- Complications of nosocomial pneumonia are the same as for community-acquired pneumonia, including lung abscess and empyema. Drug fever, sepsis with multi-organ failure, and pulmonary embolus with secondary infection are all more common in nosocomial pneumonia
- In this situation, chest ultrasound (to look for empyema) or CT scanning may demonstrate abscess, underlying tumour, or infection at extrathoracic sites.

Prognosis It has a high mortality, ranging between 20 and 50%.

Prevention Meticulous hygiene and hand washing by medical staff, in addition to careful infection control measures have been shown to reduce hospital-acquired pneumonia.

Post-operatively, early mobilization, careful cleaning and maintenance of respiratory equipment, and pre-operative smoking cessation reduce infection rates. Some intensive care units use antibiotics to selectively decontaminate the gastrointestinal tract of Gram-negative bacilli. This has been shown to reduce infection rates, but there is no proven effect on mortality or length of ITU admission.

Ventilator-acquired pneumonia (VAP)

Definition Pneumonia in a mechanically ventilated patient, which develops 48 h after intubation. It has a prevalence of up to 65% in some units. It is an independent predictor of mortality, and is the commonest nosocomial infection in ITU. Up to two-thirds of patients requiring mechanical ventilation for >48 h will develop VAP. It has a mortality of 15–50%, increasing the length of ITU stay by an average of 6.1 days.

The major cause is bacterial contamination of the lower respiratory tract from the aspiration of oropharyngeal secretions, which is not prevented by cuffed endotracheal tube or tracheostomy.

Diagnosis is suggested by

- New or progressive CXR infiltrate
- Associated with fever, high WCC, and purulent secretions

There are many non-infectious causes of fever and CXR infiltrate in ITU patients, so the diagnosis is not always straightforward.

Differential diagnosis of fever and CXR infiltrate in ITU

- Chemical aspiration without infection
- Atelectasis
- ARDS
- Left ventricular failure
- PE with lung infarction
- Pulmonary haemorrhage
- Cryptogenic organizing pneumonia (COP)
- Drug reaction
- Tumour
- Lung contusion.

Investigations

- ***CXR*** often shows a non-specific infiltrate, with air bronchograms being the best predictor of the disease
- ***Airway sampling for microbiology***
  - *Bronchoscopic sampling* Protected specimen brush (PSB) samples (with the tip of the bronchoscope placed opposite the orifice of an involved segmental bronchus, and the PSB advanced through its protective sheath into the airway) or BAL samples (from a subsegmental bronchus, with the end of the bronchoscope wedged into the airway, ideally >150 mL saline wash) are the best methods to obtain lower airway samples with minimal contamination. VAP is diagnosed when an arbitrary threshold of organisms is grown on a BAL or PSB sample. The usual cut-offs are 1000 colony-forming units/mL (cfu/mL) for PSB samples, and >10,000 cfu/mL for BAL samples. The thresholds will vary from unit to unit, and the threshold for starting treatment will also vary. Quantitative culture of bronchopulmonary secretions leads to reduced antibiotic use, and is associated with improved outcomes. Airway neutrophil counts may also aid in making the diagnosis

- *Non-bronchoscopic airway sampling*, e.g. blind bronchial sampling of lower respiratory tract secretions, is less sensitive and specific than bronchoscopic sampling. It does not need an expert operator, and is cheaper
- *Serial sampling* is favoured in some units. Regular non-invasive serial airway sampling may aid early diagnosis of VAP. It needs careful interpretation, as the microbiology of the respiratory tract changes over time in critically ill mechanically ventilated patients
- *Tracheal aspiration samples* are easy to obtain, but non-specific in diagnosing VAP, as upper airway colonization is very common

- Additional sources of fever are common in ventilated patients, including infected lines, sinusitis, urinary tract infection, and pseudomembranous colitis, and may warrant further investigation.

Antibiotic treatment Problems with the emergence of resistant bacteria mean that empirical treatment with antibiotics is used less commonly. Local policies are often in place and advice should always be sought from microbiology. The most common drug resistant pathogens are *P. aeruginosa,* MRSA, *Acinetobacter* spp. and *Klebsiella* spp. Delay in commencing antibiotics is associated with a poorer outcome.

Risk factors for resistant organisms include:

- Hospitalization in the previous 90 days
- Nursing home residence
- Current hospital admission >5 days
- Mechanical ventilation >7 days
- Prior broad-spectrum antibiotic use (e.g. third-generation cephalosporin)
- High frequency of local antibiotic resistance.

Antibiotics should be chosen on the basis of:

- Recent antibiotic treatment
- Local policy and known local flora
- Culture data.

Antibiotics should cover anaerobes and ***MRSA, Legionella*** (if long hospital stay), ***Pseudomonas aeruginosa***, and ***Acinetobacter***.

Length of treatment depends on the clinical response. Patients with *P. aeruginosa* infection have been shown to have a greater risk of recurrence following discontinuation of antibiotics at 8 days. Failure to respond should lead to a change of antibiotics, and a search for additional infection or another cause for the radiographic infiltrate. Further cultures should be sent.

Aspiration pneumonia

Definition Pneumonia that follows the aspiration of exogenous material or endogenous secretions into the lower respiratory tract.

Epidemiology Aspiration pneumonia is the commonest cause of death in patients with dysphagia due to neurological disorders and is the cause of up to 20% of pneumonias in nursing home residents. It occurs in about 10% of patients admitted to hospital with a drug overdose.

Pathophysiology Micro-aspiration is common in healthy individuals, but for an aspiration pneumonia to occur, there must be compromise of the normal defences protecting the lower airways (i.e. glottic closure, cough reflex), with inoculation of the lower respiratory tract of a significant amount of material. Most pneumonias are a result of aspiration of micro-organisms from the oral cavity or nasopharynx.

Situations predisposing to aspiration pneumonia

- ***Reduced conscious level*** (cough reflex and impaired glottic closure)
  - Alcohol
  - Drug overdose
  - Post-seizure
  - Post-anaesthesia
  - Massive CVA
- ***Dysphagia***
  - Motor neuron disease
  - Following a neurological event; those with impaired swallow reflex post-CVA are seven times more likely to develop a pneumonia than those in whom the gag reflex is unimpaired
- ***Upper gastrointestinal tract disease***
  - Surgery to the stomach or oesophagus
  - Mechanical impairment of glottic or cardiac sphincter closure, e.g. tracheostomy, nasogastric feeding, bronchoscopy
  - Pharyngeal anaesthesia
- ***Increased reflux***
  - Large volume vomiting
  - Large volume nasogastric feed
  - Feeding gastrostomy
  - Recumbent position
- ***Nursing home residents***
  - The risk of aspiration is lower in those without teeth, who receive aggressive oral hygiene
  - There is a higher incidence of silent aspiration in the otherwise healthy elderly
  - High correlation between volume of aspirate and the risk of developing pneumonia.

Aspiration pneumonia: clinical features

Three pulmonary syndromes result from aspiration. The amount and nature of the aspirated material, the site and frequency of the aspiration, and the host's response to it will determine which pulmonary syndrome occurs.

1. Chemical pneumonitis

This is aspiration of substances toxic to the lower airways, in the absence of bacterial infection.

This causes a chemical burn of the tracheobronchial tree causing an intense parenchymal inflammatory reaction, with release of inflammatory mediators, that may lead to ARDS. Animal studies show that an inoculum with a pH <2.5, of relatively large volume (about 25 mL in adults) is needed to initiate an inflammatory reaction. Animal models show rapid pathological changes within 3 min, with atelectasis, pulmonary haemorrhage, and pulmonary oedema. (This was first described by Mendelson, referring to the aspiration of sterile gastric contents and its toxic effects. The original case series was in obstetric anaesthesia.)

Clinical features

- Rapid onset of symptoms, with breathlessness (within 1–2 h)
- Low-grade fever
- Severe hypoxaemia and diffuse lung infiltrates involving dependent segments
- CXR changes within 2 h.

Treatment

- If aspiration is observed—suction and/or bronchoscopy to clear aspirated secretions or food. This may not prevent chemical injury from acid, which is similar to a flash burn
- Support of cardiac and respiratory function—with intravenous fluids, oxygen ± ventilation
- Steroids—controversial. No benefit has been shown in human studies, but there is some evidence to support their early use in ARDS
- Antibiotics—usually given, even in the absence of evidence of infection, because secondary bacterial infection is common, and may be a contributing or primary factor in the aspiration. Acid-damaged lung is more susceptible to the effects of secondary bacterial infection; up to 25% will develop secondary bacterial infection. Activity against Gram-negative and anaerobic organisms is needed, e.g. cefuroxime plus metronidazole, or penicillin plus clindamycin.

2. Bacterial infection Aspiration of bacteria normally resident in the upper airways or stomach. The normal bacterial flora are anaerobes, in a host susceptible to aspiration, and less virulent than the bacteria causing CAP.

Clinical features depend on the infecting organism:
- Cough, fever, purulent sputum, breathlessness
- The process may evolve over weeks and months, rather than hours
- May be more chronic, with weight loss and anaemia
- Absence of fever or rigors
- Foul smelling sputum
- Periodontal disease
- Involvement of dependent pulmonary lobes
- Anaerobic bacteria are more difficult to culture, so may be present, but not identified in microbiological culture
- May present with later manifestations, e.g. empyema, lung abscess.

Major pathogens are ***Peptostreptococcus, Fusobacterium nucleatum, Prevotella***, and ***Bacteroides*** spp. Mixed infection is common.

Treatment
- Antibiotics, to include anaerobic cover, e.g. co-amoxiclav or metronidazole plus penicillin
- Swallow assessment/neurological review if no obvious underlying cause found.

3. Mechanical obstruction Aspiration of matter that is not directly toxic to the lung may lead to damage by causing airway obstruction or reflex airway closure. Causative agents include:
- Saline
- Barium
- Most ingested fluids, including water
- Gastric contents with a pH >2.5
- Mechanical obstruction, such as occurs in drowning, or those who are unable to clear a potential inoculum, e.g. neurological deficit, impaired cough reflex, reduced conscious level
- Inhalation of an object, with the severity of the obstruction depending on the size and site of the aspirated particle. This is commoner in children, but does occur in adults, e.g. teeth, peanuts.

Treatment
- Tracheal suction
- No further treatment is needed if no CXR infiltrates.

Lung abscess: clinical features

Definition A localized area of lung suppuration leading to necrosis of the pulmonary parenchyma, with or without cavity formation.

Lung abscesses may be single or multiple, acute or chronic (>1 month), primary or secondary. They may occur spontaneously, but, more commonly an underlying disease exists. Lung abscess is now rare in the developed world, but has a high mortality of 20–30%. They are most common in alcoholic men aged >50.

Pathophysiology Most are the result of aspiration pneumonia. Predisposing factors for abscess are those for aspiration pneumonia (p 442).

- Dental disease
- Impaired consciousness—alcohol, post-anaesthesia, dysphagia
- Diabetes
- Bronchial carcinoma (with bronchial obstruction)
- Secondary to pneumonia (cavitation occurs in about 16% of *Staphylococcus aureus* pneumonia)
- Immunocompromise—abscesses due to *Pneumocystis jiroveci* (PCP), *Cryptococcus neoformans, Rhodococcus* species, and fungi in HIV positive patients
- Septic embolization (right heart endocarditis due to *Staphylococcus aureus* in intravenous drug abusers).

The bacterial inoculum reaches the lung parenchyma, often in a dependent lung area. Cavitation occurs when parenchymal necrosis leads to communication with the bronchus, with the entry of air and expectoration of necrotic material, leading to the formation of an air fluid level. Bronchial obstruction leads to atelectasis with stasis and subsequent infection, which can predispose to abscess formation.

Presentation

- Often insidious onset
- Productive cough, haemoptysis
- Breathlessness
- Fevers
- Night sweats
- Non-specific feature of chronic infection—anaemia, weight loss, malaise (especially in the elderly)
- Foul sputum or purulent pleural fluid.

Lemierre's syndrome (necrobacillosis) Jugular vein suppurative thrombophlebitis. This is a rare pharyngeal infection in young adults, most commonly due to the anaerobe *Fusobacterium necrophorum*. It presents with a classical history of painful pharyngitis, in the presence of bacteraemia. Infection spreads to the neck and carotid sheath, often leading to thrombosis of the internal jugular vein. This may not be obvious clinically (neck vein USS or Doppler may be needed). Septic embolization to the lung with subsequent cavitation leads to abscess formation. Empyema and abscesses in the bone, joints, liver, and kidneys can complicate.

Lung abscess: diagnosis

The diagnosis is usually made from the history along with the appearance of a cavity with an associated air-fluid level on CXR.

Investigations

- Microbiological culture, ideally before commencing antibiotics. Useful to exclude tuberculosis
    - Blood cultures
    - Sputum or bronchoscopic specimen (BAL or brushings rarely needed)
    - Transthoracic percutaneous needle aspiration (CT- or ultrasound-guided) may provide samples. Risk of bleeding, pneumothorax, and seeding of infection to pleural space, if abscess not adjacent to the pleura

In practice, blood cultures and sputum microbiology usually suffice. Samples are usually only obtained by more invasive means if appropriate antibiotics are not leading to an adequate clinical response.

- ***Imaging***—exclude aspirated foreign body, underlying neoplasm, or bronchial stenosis and obstruction
    - ***CXR*** may show consolidation, cavitation, air-fluid level (if the patient is unwell, the CXR is likely to be taken in a semi-recumbent position, so an air-fluid level may not be visible). 50% of abscesses are in the posterior segment of the right upper lobe, or the apical basal segments of either lower lobe
    - ***CT*** is useful if the diagnosis is in doubt and cannot be confirmed from the CXR appearance, or if the clinical response to treatment is inadequate. It can also help to define the exact position of the abscess (which may be useful for physiotherapy, or if surgery is being considered—rarely needed)

CT also is useful to differentiate an abscess from a pleural collection—a *lung abscess* appears as a rounded intrapulmonary mass, with no compression of adjacent lung, with a thickened irregular wall, making an acute angle at its contact with the chest wall. An *empyema* typically has a 'lenticular' shape and compresses adjacent lung, which creates an obtuse angle as it follows the contour of the chest wall.

CT can determine the presence of obstructing endobronchial disease, due to malignancy or foreign body, and may be useful in defining the extent of disease in a very sick patient who has had significant haemoptysis. Even with CT, differentiating an abscess from a cavitating malignancy can be very difficult (no radiological features differentiate them).

Microbiology Commonly mixed infection, usually anaerobes.

- The most common organisms are those colonizing the oral cavity and gingival crevices—*Peptostreptococcus, Prevotella, Bacteroides*, and *Fusobacterium* spp
- Aerobes—*Streptococcus milleri, Staphylococcus aureus, Klebsiella* spp., *Streptococcus pyogenes, Haemophilus influenzae, Nocardia*
- Non-bacterial pathogens are also reported—fungi (*Aspergillus, Cryptococcus, Histoplasma, Blastomyces*) and *Mycobacteria*

Opportunistic infections in immunocompromised—*Nocardia, Mycobacteria, Aspergillus.*

Differential diagnosis of a cavitating mass, with or without an air-fluid level

- Cavitating carcinoma—primary or metastatic
- Cavitatory tuberculosis
- Wegener's granulomatosis
- Infected pulmonary cyst or bulla (can produce a fluid level, usually thinner walled)
- Aspergilloma
- Pulmonary infarct
- Rheumatoid nodule
- Sarcoidosis
- Bronchiectasis.

Lung abscess: management

Antibiotics to cover aerobic and anaerobic infection, including β-lactamase inhibitors, e.g. co-amoxiclav and clindamycin. Long courses are needed. Risk of *Clostridium difficile* diarrhoea.

- Infections are usually mixed, therefore antibiotics to cover these
- Metronidazole to cover anaerobes
- No data to guide length of treatment. Common practice would be 1–2 weeks intravenous treatment, with a further 2–6 weeks oral antibiotics, often until out-patient clinic review.

Drainage Spontaneous drainage is common, with the production of purulent sputum. This can be increased with postural drainage and physiotherapy.

- No data to support use of bronchoscopic drainage
- Percutaneous drainage with radiologically placed small percutaneous drains for peripheral abscesses may be useful in those failing to respond to antibiotic and supportive treatment. These are usually placed under ultrasound guidance (though are rarely indicated).

Surgery is rarely required if appropriate antibiotic treatment is given. It is usually reserved for complicated infections failing to respond to standard treatment after at least 6 weeks of treatment.

May be needed if:

- Very large abscess (>6 cm diameter)
- Resistant organisms
- Haemorrhage
- Recurrent disease
- Lobectomy or pneumonectomy is occasionally needed if severe infection with an abscess leaves a large volume of damaged lung that is hard to sterilize.

Complications Haemorrhage (erosion of blood vessels as the abscess extends into the lung parenchyma). This can be massive and life-threatening (see p 43), and is an indication for urgent surgery.

If slow to respond, consider:

- Underlying malignancy
- Unusual microbiology, e.g. mycobacterium, fungi
- Immunosuppression
- Large cavity (>6 cm) may rarely require drainage
- Non-bacterial cause e.g. cavitating malignancy, Wegener's granulomatosis
- Other cause of persistent fever, e.g. *Clostridium difficile* diarrhoea, antibiotic-associated fever.

Prognosis 85% cure rate in the absence of underlying disease. Mortality is reported as high as 75% in immunocompromised patients. The prognosis is much worse in the presence of underlying lung disease, with increasing age and large abscesses (>6 cm) with *Staphylococcus aureus* infection.

Nocardiosis

Definition *Nocardia* are Gram-positive, partially acid-fast, aerobic bacilli that form branching filaments. They are found in soil, decaying organic plant matter, and water, and have been isolated from house dust, garden soil, and swimming pools. Infection typically follows inhalation, although percutaneous inoculation also occurs. The *Nocardia asteroides* species complex accounts for the majority of clinical infections.

Consider *Nocardia* infection when soft tissue abscesses and/or CNS manifestations occur in the setting of a pulmonary infection. The combination of respiratory, skin, and/or CNS involvement may lead to a misdiagnosis of vasculitis, and the respiratory manifestations may mimic cancer, tuberculosis, or fungal disease.

Epidemiology *Nocardia* occurs worldwide and the frequency of subclinical exposure is unknown. Clinically apparent infection is rare, and usually occurs in patients with immunocompromise (haematological malignancy, steroid therapy, organ transplant, diabetes, alcoholism, and HIV infection, especially IV drug users) or pre-existing lung disease (particularly pulmonary alveolar proteinosis, tuberculosis). Infection also occurs in apparently healthy people (10–25% of cases). Nosocomial infection and disease outbreaks have been reported.

Clinical features

Pulmonary disease

- The lung is the most common site of involvement
- Patients typically present with productive cough, fever, anorexia, weight loss, and malaise; dyspnoea, pleuritic pain, and haemoptysis may occur, but are less common
- Empyema occurs in up to a quarter of cases, and direct intrathoracic spread causing pericarditis, mediastinitis, rib osteomyelitis, or SVCO is also reported

Extrapulmonary disease

- Dissemination from the lungs occurs in 50% of patients
- Central nervous system is the most common site of dissemination, occurring in 25% of pulmonary nocardiosis cases. Single or multiple abscesses occur, and may be accompanied by meningitis
- Other sites include the skin and subcutaneous tissues, kidneys, bone, joints and muscle, peritoneum, eyes, pericardium, and heart valves.

Investigations

- Identification by smear and culture is the principal method of diagnosis. *Nocardia* grow on routine media usually within 2–7 days, although more prolonged culture (2–3 weeks) may be required
- Direct smear of appropriate specimens (e.g. aspirates of abscesses, biopsies) is highly sensitive and typically shows Gram-positive beaded branching filaments, which are usually acid-fast on modified ZN stain. Examination of BAL fluid may also be diagnostic

- Sensitivity testing of isolates and identification to species level is done by reference laboratories
- Biopsies typically show a mixed cellular infiltrate; granulomata occur rarely, and may result in misdiagnosis as tuberculosis or histoplasmosis
- CXR and CT may demonstrate parenchymal infiltrates, single or multiple nodules (sometimes with cavitation), or features of pleural infection
- Sputum smear is usually unhelpful. Sputum culture has a greater yield, but *Nocardia* growth may be obscured in mixed cultures. The significance of *Nocardia* growth on sputum culture in asymptomatic patients is unclear; it may represent contamination or colonization in the setting of underlying lung disease
- Blood cultures are almost always negative, although *Nocardia* bacteraemia may occur in the setting of profound immunocompromise
- Consider MRI of the brain to exclude asymptomatic CNS involvement in patients with pulmonary nocardiosis.

Management

- Discuss treatment with an infectious diseases specialist
- Drug treatment choices include sulphonamides/co-trimoxazole, minocycline, imipenem, cefotaxime, ceftriaxone, or amikacin. Sulpha drugs, in particular co-trimoxazole, have traditionally been the mainstay of therapy. Imipenem and amikacin combination therapy has been shown to be active *in vitro* and in animal models, and is recommended for pulmonary nocardiosis and for very ill patients. Extended spectrum cephalosporins such as ceftriaxone and cefotaxime have the advantages of good CNS penetration and low toxicity
- Optimal treatment duration is unclear: typically given for 6 months in non-immunocompromised patients, and for 12 months or longer for CNS involvement or immunocompromised patients
- Surgery may be required for abscess drainage.

Prognosis Clinical outcome is dependent on the site and extent of disease and on underlying host factors. Disease remissions and exacerbations are common. Cure rates are approximately 90% in pleuropulmonary disease, and 50% in brain abscess. Mortality of *Nocardia* infection is generally low, although it approaches 50% in cases of bacteraemia.

Further information

Saubolle MA, Sussland D. Nocardiosis: review of clinical and laboratory experience. *J Clin Microbiol* 2003; **41**: 4497–501

Lerner PI. Nocardiosis. *Clin Inf Dis* 1996; **22**: 891–905

Actinomycosis

Definition Actinomycosis is caused by a group of anaerobic Gram-positive bacilli, of which *Actinomyces israelii* is the commonest. These organisms are present in the mouth, gastrointestinal tract, and vagina. Clinical infection may follow dental procedures or aspiration of infected secretions. Infection is slowly progressive and may disseminate via the bloodstream or invade tissue locally, sometimes resulting in sinus tract formation.

Consider this diagnosis particularly in patients with pulmonary disease accompanied by soft tissue infection of the head and neck. The diagnosis of actinomycosis is often unsuspected, and the clinical and radiological features may mimic cancer, tuberculosis, or fungal disease.

Epidemiology Actinomycosis is rare. It can occur at any age, and is more common in men. Predisposing factors include corticosteroid use, chemotherapy, organ transplant, and HIV infection.

Clinical features

Thoracic disease Thoracic disease occurs in about 15% of cases. Symptoms of pulmonary involvement are non-specific, and include cough, chest pain, haemoptysis, fever, anorexia, and weight loss. Chest wall involvement may occur, with sinus formation or rib infection, and empyema is common. Mediastinal involvement is documented.

Extrathoracic disease Soft tissue infection of the head and neck, particularly the mandible, is the commonest disease presentation (about 50% of cases). Discharging sinuses may form. Other extrathoracic disease sites include the abdomen (particularly the ileocaecal region), pelvis, liver, bone, and CNS (manifest as single or multiple abscesses).

Investigations

- CXR and CT appearances are variable, including masses (sometimes with cavitation), parenchymal infiltrates, consolidation, mediastinal disease, and/or pleural involvement
- Diagnosis is based on the microscopy and anaerobic culture of infected material. Warn the microbiology laboratory if the diagnosis is suspected, as specific stains and culture conditions are required. Examination of infected material may reveal yellow 'sulphur granules' containing aggregated organisms. Sample sputum, pleural fluid, and pus from sinus tracts; inoculate into anaerobic transport media, and rapidly transport to lab. Endobronchial biopsies have a low sensitivity. Most infections are polymicrobial, with accompanying aerobic or anaerobic bacteria.

Management

- Discuss treatment with an infectious diseases specialist
- Drug treatment choices include penicillin, amoxicillin, clindamycin, or erythromycin. Administration should initially be intravenous. Optimal treatment duration is unclear (typically given for 6–12 months)
- Surgery may be required for abscess drainage
- Monitor response to treatment with serial CT or MRI scans
- Treat any associated periodontal disease.

Prognosis Disease relapse is common if prolonged treatment is not administered.

Further information

Mabeza GF, Mcfarlane J. Pulmonary actinomycosis. *Eur Resp J* 2003; **21**: 545–51

Anthrax

Definition and epidemiology

- *Bacillus anthracis* is an aerobic Gram-positive spore-forming bacterium that causes human disease, principally following either inhalation or cutaneous contact. Spores can survive in soil for many years. Person-to-person transmission does not occur
- Considerable recent interest has focused on the use of anthrax in bioterrorism: five envelopes containing anthrax spores were sent through the US postal service in 2001 and there were 11 confirmed cases of inhalational anthrax (including 5 deaths) and 7 confirmed cases of cutaneous anthrax. A previous outbreak occurred in Sverdlovsk in the former Soviet Union in 1979, following the release of spores from a biological weapons plant, and resulted in 68 deaths
- Anthrax infection also occurs very rarely in association with occupational exposure to *Bacillus anthracis* in animal wool or hides. The majority of occupational cases result in cutaneous disease, and a diagnosis of inhalational anthrax strongly suggests a bioterrorist attack.

Clinical features

Inhalational anthrax

- Incubation period is variable, although in the USA in 2001 it typically ranged 4–6 days following exposure from opening mail
- Patients typically experience a prodrome of flu-like symptoms such as fever and cough. Gastrointestinal symptoms (vomiting, diarrhoea, abdominal pain), drenching sweats, and altered mental status are often prominent symptoms. Breathlessness, fever, and septic shock develop several days later. Haemorrhagic meningitis is a common complication
- Large haemorrhagic pleural effusions are a characteristic feature.

Cutaneous anthrax

- Initial symptoms include itch and development of a papule at the infection site. A necrotic ulcer with a black centre and often surrounding oedema subsequently develops. Systemic symptoms such as fever and sweats may be present.

Investigations

- *Bacillus anthracis* grows on conventional media, and is readily cultured if sampling precedes antibiotic treatment; a definitive diagnosis requires specialized laboratory tests, however
- Blood tests typically reveal leucocytosis
- Blood cultures are positive in nearly all cases of inhalational anthrax when taken prior to antibiotic treatment. Staining and culture of pleural fluid may be diagnostic
- CXR in inhalational anthrax classically shows a widened mediastinum; pleural effusions and pulmonary infiltrates may be present. CT may also demonstrate mediastinal and hilar lymphadenopathy
- Gram stain and culture of the ulcer is usually diagnostic in cutaneous anthrax, although biopsy is sometimes required.

Management

- Discuss with infectious diseases and public health specialists if the diagnosis is suspected
- Antibiotic treatment should be administered immediately after taking blood cultures. Recent recommendations are for initial treatment with either ciprofloxacin or doxycycline IV, in combination with 1–2 additional antibiotics (choices include clindamycin, vancomycin, meropenem, or penicillin). Subsequent treatment should be with either ciprofloxacin or doxycycline orally for 60–100 days. Oral treatment alone may be sufficient in cases of mild cutaneous disease
- Corticosteroid treatment should be considered in patients with meningitis, or severe neck or mediastinal oedema
- Supportive care, including ventilatory support, treatment of shock with intravenous fluids and/or inotropes, and chest tube drainage of large pleural effusions may be needed.

Prognosis Inhalational anthrax is associated with a high mortality: 5 of the recent 11 cases in the USA died. The mortality of previously documented cases has been even higher, perhaps reflecting a delay or lack of antibiotic treatment.

Prophylaxis Recent USA recommendations advise prophylaxis with oral ciprofloxacin or doxycycline for individuals considered to have been exposed to anthrax spores in contaminated areas. A vaccine is available, although its value in post-exposure prophylaxis is unknown.

Tularaemia

Definition and epidemiology Tularaemia is a rare zoonosis caused by infection with the Gram negative bacteria *Francisella tularensis*. Two major subspecies are described: *biovar tularensis* (type A) is highly virulent and found in North America; *biovar palaeartica* (type B) is less virulent, and found in Europe and Asia. Small mammals (particularly rabbits and hares) acquire infection from arthropod bites and act as reservoirs; human infection follows inhalation, direct contact with infected rodents, ingestion of contaminated food, or arthropod bites. Tularaemia is most frequently encountered in rural areas, following activities such as farming and hunting, although laboratory workers are also at risk. There has been considerable interest in the development of *F. tularensis* as a biological weapon, and more recently concerns have arisen as to its possible use in bioterrorism.

Clinical features Typically abrupt onset of fever, headache, dry cough and malaise. Development of a tender ulcer and regional lymphadenopathy ('ulceroglandular tularaemia') around an infected arthropod bite is common. Tularaemia pneumonia following infection with type A is characterized by cough (productive or dry), breathlessness, and sweating, with often minimal signs on examination; may progress rapidly to respiratory failure and death. Symptoms of pneumonia are milder after infection with type B.

Investigations

- Serology is the principal method of diagnosis, although PCR-based techniques are increasingly used
- *F. tularensis* may be identified in culture of wound specimens, although the laboratory should be warned—type A is sufficiently virulent for some laboratories not to perform culture. Sputum cultures may be diagnostic
- CXR may demonstrate parenchymal infiltrates, often progressing to lobar consolidation. Pleural effusions, hilar lymphadenopathy, and lung abscess may occur.

Management

- Discuss treatment with an infectious diseases specialist
- Drug treatment choices include streptomycin or gentamicin for 10 days. Doxycycline or chloramphenicol are alternatives, although treatment failure rates are higher and a course of 14 days is recommended
- In the setting of a large-scale outbreak (e.g. following use in bioterrorism), doxycycline or ciprofloxacin may be used for treatment or following exposure.

Prognosis Mortality is 1–2% from type A; type B is benign in humans.

Further information

Tarnvik A, Berglund L. Tularaemia. *Eur Resp J* 2003; **21**: 361–73

Melioidosis

Definition and epidemiology Melioidosis is caused by *Burkholderia pseudomallei,* a Gram-negative bacillus that is found in soil and water in Southeast Asia, northern Australia, China, and India; clinical disease is particularly common in Thailand, where it may account for up to a third of all pneumonia deaths. Infection is thought to follow entry via skin abrasions or inhalation, and pneumonia is the most common clinical presentation. Most cases represent recent infection; reactivation of infection is rare but can occur many years after exposure. Risk factors for melioidosis include diabetes, alcohol excess, renal disease, and chronic lung disease (including cystic fibrosis).

Consider melioidosis in returning travellers from Asia or Australia with community-acquired pneumonia or a subacute/chronic 'tuberculosis-like' respiratory illness.

Clinical features include:

- ***Acute septicaemic melioidosis*** Patients present acutely unwell with a severe pneumonia and widespread nodular consolidation on CXR, may progress rapidly to death
- ***Localized subacute melioidosis*** Subacute cavitating lobar (often upper) pneumonia, mimicking tuberculosis
- ***Chronic suppurative melioidosis*** Chronic lung abscess ± empyema; suppurative infection may involve other organs, including skin, brain, joints, bones, liver, spleen, kidney, adrenal, prostate, lymph nodes

Diagnosis

Identification by culture is the principal method of diagnosis. Blood cultures may be diagnostic; alert the laboratory to the possibility of this infection. ELISAs are relatively insensitive.

Management

- *B. pseudomallei* is resistant to multiple antibiotics. Treat with high-dose IV ceftazidime or meropenem for at least 10–14 days (longer if severe pulmonary disease or organ abscesses), then oral antibiotic (e.g. co-trimoxazole alone or in combination with doxycycline) for at least 12 weeks to ensure eradication.
- Supportive care, with ITU admission for septic shock or severe pneumonia.

Prognosis Documented mortality rates range 19–46%.

Further information

Currie BJ. Melioidosis: an important cause of pneumonia in residents of and travelers returned from endemic regions. *Eur Resp J* 2003; **22**: 542–50

Leptospirosis

Definition and epidemiology Leptospirosis is a zoonosis transmitted from water or soil contaminated with urine of infected animals (e.g. rats, dogs, cats, pigs, cattle, hamsters, bats) through skin abrasions or mucosa. Present worldwide, more common in tropical countries, but well described in UK. Individuals most at risk in the UK include farmers, vets, sewage workers, returning travellers from the topics, military personnel, and canoeists. Incidence peaks in spring/summer. In the tropics, epidemics may occur following storms or floods.

Consider leptospirosis in all patients with diffuse alveolar haemorrhage, and in at-risk individuals with pneumonia or ARDS.

Clinical features Disease manifestations are highly variable, ranging from asymptomatic infection to multi-organ failure, pulmonary haemorrhage, and death. Patients may present solely with pulmonary haemorrhage, without other features of Weil's disease. Manifestations include:

- ***Acute (anicteric) leptospirosis*** Self-limiting flu-like illness; myalgia, rash and aseptic meningitis may occur
- ***Weil's disease (icterohaemorrhagic fever)*** Classic form of leptospirosis. Features include fever, myalgia, conjunctival haemorrhage, rash, jaundice/hepatic failure, renal failure, coagulopathy and thrombocytopaenia, shock, myocarditis/cardiac arrthymias
- ***Pulmonary disease*** Occurs in at least a third of hospitalized patients with acute leptospirosis or Weil's disease. Manifestations include mild symptoms/signs (cough, wheeze, and crackles), pneumonia, pulmonary oedema secondary to myocarditis, and ARDS or fulminant alveolar haemorrhage syndrome.

Investigations

- Serology confirms the diagnosis and is performed in a single Leptospira Reference Unit in the UK. Both ELISA and microscopic agglutination tests may be performed
- CXR and CT typically demonstrate patchy consolidation and ground-glass shadowing, commonly bilateral with lower lobe predominance.

Management

- Discuss treatment with infectious diseases and renal specialists. Antibiotic choices include penicillin, ceftriaxone, or doxycycline
- Ventilatory support required for alveolar haemorrhage and ARDS
- Ensure adequate hydration; blood products may be required
- High-dose glucocorticoids are occasionally used, although there is no convincing evidence of benefit. Plasma exchange and desmopressin infusions have been tried.

Prognosis Acute leptospirosis typically resolves spontaneously after about 14 days. Severe pulmonary disease can progress very rapidly (over hours), with reported mortality rates approaching 50%.

Differential diagnosis of zoonotic microbial causes of community-acquired pneumonia (with exposures)

- Avian influenza virus (birds, animals)
- *Bacillus anthracis* (anthrax; animals)
- Brucellosis (animals)
- *Chlamydia psittaci* (psittacosis; poultry, birds)
- *Coxiella burnetii* (Q fever; parturient cats, cattle, sheep, goats, rabbits)
- *Cryptococcus neoformans* (birds)
- *Francisella tularensis* (tularaemia; rabbits, cats, rodents)
- Hantavirus (rodents, the Americas)
- *Histoplasma capsulatum* (histoplasmosis; birds or bats, the Americas)
- Leptospirosis (water contaminated with infected animal urine)
- *Pasteurella multocida* (pasteurellosis; animals, birds)
- *Ricketsia rickettsii* (Rocky mountain spotted fever; tick bite or exposure to tick-infested habitats, USA)
- *Yersinia pestis* (pneumonic plague; rodents, cats)

Chapter 41

Respiratory infection: fungal

Aspergillus lung disease: classification

Types of disease *Aspergillus fumigatus* and other *Aspergillus* moulds are ubiquitous fungi that can be isolated from the air in most houses, and this increases with increasing indoor humidity. Inhalation of spores (conidia) can produce a range of diseases, some of which are related to each other, and some of which are not. The finding of fungal hyphae (rather than just spores) in the sputum should provoke an assessment.

Classification

1. ***IgE-mediated allergic asthma*** from inhaled *Aspergillus* spores. One of many common antigens provoking airway inflammation and bronchospasm
2. ***Exuberant IgE and IgG reaction*** to *Aspergillus* in the airways of (usually) asthmatics provoking mucous plugging with distal consolidation that may flit from area to area. This is one of the causes of pulmonary eosinophilia
3. ***Allergic bronchopulmonary aspergillosis (APBA)*** A probable evolution and progression of (2) in (usually) asthmatics with inflammatory damage to the airways and resultant bronchiectasis (but no actual invasion of *Aspergillus* into the airway walls)
4. ***Invasive Aspergillus pneumonia*** due to invasion of *Aspergillus* into lung tissue secondary to immunosuppression. This can be a multisystem disorder with *Aspergillus* invading almost any part of the body
5. ***Semi-invasive aspergillosis***, a much lower grade process than invasive aspergillus pneumonia, usually seen in older individuals with no apparent immunosuppression, but usually some underlying chronic lung disease
6. ***Aspergilloma***, where *Aspergillus* lives and grows as a separate ball of fungus in a pre-existing lung cavity. There is usually an inflammatory response to limited hyphae invasion into the tissue walls of the cavity
7. ***Hypersensitivity pneumonitis (or extrinsic allergic alveolitis)*** due to an immune inflammatory reaction to inhalation of large numbers of spores (see p 249).

The presentation and clinical setting of these various *Aspergillus*-related disorders are clearly different and thus are detailed separately.

Atopic allergy to fungal spores

Approximately 10% of asthmatics are skin prick positive to *Aspergillus* species, compared with about 70% to house dust mite. It is assumed that this allergy contributes to allergic inflammation in the airways but, in the few relevant studies, symptoms have not always correlated with exposure. However, in some studies asthma admissions to hospital correlated better with fungal spore counts than with pollen counts. Fungal spore release may explain an association between thunderstorms and asthma attacks. Particularly high exposure results from working with mouldy vegetable matter, e.g. in compost heaps during late summer/early autumn.

Asthma and positive IgG precipitins to *Aspergillus*

Definition Asthmatics with IgE responses to *Aspergillus* can also develop IgG antibodies (precipitins). Why this happens is not clear. *Aspergillus* hyphae can *sometimes* be isolated from the sputum and it has been suggested that *Aspergillus* spores are able to germinate and grow in the mucous within the airways. This may explain the mucous plugging and flitting areas of pulmonary consolidation.

Clinical features and investigations

Associated features may include:

- Serum IgE >1000 ng/mL
- Blood eosinophilia >500/mm^3
- Skin prick +ve to *Aspergillus*
- IgG precipitins to *Aspergillus* (many different allergenic proteins)
- Long history of asthma, perhaps recently deteriorated.

Therefore suspect this development in:
A patient with long-term asthma whose control deteriorates, with CXR changes, IgE & IgG to *Aspergillus*, eosinophilia, and perhaps hyphae in the sputum.

Management may only require an increase in inhaled steroids. However, there is a suggestion that courses of oral steroids are particularly effective and may prevent progression to bronchiectasis (see next section). Steroids limit the host's immunological response but do not seem to lead to *Aspergillus* invasion of the tissues. Poorly documented evidence of improvement with antifungal agents such as itraconazole.

Bronchopulmonary aspergillosis

Definition This condition is probably an extension of (2), where the inflammatory response to the *Aspergillus* in the airways provokes a more exuberant response, with damage to the bronchial walls and bronchiectasis. Some authors reserve the use of the term ABPA for when bronchiectasis is present; others may include (2), and subdivide into ABPA-S (seropositive only), and ABPA-CB (central bronchiectasis).

The prevalence of ABPA in asthmatic populations has varied considerably between studies, and clearly will depend on whether the definition includes bronchiectasis or not. It probably occurs in about 1–2% of asthmatics. A related condition occurs in patients with cystic fibrosis where it appears about 7% have evidence of colonization and potential ongoing damage.

Pathophysiology The factors promoting the evolution from atopic asthmatic to ABPA are not known. A particular HLA association has been shown, with the suggestion that a CD4/Th2 response to a particular *Aspergillus* antigen (Asp f1 antigen) with release of IL-4 and IL-5 may be critical. Proteolytic enzymes are released by *Aspergillus* as part of its exophytic feeding strategy and these enzymes may damage airway mucosa. However, most believe that the damage results from *host defence mechanisms*. Hyphae (rather than just spores) may be visible in the mucus and grown from sputum, but there does not appear to be actual invasion of the bronchial mucosa. This immune inflammatory activity produces mucoid impaction in the airways, eosinophilic pneumonitis, and bronchocentric granuloma formation.

Main criteria for diagnosis (the first four are the most important)

- Long history of asthma
- Skin prick/IgE +ve to *Aspergillus fumigatus*
- IgG precipitins to *Aspergillus fumigatus*
- Central (proximal) bronchiectasis
- Blood/sputum eosinophilia
- Total serum IgE >1000 mg/mL
- Lung infiltrates—flitting.

Other clinical features

- Long-standing asthma, recent deterioration
- Recurrent episodes of mucous plugging
- Fever/malaise
- Expectoration of dark mucous plugs, sometimes as casts of the airways
- Eosinophilia (sputum and blood)
- Occasional haemoptysis.

The major complication is poorly controlled asthma that requires repeated courses of oral steroids.

Investigations

- ***Spirometry***—degree of airways obstruction
- ***Skin prick sensitivity*** to *Aspergillus* (IgE)
- ***Sputum***—*Aspergillus* hyphae and eosinophils
- ***Blood***
    - IgG precipitins
    - IgE RAST to *Aspergillus*
    - Total serum IgE
    - Eosinophil count (suppressed if on steroids)
- ***CXR***
    - Flitting infiltrates
    - Bronchiectasis, mucous impaction (gloved finger shadows)
- ***CT*** Central (proximal) bronchiectasis with upper lobe predominance

Management The management is essentially that of severe chronic asthma, but with generous use of courses of oral steroids. Several randomized controlled trials have shown courses of itraconazole (200 mg bd for 4 months) are well tolerated, reduce steroid requirements, and improve exercise tolerance. There appears to be a sustained effect after the itraconazole is stopped, suggesting at least temporary eradication of the *Aspergillus*. Response and relapse can be monitored with IgG precipitins to *Aspergillus*. Itraconazole can cause liver dysfunction, so LFTs need monitoring.

Differential diagnosis This list revolves mainly around the pulmonary infiltrates and eosinophilia.

- Acute/chronic eosinophilic pneumonia
- Churg–Strauss syndrome
- Various parasites (e.g. filariasis, ascaris; Löffler's syndrome)
- Drug-induced eosinophilic pneumonia.

Further information

Denning DW *et al.* The link between fungi and severe asthma: a summary of the evidence. *Eur Resp J* 2006; **27**: 615–26

Wark PA *et al.* Azoles for allergic bronchopulmonary aspergillosis associated with asthma. *Cochrane database Syst Rev* 2004; **3**: CD001108

Invasive aspergillosis

Definition The term 'invasive aspergillosis' is reserved for the situation where *Aspergillus* hyphae actually invade tissue (hyalohyphomycosis). This usually occurs with severe immune suppression, particularly neutropenia and steroid use. The port of entry is probably the lungs, but spread can be to almost any area of the body. The species most commonly seen are *Aspergillus fumigatus, flavus, terreus*, and *niger*. Mortality is very high. The source of *Aspergillus* is unclear, but has been found in hospital water supplies.

Pathogenesis Alveolar macrophages probably normally destroy *Aspergillus* spores. Macrophage failure may allow more spores to germinate and any subsequent invasion with hyphae seems to be prevented by neutrophils. Inadequate neutrophil function allows invasion across tissue planes and into vessels, with infarction and further spread throughout the body. There is some evidence that CMV may inactivate macrophages, allowing spores to germinate. The fungal digestive proteases do the damage rather than the host's limited immunological responses.

Clinical features

Typical setting

Fever, chest pain, cough, haemoptysis, dyspnoea, and pulmonary infiltrate in a neutropenic patient failing to respond to broad-spectrum antibiotics.

Risk factors

- Following chemotherapy, particularly provoking severe neutropenia (<100 cells/μl)
- Bone marrow suppression for allogeneic stem cell transplants
- Advanced HIV infection and AIDS
- Immune suppression following transplant
- Infliximab (or other anti-TNFα) therapy

Spread can occur anywhere with the following well recognized:

- Sinuses (paranasal) and spread into the brain
- Endocarditis
- Eyes
- Skin (papular, ranging to ulcerative, lesions).

Careful examination and particular investigations may be needed to detect spread to these areas.

Investigations

- ***Isolate Aspergillus hyphae*** from respiratory tract by:
    - Sputum
    - Expressed sputum (3% saline via nebulizer)
    - Bronchoalveolar lavage
    - Transbronchial biopsy

(Hyphae may be present when not the primary cause of the infiltrate)

- ***Biopsies*** from other sites (most convincing when acute-angle branching, septated non-pigmented hyphae are seen)
- Circulating levels of ***galactomannan***, an exo-antigen of *Aspergillus* (commercial EIA kit not universally available, and not found so useful by all groups on account of low sensitivity and false positivity due to presence of certain antibiotics, piperacillin and tazobactam). Serial sampling is recommended
- ***CXR/CT*** CXR changes are usually non-specific. CT may show a halo of low attenuation surrounding a nodular lesion early on. An 'air crescent' sign may develop on CXR with air appearing at the edge of an area of consolidation. Usually occurs when neutrophil count rising, and probably represents gradual containment of the infection into a cavity, not unlike an aspergilloma

Ultimately, it is the clinical picture that dominates the diagnosis.

Management Prompt use of antifungals is essential.

- Intravenous amphotericin B (only about 35% response rate)
- Intravenous lipid-based amphotericin (less nephrotoxic, but very expensive)
- Itraconazole IV: 200 mg bd for 2 days, then 200 mg od for 12 days
- Voriconazole (recently available, less experience, but probably better than itraconazole, and safer than amphotericin, very expensive)
- Caspofungin (recently available, less experience, very expensive)

Some centres use oral itraconazole as prophylaxis when commencing substantial immune suppression.

Differential diagnosis

The differential will be the large number of other opportunistic infections seen in immunosuppressed patients. Another invasive mycosis, *Candida albicans*, is now less common due to its susceptibility to fluconazole.

Further information

Upton A *et al.* Invasive aspergillosis following hematopoietic cell transplantation. *Clin Infect Dis* 2007; **44**: 531–40

Patterson TF. Advances and challenges in the management of invasive mycoses. *Lancet* 2005; **366**: 1013–25

Semi-invasive aspergillosis

(also known as chronic necrotizing aspergillosis, or chronic pulmonary aspergillosis)

Definition This entity is poorly defined but it is clear that a low-grade chronic invasion of *Aspergillus* into airway walls and surrounding lung can occur. In the original descriptions, some cause of mild immuno-incompetence was present, such as diabetes, steroid therapy, chronic lung disease, poor nutrition, etc. Previous asthma is not usually present, unlike ABPA.

Pathogenesis It is assumed that this form of aspergillosis results from lowered immunity in those without a tendency to make Th2, eosinophilic, responses to antigens. There is infiltration of hyphae into lung tissue, ranging from minor patchy consolidation to multiple cavities. There is little, if any, angio-invasion. It is assumed that the fungal digestive proteases gradually do the damage, rather than the host's immunological response.

Clinical features

Suspect semi-invasive aspergillosis when

- Middle-aged
- Reason for mild immunosuppression
- A pre-existing chronic lung disease
- Fever
- Productive cough
- Patchy indolent CXR changes.

Investigations

- Sputum samples may allow isolation of hyphae
- CT will show an airway-centred type of picture with 'tree in bud' appearance. With increasing severity this gives way to denser areas and small cavities that occasionally may contain a fungus ball
- Likely to have IgG precipitins to *Aspergillus*, but not always.

Management On the assumption that mild immune suppression is the dominant cause, steroids are not usually recommended for fear of further immune suppression. This is in contrast to ABPA where the damage is due to the host's immune defence mechanisms. Oral antifungals, such as itraconazole, are recommended. Fluconazole has been used with apparent success in case series only.

Aspergilloma/mycetoma

Definition The term aspergilloma is used to describe a ball of fungal hyphae within a cavity in the lung. It is assumed that this is colonization of a prior cavity, rather than arrested invasion. Aspergillomas can occur in other organs, including the pleural space.

Pathogenesis Cavities can occur in the lung following a variety of insults such as tuberculosis, sarcoid, ordinary pneumonia/lung abscess, treated tumours, and cystic fibrosis. Fungal spores entering the cavity germinate and survive in a relatively protected environment. The ball consists of hyphae, inflammatory cells, fibrin, and debris. Around the cavity is an intense inflammatory response, often with considerable extra vascularization from bronchial arteries and occasional fungal hyphae.

Clinical features Aspergillomas are often asymptomatic. Up to 75% will present with haemoptysis, assumed to come from damaged vessels on the inner surface of the cavity wall, via a communication with a bronchus. Sometimes there are systemic symptoms, malaise, and fever, as well as chest pain. Superadded infection may provoke exacerbations.

Investigations

- ***CXR*** apical cavity with ball within that changes position if CXR is performed decubitus
- ***CT*** obvious cavity with fungus ball, and possible invasion into surrounding lung (uncommon)
- ***Sputum culture***
- ***Aspergillus IgG precipitins***. Often higher levels than seen in other *Aspergillus* diseases.

Management

- May not require treatment
- Systemic symptoms of fever and malaise may be hard to ascribe to a mycetoma and require a therapeutic trial of itraconazole
- The most significant complication is life-threatening haemoptysis. The emergency management of haemoptysis is described on p 43
- Itraconazole will not eradicate the fungus, but seems to reduce cavity size and lessen the tendency to haemoptysis. It is assumed that it kills any fungus in the walls and inhibits growth in the cavity. The place of newer agents such as voriconazole is not known.

General approach to chronic haemoptysis

- Tranexamic acid (must be taken during clot formation as binds to fibrin to prevent action of endogenous fibrinolytics)
- Treat associated bacterial infections.

Specific to aspergilloma

- Itraconazole
- Arterial embolization
- Surgical resection.

- Bronchial arteriograms should reveal a leash of vessels supplying part of the cavity wall that can be embolized, even if not actively bleeding. Short-term success rate is good; long-term, less good
- Surgery can be difficult, as mycetomas may be stuck to the chest wall. Problems of seeding the pleural space are seen less often than in the past, probably due to better antifungal agents
- A few case reports exist of successful reduction of haemoptysis with radiotherapy
- Older approaches involving intracavity injections of amphotericin are rarely used now, although a recent case series of 40 patients seemed promising.

Overview of *Aspergillus* lung disease

The essential differences between the *Aspergillus* lung diseases depends on whether the damage to the lung is mediated by host defence mechanisms (atopic asthma, flitting consolidation, ABPA, possibly aspergilloma) or by the fungus's own digestive proteolytic enzymes (invasive aspergillosis, semi-invasive, aspergilloma). These two disease states are clearly different, but there probably exists a continuum between each of the subdivisions within each group, and the dominant mechanism in aspergilloma is not entirely clear. Therefore it is likely that patients with mixed and transitional features will be encountered.

Future developments

- New antifungals—voriconazole, posaconazole, ravuconazole (the triazoles), caspofungin, micafungin, anidulafungin (the echinocandins)
- Combination therapy
- Antifungal action of older drugs—flucytosine, rifampicin, fluconazole
- Place of early surgery
- Place of prophylaxis
- Value of galactomannan and β-D-glycan blood levels in diagnosis.

Further information

Aspergillus Trust (for patients), www.aspergillustrust.org

Soubani A *et al.* The clinical spectrum of pulmonary aspergillosis. *Chest* 2002; **121**: 1988–99

Pneumocystis pneumonia (PCP): diagnosis

Definition Pneumocystis pneumonia (PCP) is the clinical syndrome of pneumonia resulting from infection with the fungus *Pneumocystis jiroveci* (previously termed *Pneumocystis carinii*). *Pneumocystis jiroveci* is widespread in the environment and most people are infected by the age of 2 years; PCP is thought, however, to follow new infection rather than reactivation of latent infection. Most cases of infection are likely to be person-to-person airborne transmission rather than environmental.

Causes Risk factors for PCP include HIV infection (particularly with CD4 count <200 x 10^6/L), treatment with chemotherapy (especially fludarabine), corticosteroids, or other immunosuppressive agents, and malnutrition in children. Neutropenia does not appear to be a particular risk factor. PCP occurring in the setting of AIDS is associated with both a greater number of organisms and fewer inflammatory cells in the lungs when compared with infection associated with other causes of immunocompromise. PCP is much less common following the routine use of co-trimoxazole prophylaxis in HIV and post-transplantation, although cases still occur, e.g. in patients presenting with advanced HIV or in those non-compliant with prophylaxis. The threshold steroid dose for predisposition to PCP is unclear, although a dose equivalent to 16 mg prednisolone or greater for 8 weeks appears to significantly increase risk; the risk is likely also to reflect the underlying condition, e.g. PCP may develop in patients with haematological malignancy taking as little as 5 mg prednisolone daily. PCP often appears to present as immunosuppressant drug doses are tapered or increased.

Clinical features Gradual onset of dry cough and exertional breathlessness, sometimes with retrosternal tightness. Fever and tachypnoea may occur; chest examination is typically normal. May present with pneumothorax. Extrapulmonary disease is very rare.

Investigations

- ***CXR*** pattern is classically of bilateral perihilar infiltrates that progress to alveolar shadowing. Less common patterns include small nodular infiltrates or focal consolidation. CXR is normal in about 10%. Pleural effusions are very rare. CT is not routinely required except in cases of a normal CXR, when it may demonstrate a bilateral ground-glass pattern or cystic lesions
- ***Hypoxia*** is common. Desaturation on exercise may suggest the diagnosis in at-risk individuals with normal saturations at rest
- ***White blood count*** is usually normal. Serum lactate dehydrogenase is typically raised (sensitive, but non-specific)
- ***Induced sputum*** (see p 769) has a diagnostic yield of about 60% in HIV infection, but is much less sensitive when performed in the setting of non-HIV immunocompromise, where the organism burden is lower. It should not be performed on the open ward or out-patient department

- ***Bronchoscopy with BAL*** is the diagnostic investigation of choice in non-HIV-infected patients and in patients with HIV in whom induced sputum analysis is non-diagnostic. BAL with silver or immunofluorescent staining has a specificity of nearly 100% and sensitivity of 80–90%. This sensitivity is lower in non-HIV-infected immunocompromised patients, reflecting their lower pathogen loads
- ***Transbronchial lung biopsy*** has a slightly higher sensitivity (around 95%), but is associated with an increased risk of complications, so is reserved for cases where BAL is non-diagnostic. Surgical lung biopsy may be required for diagnosis in a minority of HIV-negative patients.

PCP: treatment

Antimicrobial

- Liaise with infectious diseases or HIV specialist
- High-dose co-trimoxazole (trimethoprim and sulphamethoxazole) remains the drug of choice. Administer 120 mg/kg daily in 4 divided doses PO or IV (dilute 480 mg ampoules in at least 75 mL 5% dextrose; infuse over 60 min). Use IV route initially and then PO during clinical improvement; PO may be used initially in mild cases. Side-effects (e.g. rash, nausea, vomiting, blood disorders) are common, particularly in HIV-infected patients. Consider routine use of anti-emetics
- Second-line choices if intolerant or unresponsive to co-trimoxazole include intravenous pentamidine, clindamycin and primaquine, dapsone and trimethoprim, atovaquone, trimetrexate
- All treatments should be for 2–3 weeks
- If PCP is strongly suspected and the patient is unwell, treatment can be started immediately, as BAL pneumocystis stains remain positive for up to 2 weeks. Empirical treatment is also required in the occasional situation where the diagnosis is suspected but bronchoscopy is non-diagnostic or not tolerated
- In cases of HIV presenting with PCP, subsequent early introduction of HAART may rarely be associated with acute respiratory failure, perhaps due to an aggressive inflammatory response to residual pneumocystis; consider steroid trial or temporarily withholding further HAART.

Steroids

- High-dose steroids (prednisolone 40 mg twice daily PO, or IV hydrocortisone) are recommended for all patients in respiratory failure. Treat at high dose for 5 days; taper dose over 1–3 weeks (e.g. prednisolone 40 mg daily for days 6–11, then 20 mg daily for days 12–21).

Supportive therapy

- Hypoxia is common: administer supplementary high-flow oxygen, and consider use of CPAP. Mechanical ventilation, if considered appropriate, may be required; make this decision prior to initiating CPAP
- Respiratory isolation is not recommended at present.

Outcome

- Mortality <10% in the setting of AIDS, but >30% in patients with other forms of immunocompromise, probably reflecting the adverse consequences of the greater pulmonary inflammatory response to pneumocystis which is observed in non-HIV immunocompromise. Mortality from PCP requiring mechanical ventilation in HIV-infected patients is about 60%, although may be significantly higher in patients with low CD4-counts.

- Relapse rate in AIDS is high (60% in one year), so secondary prophylaxis with co-trimoxazole is recommended. Primary prophylaxis is offered to HIV-positive patients with CD4 count <200 x 10^6/L. The indications for prophylaxis in non-HIV patients are less well defined; consider prophylaxis for patients who are likely to receive high doses of prednisolone for prolonged periods

Future developments

- The effect of co-infection with CMV on the outcome of PCP in HIV-infected patients is unclear. In patients with severe PCP treated with steroids, the presence of CMV in BAL fluid is associated with a worse outcome; the role of anti-CMV therapy such as ganciclovir in such cases is unknown
- The use of PCR to detect pneumocystis may further increase diagnostic sensitivity, although in a proportion of cases detection using PCR is not accompanied by evidence of clinical infection and appears to represent colonization. It is unclear if asymptomatic carriage precedes infection in such patients, and the consequences of carriage in immunocompetent individuals are also unknown
- Pneumocystis is one of only a handful of cells known to be unable to synthesize the metabolic intermediate molecule S-adenosylmethionine (AdoMet), and as a result must scavenge this molecule from its host. In a small study, lower plasma levels of AdoMet were demonstrated in PCP when compared with healthy controls and individuals with other pulmonary infections, suggesting a possible role for AdoMet in diagnosis. This finding has not yet been replicated in a larger study, however.

Further information

Kovacs JA *et al.* New insights into transmission, diagnosis, and drug treatment of *Pneumocystis carinii* pneumonia. *JAMA* 2001; **286**: 2450–60

Thomas CF, Limper AH. Pneumocystis pneumonia. *NEJM* 2004; **350**: 2487–98

Endemic mycoses

Several types of dimorphic fungi are known to commonly cause pulmonary disease in endemic regions, particularly in North America: ***histoplasmosis, blastomycosis, coccidioidomycosis, and paracoccidioidomycosis***. Endemic fungi can rarely present in non-endemic areas, and diagnosis is often delayed because of their non-specific and varied clinical features and the failure to obtain a detailed travel history. Fungal infection may mimic other diseases such as tuberculosis and lung cancer, often leading to inappropriate investigations and treatment. Fungal infections can also cause granulomata on lung biopsy, which sometimes results in diagnostic confusion (e.g. with sarcoidosis).

Infection in immunocompetent individuals is usually either asymptomatic or mild and self-limiting, although severe infection may rarely occur in apparently immunocompetent individuals. Outbreaks of disease may occur, as well as sporadic cases. Unlike invasive candidosis and aspergillosis, where neutrophils are the key host defence mechanism, T-cell-mediated immunity is essential for defence against the endemic mycoses. Patients with impaired T-cell-mediated immunity (e.g. AIDS, lymphoma, steroid use) are therefore at particular risk of developing severe or disseminated infection.

Histoplasmosis

Epidemiology *Histoplasma capsulatum* is found in bird and bat dropping contaminated soil in the mid-west and south-east USA, particularly the Ohio and Mississippi valleys, as well as in Mexico and parts of South America. The mycelial form is inhaled and subsequently develops into the yeast form ('dimorphism') within the lung, before spread via the lymphatics and the activation of T-cell-mediated immunity with granuloma development.

Clinical features Manifestations of infection are highly variable.

- ***Asymptomatic*** infection occurs in the majority of cases. CXR may be normal or demonstrate single or multiple nodules, which may calcify in a characteristic 'target lesion' pattern. Lymphadenopathy may occur with eggshell calcification
- ***Acute*** symptoms may follow heavy or recurrent exposure (e.g. pigeon fanciers, cavers). Range from a self-limiting flu-like illness of fever, cough, and malaise to fulminant disease with respiratory failure. CXR may be normal or show consolidation, bilateral alveolar shadowing, multiple small nodules, and sometimes lymphadenopathy
- ***Chronic***s progressive lung disease occurs particularly in patients with underlying COPD; lung cavitation is common, sometimes leading to an incorrect diagnosis of tuberculosis or cancer
- ***Disseminated*** disease may affect the immunocompromised (particularly AIDS) and the elderly. Presentation may be acute or chronic, and manifestations include fever, weight loss, and diffuse lung involvement, although almost any organ system may be affected; other features may include hepatosplenomegaly, gastrointestinal symptoms, headache and meningism, cytopenias, endocarditis, and adrenal failure

- Other unusual manifestations include broncholithiasis, mediastinal fibrosis (with compression of large airways, oesophagus, or superior vena cava), or isolated extrapulmonary disease (e.g. arthritis, pericarditis, erythema nodosum, erythema multiforme)

Diagnosis

- Smears or culture of infected material, e.g. sputum or BAL fluid (for chronic pulmonary disease, insensitive for acute disease), blood, urine, or bone marrow (for disseminated disease). May take several weeks
- Serology in acute disease—typically negative at presentation, and becomes positive after several weeks. A variety of serological tests are in use, including:
  - Complement fixation, designed to detect antibodies to *Histoplasma* mycelial antigen or *Histoplasma* yeast antigen. A positive result (serum titre ≥ 1: 16 for mycelial antigen, ≥ 1: 32 for yeast antigen) for either antigen, in a compatible clinical setting, is considered diagnostic of active disease
  - Immunodiffusion may distinguish active disease from previous exposure, but is less sensitive than complement fixation, and a negative result does not exclude the diagnosis
- Serum or urine *Histoplasma* polysaccharide antigen test—useful for diagnosis of disseminated disease and also pulmonary disease. Positive in 85–95% cases in AIDS patients. Antigenuria is seen in 90%, and antigenaemia in <50% of non-AIDS patients

Treatment

- Infection in immunocompetent individuals is typically self-limiting, and symptoms usually resolve within 2–4 weeks without treatment
- Indications for antifungal treatment are:
  - Persistent symptoms (usually lasting > 1 month)
  - Progressive disseminated disease
  - Heavy exposure leading to ARDS
  - Infection in the setting of immunocompromise
- Oral itraconazole is appropriate for persistent symptoms in mild–moderate disease and for disseminated disease, including patients with AIDS who have mild disease. Treat for 6–12 weeks in acute histoplasmosis, and for 1–2 years in chronic disease. In the setting of AIDS, treatment should be lifelong or until CD4 count >200 for at least 6 months after starting HAART. Check itraconazole drug interactions and monitor liver function (ideally monthly) if taking for >1 month. Hypokalaemia may be associated with long-term use
- Intravenous amphotericin B should be used to treat severe infection in the setting of ARDS or immunocompromise.

Blastomycosis

Epidemiology Infection with *Blastomyces dermatitidis* follows the inhalation of spores from contaminated soil, and clinical infection may follow outdoor activities. Blastomycosis is endemic in a distribution similar to that of histoplasmosis in the USA, although extending further north: it is endemic in the south-east USA, and the Mississippi, Ohio, and St Lawrence river valleys. Blastomycosis also occurs in Africa, India, and the Middle East. It is significantly less common than histoplasmosis.

Clinical features Clinical presentation is variable, and may mimic other diseases such as bacterial pneumonia, tuberculosis, and lung cancer. Clinical manifestations include:

- ***Asymptomatic*** in at least 50% of those infected
- ***Acute*** presentation is typically with fever, cough, productive of mucopurulent sputum, and sometimes pleuritic chest pain; misdiagnosis as bacterial pneumonia is common. Acute presentation of fulminant respiratory disease with ARDS may occur. Other acute presentations include a flu-like illness with fever, myalgia, arthralgia, and erythema nodosum
- ***Chronic*** presentation may occur with fever, productive cough, and weight loss
- ***Disseminated*** disease occurs in a minority of patients (especially in the immunocompromised), and most commonly involves the lungs, skin, bone, joints, and CNS.

CXR Airspace infiltrates are the most common finding, but a very wide range of appearances are seen, including nodular pattern, lobar consolidation, diffuse infiltrates, or large peripheral masses (often with air bronchograms). Lymphadenopathy and pleural effusions may rarely occur.

Diagnosis

- Diagnosis is by the staining or culture of infected material. A pyogenic inflammatory response to the fungus is common (unlike in histoplasmosis) and facilitates diagnosis
- Culture of sputum has a high yield and is diagnostic in most cases of acute pulmonary disease. Multiple specimens may be required, however. A drawback of sputum culture is that several weeks may be required before the fungus is identified. Cytological examination of sputum may provide a rapid diagnosis if the examiner is trained appropriately and alerted to the possible diagnosis
- Bronchoscopy has a similar diagnostic yield to sputum culture (92% in one study), and is recommended for patients with negative sputum results; note that lidocaine may inhibit the fungal growth and minimal concentrations should be used
- More invasive procedures such as surgical lung biopsy or thoracoscopy are only rarely needed. Histological specimens require particular stains (e.g. silver stain) to facilitate identification of the fungus
- Currently available serological tests lack sensitivity and are rarely helpful.

Treatment is usually with itraconazole for at least 6 months. Observation without treatment is not generally recommended, although this is controversial and symptoms are usually self-limiting in immunocompetent individuals. Amphotericin B should be used to treat very ill patients.

Coccidioidomycosis

Coccidioidomycosis is endemic in parts of south-west USA (Arizona, California, Texas, New Mexico, Utah, Nevada), northern Mexico, and Central and South America. Infection follows inhalation of *Coccidioides immitis* spores from soil. Manifestations of infection are variable, including:

- ***Asymptomatic*** infection, which appears to be common in endemic regions
- ***Acute*** pulmonary disease. Presents in a similar manner to bacterial pneumonia, with fever, cough, pleuritic chest pain, and often skin rash (e.g. erythema nodosum or erythema multiforme). Eosinophilia may be present. CXR appearance is variable, and may show areas of consolidation, lymphadenopathy, and pleural effusion, or be normal. The disease is self-limiting in most cases; a minority progress to ARDS or chronic disease
- ***Chronic*** pulmonary disease. Uncommon, may be asymptomatic. CXR typically shows single or multiple nodules that may cavitate; upper lobe infiltrates similar to those seen in tuberculosis may develop
- ***Disseminated*** disease. Rare, occurs particularly in the immunocompromised. Presentation may be acute or chronic. Pulmonary disease occurs in association with involvement of the skin, bones, joints, genitourinary system, or CNS.

Diagnosis is with stains or culture of infected tissues. Sputum cultures are often positive in cavitating disease. BAL fluid culture and lung biopsies may also be diagnostic. Serological tests are also available.

Treatment is not required in the majority of patients, who have mild self-limiting disease. Fluconazole is the antifungal of choice, when required.

Paracoccidioidomycosis

- Paracoccidioidomycosis is endemic in parts of Central and South America and Mexico
- Typically presents as chronic pulmonary disease, although acute disseminated disease may occur in the immunocompromised
- Diagnosis is made on culture of sputum or BAL fluid, or following staining of lung biopsy samples
- Treatment is with itraconazole, and long courses of up to 6 months may be needed.

Other fungi: cryptococcosis

Epidemiology

- *Cryptococcus neoformans* is found worldwide in bird droppings. Following inhalation, yeasts propagate within the alveoli without usually causing symptoms. Migration to the central nervous system may then occur, and meningoencephalitis is the most common clinical manifestation of infection
- Patients with impaired cell-mediated immunity (e.g. AIDS, sterioid use, lymphoma) are particularly vulnerable to cryptococcal infection

Clinical features

- Clinically evident cryptococcal lung disease is rare but well described, even in HIV-negative patients. Symptoms are non-specific, including fever and cough, and presentations may be acute or chronic. The CXR nods to interstitial or pleural involvement
- Pulmonary involvement is often associated with meningitis, and clinical signs of meningism are characteristically absent. CT head (to exclude a space-occupying lesion) followed by lumbar puncture should therefore be considered in all patients with pulmonary cryptococcal disease.

Diagnosis Diagnostic techniques include:

- India ink stain on CSF, or latex agglutination test for capsular antigen in BAL or pleural fluid, blood, or CSF
- Stains and culture of sputum, blood, urine, or BAL fluid. Positive culture from sputum may indicate colonization rather than active disease, and should be interpreted in the clinical context
- Serum cryptococcal antigen test is extremely sensitive and specific for the diagnosis

Treatment of cryptococcal infection in the immunocompromised is with amphotericin B IV and flucytosine IV for 2–3 weeks, followed by fluconazole. The natural history of disease in immunocompetent patients is poorly understood, and observation alone is often recommended; disseminated disease may occur, however, and some experts advise treatment with fluconazole.

Candidal pneumonia

- *Candida* occurs as part of the normal human flora, and is found in the gastrointestinal tract and on the skin. Invasive disease may occur in the immunocompromised, particularly in neuropenic patients. Prophylaxis with fluconazole is used following bone marrow transplantation
- *Candida* is often isolated from respiratory secretions, but very rarely causes respiratory disease. Seeding of the lungs leading to infiltrates or enlarging nodules may occur with disseminated candidal infection
- Risk factors for candidaemia include immunocompromise, central venous lines, parenteral nutrition, and gastrointestinal surgery. In lung transplant recipients a positive donor tracheal culture for *Candida* is a marker for post-transplant candidal infection
- The clinical and radiological features of pulmonary involvement are non-specific. Extrapulmonary manifestations of infection are common, e.g. skin, eye, hepatic, or CNS involvement. Candidaemia is typically associated with a high fever
- Definitive diagnosis of pulmonary disease requires identification of tissue invasion by *Candida* on TBB or surgical lung biopsy
- Treat with amphotericin B 0.7 mg/kg/day IV or fluconazole 400 mg/day PO, and remove any central lines
- Candidaemia carries a mortality of 30–40%.

Chapter 42

Respiratory infection: mycobacterial

Tuberculosis: epidemiology and pathophysiology

Tuberculosis (TB) is the second leading infectious cause of death worldwide (after AIDS), killing around 2 million people per year, despite being a potentially curable disease. Rising rates of HIV and immigration mean that TB remains a large proportion of the workload for respiratory physicians in some parts of the UK. The disease is a great mimicker and should often be considered as a differential diagnosis.

Epidemiology The highest incidence is in sub-Saharan Africa (290 cases per 100 000 population). High population density countries in Asia (India, China, Pakistan, and Indonesia) account for half the global burden. The countries comprising the former Soviet Union have rapidly increasing rates because of economic decline and failing health services, with around 10% multi-drug resistance in this area. Globally, around 11% of TB cases are co-infected with HIV, with this number increasing to 38% in sub-Saharan Africa, and less than 1% in India and China.

In the UK, 37% of TB cases are in Caucasians (usually over the age of 50), with 60% in people born abroad (median age of 30). At least 3% of cases are co-infected with HIV. TB is concentrated in the major cities, with 40% of cases in London.

Pathophysiology The disease is spread by airborne droplets containing *Mycobacterium tuberculosis* (MTB). Droplets can remain airborne for hours after expectoration, because of their small size. Infectious droplets are inhaled and become lodged in the distal airways.

MTB is taken up by alveolar macrophages, with either successful containment of the infection, or progression to primary disease (primary progressive TB).

MTB replicates following ingestion by alveolar macrophages, with spread via the lymphatics to hilar lymph nodes. Cell-mediated immunity leads to granuloma formation by activated T lymphocytes and macrophages, which limits further bacterial replication and disease spread. Unless there is a deficiency in cell-mediated immunity, active disease may never occur.

Active disease occurs when the host's immune response is unable to contain MTB replication, occurring most often in the lung parenchyma and hilar lymph nodes. It can occur in any organ, from haematogenous spread. This is most common in young children and in immunosuppressed adults.

Many factors influence whether or not infection leads to active disease, including age, host immunity, and time since infection. The estimated lifetime risk of clinical disease of a child newly infected with MTB is about 10%.

Most disease in adults is due to reactivation of childhood disease, so-called 'post primary disease', from activation of latent TB lying dormant in the lung Gohn's focus.

Main risk factors for active TB in the UK

1. Place and date of birth:
   - Caucasian population, increasing prevalence with age (M >F)
   - Black immigrants, highest prevalence in the young (M = F)
   - Indian subcontinent, highest prevalence in middle age (M = F)
2. HIV/AIDS
3. Poverty—1 in 50 homeless people in London have TB
4. Medical factors—diabetes, renal disease, malignant disease, systemic chemotherapy, steroids and new TNFA antagonists e.g. infliximab. Also smoking and vitamin D deficiency (a relationship between the vitamin D receptor and interleukin-1 levels is postulated)

Smear positive TB

Acid-fast bacilli (AFB) seen on sputum smear (Ziehl–Neelsen stain), potentially infectious. Patient may need to be isolated.

Culture positive TB

AFB not seen on smear. TB grown on culture (may take up to 9 weeks). Much less infectious.

TB: pulmonary disease

Symptoms

Most cases present with pulmonary disease, classically:
- Productive cough
- Haemoptysis
- Breathlessness
- Systemic symptoms—weight loss, night sweats, and malaise
- Chest pain

Haemoptysis is more common with cavitatory disease, and up to two-thirds will be smear positive. Most haemoptysis is small volume. Massive haemoptysis is rare, and is most common as a consequence of destruction of a lobe, with consequent bronchiectasis formation (possibly with secondary aspergillus infection or mycetoma in a healed TB cavity). This is seen in those untreated in the pre-chemotherapy era. Most haemoptysis will resolve with antituberculous chemotherapy.

Signs are often non-specific.
- Examination may be normal
- Lymphadenopathy (particularly cervical)
- Crackles
- Signs of a pleural effusion
- Signs of consolidation (with extensive disease)
- Signs of weight loss/underlying immunocompromise
- Look for evidence of extrapulmonary disease, e.g. skin, joints, CNS, retina, and spinal disease

Complications Long-term sequelae of inadequately treated infection include:
- ***Bronchiectasis***, bronchial obstruction, and airway stenosis (uncommon) may result from endobronchial disease, though this is much less common in the post-chemotherapy era. It is more common in the presence of extensive parenchymal disease, and is associated with lymph node enlargement with compromise of airway size
- ***Pleural disease*** is due to either primary progressive disease or reactivation of latent infection. It probably represents an increased immune response—a delayed type hypersensitivity reaction to mycobacterial antigens, rather than a diminished one, which is the case in other forms of TB infection. Culture is more likely from pleural tissue than fluid (where the organism burden is lower). See p 294
- ***Pneumothorax*** is rare (<1% in the developed world) and results from the rupture of a peripheral cavity. Can lead to the formation of a bronchopleural fistula
- ***Draining abscess***
- ***Right middle lobe syndrome***—compression of the right middle lobe bronchus by hilar lymph nodes leads to lobar collapse
- The previous treatment with ***thoracoplasty*** can lead to respiratory failure in later life due to compromised vital capacity

TB: extrapulmonary disease

Extrapulmonary disease is seen in about 20% of HIV seronegative patients. This proportion is higher in HIV positive patients.

The tuberculin skin test (see p 492) is more frequently positive in extrapulmonary disease, as this most commonly represents reactivation disease, and less commonly primary disease. Anergy is more likely in those with poor nutritional status, underlying disease (including HIV), and the elderly.

CNS disease This is the most serious manifestation, and includes meningeal involvement and space-occupying lesions (tuberculoma) that lead to cranial nerve lesions. The clinical manifestations are due to the presence of MTB, and the host's immune response to it.

TB meningitis presents with headache, fever, altered conscious level, and focal neurological signs, including cranial nerve palsies. Fits are common.

CSF contains lymphocytes, high protein, and low glucose. PCR of CSF may be useful, but is not 100% sensitive.

Pericardial TB The yield is low from pericardial fluid and biopsy. 85% have a positive tuberculin test. A large effusion may lead to cardiac tamponade, and may need to be drained.

Spinal disease can affect any bone or joint; spine involvement (Pott's disease) is most common in the thoracic spine. Surgery may be needed if there is evidence of cord compression or instability.

GU disease from seeding during haematogenous spread. Involvement of the renal and genital tracts is uncommon.

In men—may cause prostatitis and epididymitis.

In women—genitourinary TB is a cause of infertility. Sterile pyuria (white and red blood cells in the urine, in the absence of bacterial infection) may indicate TB infection.

Peripheral cold abscess can occur at almost any body site.

Disseminated disease is more common in immunosuppressed individuals. Pulmonary disease is typically a miliary (millet seed) pattern, but pulmonary disease is not universal in disseminated disease. This has a higher mortality than localized disease.

TB: investigations

The diagnosis is usually made in one of three ways: sputum (or other sample, e.g. pus, CSF, urine, a minimum of three samples) ***smear or culture***, or the identification of tissue ***caseating granulomas***.

- ***CXR*** classically shows upper lobe infiltrates with cavitation.
  - May be associated with hilar or paratracheal lymphadenopathy
  - May show changes consistent with prior TB infection, with fibrous scar tissue and calcification
  - HIV infected patients typically have less florid CXR changes, and are less likely to have cavitatory disease. Miliary pattern is more common in later stages of AIDS
  - All patients with non-pulmonary TB should have a CXR, to exclude or confirm pulmonary disease
- ***Sputum Ziehl–Neelsen (ZN) stain and culture*** is required for definitive diagnosis, and is vital for drug resistance testing. ZN is only 50–80% sensitive
  - Smear negative disease accounts for about 20% of disease transmission; smear positive cases are more infectious
  - Induced sputum is as effective as BAL, especially if the CXR shows changes consistent with active disease (but should not be used for potential MDR-TB, due to the danger to health workers)
  - Conventional culture takes 6 weeks or longer
  - Nucleic acid amplification techniques and DNA finger printing may be used to confirm mycobacteria serotype and drug susceptibility. May also be useful in elucidating the epidemiology of TB outbreaks
  - Non-mycobacterial TB (opportunistic mycobacteria) tend to be present in much lower concentrations than MTB, and are therefore seen on a smear much less commonly, but many grow much faster, and are therefore seen on culture much earlier
- ***Tuberculin skin test*** is only useful if strongly positive (suggesting active disease) or if negative. The skin test must be interpreted with the clinical picture, and with knowledge of the patient's ethnic origin, exposure, and BCG vaccination history. Novel immune-based rapid blood tests for the diagnosis of latent TB are probably more sensitive and specific and some now favour their use (p 510)
- ***Bronchoscopy*** may be needed to obtain BAL samples if there is a high index of clinical suspicion, but a non-productive cough or unhelpful sputum culture. In extensive disease, macroscopic bronchoscopic abnormality may be present, with erythematous or ulcerated airways. Granulation tissue or enlarged lymph nodes may be visible. Nodes can perforate or protrude into the bronchial lumen, extruding caseous material into the airway. This is rare in the developed world
- ***Biopsy from extrapulmonary*** sites, e.g. neck lymph nodes, or mediastinoscopy may be warranted. Lymph node biopsy samples, pleural biopsies, and pus aspirated from lymph nodes should be transported to the laboratory in a dry pot (not formalin). Bone marrow or liver biopsy may aid diagnosis in miliary TB. The bone marrow culture yield is higher in pancytopenia

- ***Gastric washings*** reflect TB swallowed overnight. Rarely performed if bronchoscopy is readily available. Used more commonly in children
- ***Blood tests*** Baseline FBC, renal, and liver function tests. Useful to document normal baseline levels before starting antituberculous chemotherapy. HIV test is mandatory in all
- ***Urine*** Early morning urine (EMU) if renal disease suspected
- ***CT scan*** is more sensitive than CXR, especially for smaller areas of disease. It may show cavitatory disease, and signs of airway disease—the 'tree in bud' appearance, useful for differentiating between active disease and non-active old disease. Less commonly needed.

A tuberculoma is an encapsulated focus of reactivated TB. These lesions rarely cavitate, and the differential diagnosis is wide, including malignancy and vasculitis. Diagnosis may only be possible by percutaneous biopsy as, in the absence of a main airway component, cultures may be negative.

Skin tests

- Mantoux
  - Read at 48 h
  - Intradermal. Use 0.1 mL of 1 in 1000 (= 0.1 mL of 100 TU/mL = 10 tuberculin units)
  - Graded:

<5 mm	negative
5–14 mm	positive
>15mm	strongly positive

- Heaf test. This has been phased out in the UK. Mantoux testing is the method of choice
  - Read at 1 week
  - 100 000 TU/mL (multipuncture)
- Graded:
  - Grade 0 no reaction
  - Grade 1 4–6 small dots
  - Grade 2 coalesces, normal skin in centre
  - Grade 3 coalesces, central skin filled (5–10 mm wide)
  - Grade 4 solid induration >10 mm ± vesiculation or ulceration
  - An excessive response can be treated with topical betnovate (PPD is dead material)

TB: management 1

Treatment aims to cure disease without relapse, prevent transmission, and prevent emergence of drug resistance.

Long-term treatment with a number of drugs is required as, before treatment is started, TB can remain dormant for long periods, making the emergence of naturally resistant mutants possible.

- Never treat with a single drug
- Never add a single drug to a failing regime
- Send material for bacteriological diagnosis prior to initiating treatment.

The majority of patients can be treated as out-patients.

Smear-positive HIV-negative patients should become smear-negative within 2 weeks of starting treatment (this does not apply to MDR-TB). These patients should be isolated either at hospital (if they are admitted) or at home for this time period.

Notification All new cases must be notified (including those diagnosed after death), as this initiates contact tracing. In some districts notification triggers specialist nursing input. The doctor making the diagnosis has a legal responsibility to notify. It also provides epidemiological and surveillance data, enabling treatment and screening services to be planned. A patient can be denotified if the mycobacterium cultured turns out to be an opportunistic mycobacterium, for example.

Drug treatment It is vital to send material for laboratory diagnosis if possible (to allow for subsequent drug susceptibility testing) prior to the initiation of treatment. In practice, if there is a high clinical suspicion of TB, treatment should be started before culture and full sensitivities are available.

Drug treatment is usually in 2 phases:

Initial intensive phase (designed to kill actively growing bacteria), followed by a *continuation phase* (designed to eliminate residual bacteria).

- The intensive phase (8 weeks) shortens the duration of infectiousness At least three drugs are needed, e.g. isoniazid (bactericidal), rifampicin (bacteriostatic), and pyrazinamide (bacteriostatic/partially bacteriocidal). Three drugs reduces the treatment time from 9 to 6 months
- Ethambutol added if there is a likelihood of drug resistance (in practice this is standard therapy for non-Caucasian patients, who are more likely to have come from an area with a high prevalence of resistance)
- The continuation phase is usually with two drugs. Fewer bacteria are present at the start of this phase, and there is therefore a lower chance that drug-resistant mutants will emerge, making drug resistance less of a problem.

Compliance is of major importance and all patients should have a risk assessment for treatment adherence. If the clinical response is not satisfactory, check sputum 2 months before the end of the planned treatment period.

Compliance can be monitored with urine colour testing (turns red with rifampicin) and tablet counts. If concerns about compliance, consider directly observed treatment (DOT). Every TB patient should have a key worker, who should be easily contactable.

From September 2007 there are no prescription costs for TB drugs in the UK.

Table 42.1 Annual risk of TB/100 000 in England and Wales based on age and place of birth

Age	**Place of birth**	**Years after first entry**	**All patient rate**	**Indian subcontinent rate**
0–14	UK		3	21
	Abroad		31	88
>15	UK		4	59
15–34	Abroad	0–4	180	540
		>5	53	87
>35	Abroad	0–4	146	593
		>5	39	108

TB: management 2

Directly observed therapy (DOT) aims to increase compliance, by nurse-supervised and observed daily or weekly tablet swallowing. This has been shown to increase treatment completion, reduce relapses, and reduce development of drug resistance, as the ingestion of each dose is witnessed. This is recommended for patients unlikely to comply, including alcoholics, drug abusers, the homeless, those with serious mental illness, and those with MDR-TB. Consider other incentives to improve adherence such as providing food and transport costs.

Compulsory detention under Sections 37 and 38 of the Public Health Act (England) is allowed for infectious pulmonary TB, but compulsory treatment is not allowed. This is only used in extreme circumstances to protect public health.

Standard treatment regimes **(see p 498)**

- The standard regime is for 6 months—four drugs in the initial 2-month phase (rifampicin (R), isoniazid (H), pyrazinamide (Z), and ethambutol (E) (or streptomycin) and 2 drugs in the last 4 months (rifampicin and isoniazid) in patients with fully sensitive organisms
- If drug sensitivity is unavailable at 2 months, continue the 4-drug regime until it is available (even if this is for more than 2 months)
- The fourth drug (usually ethambutol) can be omitted in those at low risk of isoniazid resistance (non-previously treated, HIV-negative, UK-born Caucasians, with no drug-resistant contacts). There is a higher risk of isoniazid resistance in ethnic minority groups, immigrants, refugees, those who have had previous treatment, and those who are HIV positive. This depends on local policy and the ethnic make-up of the local area. If in doubt, start treatment with 4 drugs
- Other treatment regimes are also effective (e.g. daily for 2 months, then 2 or 3 times weekly for 4 months, or 3 times weekly for the whole 6 months), though are used less commonly
- Check baseline renal and liver function in all patients. If normal, and not at high risk of adverse drug reaction, they do not need to be re-checked
- Dosages are weight dependent, and may need to be changed for weight loss or gain during the treatment course
- A 6-month treatment course is effective for all other forms of non-CNS extrapulmonary TB (including lymph node and spinal disease), with the same drugs as for respiratory disease. Surgery may be needed in addition, for spinal disease
- CNS disease needs a 12-month treatment course
- Steroids may be useful for large pleural effusions, pericardial effusions (60 mg/day for constrictive pericarditis), and CNS disease, especially if associated with neurological impairment. Steroids may also be indicated in ureteric disease, and to suppress hypersensitivity reactions to the TB drugs.

- Peripheral lymph nodes may enlarge and abscesses may form during treatment; this does not imply failure of treatment, but should prompt a compliance check
- Pyridoxine is not required, unless subjects are at higher risk of pyrazinamide-related peripheral neuropathy—in diabetes, renal failure, HIV, and alcoholics.

Meningitis A 12-month course of rifampicin and isoniazid, with pyrazinamide and a fourth drug (e.g. ethambutol) for at least the first 2 months, is effective. If pyrazinamide not used, extend treatment period to 18 months. Steroids may be needed for severe disease, equivalent to prednisolone 20–40 mg OD if on rifampicin, otherwise 10–20 mg OD. Steroids can usually be tapered after the initial 2–3 weeks of treatment. Ethambutol should be used with caution in unconscious patients, as visual acuity cannot be tested and there is a small risk of ocular toxicity.

Cerebral tuberculoma without meningitis 12-month regime.
Disseminated TB/miliary TB 6-month regime unless CNS involvement. Exclude CNS disease in miliary TB with CSF examination, whether or not symptoms are present. Start treatment even if LFTs are abnormal (this may be due to intrahepatic granulomas). Seek advice if LTFs deteriorate significantly on treatment. See p 505.
Bone and spinal TB 6-month standard regime. A CT or MRI should be performed in patients with active spinal disease who have neurological symptoms and signs. If there is direct spinal cord involvement (e.g. a spinal cord tuberculoma), treatment should be as for meningeal TB. There is no place for routine spinal surgery (e.g. anterior spinal fusion) in the absence of spinal instability.
Pericardial TB standard 6-month regime. Steroids, e.g. prednisolone 60 mg OD, tapered after 2–3 weeks of treatment may be required.
Peripheral lymph node TB standard 6-month regime, which should be used even if the infected node has been surgically removed. Stop treatment at the end of the 6-month course, regardless of the appearance of new nodes, residual nodes, or draining sinuses.

Patient advice to document on starting standard anti-TB chemotherapy
- Possibility of nausea and abdominal pain
- Persistent vomiting and/or jaundice—stop drugs *immediately* and contact doctor
- Red urine with rifampicin
- Red contact lenses with rifampicin
- Contraception advice, if on the oral contraceptive pill as efficacy reduced
- Visual acuity (Snellen chart) (ethambutol)
- Visual disturbance (ethambutol)—stop drugs *immediately* and contact doctor
- Potential drug interactions.

First-line antituberculosis drugs

Isoniazid (H) Bactericidal. Single daily dose, well tolerated. Major side-effect is age-dependent hepatitis. Increased toxicity with alcohol. Peripheral neuropathy is uncommon; although increased risk with diabetes and pregnancy; reduce incidence with 10 mg pyridoxine daily
Rifampicin (R) Bactericidal. Single daily dose, well tolerated. Increases hepatic microsomal enzymes; therefore increases clearance of hepatic metabolized drugs, including prednisolone and the oral contraceptive pill, thus the risks of pregnancy must be highlighted. Red discoloration of urine and contact lenses also occurs, and GI upset.
Pyrazinamide (Z) Bactericidal. Single daily dose. GI upset common. Major side-effect is hepatic toxicity. Renal excretion leads to hyperuricaemia.
Ethambutol (E) has some bactericidal effect, mostly bacteriostatic at usual doses. Single daily dose, well tolerated. Side-effect—optic neuritis, uncommon. Document visual acuity (Snellen chart) before starting.
Streptomycin Bactericidal. Given parenterally. Increased risk of ototoxicity in the fetus and the elderly.

Combined preparations
Rifinah® 150 (contains rifampicin 150 mg and isoniazid 100 mg), **Rifinah® 300** (contains rifampicin 300 mg and isoniazid 150 mg).
Rifater® (contains 120 mg rifampicin, 50 mg isoniazid, and 300 mg pyrazinamide).

Table 42.2 Recommended doses of standard antituberculosis drugs

Drug		Daily dose	Intermittent dose
Isoniazid (H)		300 mg	15 mg/kg 3 times weekly
Rifampicin (R)	<50 kg	450 mg	600–900 mg 3 times weekly
	≥50 kg	600 mg	
Pyrazinamide (Z)	<50 kg	1.5 g	<50 kg 2.0 g
	≥50 kg	2.0 g	≥50 kg 2.5 g 3 times weekly or 3.5 g twice weekly
Ethambutol (E)		15 mg/kg	30 mg/kg 3 times weekly or 45 mg/kg twice weekly

For example, a 75-kg adult commencing quadruple therapy would be given:
- Isoniazid 300 mg od
- Rifampicin 600 mg od
- Pyrazinamide 2.0 g od
- Ethambutol 1.2 g. od ± pyridoxine 10 mg od

If using a combined preparation e.g. Rifater® with ethambutol,
- 45 kg adult: Rifater® 4 tablets and ethambutol 700 mg od
- 60 kg adult: Rifater® 5 tablets and ethambutol 900 mg od
- 80 kg adult: Rifater® 6 tablets and ethambutol 1.2 g od

Drug regimes are often abbreviated to the number of months each phase of treatment lasts, followed by the letters for the drugs being administered during that treatment phase, e.g. 2HRZE/4HR is the standard 6-month recommended regime, 2HRE/7HR is 2 months of isoniazid, rifampicin, and ethambutol, followed by 7 months of isoniazid and rifampicin.

Table 42.3 Interactions of TB drugs

Drug	Increases level of	Decreases level of
Rifampicin	(Level decreased by ketoconazole & PAS)	Warfarin OCP Phenytoin Glucocorticoids Theophyllines, Digoxin Methadone Sulphonylureas ciclosporin
Isoniazid	Phenytoin carbamazepine Warfarin Diazepam	Azoles, e.g. ketoconazole
Pyrazinamide	Probenecid	

TB: in-patient admission

- This is rarely needed but, if necessary, patients with suspected pulmonary TB should initially be admitted to a side room vented to the outside air (until proven non-infectious)
- Patients with smear-positive non-MDR-TB should be managed as infectious (in a side room, with face mask). This especially applies if they are on a ward with immunosuppressed patients (who may be at higher risk)
- A risk assessment (including an assessment of the immune status of other ward patients) can be made once the infectiousness and likelihood of drug resistance of the patient are known
- Patients with non-pulmonary TB can be nursed on a general ward (but aerosol-generating procedures, e.g. abscess irrigation, may need patient isolation)
- Staff should wear face masks if the patient is potentially infectious
- In-patients with smear-positive pulmonary TB should be asked to wear a face mask whenever they leave their room, unless they have received 2 weeks' drug treatment
- Barrier nursing is unnecessary for smear-negative non-MDR-TB
- Liaise closely with infection control/microbiology/public health specialists
- If a patient on an open ward is found to have infectious TB, the risk to the other patients is small. Patients whose exposure is considered comparable to that of a household contact should be screened. Only those in the same bay as a coughing infectious case, for at least 8 h, are considered at risk. Exposure should be documented and the patient and the GP contacted
- Non-MDR-TB HIV-negative patients usually become non-infectious after 2 weeks chemotherapy. Any bacilli seen in smears after that time are likely to be dead
- Patients with HIV and those with TB should not be nursed in close proximity
- All patients with known or suspected MDR-TB should be admitted to negative pressure ventilated side room. Staff should wear protective face masks (FFP3)
- At discharge, a clear plan must be in place for the administration and supervision of all chemotherapy; this is particularly important for patients with MDR-TB, where close liaison with the infection control team and consultant in communicable disease control is paramount.

Treatment failure/disease relapse

- This is usually due to poor compliance
- Drug resistance may have developed
- Never add a single drug to a failing regime. Add only 2 or 3, ideally those to which the patient has not been previously exposed
- Assume drug resistance to all or some of the drugs in the failed regime
- Repeat cultures and sensitivity testing in this situation. Consider specific molecular tests for rifampicin resistance. If found, then treat as for MDR-TB (see p 508).

TB: treatment follow-up

- CXR is advised at the end of therapy for pulmonary disease
- Relapse is uncommon in those compliant with standard treatment regimes in the UK (0–3%); therefore long-term follow-up is not recommended
- Follow-up at 12 months after treatment completion is recommended for patients treated for drug-resistant TB
- Relapse after good compliance is usually due to fully sensitive organism; therefore treatment can be with the same regime again
- Relapse due to poor compliance needs a fully supervised regime.

MDR-TB follow-up

Prolonged follow-up is recommended; lifelong for HIV-positive patients.

TB in pregnancy

There is no increased risk of developing clinical disease in pregnancy. Presentation is the same as in non-pregnant individuals, but the diagnosis may be delayed by the non-specific nature of the symptoms in the early stages of disease, with malaise and fatigue being common in the early stages of pregnancy. A CXR is more likely to be delayed.

The tuberculin skin test result is not affected by pregnancy; this applies to HIV positive and negative subjects. A negative skin test should not lead to BCG vaccination, as live vaccines are contraindicated in pregnancy. In this situation, the skin test should be repeated after delivery, and BCG given then, after a second negative test.

TB outcome in pregnancy

- If diagnosed in the first trimester, the disease has the same outcome as for non-pregnant women
- If diagnosed in the second or third trimester, studies give more variable outcomes (some studies show a good fetal outcome; some show higher rates of small-for-dates babies, pre-eclampsia, and spontaneous abortion), but these effects tend to be related to late diagnosis and incomplete drug treatment. Some studies also show a poorer fetal outcome in extrapulmonary disease
- Late diagnosis of pulmonary TB can lead to a 4-fold increased obstetric mortality and 9-fold increased pre-term labour in some developing countries.

Treatment in pregnancy

- Isoniazid, rifampicin, and ethambutol are not teratogenic, and can be used safely in pregnancy. The 'standard' short course therapy is recommended (i.e. 6-month treatment)
- Limited pyrazinamide data on the risk of teratogenicity
- Streptomycin may be ototoxic to the fetus
- Active TB must be treated in pregnancy, because of the risk of untreated disease to the mother and fetus
- Reserve drugs may be toxic, and the risk/benefit ratio of each case must be assessed individually if second-line drugs are needed
- Babies of sputum-positive mothers, who have had less than 2 weeks treatment by delivery, should be treated with isoniazid and have a skin test at 6 weeks. If the skin test is negative, the chemoprophylaxis should be stopped and BCG given 1 week later (as BCG is sensitive to isoniazid)
- Congenital infection is very rare (less than 300 reported cases). The child can be infected at delivery (this is rare).

Breast feeding

- Most antituberculosis drugs are safe. Isoniazid—monitor infant for possible toxicity, as there is a theoretical risk of convulsions and neuropathy. Give prophylactic pyridoxine to the mother and infant
- Concentrations of drugs reaching breast milk are too low to prevent or treat infection in the infant

TB chemotherapy with comorbid disease

Liver disease

- Drug-induced hepatitis can be fatal. A raised ALT is more common in those who regularly consume alcohol, have viral hepatitis or other chronic liver disease, take concomitant hepatotoxic drugs, are pregnant, or are within 3 months post partum
- About 20% of those treated with isoniazid alone will have an asymptomatic transient rise in ALT. In the majority, this represents hepatic adaptation. Acetylator status (fast or slow) may influence this
- Isoniazid-induced hepatitis can be symptomatic or asymptomatic usually occurs within weeks or months of treatment, and is age related
- Isoniazid inhibits several cytochrome P450 enzymes, potentially increasing the plasma concentrations of other hepatotoxic drugs
- Rifampicin can cause subclinical hyperbilirubinaemia without hepatocellular damage. It can also cause direct hepatocellular damage and potentiate the hepatotoxicity of other TB drugs
- Pyrazinamide should not be used in patients with known chronic liver disease
- Decompensated liver disease—use a drug regime without rifampicin
- Baseline and regular monitoring of liver function is necessary (weekly LFTs for the first 2 weeks, then at 2-weekly intervals).

Renal failure

- Isoniazid and rifampicin have biliary excretion, so can be given in normal doses in renal disease
- Pyrazinamide metabolites are renally cleared; the dose may need to be less frequent in those with renal insufficiency
- Give pyridoxine in addition to isoniazid in those with severe renal disease to prevent isoniazid-induced peripheral neuropathy
- Ethambutol can accumulate causing optic neuropathy; therefore use a lower dose
- Dialysis patients should receive drugs after dialysis.

HIV infection

- Regimes are similar for HIV-positive and HIV-negative patients; give a standard 4-drug regime. Liaise closely with HIV specialists
- Better outcome with regimes including rifampicin
- Death during tuberculosis chemotherapy is more common in HIV-infected patients, who also have higher relapse rates than non-HIV-infected subjects
- Higher incidence of miliary disease in those with low CD4 counts
- Protease inhibitors and non-nucleoside reverse transcription inhibitors should not be used with rifampicin (they interfere with each other's metabolism)
- Paradoxical worsening of disease (worsening fever, CXR infiltrates, or new manifestations of the disease) at the initiation of HIV treatment are more common in HIV-positive patients. This is probably due to

immune reconstitution, and the increased recognition of mycobacterial antigens with improvement of the subject's immune response
- Patients co-infected with TB and HIV should be considered potentially infectious at each admission, until proved otherwise, and should be segregated from others. Review the immune status of other patients and their likely drug resistances, and their potential infectiousness
- In HIV-infected individuals (in whom the HIV diagnosis is new), usual practice is to start tuberculosis chemotherapy before HIV chemotherapy. Antiretroviral therapy is usually started later (but there is no consensus as to when). Liaise closely with HIV specialists.

Diabetes

Increased risk of TB, and the disease may be more extensive. Rifampicin reduces the efficacy of sulphonylureas.

TB drugs and abnormal liver function tests

- Chronic liver disease—regular monitoring of LFTs, weekly for the first 2 weeks, then at 2-weekly intervals
- New drug-induced hepatitis
  - Virological tests to exclude concomitant viral hepatitis
  - AST/ALT rise 2× normal—monitor LFTs weekly for 2 weeks, then 2-weekly until normal.
  - AST/ALT rise under 2× normal—repeat LFT at 2 weeks.
  - AST/ALT rise 5× normal or bilirubin rise—cease rifampicin, isoniazid, and pyrazinamide unless the patient is unwell. If the patient is unwell, or sputum still positive, consider admission for parenteral therapy, e.g. streptomycin and ethambutol with appropriate monitoring
- Drug re-challenge once LFTs are normal:
  - Re-introduce sequentially, in order:

    Isoniazid: at 50 mg/day, sequential increase to 300 mg/day after 2–3 days if no reaction

    Rifampicin: at 75 mg/day, increase to 300 mg/day after 2–3 days if no reaction, then to maximum dose/kg

    Pyrazinamide: start at 250 mg/day, increase to 1 g/day after 2–3 days, and to maximum dose/kg if no reaction
  - Daily monitoring of LFTs and clinical condition
  - If no further reaction, continue chemotherapy
  - If there is a further reaction, exclude the offending drug, and change to an alternative regime
  - If intolerant of pyrazinamide, use rifampicin and isoniazid for 9 months, with ethambutol for 2 months.

TB: adverse drug reactions

These occur in around 10% of patients, often requiring a change of therapy. Reactions are more common in those on non-standard therapy and in HIV-positive individuals.

Isoniazid peripheral neuropathy can be prevented by pyridoxine 10 mg daily (recommended in those at highest risk—diabetes, renal failure, alcoholics, HIV-positive).

Rifampicin causes shock, acute renal failure, thrombocytopenia. Withdraw and do not reintroduce the drug. Double maintenance steroid doses at the start of treatment (because of enzyme induction).

Ethambutol causes rare optic toxicity; recommend baseline visual acuity assessment with a Snellen chart. Use only in those with adequate visual acuity, and those able to report changes in visual acuity or new visual symptoms. Document that the patient has been told to cease the drug **immediately** at the onset of new visual symptoms.

Check baseline renal function before starting ethambutol, and avoid in renal failure.

HIV-positive patients Rifampicin and isoniazid lead to reduced serum concentrations of antifungals. Ketoconazole can inhibit rifampicin absorption. Rifampicin may reduce drug levels of protease inhibitors (as they are metabolized via the cytochrome P450 pathway, which is induced by rifampicin). Rifabutin can cause a severe iritis. Liaise closely with HIV specialist.

Drug resistance occurs in less than 2% of Caucasian cases in the UK, with higher levels in ethnic minority groups.

- Isoniazid resistance is seen in up to 6% in patients of African and Indian subcontinent origin.
- Increased drug resistance is seen in HIV-positive patients (fourfold increased risk).
- Second-line drugs are generally more toxic and less effective than first-line drugs, and the treatment of drug resistance can therefore often be complex and difficult
- The regime must include at least three drugs to which the organism is known to be susceptible. An injectible drug is often added, as this has shown improved outcomes
- The initial regime will depend on the incidence of drug resistance in the community, and should be altered depending on local drug susceptibility patterns
- In general, always add at least two drugs to which the MTB is susceptible
- Parenteral treatment is usually recommended when there is resistance to two or more drugs.

Table 42.4 Recommended drug regimes for non-MDR drug resistant TB

Drug resistance	Initial phase	Continuation phase
S	2RHZE	4RH
H known before treatment	2RZSE	7RE
H known after treatment	2RZE	10RE
Z	2RHE	7HR
E	2RHZ	4RH
R (only if confirmed as isolated resistance)	2HZE	16HE
S and H	2RZE	10RE

Isoniazid (H), rifampicin (R), pyrazinamide (Z), ethambutol (E)

Rifampicin monoresistance is uncommon, but does require regime modification. In most cases, rifampicin resistance is a marker of MDR-TB, and should be treated as such until full sensitivities are known.

Multiple drug resistant TB (MDR-TB)

Defined as MTB resistant to two or more first-line agents, usually isoniazid and rifampicin.

- Treatment is complex and time-consuming
- MDR-TB is not more infectious than other forms of TB, but the consequences of acquiring it are more serious
- Seek specialist advice; patients should be managed by experts with experience of managing resistant cases, in a hospital with isolation facilities. The mdrtbcentre@ctc.nhs.uk email address, based in Liverpool, can be used to seek advice from experts in the management of MDR disease. An MDR-TB UK database is run from the Cardiothoracic Centre in Liverpool
- Rapid molecular tests for rifampicin resistance should be carried out in all patients suspected of having MDR-TB. Liaise closely with the reference laboratory
- Close monitoring (because of increased drug toxicity) is needed
- Compliance is paramount
- MDR-TB comprised 1.3% of all UK cases in 1998
- Start treatment with 5 or more drugs to which the organism is likely to be susceptible. Continue until sputum cultures are negative. Continue with at least 3 drugs to which TB is sensitive, for a minimum of 9 months, sometimes for 24 months
- Surgery may be indicated.

Contacts of MDR-TB Chemoprophylaxis for contacts should include at least 2 drugs. Base the drug choice on the sensitivities of the index case for a minimum of 6 months (although there are no data to support this treatment period). If there is extensive resistance, no regime may be suitable, and regular follow-up needed instead.

Risk factors for resistant disease

- Previous anti-TB treatment, prior treatment failure
- HIV infection
- Contact with drug-resistant disease
- Residence in London
- Male gender, age 25–44
- Treatment failure.

XDR-TB 'extensively drug-resistant TB' is disease resistant to at least three classes of second line drugs. 347 infected patients are described worldwide so far, and the disease appears to be emerging in regions with high HIV prevalence, where it has a mortality of nearly 100%. 2004 data estimates that 0.4% of the global burden of TB is XDR-TB, about 30 000 cases. Genotyping data suggest the emergence of XDR-TB is due to the transmission of XDR strains between individuals, and is not a consequence of previous unsuccessful treatment. 85% of South African XDR isolates are from the KZN family of tuberculosis strains, which were mostly fully susceptible when first described in 1996.

Table 42.5 Second-line tuberculosis chemotherapy

Drug	Dose	Potential side-effects
Amikacin	15 mg/kg	Tinnitus, ataxia, renal impairment, vertigo
Azithromycin	500 mg od	GI upset
Capreomycin	15 mg/kg	As for amikacin
Ciprofloxacin	750 mg bd	Abdominal upset, headache, drug interactions
Clarithromycin	500 mg bd	GI upset
Ethionamide (or protionamide)	<50 kg: 375 mg bd ≥50 kg: 500 mg bd	GI upset, hepatitis. Avoid in pregnancy
Kanamycin	15 mg/kg	As for amikacin
Ofloxacin	400 mg bd	Abdominal upset, headache
PAS	10 g od or 5 g bd	GI upset, fever, rash, hepatitis
Rifabutin	300–450 mg od	As for rifampicin. Uveitis (particulary with HIV infection) with drug interactions, e.g. with macrolides
Streptomycin	15 mg/kg (max dose 1 g od)	As for amikacin
Thiacetazone	150 mg	GI upset, rash, conjunctivitis,vertigo. Avoid if HIV-positive (risk of Stevens–Johnson syndrome)

If the drug choice is limited by drug resistance and intolerance, consider desensitization and reintroduction of the offending drug. Desensitization must be carried out with concurrent treatment with 2 other drugs (to minimize emergence of resistant strains).

Immunotherapy Additional treatments aimed at immunomodulation may facilitate bacillary clearance and increase cure rates, particularly in MDR disease. Small studies suggest that IL-2 and nebulized interferon-gamma may have some benefit in this setting, and in patients with HIV co-infection. A larger study in HIV-negative patients with pulmonary TB has not shown improved bacillary clearance, suggesting that single cytokine therapy in individuals with drug-susceptible TB is unlikely to improve the outcome. In MDR-TB, however, there may be greater benefits of treatment. Administration of *M. vaccae* has been postulated to enhance the Th1 response and suppress Th2 responses to MTB, but clinical trials of this agent have been disappointing, despite promising *in vitro* studies.

Latent TB infection

Defined as a positive skin test, with a normal CXR and no symptoms. This represents the presence of a small total number of bacteria.

Tuberculin skin test A positive skin test results from the development of cell-mediated immunity against TB. The multiple puncture method (Heaf) is being phased out. Mantoux testing is used more commonly in the UK.

Potential problems with skin testing:

- Low sensitivity in the immunocompromised, and cross-reactivity with BCG
- The patient has to return to have the test read after 48–72 h
- Criteria for a positive test depend on the population in which it is being used.

Interferon gamma tests Two blood tests (T-SPOT.TB, Oxford Immunotec Ltd. and QuantiFERON-TB Gold, Cellestis Ltd.) are now commercially available, and are based on the detection of IFNγ released by T cells in response to *M. tuberculosis* specific antigens. The T-SPOT.TB test is an ELISpot test, counting individual T cells producing IFNγ; the QuantiFERON test is based on a whole-blood ELISA, and measures the IFNγ level in the supernatant of the stimulated whole blood sample. Both assays use two proteins (ESAT-6 and CFP10) encoded by a unique genomic sequence of MTB, which is absent from *M. bovis* BCG and the majority of opportunistic mycobacteria. These proteins are the main targets for IFNγ-secreting T lymphocytes in individuals infected with MTB. These tests have several advantages over the tuberculin skin test: no return visit for test reading is required, the result is available the next day, and repeated testing does not cause boosting. With both tests, blood must be collected in a heparinized tube, and processed within 6–8 h of venepuncture. The blood should be transferred to the laboratory at room temperature. Validation of these new tests has been difficult in the absence of a gold standard, although data suggest that the T-SPOT.TB test is more sensitive for the diagnosis of latent TB than the tuberculin skin test, particularly in children and HIV-positive individuals, and is probably more sensitive than the QuantiFERON test in the diagnosis of active TB.

Latent infection versus active disease

It is important to differentiate between active and latent disease.

Active disease is a positive skin test (usually), abnormal CXR, and symptoms.

Latent infection (small numbers of bacilli present) is usually treated with chemoprophylaxis (see below). Treatment of latent TB reduces the risk of subsequent development of active disease by about 90%.

HIV infection The tuberculin skin test may be falsely negative, and radiological changes may be atypical. Current guidelines recommend close monitoring and no chemoprophylaxis, because of the difficulties in identifying active from latent disease, and because of the risk of emergence of resistant strains. Exposure to smear-positive disease should lead to chemoprophylaxis in the absence of clinical disease. Recommended follow-up is at 3 and 12 months for those not receiving chemophrophylaxis (but who were eligible for it).

HIV-positive patients should receive long-term follow-up as part of their ongoing HIV management.

Chemoprophylaxis is given to contacts with strongly positive Heaf reactions, who have no radiological or clinical evidence of active disease. The risk of developing disease after exposure depends on a number of factors, including BCG and HIV/immune status, and whether infection was recent. Younger patients must have had relatively recent infection, and have a longer life expectancy from which to gain the benefits of chemoprophylaxis. Chemoprophylaxis is recommended for:

- Those with recent documented tuberculin conversion
- HIV-infected contacts of smear-positive cases
- Children aged <16 with a strongly positive Heaf (grade 2–4 if no prior BCG, grade 3–4 if prior BCG)
- Individuals with HIV, injecting drugs, with haematological malignancy, chronic renal failure or on dialysis, with silicosis, gastrectomy, solid organ transplant or receiving anti-TNFα therapy have a higher risk of developing active TB

Drug regimes

- Rifampicin and isoniazid daily for 3 months (3RH). Best compliance, but slightly higher side-effect profile
- Isoniazid daily for 6 months (6H). Lowest toxicity regime. Has a 60–90% effectiveness in reducing progression of latent infection to clinical disease
- 6H is recommended for people with HIV
- 6R is recommended for contacts of patients with isoniazid resistant disease
- Individuals who decline chemoprophylaxis should be given the 'Inform and advise' information leaflet, and have a CXR at 3 and 12 months.

TB and anti-TNFα treatment

Humanized monoclonal anti-TNFα antibody has recently been approved for the treatment of rheumatoid arthritis (RA), Crohn's disease, psoriatic arthropathy, and juvenile idiopathic arthritis. Etanercept (Enbrel) is a fusion protein that binds free TNFα using a soluble portion of the TNFα receptor, and is licensed for use in rheumatoid arthritis. Adalimumab (Humira) is a recombinant humanized monoclonal antibody against TNFα, also licensed for use in RA. Infliximab (Remicade) is a human chimera monoclonal antibody, licensed for the treatment of RA, Crohn's disease, and ankylosing spondylitis.

These drugs cause profound immunosuppression, and patients treated with them have an increased risk of developing TB. Most TB cases have been seen with infliximab (242 at time of publication), with most occurring within three treatment cycles (within a mean of 12 weeks of starting treatment). TB is the most frequently described opportunistic infection in this context. 50% of the reported cases are extrapulmonary disease. The initial high incidence of cases has now plateaued, presumably due to improved assessment and awareness and the use of isoniazid chemoprophylaxis. The calculated TB prevalence in etanercept/infliximab-treated RA patients in America is 41 per 100 000, 9 per 100 000 for Crohn's disease. Overall, there is an average 5-fold increased risk of developing TB with anti-TNFα.

All patients due to start anti-TNFα antibody treatment should be screened for active and latent TB

- All patients should have a clinical examination, with history of previous TB treatment and exposure carefully documented. All should have a CXR and tuberculin test
- Those with an abnormal CXR consistent with previous TB or those who have a history of extrapulmonary TB, who have received adequate treatment (as assessed by an expert), can start anti-TNFα therapy, but need monitoring every 3 months with a CXR and symptom assessment. The onset of any new respiratory symptoms, especially within 3 months of starting anti-TNFα therapy, should be investigated promptly
- Those with an abnormal CXR consistent with previous TB or those who have a prior history of extrapulmonary TB, who have NOT had adequate treatment, need to have active tuberculosis excluded by appropriate investigations. They should receive chemoprophylaxis before anti-TNFα therapy commences (assuming active disease is not identified). If there is clinical concern because of the delay in starting anti-TNFα treatment, a shorter course of chemoprophylaxis can be given, but this may be more toxic
- Any TB diagnosed (pulmonary or extra-pulmonary) should be treated with standard chemotherapy
- If active TB is present, patients should receive a minimum of 2 months anti-TB chemotherapy before starting anti-TNFα therapy
- If the CXR is normal, the tuberculin test may be helpful if the patient is not on immunosuppressants, and must be interpreted knowing the BCG history. A tuberculin skin test is unhelpful if the patient is on immunosuppressants. In this situation, an individual assessment should be made: if the risk of drug-induced hepatitis is less than the annual risk of developing TB, chemoprophylaxis should be given. However, if the

risk of hepatitis is greater, the patient should be monitored regularly and any suggestive symptoms investigated promptly. See Table 42.6
- No chemoprophylaxis regime is 100% effective: the protective efficacy of 6H is reported at 60 and 50% for 3HR
- In those without previous BCG, Heaf grades 0–1 (Mantoux 1 in 10 000, 0–5 mm) are negative, and Heaf grades 2–4 (Mantoux 1 in 10 000, >6 mm) are positive and should lead to a risk assessment
- In those with prior BCG, Heaf grades 0–2 (Mantoux 1 in 10 000, 0–14 mm) are negative, and Heaf grades 3–4 (Mantoux 1 in 10 000, >15 mm) may represent either latent infection or BCG effect, and therefore need further investigation
- In general, all black African patients aged >15 and all South Asians born outside the UK should be considered for chemoprophylaxis with 6 months isoniazid
- If a patient develops TB, whilst on anti-TNFα therapy, treat with the full standard course of antituberculous chemotherapy. The anti-TNFα can be continued if indicated
- Close liaison between the prescriber of the TNFα antibody treatment and TB specialists is needed.

Table 42.6 Sample calculations for aiding TB risk assessment for patients starting anti-TNF-α treatment.

Case type	Annual risk of TB disease/ 100 000	TB risk adjusted ×5 for anti-TNFα effect	Risk of hepatitis following 6H chemoprophylaxis/100 000	Risk/benefit conclusion
White, UK born, age 55–74	7	35	278	Observation
ISC, in UK >3 years, age >35	593	2965	278	Prophylaxis
Black African age 35–54	168	840	278	Prophylaxis
Other ethnic group, in UK >5 years, age >35	39	195	278	Observation

ISC = Indian subcontinent.
The risk of hepatitis with 3RH chemoprophylaxis is 1766/100, 000

Further information

BTS recommendations for assessing risk and for managing *Mycobacterium tuberculosis* infection and disease in patients due to start anti-TNF-α treatment. *Thorax* 2005; **60**: 800–5.

TB: screening and contact tracing

Immigrant screening Immigrants are screened, as ethnic minority groups in the UK constitute 50% of TB cases. New entrants are screened at port of arrival. The incidence of TB is highest in the first few years after arrival to the UK. Return visits to countries with a high background prevalence are a risk factor for acquiring disease. Immigrants with symptoms suggestive of TB, and those who are asymptomatic with a grade 3 or 4 tuberculin skin test, should be referred to the local chest clinic for CXR and assessment. BCG vaccination is recommended for tuberculin-negative immigrants (but not in those who are HIV-positive, because of the risk of generalized BCG infection).

Contact tracing identifies those with TB, and those who are infected but without evidence of disease. It also identifies those suitable for BCG vaccination.

Close contacts are usually those within the same household, sharing kitchen facilities, and frequent household visitors.

Casual contacts usually include most occupational contacts. Examination is usually only needed if the index case was smear-positive, or if the contacts are at high risk. This also applies if more than 10% of the close contacts have been infected, i.e. the index case is considered highly infectious.

- 10% of TB is diagnosed by contact tracing, with disease occurring in about 1% of contacts
- Smear-negative patients are much less infectious, but contact tracing is still recommended in these patients
- Contacts should be traced for the period the index case has been infectious, or for 3 months prior to the first positive sputum or culture, if the time period is uncertain
- Most disease in contacts is found at the first screening visit
- Subjects should be advised to report suspicious symptoms
- Follow-up is recommended at 3 and 12 months for those not receiving chemoprophylaxis.
- School index cases. If a pupil is diagnosed with smear-positive TB, the rest of the class and year group who share classes should be assessed as part of routine contact tracing. If a school teacher is diagnosed with smear-positive TB, the pupils in their class during the previous 3 months should be assessed as part of routine contact tracing. The extension of contact tracing to include non-teaching staff etc. will depend on the infectivity and proximity of the index case, and whether the contacts are likely to be especially susceptible to infection.

Airplane transmission Transmission rates are low, even on long haul flights. Contract tracing of passengers and crew is only necessary if the index case was smear-positive and coughing during a flight of at least 8 h. In this situation, screening is only recommended in those at high risk—immunocompromised travellers and children, or if the index case was unusually infectious or had MDR-TB.

M. bovis Cattle TB is due to *M. bovis*. Humans are at low risk, as the majority of milk consumed is pasteurized. *M. bovis* is distinguishable from *M. tuberculosis* in the laboratory, although initial diagnosis can be difficult (only distinguishable on culture, not using DNA or RNA testing). Around 40 cases are isolated per year. BCG is live attenuated *M. bovis*.

Extrapulmonary disease Contact screening is not recommended.

Contact examination This usually involves symptom enquiry, BCG vaccination status, Mantoux test, and CXR.

***Contacts of smear-positive index** case* If symptoms are present, and if the contact was not previously vaccinated, those with negative Mantoux should be retested after 6 weeks to allow for tuberculin conversion. If retesting is not possible, give BCG after the first negative Mantoux.

HIV-infected contacts CXR is indicated, as a negative Mantoux test may be due to anergy, and may therefore be a false negative. Mantoux testing is not contraindicated in HIV (PPD is dead). BCG is contraindicated (it is a live vaccine).

BCG vaccination

The UK national schools' vaccination programme ceased in 2005 and now aims to target vaccination to selected 'at risk' groups. Vaccination is offered to:

- All infants whose parents or grandparents originate from a country with a TB incidence of 40/100 000 or higher, or those living in areas with a TB incidence of 40/100 000 or higher
- All Mantoux-negative contacts of patients with respiratory TB, if they are previously unvaccinated and aged <35 years. Laboratory and health care workers who are contacts meeting the same criteria should be vaccinated if they are aged >36.
- All Mantoux-negative new entrants from high-incidence countries if previously unvaccinated, if aged <16. If originating from sub-Saharan Africa or a country with a TB incidence of 500 per 100 000, those aged 16 to 35 should also be offered vaccination
- All Mantoux–negative health care workers, irrespective of age, who are previously unvaccinated and who will be exposed to patients and clinical materials
- Mantoux-negative, previously unvaccinated individuals aged <35, if potentially at risk of TB exposure because of their occupation, including veterinary and abattoir workers, prison staff, staff in care homes for the elderly, staff of accommodation for refugees and the homeless, and those going to work in a high-incidence country for more than one month
- BCG has an efficacy of around 70% against TB in children, but difficulties with vaccine supply and regional policies have meant that not all children in the UK have been vaccinated in the past. It is less effective in adults, and is not used in America
- Adverse events include pain and suppuration at the injection site, and localized lymphadenitis. A course of rifampicin and/or isoniazid for 3–6 months, depending on response, may be needed

Disseminated BCG infection (BCGosis)

Live attenuated BCG immunotherapy is the most effective intravesical agent for the treatment and prophylaxis of superficial bladder cancer. It prevents tumour recurrence and prolongs disease-free survival, and may be more effective than chemotherapy in this setting. BCG can penetrate deep within the detrusor muscle and has been identified in pelvic lymph nodes after instillation, so has a potentially much longer duration of action than standard intravesical chemotherapy. BCG leads to a T-cell-mediated immune response, which has anti-tumour activity. After intravesical instillation, live mycobacteria attach to the urothelial lining. BCG organisms are internalized by bladder epithelial cells, leaving bacterial cell surface glycoproteins attached to the epithelial cell membrane. These antigens are thought to mediate the immune response.

- The standard treatment regime is 6 weekly instillations of 100 million to 1 billion colony-forming units of BCG (cfu). Some advocate a further 3-week course, 6 weeks after cessation of the first cycle. The dose–response curve is bell shaped, with excess BCG probably promoting increased tumour activity
- Local side-effects are common, with cystitis reported in around 90% of patients; low-grade fever and malaise are frequent. Cystitis persisting >48 h after treatment should be treated with a fluoroquinolone or isoniazid 300 mg od, rifampicin 600 mg od should be added if the symptoms persist at one week
- Breaks in the uro-epithelium are a risk factor for systemic infection, and therefore patients with persistent cystitis or haematuria should have their treatment delayed
- Significant reactions are reported in around 5%, with high fever commonest. A high fever post treatment (>39°C) may represent the onset of systemic BCG infection or hypersensitivity, and hospital admission is recommended
- BCG sepsis is reported in around 0.4–0.7%, with 10 deaths attributed to intravesical BCG to date. The major differential diagnosis is Gram-negative sepsis; thus patients should be treated with broad-spectrum antibiotics
- Later onset symptoms (at up to 8–12 weeks, though may occur much earlier) including fever, malaise, arthralgia, and breathlessness may represent systemic BCG infection, though there is debate as to whether these sorts of systemic symptoms are due to systemic BCG infection or hypersensitivity to BCG. Non-caseating granulomas can be identified on lung and liver biopsy. Culture of organisms is rarely reported, but tissue *M. bovis* can be identified by PCR
- Disseminated infection—treat with rifampicin 600 mg od and isoniazid 300 mg od for 6 months. Some advocate the addition of ethambutol. Prednisolone 40 mg od may be added, and response to corticosteroids is said to support the diagnosis of hypersensitivity. There are no trial data to support these treatment regimes or length of treatment, but *M. bovis* is susceptible to most anti-TB drugs, except pyrazinamide and cycloserine. There is no evidence that isoniazid reduces the anti-tumour effects of BCG

- BCG hypersensitivity pneumonits is suggested by pulmonary infiltrates; micronodular and miliary appearances are reported with or without eosinophilia
- Granulomatous hepatitis is reported. Standard TB treatment (6 months) is suggested, with prednisolone if symptoms of hypersensitivity predominate
- Systemic BCG infection is reported in HIV-positive infants and infants with severe immune deficiency, undiagnosed at the time of BCG vaccination. Systemic BCG infection is reported after BCG injection into melanoma.

Future developments in TB

- New TB vaccine (MVA85A)—heterogolous prime boost immunization regimes have been shown to induce higher levels of cellular immunity than homologous boosting with the same vaccine. Initial data on a BCG prime-recombinant modified vaccinia virus Ankara, expressing Ag 85A, are promising. This is now in clinical trials in the UK and Africa. The TB Vaccine Cluster Project (EU funded) aims to provide novel vaccines for human use, and boost BCG effect using modified BCG.
- Compound R207910 is a new antibiotic which has shown *in vitro* anti-TB activity in mice models
- Nebulized gamma interferon used in the USA as additional treatment in MDR-TB in those failing multiple agent chemotherapy.

Further information

Chemotherapy and management of tuberculosis in the UK: recommendations 1998. Drug doses and regimes as recommended in this document. *Thorax* 1998; **53**: 536–48.

Control and prevention of tuberculosis in the UK: Code of practice 2000. *Thorax* 2000; **55**: 887–901

NICE Guideline: Clinical diagnosis and management of tuberculosis, and measures for its prevention and control 2006. See www.nice.org.uk/CG033.

BTS recommendations for assessing risk and managing *Mycobacterium tuberculosis* infection and disease in patients due to start anti-TNFα treatment. *Thorax* 2005; **60**: 800–5.

UK's national tuberculosis charity. www.tbalert.org

Non-tuberculous mycobacteria (NTM)

NTM is also called atypical mycobacteria, opportunistic mycobacteria, environmental mycobacteria, mycobacteria other than tuberculosis (MOTT).

Aetiology

- Found in the environment: in soil, water (including tap water), dust, milk, animals, and birds
- Many different species. The four most important are *Mycobacterium avium complex (MAC), Mycobacterium kansasii, Mycobacterium malmoense*, and *Mycobacterium xenopi*
- They are low-grade pathogens in humans
- Most commonly cause pulmonary infections in middle-aged and older adults, and in those with pre-existing lung disease, such as bronchiectasis, CF, emphysema, or old healed TB, or in immunodeficiency
- *Disseminated infection* may occur, especially in the immunocompromised
- *Lymphadenitis* typically occurs in children aged 1–5 years. This presents with enlarged non-tender cervical lymph nodes and a normal CXR. The node should be surgically resected. Antibiotic treatment is only required if there is recurrence. Large nodes may need antituberculous chemotherapy to shrink the node prior to resection
- *Local invasion* may occur from skin lesion (e.g. *M. marinum, M. ulcerans, M. fortuitum, M. abscessus, M. chelonae, M. avium* complex).

Clinical features The symptoms are generally non-specific, hence the difficulty in diagnosis.

- Sub-acute illness with weight loss, productive cough, dyspnoea, fever, and occasionally haemoptysis
- May present in a patient with known underlying lung disease, such as COPD, in whom disease progression is atypical
- Colonization of abnormal lung may not cause symptoms, but can progress to cause disease later
- May be similar to symptoms caused by *Mycobacterium tuberculosis*
- 'Lady Windermere syndrome' is habitual voluntary cough suppression, which may lead to failure to clear airway secretions, predisposing to lingula or RML consolidation, bronchiectasis, and MAC infection. Found in otherwise healthy middle-aged women (Reich JM, *Chest* 1992;**101**:1605–9).

Investigations

- ***CXR*** can be indistinguishable from that of MTB, with upper zone infiltrate with cavitation. Airway nodularity and associated bronchiectasis are recognized. The CXR may be difficult to interpret in the presence of pre-existing lung disease. HRCT may help. It is impossible to identify which atypical mycobacterium is causing infection from the CXR appearance

- **Sputum samples** Microbiology for ZN stain, culture, and further testing. If there is growth of an atypical acid-fast bacillus:
  - *Where was the isolate from?* Culture from lung biopsy, BAL, pleural fluid, or blood culture is more significant than culture from sputum
  - *What is the isolate and what is the degree of growth?*
  - *How many samples have been positive?*
- A single isolate from a non-sterile site may not be significant. Contamination can occur, especially from bronchoscopes when BAL is performed. Multiple isolates (>2) from non-sterile sites are needed to establish disease, or >1 from a sterile site, especially if there is supportive histopathology. Liaise with microbiologists to help to determine the significance of a positive result
- May need ***lung biopsy*** to help differentiate
- ***No skin test*** is available.

Diagnosis Pulmonary disease is likely if:

- CXR is suggestive and 3 or more positive sputum cultures are obtained 1 week apart, with or without symptoms
- Or 1 positive culture from a sterile site, such as pleural fluid or biopsy
- Or 2 positive cultures from bronchoalveolar lavage on separate occasions.

In the UK, pulmonary infection is most commonly caused by *Mycobacterium kansasii*, *Mycobacterium avium* complex, *Mycobacterium malmoense*, and *Mycobacterium xenopi*.

NTM: management

- The decision to treat is based on the likelihood of active infection
- No need to notify or contact trace as there is low risk of cross-infection
- De-notify if the MTB grown turns out to be an atypical mycobacterium, and change treatment accordingly
- Treatment considerations according to BTS guidelines:
  - *M. kansasii*—progresses without treatment. Treat with rifampicin and ethambutol for a minimum of 9 months. A longer treatment period is required if immunocompromised (2 years or until sputum is clear of infection for 12 months). Good response to treatment. Indefinite treatment if non-compliant. 100% response rate, >90% 5-year cure, with <10% relapse with full compliance
  - *M. avium* complex (MAC)—may be asymptomatic. Can be antibiotic resistant. Treat with triple therapy: rifampicin with ethambutol with or without isoniazid for 2 years. 50% response rate and 20% relapse rate. Clarithromycin or azithromycin may be effective
  - *M. malmoense*—treat with ethambutol and rifampicin for 18–24 months
  - *M. xenopi*—often resistant. Disease may progress despite treatment. Treat with ethambutol, isoniazid, and rifampicin for at least 2 years
  - *M. malmoense*, and *M. xenopi*—90% response rate, and 10% relapse rate at 2 years.

It is recognized that laboratory antibiotic sensitivities and resistance may not correlate with the clinical therapeutic response. Antibiotic choice is best judged on clinical response.

HIV-positive patients

- HIV is a risk factor for NTM
- *Mycobacterium avium* complex is the cause of infection in 90% of cases
- Infections may occur late in the disease, when CD4 count <50
- Infections may develop during the first 2 months of highly active anti-retroviral treatment (HAART)
- Disease is rarely confined to the lungs. Lymphadenitis and disseminated infection are recognized
- Lung disease causes similar symptoms to those seen in the non-immuno-compromised
- CXR shows diffuse interstitial, reticulonodular, or alveolar infiltrates
- A single isolate may represent colonization
- If an organism is repeatedly isolated in the presence of symptoms and/or an abnormal CXR, start treatment
- Lifelong antibiotic treatment is recommended for pulmonary or disseminated disease, with a 3–4 drug regimen
- Disseminated MAC incidence is decreased by antibiotic prophylaxis (with azithromycin weekly) and HAART restoring immunocompetence
- There are potential drug interactions between rifampicin, macrolides, and protease inhibitors and NNRTIs.

Further Information

Management of opportunistic mycobacterial infections. *Thorax* 2000; **55**: 210–18.

Griffith DE *et al.* ATS/IDSA Statement: diagnosis, treatment and prevention of NTM. *Am J Respir Crit Care Med* 2007; **175**: 367–416.

Chapter 43

Respiratory infection: parasitic

A wide variety of parasitic organisms may infect the lungs, although clinical disease is rare in the UK. In general, parasites may cause lung disease by two different mechanisms:

- Hypersensitivity reactions, e.g. Löffler's syndrome and eosinophilic lung disease, most commonly from helminths such as *Ascaris*, *Toxocara*, and liver flukes
- Direct infection and invasion, e.g. amoebic disease, pulmonary hydatid disease.

Some of the more important examples are noted below.

Pulmonary hydatid disease

- Hydatidosis is the commonest parasitic lung disease worldwide
- Human infection follows ingestion of parasite eggs, with the adult worm found in dogs, sheep, goats, horses, camels, and moose; infection is common in sheep-raising regions, particularly Central Europe and the Mediterranean, as well as Alaska and Arctic Canada
- Two main forms:
    - *Echinococcus granulosus*, which causes cystic hydatid disease as the larvae grow in the lungs. Common. Symptoms include cough (sometimes productive of cyst contents, 'hydatidoptysis'), haemoptysis, and chest pain. CXR shows rounded cysts, sometimes with calcified walls, most commonly in lower lobes; CT may show 'daughter cysts'. Cyst rupture may occur, with wheeze, eosinophilia, and bronchial or pleural spread
    - *Echinococcus multilocularis*, which leads to alveolar hydatid disease following tissue invasion. Rare. Lung masses are less clearly delineated on CT than in cystic disease
- Diagnose from serology or sputum analysis. Serology is insensitive for the diagnosis of pulmonary disease (around 50%). Demonstration of liver cysts supports the diagnosis. Avoid needle aspiration of cysts, which may result in hypersensitivity or dissemination
- Treatment is with surgical excision in most cases. Medical treatment with albendazole if the patient is unfit for surgery or following cyst rupture and dissemination.

Amoebic pulmonary disease

- Intestinal and liver infection is common, with lung involvement in a minority
- Lung disease can develop either directly from the liver or via the bloodstream or lymphatics
- Pulmonary manifestations include right lower lobe consolidation, empyema, lung abscess, or hepatobronchial fistulae (resulting in large volumes of brown or 'anchovy' sputum). May be associated pericardial disease
- Diagnose using serology or following identification of trophozoites in stool, sputum, or pleural fluid
- Treatment is with metronidazole plus iodoquinol or diloxanide.

Pulmonary ascariasis

- Distributed worldwide
- Lung involvement occurs during maturation of *Ascaris lumbricoides*, and is typically manifest as a hypersensitivity reaction with cough, wheeze, fever, CXR infiltrates, and peripheral eosinophilia
- Examination of stool for eggs may confirm the diagnosis
- Usually resolves spontaneously after 1–2 weeks. Consider treatment with mebendazole for gastrointestinal infection.

Strongyloidiasis

- Caused by *Strongyloides stercoralis*, found in Central and South America and Africa
- Pulmonary involvement may lead to a Löffler-type syndrome with wheeze, skin rash, eosinophilia, and CXR infiltrate. In the setting of immunocompromise, disseminated infection may occur leading to the 'hyperinfection syndrome'. ARDS may develop, and secondary bacterial sepsis is common
- Diagnose using serology or following microbiological analysis of stool or duodenal fluid
- Treatment is with thiabendazole.

Toxocariasis

- Caused by *Toxocara canis*, distributed worldwide. Dogs are the primary host
- Ingestion of eggs from contaminated soil may result in visceral larva migrans. Migration of larvae through the lungs results in an immune response, with wheeze, cough, and eosinophilia
- Diagnosis may be made from serology
- Treatment often not required; steroids may be beneficial in severe cases.

Dirofilariasis

- Found in USA, Japan, South America
- Infection is caused by *Dirofilaria immitis* following mosquito transfer from animals, especially dogs. Worms lodge in the pulmonary arteries and elicit an inflammatory response, leading to a necrotic nodule
- Presentation is classically asymptomatic with a single peripheral nodule on CXR, mimicking cancer. Patients may present with cough, chest pain, and haemoptysis, presumably due to pulmonary infarction
- Definitive diagnosis requires lung biopsy. Serology lacks sensitivity and specificity
- Treatment is not usually needed.

Schistosomiasis

- Found in the Middle East, South America, South-east Asia, Africa, and the Caribbean
- *Schistosoma* species are carried by snails, and infection follows skin penetration, often during swimming
- Pulmonary involvement may reflect acute tissue migration, causing cough, wheeze, and CXR infiltrates, or chronic infection, leading to interstitial infiltrates, pulmonary hypertension, or AV fistulae
- Diagnosis from observation of ova in sputum, BAL, urine, or stool, or from lung biopsy
- Treatment is with praziquantel.

Paragonimiasis

- Caused by *Paragonimus westermani*, distributed in West Africa, the Far East, India, and Central and South America
- Following ingestion, flukes migrate to the lung or pleura. Clinical features may be acute or chronic, and include chest pain, pneumothorax, pleural effusion, Löffler's syndrome, and recurrent haemoptysis. Serum eosinophilia is common
- Diagnose with serology or observation of eggs in sputum, TBB, BAL, or pleural fluid
- Treatment is with praziquantel.

Tropical pulmonary eosinophilia

- Follows infection with *Wuchereria bancrofti* or *Brugia malayi* in the tropics
- Pulmonary involvement is common and represents a hypersensitivity reaction to the organism, with cough, wheeze, CXR infiltrates, and raised serum IgE
- Treatment is with diethylcarbamazine.

Chapter 44

Respiratory infection: viral

Viral pneumonia: overview

- Viral upper respiratory tract infections are common, but typically self-limiting, and are usually managed in the community. Viral pneumonia is much less common but is more serious and usually requires hospitalization. Viral pneumonia in the immunocompetent is rare and typically affects children or the elderly; influenza strains are the commonest cause in adults
- Viruses may cause serious respiratory infection in the immunocompromised (particularly patients with depressed T-cell function, e.g. following organ transplantation). CMV is the commonest serious viral pathogen that affects immunocompromised patients. Influenza, parainfluenza, RSV, measles, and adenovirus may also cause pneumonia in the immunocompromised, although diagnosis of these viruses is difficult and infection is commonly undetected
- The clinical and radiological features of viral pneumonia are non-specific. Worsening cough and breathlessness following an upper respiratory tract infection suggest the development of pneumonia; wheeze may accompany bronchiolitis. CXR typically shows non-specific diffuse interstitial infiltrates, and hypoxia may occur. Secondary bacterial infection may complicate viral pneumonia
- A variety of diagnostic techniques are available, including viral culture and immunofluorescence staining (e.g. of BAL fluid) and serology
- Treatment consists of supportive care and in some cases antivirals. Infection with certain viruses may require isolation. Treat secondary bacterial infection with antibiotics
- Specific features of the common and/or important viruses are noted in the remainder of the chapter.

Influenza: diagnosis

- Commonest cause of viral pneumonia in immunocompetent adults. It is transmitted via respiratory secretions and is extremely contagious. Seasonal influenza is very well recognized in the UK, particularly during the winter months, and recently outbreaks of H5N1 avian influenza have occurred in many countries, raising fears of the development of sustained human-to-human transmission and a new global pandemic
- Three pathogenic serotypes: A, B, and C. Type A causes more severe disease and occurs in annual epidemics and intermittent pandemics. Types B and C cause epidemics
- The surface antigens haemagglutinin and neuraminidase determine influenza serotype. Genetic mutations may result in antigenic shifts (major genetic rearrangements between strains, associated with pandemics) and antigenic drifts (more minor genetic variations associated with epidemics). Genetic rearrangement of virus occurs in animal and bird reservoirs, and the virus may then be transferred to humans
- Seasonal influenza may affect previously well individuals, although it occurs more commonly in the elderly, particularly in the setting of chronic heart or lung disease or immunocompromise. Pandemic influenza differs in that it is also associated with significant mortality in younger adults.

Regularly updated information on seasonal, avian, and pandemic influenza is available from the Health Protection Agency website:
http://www.hpa.org.uk/infections/topics_az/influenza
Additional guidelines are available for the management of suspected influenza in the setting of a pandemic with UK Pandemic Alert Level 2 (cases of pandemic influenza identified in UK):
http://www.brit-thoracic.org.uk/PandemicFlu.html
http://www.dh.gov.uk/en/PandemicFlu/index.htm

Clinical and laboratory features Incubation period typically 1–4 days; adults contagious for 7 days and children for 21 days from illness onset. The clinical picture following infection is variable and may be influenced in part by the influenza subtype. Features include:

- **Asymptomatic** infection
- **'Flu'** (acute onset of fever, cough, headache, coryzal symptoms, myalgia, sore throat)
- Complications include:
  - Bronchitis/bronchiolitis
  - **Primary influenza viral pneumonia** (onset typically within 48 h of initial fever; cough dry or productive, haemoptysis may occur, bilateral crackles and/or wheeze; may progress very rapidly to respiratory failure and death; described in majority of patients infected with avian influenza H5N1, often associated with lymphopenia, thrombocytopenia, abnormal liver function, and multi-organ failure)

- **Secondary bacterial pneumonia** (significantly more common than viral pneumonia; onset typically 4–5 days after initial fever, during early convalescence, although may occur earlier; pathogens include *S. pneumoniae*, *S. aureus*—particularly associated with lung abscess—and *H. influenzae*; mixed bacterial/viral pneumonia may occur)
- Gastrointestinal symptoms (e.g. watery diarrhoea; more frequently described during avian influenza A H5N1 than seasonal infection)
- Otitis media (particularly in children), conjunctivitis; rarely parotitis
- Myositis (creatine kinase may be elevated; rarely myoglobinuria with renal failure)
- Neurological (encephalitis, acute necrotizing encephalopathy, transverse myelitis, Guillain–Barré syndrome all rare; Reye's syndrome with encephalopathy and fatty liver following aspirin use is well described in children and adolescents)
- Cardiovascular (ECG abnormalities common, myocarditis or pericarditis rare).

Imaging

- ***CXR*** typically shows bilateral mid-zone interstitial infiltrates in primary viral pneumonia, although focal consolidation is also well described. Lobar consolidation occurs in secondary bacterial pneumonia.

Differential diagnosis of 'flu-like' illness includes adenovirus, RSV, rhinovirus, parainfluenza, *Chlamydia pneumoniae*, *Legionella*, *Mycoplasma*, and *S. pneumoniae*. A very high fever is said to favour a diagnosis of influenza. Consider SARS (p 542) in patients with an appropriate travel history.

Diagnosis is often suggested by knowledge of a local outbreak. Diagnostic investigations include:

- **Virology** (not routinely required if pandemic established with widespread infection across the UK—Alert Level 4—when diagnosis will be clinical)
  - Presentation <7 days after illness onset: nose and throat swabs in virus transport medium (for direct immunofluorescence, ELISA, virus culture, and/or PCR)
  - Presentation >7 days after illness onset: 'acute' serum and subsequently 'convalescent' serum after 7 days (for influenza serological testing)
- **Bacteriology** (in patients with influenza-related pneumonia)
  - Blood culture
  - Pneumococcal and *Legionella* urinary antigen
  - Sputum M,C&S (if purulent sputum and either no prior antibiotics or failure to respond to empirical antibiotics)
  - 'Acute' serum and subsequently 'convalescent' serum after 7 days for influenza/other agents serological testing

Influenza: management

Severity assessment

- Patients with uncomplicated influenza do not require admission
- For influenza-related pneumonia, a CURB-65 score (p 424) of ≥3 indicates severe pneumonia and a high risk of death; patients with a score of 0 or 1 may be considered for home treatment
- Bilateral CXR infiltrates consistent with primary viral pneumonia should be considered as severe pneumonia, irrespective of CURB-65 score.

Infection control

- Outside the setting of a UK pandemic, most suspected cases of influenza are likely to be seasonal, although H5N1 avian influenza should be seriously considered in patients with:
  - Fever or history of fever and breathlessness or cough
  - *and* travel in the previous 2 weeks to a region known to have cases of H5N1 in birds (e.g. China, Egypt, Indonesia, Thailand, Vietnam, many more; see Health Protection Agency website on p 532 for updated list)
  - *and* close contact (within 1 m) with live or dead poultry (not meat or eggs) or other H5N1-confirmed animal (e.g. pigs) within 7 days of symptom onset
  - Consider also in patients with febrile respiratory illness and contact with sick, dying, or dead poultry in absence of travel history, and in health care and laboratory workers with exposure to confirmed or possible avian influenza cases

In such cases, the patient should be assessed either at their home or in a hospital side-room, with both patient and staff wearing surgical masks and staff wearing gown and gloves. Immediately inform local Health Protection Unit, as well as hospital infection control and occupational health. If hospitalization is required, patients should be in strict respiratory isolation, preferably in a negative pressure room (although patients should not be transferred for this reason alone), and staff should wear high filtration mask (FFP3), gown, gloves, and eye protection (consider also cap and plastic apron, depending on situation). Mark all laboratory samples as 'high risk' and inform local laboratory of the sample status.

Treatment

- **Supportive care:** oxygen, intravenous fluids, nutritional support. Consider ITU/HDU admission for patients with one of more of: primary viral pneumonia; CURB-65 score of 4 or 5; PaO_2 <8 Kpa despite high-flow oxygen; progressive hypercapnia; pH <7.26; septic shock. NIV may be used for patients with COPD and decompensated type II respiratory failure, although infection control measures should be in place and protective equipment worn by staff to minimize any spread of infection from respiratory droplets

- **Antiviral** treatment with neuraminidase inhibitors is indicated for patients with an influenza-like illness and fever >38°C within 48 h of symptom onset; consider also treating immunocompromised or very elderly patients in the absence of fever, and severely ill or immunocompromised patients if >48 h from disease onset. Treat with oseltamivir (Tamiflu) 75 mg bd for 5 days (75 mg od if creatinine clearance <30 ml/min); anti-emetics may be needed for nausea. Antivirals appear to reduce illness duration (by 1 day), hospitalization, and subsequent antibiotic requirements; possible effects on mortality have not been adequately studied, and the efficacy of neuraminidase inhibitors in pandemic influenza is unknown. The neuraminidase inhibitor zanamivir may be given intravenously (e.g. for ventilated patients), but its effectiveness in this situation is unproven. Antiviral prophylaxis may be considered for health care workers caring for patients with suspected avian influenza, as well as the patient's household contacts
- Treat influenza-related pneumonia with **antibiotics** according to severity, e.g. oral co-amoxiclav, a tetracycline (e.g. doxycycline), or a macrolide if non-severe; intravenous co-amoxiclav or cefuroxime or cefotaxime together with a macrolide if severe.

Outcome Uncomplicated influenza typically resolves within 7 days, although cough and malaise may persist for several weeks. The reported mortality from primary influenza viral pneumonia is >40% and up to 24% from secondary bacterial pneumonia.

Vaccination

- The influenza inactivated vaccine is modified annually based on recent viral strains, and provides partial protection against influenza illness, hospitalization, and death. Vaccination if age >65, chronic comorbidity, nursing home residents, or health workers. Vaccination will not protect against H5N1 avian influenza, but may make simultaneous co-infection with human and avian influenza less likely, and so reduce the likelihood of viral genetic re-assortment
- Administration of oseltamivir 75 mg od to high-risk individuals throughout periods of exposure may also prevent infection
- Live attenuated influenza vaccines are currently under investigation.

Cytomegalovirus pneumonia

Epidemiology

- CMV is the commonest serious viral pathogen in the immunocompromised, and is a particular problem following transplantation, where prophylaxis is now widely used
- Individuals are described as 'seropositive' for CMV if they have evidence of IgG antibodies indicating latent infection following previous exposure; seropositivity increases with age. Infection in transplant recipients results from either transmission from a CMV-positive donor to a CMV antibody-negative recipient (via the organ or a blood transfusion) or reactivation of latent CMV in a seropositive recipient as a result of immunosuppression
- Infection occurs most frequently during the first 4 months following organ or bone marrow transplantation, corresponding to the period of maximal T-cell suppression. Graft-versus-host disease increases the risk of CMV infection.

Clinical and laboratory features

- 'Flu-like' symptoms in immunocompetent patients
- Symptoms of CMV pneumonia in the immunocompromised are non-specific: fever, dry cough, dyspnoea, and malaise
- Extrapulmonary manifestations of CMV infection (e.g. gastro-oesophagitis; hepatitis) may suggest the diagnosis
- Hypoxia may occur. Leucopenia, thrombocytopenia, and abnormal liver function tests are characteristic.

Imaging

- ***CXR*** typically bilateral diffuse interstitial infiltrate, although lobar consolidation and localized haziness also described; can be normal. A nodular infiltrate may suggest co-infection with *Aspergillus*
- ***CT*** features include localized or diffuse ground-glass and nodular shadowing that may progress to airspace consolidation.

Diagnosis Antibody tests are used to estimate risk following transplantation, but diagnosis of active disease requires evidence of either viraemia (by antigen or PCR testing of blood) or tissue invasion (by biopsy). A wide range of diagnostic tests are available, and the choice of tests varies between centres—discuss with your local virologist. The nature of the transplant and immunosuppression also influence the interpretation of test results. Methods include:

- Early antigen fluorescence test on BAL fluid (high sensitivity, low specificity)
- Qualitative PCR on blood or BAL fluid (highly sensitive, but unable to differentiate between latent and replicating CMV; negative result practically excludes the diagnosis, positive result is unhelpful)
- CMV antigenaemia on blood (rapid, differentiates between latent and replicating virus)
- Quantitative PCR on blood or BAL fluid (rapid, differentiates between latent and replicating virus).

- Indirect immunofluorescence with monoclonal antibodies to CMV in BAL fluid (rapid, highly sensitive, and specific)
- Histology of lung tissue from transbronchial or surgical biopsies (demonstrate CMV inclusion bodies—the 'owl's eye' appearance—within infected cells; considered gold standard investigation).

In some cases a definitive diagnosis is not possible, and treatment is empirical.

Treatment Ganciclovir 5 mg/kg IV bd for 2–4 weeks (side-effects include neutropenia, anaemia). Consider additional treatment with anti-CMV hyperimmune globulin or prolonged oral valganciclovir in cases of severe or relapsed disease. Foscarnet 60 mg/kg tds for 2–3 weeks is an alternative to ganciclovir for resistant cases, but toxicity (nephrotoxicity, metabolic disturbance) can limit treatment.

Complications

- Opportunistic infection (e.g. PCP, aspergillosis) due to further suppression of T-cell function by the CMV infection itself
- Increased risk of organ rejection, as allografts are more susceptible to CMV infection than native organs.

Outcome The reported mortality from CMV pneumonia varies, although may be as high as 85%. Relapse occurs in up to one-third of patients.

Varicella pneumonia

- Pneumonia occurs in a small proportion of adults with chickenpox or shingles. Risk factors for its development include smoking, increased number of skin spots (>100), pregnancy (third trimester), steroid treatment, and immunocompromise
- There is typically a history of recent exposure to a contact infected with chickenpox or shingles. Chest symptoms tend to occur several days after the onset of rash (erythematous macules progressing to papules and then vesicles), although rarely may precede the rash. Cough and breathlessness are common, and pleuritic pain and haemoptysis may occur
- CXR typically shows a diffuse small nodular infiltrate; hilar lymphadenopathy and pleural effusions may uncommonly occur. Nodules may subsequently calcify and persist
- Multi-organ involvement may occur
- Diagnosis is usually suspected on the basis of the history of exposure, presence of rash, and CXR features. Cytological examination of smears from skin lesions, serology, or viral culture or PCR on BAL fluid may confirm the diagnosis
- Treatment of varicella pneumonia is with early administration of aciclovir 10–12.5 mg/kg, IV tds for 7–10 days. Aciclovir is not licensed for use in pregnancy, but does not appear to be associated with increased fetal abnormalities and the benefits of treatment almost certainly outweigh any risk. Varicella is very infectious until lesions enter the 'crusting' stage; in-patients should be isolated. Extracorporeal membrane oxygenation/life support has been used successfully in individuals with fulminant respiratory failure. Consider early administration of varicella-zoster immune globulin for immunocompromised and pregnant patients exposed to varicella
- Most cases resolve spontaneously, but a minority progress to respiratory failure and death. Mortality may be significantly higher in pregnancy.

Respiratory syncytial virus

- Very common cause of bronchiolitis and pneumonia in children. Role in adult respiratory disease is more significant than previously appreciated, and infection often goes unrecognized
- Adult infection occurs particularly in the setting of underlying cardiac or respiratory disease or malignancy; outbreaks affecting adults in hospitals and nursing homes also occur. RSV may be a relatively common viral cause of pneumonia in patients who have recently undergone bone marrow transplantation
- Bronchoscopy with BAL is often diagnostic: detection of RSV antigen in BAL fluid has a sensitivity of nearly 90%. PCR-based diagnostic techniques and serological testing may have a role
- Bacterial superinfection may be a frequent complication
- Treatment is principally supportive. Role of aerosolized ribavirin and steroids in the treatment of severe disease in adults is unclear. Reports of successful outcomes in bone marrow transplant recipients following treatment with ribavirin and immunoglobulin.

Measles

- Very rare in adults. Bronchiolitis and pneumonia affect 50% of patients infected with measles and are a common cause of mortality in children
- Symptoms of fever and upper respiratory tract infection are followed by a diffuse maculopapular rash. Leucopenia is common
- CXR may show reticulonodular infiltrates, hilar lymphadenopathy, and pleural effusions
- Secondary bacterial infection is common
- Treatment is supportive. Treat secondary bacterial infection with antibiotics.

Hantavirus pulmonary syndrome

- First described following an outbreak in the south-western USA in 1993. Several different hantaviruses (e.g. Sin Nombre virus) have been associated with this syndrome. Previously described hantavirus-associated diseases occurred more commonly in Scandinavia and north-eastern Asia, and tended to cause haemorrhagic fever and renal failure with relative sparing of the lung
- Very rare, and affected individuals are almost exclusively from the USA, particularly from the Four Corners Region where Arizona, Colorado, Utah, and New Mexico meet
- Disease develops following inhalation of aerosolized viruses from rodent faeces, urine, or saliva
- Typically affects previously well young adults
- Common presenting symptoms are fever, chills, cough, myalgia, and gastrointestinal symptoms, such as vomiting and abdominal pain. Breathlessness occurs later in the disease course, and is often quickly followed by respiratory failure and the development of ARDS. Shock may occur and is associated with a poor prognosis
- Laboratory testing classically reveals neutrophilia and thrombocytopenia, sometimes renal impairment and mildly abnormal LFTs
- CXR typically shows initially bilateral basal infiltrates that progress to involve all regions of the lung; a minority are normal
- Diagnosis may be confirmed using serology, PCR for the virus, or by detection of viral antigen using immunochemistry
- Treatment is supportive within an intensive care unit. It is unclear if person-to-person transmission occurs, and patients should be in respiratory isolation. Intravenous ribavirin is commonly administered, although it is unclear if this improves outcome
- Mortality 30–50%, with death usually occurring within several days of presentation

Severe acute respiratory syndrome (SARS): epidemiology and pathophysiology

This rapidly progressive acute respiratory illness was first recognized in November 2002 in the Guangdong Province of China. By late February 2003 it had spread internationally. It was termed SARS by the World Health Organization (WHO), whose involvement was (in association with health authorities from the United States, Canada, Singapore, Hong Kong, and other Asian countries) to determine an aetiology, establish infection control measures to prevent further spread, establish a laboratory test for diagnosis, and evaluate treatments.

Epidemiology Cases of SARS were first recognized in the Guangdong province of China in November 2002, with 792 cases reported by February 2003. This first outbreak mainly affected health care workers and their contacts. The disease spread to Hong Kong via a Guangdong province physician, who infected individuals in a Hong Kong hotel lift. The disease rapidly spread to Singapore, Thailand, Vietnam, and Canada via travellers from Guangdong province and Hong Kong. Case numbers fell by mid May 2003, and by July 2003 the worldwide epidemic had ended. Further cases have subsequently been reported. An isolated case of laboratory-acquired SARS was reported in Singapore in September 2003. A further laboratory outbreak occurred in March 2004, with serologically proven infection in four individuals working at the same institute in Beijing.

A total of 8098 cases were reported to the WHO by August 2003, with 774 deaths, giving a case fatality rate of 9.5%. The fatality rate for those aged ≥60 was 43%. 29 countries on all five continents were affected. 83% of the worldwide cases were in China and Hong Kong. No deaths occurred in the United States or the UK. 41 deaths (of 251 cases) were in Canada.

Case definition The WHO defined criteria for those presenting with the disease after July 2004:

- Fever >38°C *plus*
- One or more symptom of lower respiratory tract illness (cough, difficulty breathing, shortness of breath) *plus*
- Radiographic evidence of lung infiltrate consistent with pneumonia or ARDS, *or* autopsy findings consistent with the pathology of pneumonia *or* ARDS without identifiable cause *plus*
- No alternative diagnosis to explain the illness

Laboratory case definition

- A person with symptoms or signs suggestive of SARS *plus*
- Positive laboratory findings for SARS-CoV based on one or more of:
  - PCR positive for SARS-CoV
  - Seroconversion by ELISA or IFA
  - Virus isolation

Testing should only be undertaken in a national or regional reference laboratory, as per WHO recommendations.

Pathophysiology A novel, previously undescribed coronavirus (SARS-CoV) is thought to be the causal agent. It is still to be ascertained whether microbiological and other cofactors enhance severity or transmissibility. The complete genetic sequence of the SARS-CoV has now been determined. It is currently thought that animals act as the main reservoir.

SARS is mostly spread by large droplets and person-to-person contact. There have been no reports of food- or water-borne transmission. However, SARS-CoV is shed in large quantities in stool, and profuse watery diarrhoea is a common symptom. Nosocomial transmission of SARS-CoV has been a striking feature in most outbreaks. The use of aerosol generating procedures (endotracheal intubation, nebulization, bronchoscopy) may amplify transmission.

Lung post mortem studies show diffuse alveolar damage, secondary bacterial pneumonia, and interstitial giant cell and macrophage infiltration. Pathological findings similar to those of bronchiolitis obliterans are recognized. There are no specific diagnostic features.

Incubation period is 2–10 days prior to the onset of the first symptom, which is typically fever.

SARS: clinical features and management

Clinical features The disease is a two-stage illness, commencing with a prodrome of fever (>38°C), with or without rigors, with non-specific systemic symptoms, e.g. malaise, headache, and myalgia.

The respiratory stage of the illness starts 3–7 days after the prodromal phase with dry cough and breathlessness. Progression to respiratory failure needing ventilation is well recognized. Up to 70% of patients develop large volume watery diarrhoea without blood or mucus.

Destruction of lung tissue is thought to result from an excessive immune response to the virus, rather than from the direct effects of virus replication. Peak viral load is at day 12–14 of infection, with virus shed not only in respiratory secretions, but in faeces and other body fluids.

Retrospectively devised but non-validated scoring systems show that the presence of cough, myalgia, diarrhoea, and rhinorrhoea or sore throat are 100% sensitive and 76% specific at identifying a patient with SARS.

Children experience a milder form of the disease, with a low death rate.

Investigations The illness is a symptom complex and the case definition is broad. Diagnosis is made on the basis of the clinical syndrome and absence of positive bacteriology and virology. SARS is a diagnosis of exclusion.

Recommended investigations in a suspected case include

- Blood tests
  - White blood count is normal or reduced, with a low total lymphocyte count (in 98% in the Hong Kong case series)
  - Leucopenia and thrombocytopenia are also recognized, with raised creatine kinase (CK) and alanine transferase (ALT). A raised lactate dehydrogenase (LDH) is associated with a poorer outcome
- CXR ranges from normal to diffuse bilateral interstitial infiltrate. Areas of focal consolidation, initially peripherally and lower zone in distribution, are also described. Cavitation, hilar lympadenopathy, and pleural effusion are uncommon at presentation.
- CT may reveal areas of interstitial infiltrate, ground-glass opacities, and interlobular septal thickening in those with a normal CXR. Spontaneous pneumothorax, pneumomediastinum, subpleural fibrosis, and/or cystic changes can occur in later stages
- SARS-CoV can be detected by RT-PCR (sensitivity 70%, dependent on specimen type and duration of illness). Useful specimens include nasopharyngeal aspirate, throat swab, urine, and faeces. An initial positive result on PCR must be confirmed by another clinical sample, re-extracting and testing the original sample, and using assays that target different parts of the genome. However, identification of seroconversion on a whole virus immunoassay remains the gold standard for the retrospective virological confirmation of the disease. The antibody response peaks at 10–14 days after the onset of fever. Agreement has been reached between international agencies to share specimens and laboratory data to develop a diagnostic test as soon as possible. Work to standardize PCR and ELISA testing for the SARS virus is ongoing

Treatment

- There is no specific treatment for SARS other than general supportive care. No RCT treatment data exists
- Some patients have been treated with oseltamivir and/or intravenous ribavirin. Immunoglobulin, anti-TNFα, highly active retroviral therapy (HAART), anti-platelet agents, and convalescence serum from SARS patients have all been all tried
- Patients treated with Kaletra® (400 mg ritonivir and 100 mg lopinavir) with ribavarin for 14 days had a lower incidence of ARDS and death, and this combination should be considered early for SARS patients, ideally in a randomized controlled trial
- Interferon β limits SARS-CoV replication *in vitro*, and patients treated with interferon alfacon-1 with corticosteroid had a better clinical course, with lower death rates
- Steroids lead to reduced fever, and improved oxygenation and CXR appearance, but do not alter need for ITU, or the death rate at 3 weeks. Some data suggest that high dose IV methylprednisolone (500 mg qds for 3–6 days) may be life-saving for patients with deteriorating radiographic consolidation and increasing oxygen requirements ('critical SARS')
- A series from Toronto showed a trend towards worsening outcome in those treated with ribavirin, due to elevated transaminases and haemolysis. There are no *in vitro* data to show any anti-SARS virus activity of ribavirin
- Experimental animal models show reduced viral replication with pegylated interferon α, and human studies using interferon and corticosteroids have shown no adverse effects
- Some studies show benefit from therapy with high-dose methylprednisolone given in the later stages of the illness; however, randomized placebo-controlled trials are awaited
- Vaccinations are being developed

Hospital admission Nosocomial transmission of SARS-CoV has been a striking feature in most outbreaks. Infected and suspected cases should be managed in negative pressure side rooms. Full protective clothing, including protective eye wear and face masks, are recommended for all visitors and health care workers. The use of aerosol generating procedures should be avoided where possible.

Prognosis Older age is associated with a poorer outcome. Diabetes and other comorbid illness are independent risk factors for death.

Prevention focuses on avoidance of exposure and effective infection control measures. Closure of hospitals and schools in affected areas and the use of quarantine measures helped to limit the spread of the disease in a number of countries.

Further information

Peiris JSM, Yuen KY *et al.* The severe acute respiratory syndrome. *NEJM* 2003; **349**: 2431–41

WHO website for continuously updated information: www.who.int/csr/sars/en

Diagnosis and pharmacotherapy of severe acute respiratory syndrome: what have we learnt? ERJ 2004: **24**: 1025–32.

Chapter 45

Sarcoidosis

Aetiology and pathology

Definition

- A multisystem inflammatory disorder of unknown cause, likely resulting from the interplay of environmental and genetic factors
- Characterized by non-caseating granulomata and CD4 Th1-biased T-cell response in affected organs
- Commonly involves the respiratory system, but can affect nearly all organs
- 50–60% of people have spontaneous remissions; others may develop chronic progressive disease

Aetiology Incidence varies with population studies, from 5 to 100/100 000, according to geographic distribution. UK incidence is about 5–10/100 000. Commoner in African-Americans, West Indians, and the Irish. Commonly presents between ages of 20 and 40. Unusual in children and the elderly. Typically more aggressive disease in Black populations than in Caucasians—especially with skin disease, peripheral lymphadenopathy, bone marrow, and liver involvement; higher relapse rates and worse long-term prognosis

Genetics Familial and ethnic clustering of cases suggest a genetic predisposition. Siblings of an affected person have a 5x increased risk of developing sarcoidosis. Best evidence of HLA association comes from recent large multicentre ACCESS study, showing HLA-DRB1*0301 is associated with susceptibility to disease in Blacks and Whites. Also a genome-wide scan for susceptibility genes in familial sarcoidosis has been performed, pointing to a locus on chromosome 5 in African-Americans and chromosome 6 in German Caucasians.

Pathology Sarcoidosis is caused by an immunological response:

- Unknown antigenic stimulus triggers CD4 (helper) T-cell activation and expansion. This response is exaggerated and Th1-biased, with resultant interferon gamma and IL-2 production from these T-cells
- Activated T cells proliferate and release mediators, attracting additional inflammatory cells with concomitant macrophage activation and aggregation
- This leads to immune granuloma formation, which is enhanced by interferon gamma
- Granulomata themselves cause increased local fibroblast stimulation and hence fibrosis
- Metabolic activity of macrophages causes raised ACE (angiotensin-converting enzyme) levels in serum, lung tissue, and bronchoalveolar fluid. Increase in T-cell activity causes B-lymphocyte stimulation, which can cause raised serum immunoglobulins and immune complexes
- In most patients, response resolves over 2–5 years

Delayed-type hypersensitivity reactions are depressed in sarcoidosis. This is thought to be due to the migration of lymphocytes to the active compartment (lungs), with resultant peripheral blood lymphopenia. Seen as a decreased response to tuberculin, mumps virus, and *Candida albicans* antigens. This is not thought to be clinically significant.

Sarcoid-like reactions are reported in association with malignancy and also in HIV patients starting on antiretroviral therapy (very rare). Non-caseating pulmonary granulomas are found, but there are no other symptoms or signs of sarcoidosis.

Differential diagnosis of granuloma on lung biopsy

- Sarcoidosis
- Tuberculosis
- Extrinsic allergic alveolitis
- Wegner's granulomatosis
- Primary biliary cirrhosis
- Granulomatous orchitis
- Langerhans cell histiocytosis
- Leprosy
- Tertiary syphilis
- Brucellosis
- Berylliosis
- Silicosis
- Hypogammaglobulinaemia
- Fungal infections—coccidioidomycosis
- Schistosomiasis
- Cat scratch fever
- Lymphoma
- Giant cell arteritis
- Polyarteritis nodosa
- Takyasu's arteritis
- Crohn's disease
- De Quervain's thyroiditis

Further information

Iannuzzi MC. Advances in genetics of sarcoidosis. *Proc Am Thorac Soc* 2007; **4**: 457–60.

Schurmann M, Lympany PA *et al.* Familial sarcoidosis is linked to the major histocompatability complex region. *Am J Respir Crit Care Med* 2000; **162**: 861–4.

Schurmann M, Bein G *et al.* HLA-DQB1 and HLA-DPB1 genotypes in familial sarcoidosis. *Respir Med* 1998; **92**: 649–52.

Chest disease: clinical features

More than 90% of patients with sarcoidosis have thoracic involvement, with an abnormal CXR. Pulmonary sarcoidosis can be an incidental CXR finding in approximately 30% of patients. There is spontaneous remission in two-thirds and 10–30% have a chronic course.

Clinical features There are probably at least 2 distinct clinical courses:

- **Löfgren's syndrome** Mild acute disease, which is usually non-progressive. Presents with fever, bilateral hilar lymphadenopathy, erythema nodosum, and arthralgia. Occurs particularly in Caucasians. Has a good prognosis and resolves completely and spontaneously in 80% within 1–2 years. A minority may develop lung disease
- **Persistent progressive** infiltrative lung disease

Hilar/mediastinal lymphadenopathy May be asymptomatic or cause cough or chest pain. Often bilateral and symmetrical, but can be unilateral and asymmetrical. Can be associated with systemic symptoms of malaise and arthralgia, which are helped by non-steroidal anti-inflammatory drugs. Benign course.

Important to exclude other causes of lymphadenopathy, such as TB and lymphoma. May need HRCT and lymph node aspirate or biopsy.

Does not require systemic steroid treatment.

Stage I: 85% resolve spontaneously over 2 years, 15% develop lung infiltrates. The average time for bilateral hilar lymphadenopathy resolution is 8 months

Interstitial lung involvement May be asymptomatic or cause morbidity and mortality, with dyspnoea, cough, chest ache or frank pain, malaise, fatigue, and impaired quality of life. Rarely have crackles or clubbing on examination. Pulmonary infiltrates on CXR. Can return to normal over time, or progress to fibrosis and respiratory failure. Lung function tests may be normal, or may show a restrictive defect with reduced transfer factor.

Differential diagnosis Other interstitial lung disease, malignancy, infection.

Radiological classification of thoracic sarcoidosis

Stage 0	Normal
Stage I	Hilar lymphadenopathy
Stage II	Hilar lymphadenopathy and parenchymal infiltrate
Stage III	Parenchymal infiltrate
Stage IV	Fibrosis

Seeing a patient with possible sarcoidosis in clinic

- Make diagnosis—clinically, HRCT ± histology
- Assess extent/severity/presence of extrapulmonary involvement—CXR, PFT, ECG, eyes, rash, renal function, serum calcium, liver function, immunoglobulins, and ACE (latter two can be raised in active sarcoidosis)
- Stable or progressive?—CXR, PFT (VC ± KCO), oximetry, ACE, urea (if renal involvement)
- Treatment?

Differential diagnosis of bilateral hilar lymphadenopathy on CXR

- Sarcoidosis
- Tuberculosis
- Lymphoma
- Coccidioidomycosis and histoplasmosis
- Leukaemia
- Berylliosis
- Hypogammaglobulinaemia and recurrent infections.

Further information

Judson MA, Baughman RP *et al.* Two year prognosis of sarcoidosis: the ACCESS experience. *Sarcoidosis Vasc Diffuse Lung Dis* 2003; **20**: 204–11.

Chest disease: management

Diagnosis is based on a characteristic clinical picture, plus:
- Histological evidence of non-caseating granuloma in any tissue
- Characteristic picture on imaging (thoracic HRCT scan or gallium scan)
- Lymphocytosis on bronchoalveolar lavage (BAL)

Other diseases capable of producing similar clinical and histological picture, particularly tuberculosis and lymphoma, should be excluded.

Investigations

- ***HRCT*** Micronodules in a subpleural and bronchovascular distribution. Fissural nodularity and bronchial distortion. Irregular linear opacities, ground-glass shadowing related to bronchovascular bundles, and nodular or ill-defined shadows. Air-trapping due to small airway granulomata common. Endobronchial disease in 55%. Possible honeycomb lung. Hilar and mediastinal lymphadenopathy. CT-guided FNA of subcarinal or mediastinal nodes may be possible and yield a tissue diagnosis
- ***Bronchoscopy (transbronchial biopsy, TBNA, bronchial biopsy, or bronchoalveolar lavage)*** may not be necessary if there is no diagnostic doubt clinically and radiologically. Positive yield of bronchial biopsy is 41–57%. Higher if visible abnormal mucosa. Positive yield of transbronchial biopsy is 40–90% (still high yield even if lungs appear normal on HRCT). This is the initial procedure of choice in a patient with suspected pulmonary sarcoidosis. Transbronchial needle aspiration (TBNA) of the mediastinal lymph nodes will yield a diagnosis in 63–90% of cases. Transbronchial biopsy and TBNA have a higher yield together than either alone. Experience is limited in endoscopic ultrasound FNA (EUS-FNA) in sarcoidosis. BAL in sarcoidosis shows a CD4:CD8 ratio of >3.5. If this test is not available, a lymphocytosis of $>2 \times 10^5$cells/mL supports the diagnosis, but is not diagnostic. (Lymphocytosis is also seen in UIP, COP, hypersensitivity pneumonitis, and smokers)
- ***Mediastinoscopy*** for central or paratracheal nodes or open lung biopsy: 90% positive yield. May be necessary to exclude lymphoma. Surgical biopsy is not usually necessary, but if other procedures have not yielded a definitive diagnosis, it may be required. Lymph node ± lung (usually via VATS) can be biopsied.
- ***Biopsy other affected areas*** such as skin, liver, etc. if indicated, as these may be easier to biopsy in order to make a diagnosis
- ***Mantoux/Heaf test*** may show minimal reaction/grade 0 in sarcoid (peripheral cutaneous anergy to tuberculin due to migration of T cells to active sites of disease). A positive Mantoux or Heaf test therefore make sarcoidosis less likely as a diagnosis, although does not necessarily make tuberculosis more likely as the diagnosis. Heaf testing not widely used now.
- ***Kveim test*** No longer performed clinically, due to risks of transmissible diseases. It involved injecting homogenized splenic tissue from a patient with sarcoidosis to see if a granulomatous reaction occurred.

Monitoring disease There is no single measurement to assess all the aspects of patients with sarcoidosis. Clinical examination and serial measurements are key.

- ***PFT*** Pulmonary sarcoidosis gives a restrictive defect with decreased TLC and VC. TLCO provides the most sensitive measurement of change, although a properly performed VC is probably adequate for clinical purposes. Likely to improve with steroids. Airflow obstruction may also occur
- ***CXR*** may improve with time or treatment
- ***ACE*** (angiotensin-converting enzyme) levels increased in up to 80% of patients with acute sarcoidosis, although can be normal in active disease. It may be a surrogate marker of the total granuloma burden. Levels become normal as disease resolves. Can be useful to monitor the clinical course, if activity is uncertain, but levels should not be used in isolation to determine treatment. Levels suppressed by steroids and when steroids are stopped levels usually increase, unrelated to sarcoidosis activity. This is not a specific test. False positives include TB
- ***Calcium*** may rise with active sarcoidosis or in the summer months. This may cause renal impairment, so urea or creatinine should also be checked
- ***BAL*** not performed routinely to assess progress of sarcoidosis, but changes in proportions of cells seen in lavage would indicate improvement
- ***PET*** scan may be positive in areas of disease activity. Not reliable for studying brain or heart. Limited studies of serial data
- ***Gallium scan*** rarely used now, as non-specific and expensive. Areas of active inflammation are positive, with a classic 'panda pattern'. Positive areas soon become negative with steroid use. Bowel and liver positive anyway, so disease cannot be charted in these areas.

General management

Most patients with pulmonary sarcoidosis do not require treatment. Asymptomatic CXR infiltrates are usually monitored.

Indications for immunosuppressive treatment

- Increasing symptoms, deteriorating PFTs, and worsening CXR infiltrates
- Cardiac sarcoidosis
- Neurosarcoidosis
- Sight-threatening ocular sarcoidosis
- Hypercalcaemia
- Lupus pernio
- Splenic, hepatic, or renal sarcoidosis.

Starting drug treatment

- When required, treatment is usually with steroids initially. Good evidence for short to medium term improvement in symptoms, respiratory function, and radiology, but long-term benefits less clear
- Give high doses, such as 40 mg prednisolone/day, to control active disease. Rarely need more than 40 mg/day. Usually give this high dose for 4 weeks and then reduce if there has been a response
- **Maintenance dose** of around 5–20 mg, to control symptoms. Leave on this dose for a few months and then slowly reduce steroid dose further. Maintain on low dose of prednisolone (5–7.5 mg/day or alternate days) for prolonged period of up to 12 months to consolidate resolution, before considering complete withdrawal.
- Some patients, especially those with progressive pulmonary sarcoidosis, may require longer treatment (years) of low-dose prednisolone to prevent relapse
- **Inhaled steroids** are of limited efficacy in sarcoidosis, but may be useful if there is cough or bronchial hyperreactivity
- **Relapses** often occur when treatment is stopped and may require the reintroduction of steroids, or the increase of steroid dose. Duration and dose of steroids is dictated by site and response to treatment
- Avoid futile steroid treatment for end-stage disease, such as honeycomb lung
- **If steroid treatment fails**, or sarcoidosis is life-threatening, other immunosuppressive regimes may be indicated. Pulsed high-dose intravenous methylprednisolone is an option, which can be particularly useful for neurosarcoidosis
- In cases where **prolonged immunosuppression** is required, or if steroid side-effects cannot be tolerated, other immunosuppressive drugs should be considered. Possibilities include azathioprine and methotrexate. There are limited data for their use in sarcoidosis
- Patients who have troublesome symptoms related to sarcoidosis, such as arthralgia, skin disease, fever, sweats, ocular symptoms, systemic symptoms such as fatigue, may require symptomatic steroid treatment.

Lower initial doses such as 20 mg/day are likely to be sufficient to gain symptomatic control and doses can then be reduced
- Prescribe gastric and bone protection with steroids when necessary

Other drugs used in sarcoidosis

(See p 601 for more information regarding immunosuppressive drugs.)
If there is progressive pulmonary sarcoidosis, refractory to steroids, consider:
- **Methotrexate** Given once/week 15–25 mg PO for 6-month trial. Use instead of or in addition to low-dose prednisolone. Avoid if hepatic or renal failure. Side-effects: GI upset, stomatitis, pneumonitis, myelosuppression. Teratogenic. Low oncogenic potential. Monitor FBC and MCV, AST, ALT every 2 weeks for 3 months, then monthly. Do not use for >2 years. Useful for chronic sarcoidosis and cutaneous disease
- **Azathioprine** Used in neurosarcoidosis and stage II/III pulmonary sarcoidosis with partial/no steroid response. 100–150 mg/day. Use instead of or in addition to low-dose prednisolone. Side-effects: myelosuppression, GI upset, stomatitis, idiosyncratic reaction–fever, rash. Low oncogenic potential. No gonadal toxicity. Check FBC every 2 weeks for 3 months, then monthly. TPMT (thiopurine methyltransferase) testing should be performed prior to commencement (see p 678)
- **Cyclophosphamide** IV pulsed, for neurosarcoidosis unresponsive to steroids. Toxicity profile limits use. (See p 681)
- **Anti-malarials** Chloroquine and hydroxychloroquine 200 mg od/bd. For skin and hypercalcaemia. Steroid sparing. Can be given with steroids and other immunosuppressant in severe sarcoidosis. Side-effects: rarely, ocular toxicity
- **Others** New unproven efficacy: ciclosporin, thalidomide, TNFα inhibitors (etanercept, infliximab)

Prognosis There are no prognostic markers in sarcoidosis, apart from:
- *Good prognosis* Löfgren's syndrome has complete resolution in 80% of people
- *Poorer prognosis with chronic disease* Lupus pernio, nasal mucosa involvement, chronic uveitis, chronic hypercalcaemia, nephrocalcinosis, neural involvement, age greater than 40 and Black race
- Prognosis according to CXR appearance:
  - Stage II: 50% cases recover spontaneously in 2 years, 30–40% require systemic steroids, 10–15% require long-term steroids
  - Stage III: Worse prognosis. Only 30% show significant improvement with steroids

Transplant Consider if patient has end-stage lung disease, rapidly progressive disease despite treatment, or if they are oxygen dependent. Sarcoidosis is a rare indication for lung transplant. Granulomata recur in transplanted lung, but do not cause higher rates of graft failure.

Extra-thoracic disease 1

Varies according to ethnic origin and sex of patient.

Systemic symptoms are common, such as fever, sweats, loss of appetite, weight loss, fatigue, malaise, chest pain, dyspnoea, and cough. Polyarthralgia often affects the knees, ankles, wrists, and elbows, and can be improved by NSAIDs.

Hypercalcaemia Granulomata convert vitamin D_3 to active 1,25-dihydroxycholecalciferol. This causes enhanced calcium absorption from intestine. Sunlight also increases levels of vitamin D and calcium. High calcium may cause systemic effects and is often associated with renal damage and hypercalciuria. Commoner in Caucasians and in men.

Treatment If mildly raised, limit dietary calcium intake, avoid sun exposure and drink plenty of fluids. Otherwise, steroids, often low dose once calcium level controlled (should be within 2 weeks—if not investigate for other cause for hypercalcaemia). Decrease dose when calcium level satisfactory. Some patients may only need steroids during the summer months. Hydroxychloroquine can also be used.

Skin 25% of patients have skin involvement. More common in women.
Erythema nodosum Raised papules, nodules, or plaques, usually on shins. Also tender, indurated, or bruised appearance. Firm and often have shiny appearance. Nodular change involving different tattoo colours recognized and is characteristic of sarcoidosis. Sarcoid tissue may arise in old scars, or cause scar hypertrophy.
Lupus pernio is a bluish tinge that occurs on nose, cheeks, and ears. It is associated with chronic disease.

Diagnosis Usually easily biopsied

Treatment Initially with topical preparations. Lupus pernio should be treated with systemic steroids. Hydroxychloroquine or methotrexate may be necessary. Role of long-term tetracyclines for cutaneous sarcoidosis under investigation

Eye Common, occurring in 25% plus of cases, especially women and African-Caribbeans
Uveitis (acute or chronic), episcleritis, scleritis, glaucoma, conjunctivitis, and retinal involvement can occur. May be asymptomatic, or cause painful red eye, with photophobia, lacrimation, and blurred vision. Pupil irregular or constricted. Untreated, can cause visual impairment.
Lacrimal involvement in sarcoidosis gives keratoconjunctivitis sicca—dry eye with diminished tear secretion. Painful red eyes. Treat with artificial tears.

Diagnosis Assessment by an ophthalmologist with slit lamp examination if any ocular symptoms. Some recommend that all newly diagnosed patients with sarcoidosis have slit lamp examination. Mild asymptomatic eye involvement is common. May need conjunctival biopsy, if no evidence of sarcoid elsewhere.

Treatment Local steroids are commonly used if there is no other indication for systemic steroids. However, if it does not respond, systemic steroids should be used.

Heart Cardiac sarcoidosis occurs in 5% of patients with pulmonary disease. Post mortem studies show cardiac sarcoidosis is present in 25%, so is often undiagnosed. Patients may present with chest pain or, more commonly, are found to have conduction defects on the ECG. These may be benign and asymptomatic, like first-degree heart block, but more significant arrhythmias can occur, the first indication of which may be sudden death. Myocardial granulomata can occur in any part of the heart. Commonly they occur in the interventricular septum, where they can affect nodal and conducting tissue. The left ventricular wall can be affected, with fibrosis causing reduced compliance and contractile difficulties, leading to cardiac failure. Aneurysms can form, and pericarditis can occur. Valvular dysfunction due to infiltration of the papillary muscles is rare. The clinical course can be uncertain.

Diagnosis Echocardiogram may show signs of cardiomyopathy—usually restrictive. MRI, technetium scan, or gallium scan show non-segmental fixed defects. Biopsy is diagnostic, but can be difficult as sarcoidosis is patchy. Not recommended in general. ECG and 24-h tape may be helpful in investigation.

Treatment Must be treated with systemic steroids 20–40 mg prednisolone/day, which improve symptoms and ECG and Echo features. These should be slowly reduced, but intractable arrhythmias may need continued high dosage. May need other immunosuppressants. Investigate with 24-h tape if uncertain. Amiodarone, a pacemaker, implantable defibrillator, or heart transplant may be necessary.

In clinic Perform a screening ECG on all patients with sarcoidosis perhaps every 6 months.

Extra-thoracic disease 2

Kidney A degree of renal involvement is found in 35% of patients with sarcoidosis. Rarely can present with renal failure, obstructive uropathy, nephrolithiasis, or urinary tract disorder. Nephrocalcinosis is a common cause of chronic renal failure. Often associated hypercalcaemia or other manifestation of sarcoidosis.

Diagnosis Renal biopsy with granulomata found in interstitium, but this is rarely needed in this context. Search for pulmonary sarcoidosis.

Treatment Steroids ± hydroxychloroquine for hypercalcaemia.

CNS Involved in 4–18% of patients. Can affect any part of the peripheral or central nervous system. Can present as a peripheral nerve or cranial nerve lesion. Most common is lower motor neuron facial nerve palsy, with optic nerve involvement being next commonest. Mononeuritis multiplex recognized. May be less specific, with psychiatric features. Hypothalamic granulomata may cause diabetes insipidus, appetite disturbance, or hypersomnolence.

Diagnosis Difficult, but may be made easier if there is another sign of systemic sarcoidosis, for example bilateral hilar lymphadenopathy. Lumbar puncture may show a raised CSF ACE and an increased lymphocyte count. Confirm with biopsy if possible—cerebral or meningeal tissue if no pulmonary involvement.

Treatment Must be treated with steroids, but often quite resistant to treatment. May need to try further immunosuppressants.

Musculoskeletal Arthralgia is common in sarcoidosis, but arthritis is unusual. Arthralgia commonly affects the ankles and feet, but also hands, wrists, and elbows. A subacute proximal myopathy can occur, as well as bone cysts, especially of terminal phalanges. The latter show little response to systemic steroids.

Diagnosis Granuloma seen on muscle biopsy.

Treatment NSAIDs; steroids may be necessary.

GI 60% of liver biopsies on patients with sarcoidosis show granuloma. Frequently asymptomatic. Hepatomegaly unusual, but can get portal fibrosis and cirrhosis. LFTs suggestive if 3× normal, especially ALP and γGT.

Diagnosis Biopsy.

Treatment Steroids—may reduce size of liver and improve LFTs.

Haematological Splenomegaly can occur and may be massive, causing abdominal discomfort. A massive spleen may require splenectomy to avoid rupture. Associated anaemia, neutropenia, and thrombocytopenia. Lymphopenia often seen.

ENT Nasal or laryngeal granuloma. Sinus invasion. Parotid and other salivary gland enlargement, dry mouth.

Rarely Breast disease, ovarian or testicular masses.

Further information

Judson MA, Iannuzzi MC (Eds). Sarcoidosis: evolving concepts and controversies. *Sem Respir Crit Care Med* 2007; **28**.

American Thoracic Society/European Respiratory Society/World Association of Sarcoidosis and other Granulomatous Disorders statement on sarcoidosis. *Eur Respir J* 1999; **14**: 735–7.

Guidelines for the diagnosis and assessment of diffuse parenchymal lung disease. *Thorax* 1999; **54**(suppl. 1): S1.

Judson MA, Baughman RP *et al.* Two year prognosis of sarcoidosis: the ACCESS experience. *Sarcoidosis Vasc Diffuse Lung Dis* 2003; **20**: 204–11.

World Association of Sarcoidosis and other Granulomatous Disorders website, www.pinali.unipd.it/sarcoid

Chapter 46

Sickle cell disease: pulmonary complications

Overview

Background

Sickle cell disease is an autosomal recessive condition resulting in a substitution of a valine for glycine in the beta-globin subunit of haemoglobin (Hb), forming HbS. HbS is less soluble under reduced oxygen tensions and leads to deformation of red blood cells (sickling) when deoxygenated (for example, in atelectatic lung), resulting in chronic haemolysis and vascular occlusion with tissue infarction in individuals homozygous for the beta-globin gene mutation (sickle cell anaemia/disease). Haemoglobin electrophoresis or high-performance liquid chromatography (HPLC) in sickle cell disease demonstrates HbS ~80–99% and no normal haemoglobin HbA; anaemia Hb 6–9 g/dl is usual. Heterozygote carriers of the beta-globin gene mutation are referred to as having 'sickle cell trait' and are largely asymptomatic, although sickle crises may occur during extreme hypoxia (e.g. during anaesthesia); HPLC analysis demonstrates HbS ~35–40% and HbA (normal haemoglobin) ~50%. Sickle haemoglobin solubility testing does not distinguish between trait and homozygous disease.

Pulmonary complications

- ***Obstructive airways disease*** and airway hyper-reactivity is often noted on pulmonary function testing; pathogenesis unclear
- ***Nocturnal oxyhaemoglobin desaturation*** is common, pathogenesis unclear—tonsillar hypertrophy is common, and OSA may be a contributing factor
- ***Pneumonia*** is more common, particularly from *Chlamydia pneumoniae, S. pneumoniae, H. influenzae,* Mycoplasma, Legionella and respiratory viruses; may precipitate acute chest syndrome. Invasive pneumococcal disease is significantly more common. Patients should take lifelong prophylactic penicillin, as functionally asplenic
- ***Pulmonary thromboembolism*** appears to be more common; may precipitate acute chest syndrome
- ***Acute chest syndrome***
- ***Sickle cell chronic lung disease***

Acute chest syndrome

Definition and clinical features Defined as new pulmonary infiltrates on CXR, associated with symptoms such as fever, cough, chest pain and breathlessness. A form of acute lung injury; may progress to ARDS. Leading cause of death in sickle cell disease; occurs in up to half of all patients during their lifetime. Risk factors include young age, high steady state leukocyte counts and haemoglobin levels, and past history of acute chest syndrome. May follow surgery and anaesthesia.

Causes may not be apparent, and include one or more of infection, pulmonary fat embolism (preceded by bony pain), *in situ* thrombosis or pulmonary embolism, atelectasis following hypoventilation (from acute painful crisis of chest wall or excessive opiates), and possibly pulmonary oedema due to excessive hydration. Each leads to hypoxia with increased sickling and vascular occlusion, and initially mild disease can escalate rapidly to ARDS and death. All patients with a painful vaso-occlusive crisis should be monitored closely for the development of the acute chest syndrome; routine use of incentive spirometry may help prevent its development in these patients.

Investigations

- ***Blood tests*** Raised white cell count, anaemia; check HbS %
- ***Hypoxia*** is common and may be underestimated using pulse oximetry; A–a gradient predicts clinical severity; consider ITU transfer if worsens
- ***Culture*** blood and sputum
- ***CXR*** shows multifocal pulmonary infiltrates, sometimes with pleural effusion
- ***BAL*** may be considered in patients not responding to treatment.

▶▶ Management of sickle cell acute chest syndrome

Supportive care on ITU may be required. Liaise with haematology team. Treatment comprises:

- ***Oxygen*** to correct hypoxia; monitor ABGs
- Empirical broad-spectrum ***antibiotics*** (including a macrolide)
- ***Rehydration*** (IV fluids may be needed; care to avoid overhydration)
- ***Bronchodilators*** are often used; airflow obstruction is common, may contribute to high airway pressures during mechanical ventilation
- Ensure adequate ***analgesia*** for bony pain (consider NSAIDs; IM or SC opiates often required)
- ***Incentive spirometry*** and chest physiotherapy to prevent atelectasis. Pain may limit their use, and CPAP may be better tolerated
- ***Simple and exchange blood transfusion*** both reduce the HbS concentration and improve oxygenation in acute chest syndrome. Indications for transfusion include persistent or worsening hypoxia, severe disease, multilobar involvement, neurological complications, multi-organ failure, or history of cardiac disease. Simple transfusion is recommended if severely anaemic, although Hb should not be raised above 10.5 g/dl as the increase in blood viscosity exacerbates sickling. Exchange transfusion should be used in patients with a relatively high Hb, aiming for HbS <20% and maintaining total Hb <14.5 g/dl
- Other treatments. Successful use of inhaled ***nitric oxide*** for the treatment of a handful of refractory cases has been reported. Corticosteroids may be of benefit in children, but rebound pain crises may occur and routine use of corticosteroids is not recommended. Hydroxyurea increases fetal Hb and reduces sickling, and significantly reduces the incidence of acute chest syndrome; it is recommended for patients with recurrent episodes.

Prognosis Approximately 13% of patients with acute chest syndrome require mechanical ventilation; overall mortality 4–9%.

Sickle cell chronic lung disease

Sickle cell chronic lung disease is a poorly described entity, characterized by progressive breathlessness and abnormal pulmonary function, sometimes with pulmonary hypertension. Thought to follow recurrent episodes of lung infarction/infection, although there may not be a history of previous acute chest syndrome. Prevalence in sickle cell disease estimated at 4%. Radiologically, characterized by multifocal interstitial infiltrate. **PFTs** typically restrictive, although airways obstruction also described.

Severe *pulmonary hypertension* may occur in up to a third of patients with sickle cell disease. Management is largely as for idiopathic pulmonary arterial hypertension, with anticoagulation and vasodilators in a specialist centre (p 392). Hydroxyurea reduces episodes of acute chest syndrome and may be of benefit. Inhaled nitric oxide may have a role; studies are ongoing. Pulmonary thromboendarterectomy may be considered in patients with proximal pulmonary artery occlusion.

Further information

Siddiqui AK, Ahmed S. Pulmonary manifestations of sickle cell disease. *Postgrad Med J* 2003; **79**: 384–90.

Mak V, Davies SC. Acute chest syndrome of sickle cell anaemia. *Thorax* 2003; **58**: 726–8.

Chapter 47

Sleep apnoea and hypoventilation

Obstructive sleep apnoea (OSA)

Definition and epidemiology OSA, or obstructive sleep apnoea/hypopnoea (OSAH) are currently the preferred terms for the problem of dynamic upper airway obstruction during sleep.

- OSA is part of a spectrum, with trivial snoring at one end and repetitive complete obstruction throughout the night (such that the patient cannot sleep and breathe at the same time) at the other
- Along this spectrum is a point at which the degree of obstruction and recovery fragments sleep enough to cause daytime symptoms
- Distinction should be made between the sleep study findings alone (i.e. presence of sleep apnoea episodes), and an abnormal sleep study *plus* the presence of symptoms (i.e. *obstructive sleep apnoea syndrome*, OSAS).

Thresholds defining 'abnormality' are arbitrary (e.g. 10 s to define an apnoea). Numerical definitions of OSA, based on counting individual events during a sleep study, are not very helpful. The current definition of the clinical syndrome should be:

> Upper airway narrowing, provoked by sleep, causing sufficient sleep fragmentation to result in significant daytime symptoms, usually excessive sleepiness.

- Prevalence depends on the chosen thresholds for defining both an abnormality on the sleep study, and significant symptoms
- 0.5–1% of adult men in the UK (and about a fifth as many women) have OSA syndrome sufficient to be candidates for treatment with nasal continuous positive airway pressure (CPAP) treatment
- Prevalence figures depend on levels of obesity and will be higher in the USA, and probably rise inexorably in the UK in the future
- The prevalence in women is thought to be lower due to their different fat distribution. Upper body obesity (and thus neck obesity) is more a male pattern
- OSA is the third most common serious respiratory condition after asthma and COPD. In some respiratory units it has now become the commonest reason for specialist referral

Pathophysiology and associated conditions Control of the upper airway musculature is complex; upper airway patency depends on dilator muscle activity. All postural muscles relax during sleep (including pharyngeal dilators); some narrowing of the upper airway is normal. Excessive narrowing with the onset of sleep is due to the following factors.

Causes of a small pharyngeal size when awake (such that normal muscle relaxation with sleep is enough to provoke critical narrowing).

- Fatty infiltration of pharyngeal tissues and external pressure from increased neck fat and/or muscle bulk
- Large tonsils
- Subtle 'abnormalities' of craniofacial shape, e.g. minor micrognathia or retrognathia
- Extra submucosal tissue, e.g. myxoedema, mucopolysaccharidoses

Causes of excessive narrowing of the airway occurring with muscle relaxation at sleep onset

- Mass loading from an obese or muscular neck may simply 'overwhelm' residual dilator action, as well as reduce the starting size
- Neuromuscular diseases with pharyngeal involvement may lead to greater loss of dilator muscle tone, e.g. stroke, myotonic dystrophy, Duchenne dystrophy, motor neuron disease
- Muscle relaxants, such as sedatives and alcohol
- Increasing age

Predisposing conditions OSA is found more commonly in certain conditions, such as acromegaly and hypothyroidism, but the reasons are not well understood. It is unclear whether there need to be any other non-anatomical factors (such as unstable ventilatory control, or pharyngeal sensory abnormalities) to provoke OSA. Most associated abnormalities that have been described are likely to be *secondary* to long periods of snoring and OSA, rather than primary causal factors.

Short-term consequences of OSA In severe OSA, repetitive collapse of the upper airway, with arousal required to re-activate the pharyngeal dilators, occurs approximately every minute throughout the sleeping period (60 events/h, or over 400 per night); they are usually attended by hypoxia and hypercapnia that are corrected during the inter-apnoeic hyperventilatory period. Obstructive events short of complete obstruction also provoke arousal, as it is usually the compensatory reflex increase in inspiratory effort, rather than the blood gas deterioration directly, that wakens the brain. In this situation the drops in oxygen saturation may be very much less and, in younger thinner individuals, almost imperceptible on oximetry tracings. This is because the compensation afforded by the increased inspiratory effort may be adequate, and the bigger oxygen stores in the lungs of the less obese will buffer any brief hypoventilation.

- Recurrent arousals lead to highly fragmented and unrefreshing sleep
- Excessive daytime sleepiness results
- The correlation between the sleep fragmentation and the resultant degree of sleepiness is not tight, with some patients being sleepy with low levels of fragmentation, and vice versa
- This is thought to result partly from inter-individual differences in sensitivity to the effects of sleep fragmentation
- With every arousal there is a rise in blood pressure, often over 50 mmHg. It is unclear if these BP rises do any damage to the cardiovascular system. There is also a carry-over of hypertension (average of 3 mmHg) into the waking hours which falls after treatment at 1 month
- There is true nocturia, mechanism unclear; there may be raised atrial natriuretic peptide (ANP) levels from increased central blood volume, brought about by the subatmospheric intrathoracic pressures during the obstructed breathing; or it may be simply a reflection of highly fragmented sleep preventing the normal reduction in urine flow associated with sleep.

OSA: clinical features

Chapter 14 (p 85) covers many of the essential features in the history and discusses the differential diagnosis of excessive daytime sleepiness.

Most patients present with:

- Excessive sleepiness, measured using the Epworth Sleepiness Scale; >9 is considered abnormally sleepy (p 89)
- Loud snoring, and apnoeic episodes recognized by the bed partner
- The patient recognizes that he wakes up choking from time to time
- Poor concentration
- Unrefreshing sleep and waking unrefreshed
- Nocturia (true nocturia with reversal of the usual day/night ratio)

Less often there will be:

- Nocturnal sweating
- Reduced libido
- Oesophageal reflux
- Increasingly common are patients arriving with spouses worried by the apnoeic pauses they have observed

Sleepiness

- Sometimes difficult to assess: failure by the patient to recognize the problem, or denial due to concerns over driving and licensing
- The Epworth scale (p 89) assesses *tendency to fall asleep*, rather than *perceived sleepiness per se*, as some patients may regard their situation as normal
- It is important to separate the symptom of tiredness from sleepiness (p 86), the latter being much more typical of OSA, although sometimes complained of (rather than sleepiness) by women with OSA

Examination and investigations

The examination (often unrewarding) and the investigations are detailed in Chapter 14 (p 88). Look for the presence of additional lower airways obstruction, with associated CO_2 retention, so-called 'overlap syndrome'. CO_2 retention in pure OSA is very uncommon (except in the very, very obese). It appears that the additive effect of some lower airways obstruction (often not enough in its own right to precipitate CO_2 retention) is required, which perhaps limits the inter-apnoeic hyperventilation and thus gradually encourages tolerance to raised levels of CO_2.

The majority of patients with significant OSA are male, tend to have a combination of upper body obesity (neck circumference >17 in), and a relatively undersized or set back mandible. Airway size can be assessed with scoring systems, e.g. p 591.

Sleep study

The sleep study assesses if there is anything likely to be the cause of the patient's symptoms. The considerable grey area between normality and abnormality means that sometimes it is unclear whether the symptoms can be blamed on the sleep study findings. There is also considerable night-to-night variation in sleep study indices that further blurs the distinction between normality and abnormality. In this situation it may be necessary to undertake a therapeutic trial of nasal CPAP and let the patient decide if the benefits of treatment outweigh the disadvantages.

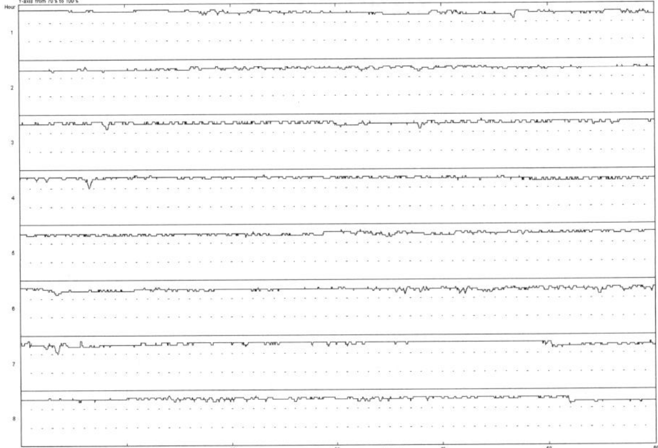

Fig. 47.1 Normal overnight oximetry. Normal baseline and a few dips. Vertical axis, 70-100% SaO_2 for each panel; horizontal axis, 60 minutes each panel.

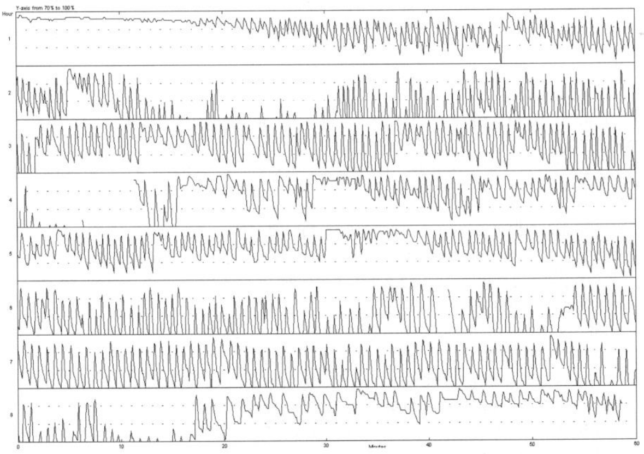

Fig. 47.2 Severe OSA. Large numbers of regular dips, sawtooth shaped (faster rise in SaO_2 than fall).

OSA: types of sleep study

- Overnight oximetry alone
- More than just oximetry, with other channels such as snoring, body movement, heart rate, oronasal airflow, chest and abdominal movements, leg movements: so-called 'limited' sleep studies, or 'respiratory PSG'
- Full polysomnography, with EEG, EOG, and EMG, to stage sleep electrophysiologically, in addition to the channels listed above

There is no evidence that OSA diagnosis needs full polysomnography (PSG with EEG) and it is not indicated for most patients. Oximetry will identify most cases, allowing onward referral for CPAP treatment. False-positive oximetry occurs with Cheyne–Stokes breathing (heart failure, post-stroke) and when there is a low baseline SaO_2 (e.g. COPD); this allows the SaO_2 to oscillate more, with small changes in PaO_2 due to the increasing steepness of the Hb dissociation curve at lower SaO_2. False negatives, discussed earlier, can occur with younger and thinner patients.

With appropriate expertise, and recognition of its limitations, oximetry alone is a very valuable tool in the diagnosis and management of OSA.

Limited sleep studies (respiratory PSG) are the usual routine investigation. Different units have expertise in interpreting different sorts of sleep studies. Experience is more important than the particular sleep study equipment used. Any system should assess the degree of sleep fragmentation and the degree of upper airway narrowing: this can be done using many different direct and indirect techniques.

Management

Not all patients need treatment. The evidence for significant treatment benefits rests on *symptoms*, which drive treatment, rather than the degree of OSA on a sleep study. Treatment decisions require a close dialogue between physician and patient.

Key features in making a treatment choice

- How sleepy is the patient? Does it affect quality of life? Is it critical to the patient's livelihood (e.g. HGV driving)? Are they motivated to do anything about it?
- Has the patient underestimated the impact of their sleepiness or misled the doctor because of concerns over driving issues?
- Is there any evidence of the 'overlap' syndrome, where additional lower airways obstruction has contributed to pushing the patient into type II ventilatory failure? If so, is this a stable state or part of an acute decline with a respiratory acidosis?
- Is obesity the dominant risk factor or is there a surgically remediable component (e.g. tonsillar hypertrophy)?

There is no RCT evidence that CVD, nocturnal angina, or poorly controlled hypertension should influence the decision to treat. Many, however, would lower the treatment threshold. There is some evidence that treating OSA when there is left heart failure improves ejection fraction and possibly survival.

Simple approaches

- Weight loss. This is difficult; slimming clubs have the best record for non-surgical approaches
- Reduce evening alcohol consumption
- Sleep decubitus, rather than supine, and with the bedhead elevated

For snorers and mild OSA

- Mandibular advancement devices, assuming adequate dentition
- Pharyngeal surgery as a last resort (poor RCT data and what there is suggests poor outcomes)

For significant OSA

- Nasal continuous positive airway pressure therapy (CPAP)
- Bariatric surgery (e.g. gastroplasty or gastric bypass operations)
- Tracheostomy (rarely indicated)
- Mandibular/maxillary advancement surgery in highly selected cases

Severe OSA with CO_2 retention

- May require a period of non-invasive positive pressure ventilation (NIPPV) prior to CPAP if acidotic
- Compensated CO_2 retention may reverse with CPAP alone

If there are large tonsils then their removal may be appropriate, although this seems to be much more successful in children than in adults. In reality pharyngeal surgery is a poor option for either snoring or OSA; what little evidence there is suggests that the outcomes are little better than placebo. There is no place for alerting agents (such as modafinil) in the routine management of sleepiness in OSA. It is unclear if these drugs help; they may reduce the perception of sleepiness more than the sleepiness itself, and have only been studied in the residual sleepiness sometimes found in patients, even when treated successfully with nasal CPAP.

Mandibular advancement devices

- Worn in the mouth at night, holding the lower jaw forward: similar to 'jaw thrust' in an unconscious patient
- Many designs, but essentially one half clips to the upper teeth and the other half to the lower, and connected together with the lower jaw misaligned forward by 5–10 mm
- Some give adjustable forward displacement; some are fixed
- They need to be customized to match the patient's dentition, which usually requires the services of a dentist
- DIY devices exist that are heated and moulded to the teeth directly
- Control snoring and OSA at the milder end of the spectrum
- Side-effects include tooth pain and jaw ache, which often lessen with time
- Long-term use may be associated with movement of the teeth and alterations to the bite
- The initial cost (usually over £300) is similar to that of a CPAP machine (£250) and they usually only last about a year.

OSA: nasal CPAP

Nasal CPAP consists of a blower/pressure generator that sits by the patient's bed and is connected to a mask by a length of large-bore tubing. The masks are usually just nasal, but nose and mouth masks are also used. The blower raises the pressure at which the patient is breathing (to about 10 cmH_2O) and splints open the pharynx, preventing its collapse, sleep fragmentation, and the consequent daytime sleepiness. *Nasal CPAP is a highly effective therapy with resolution of the sleepiness and large gains in quality of life*. It is a sufficiently curious and initially uncomfortable therapy to require a *careful induction programme*. Without this, the take-up and compliance rates are poor. Most centres have found that a dedicated CPAP nurse or technician is required. Many centres use special patient education aids, such as video presentations, and provide help lines manned by previous patients established on CPAP. The best method of establishing a patient on CPAP and deriving the required mask pressure is not known, and many different approaches appear to work. Recent innovations include CPAP machines that automatically hunt for the required pressure, and do not require a formal overnight titration with a technician present. New mask designs appear at regular intervals with a slow improvement in their comfort and fit (important to prevent air leaks). Patients require subsequent long-term follow-up to maintain their CPAP equipment and attend to problems.

The commonest problems encountered include:

- Mouth leaks lead to increased air through the nose and out of the mouth, with excessive drying of the mucosa, nasal congestion, rhinitis, and sneezing. Use either a chin support to close the mouth or the addition of a heated humidifier
- Pain and ulceration of the skin on the nasal bridge. Try different masks or patient 'interfaces'
- Claustrophobia. This usually settles but may require a different interface
- Temporary nasal congestion, usually during a cold. Try nasal decongestants for these short periods only, such as xylometazoline

Alternative diagnoses

Most patients who snore, are sleepy, and have an abnormal sleep study, will have ordinary obstructive sleep apnoea and respond to nasal CPAP. Sometimes, differentiating obstructive sleep apnoea from central apnoeas (p 582) can be difficult because some patients with Cheyne–Stokes breathing, for example, may have a few obstructed breaths at the end of each apnoeic cycle, even though the problem is primarily central. Poor response to CPAP should at least prompt a reappraisal of the diagnosis. Not all obstructive sleep apnoea is due to pharyngeal collapse; a very small number of patients have laryngeal closure. This can occur with:

- Shy–Drager syndrome (multisystem atrophy). This causes laryngeal abductor weakness with laryngeal closure during sleep, with stridulous obstruction rather than the usual noise of snoring
- Rheumatoid arthritis can damage the larynx with resultant OSA
- Arnold–Chiari malformation can compress the brainstem and interfere with the control of the larynx and pharynx, as well as the control of ventilation, with mixed findings on the sleep study
- These forms of obstruction also respond to nasal CPAP therapy as the larynx is also 'blown open' by raising airway pressure.

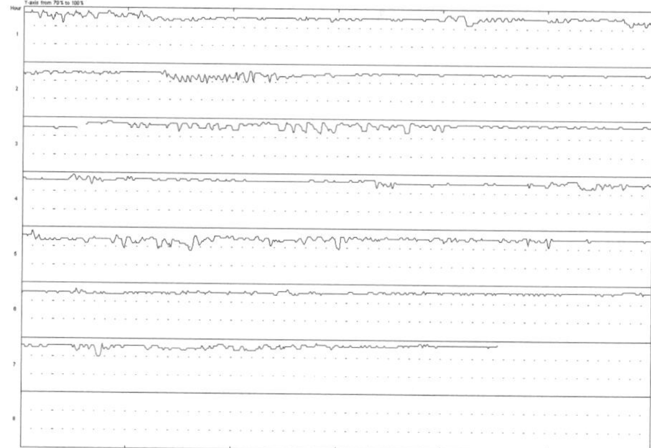

Fig. 47.3 Sleep onset periodic ventilation. Short bursts of dipping, otherwise normal.

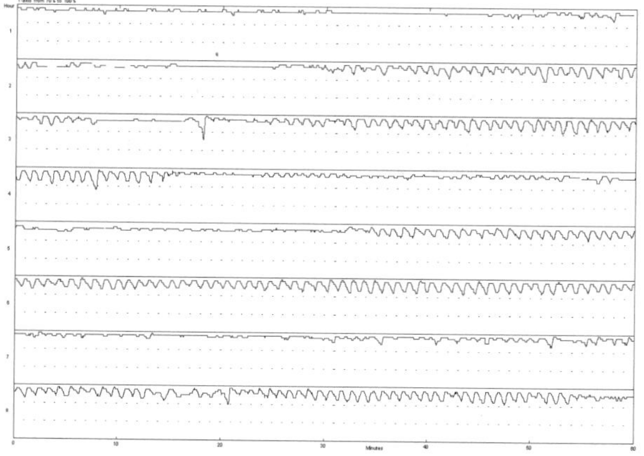

Fig. 47.4 Cheyne–Stokes ventilation. Prolonged periods of dipping, often sinusoidal rather than sawtooth.

OSA: driving advice to patients

In UK law one is responsible for one's vigilance levels while driving. We know when we are sleepy and should stop driving. Driving while sleepy has been likened to driving whilst drunk, and a prison sentence can result from sleep-related accidents on the road. No one should drive while they are sleepy, and the same applies to pathological causes of sleepiness.

Advice to all patients with OSA. Do not drive while sleepy; stop and have a nap. On diagnosis, patients with OSA *syndrome* (i.e. with daytime hypersomnolence) should notify the DVLA who will send them a questionnaire. If they admit to excessive daytime sleepiness their licence is revoked. If already treated and the sleepiness has resolved, then the licence is not revoked. It is the doctor's duty to tell the patient of the diagnosis of OSAS and of the requirement to inform the DVLA. Patients who are not sleepy and only have OSA on their sleep study do not have OSA *syndrome* (OSAS), and thus do not need to inform the DVLA. According to US epidemiological studies, 1/20 men have OSA on a sleep study, which would rather overwhelm the DVLA.

The doctor can advise the patient whether they should stop driving entirely (wise if the patient is very sleepy and/or drives a heavy goods vehicle or public service vehicle—class 2 licence holders), or to continue driving only with extreme caution for short distances. The advice given to the patient should be recorded in the notes.

Driving can be restarted as soon as the sleepiness has resolved and been confirmed by medical opinion, but in the case of class 2 licence holders the success of the treatment must be verified by a specialist clinic. This means a normal ESS and evidence of adequate nasal CPAP usage from the hour metres built into most nasal CPAP machines. A minimum usage has not been defined, but 3 h per night on average is often the arbitrary threshold used. Non-usage for even one night can lead to a return of sleepiness, so patients have to continue to act responsibly.

OSA in children

Adult respiratory physicians interested in sleep apnoea may be asked to investigate children with OSA due to poor sleep services for children.

- Mainly due to enlarged tonsils and adenoids; varying degrees of OSA are present in up to 4% of children around the age of five; prevalence tails off as tonsils atrophy
- These children present with snoring, restless sleep, and different daytime symptoms to those of adults. Obvious sleepiness is less common
- Sleep-deprived children tend to become hyperactive with reduced attention spans, and be labelled as difficult or disruptive
- Symptoms will fluctuate with the size of the tonsils and this depends on the presence of upper respiratory infections
- Mild intermittent sleep disturbance may not matter, but every-night sleep fragmentation for months interferes with development in a variety of ways
- The clinical decision is mainly whether to recommend removal of tonsils, or a wait and see policy, remembering that there is a significant morbidity from adenotonsillectomy, and even the occasional death
- A halfway house is the use of nasal steroids, which can reduce tonsillar size sufficiently to improve symptoms until natural tonsillar atrophy occurs.

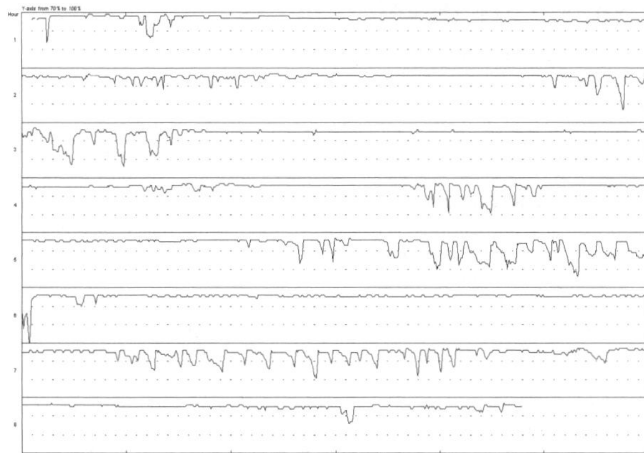

Fig. 47.5 REM sleep hypoventilation in scoliosis. Substantial dips, in bursts, compatible with the occurrence of REM periods.

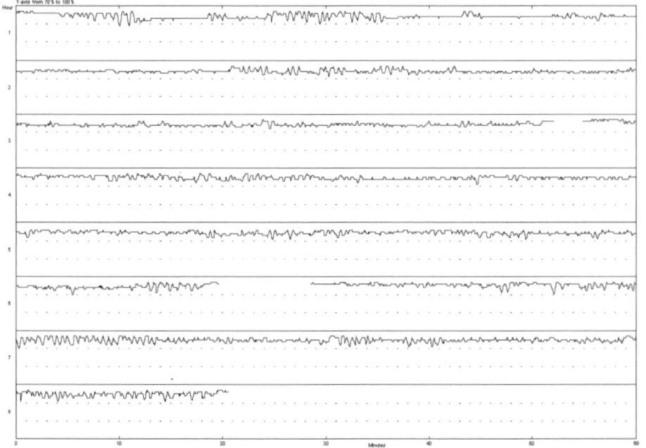

Fig. 47.6 Moderate OSA with many <4% dips in SaO_2.

OSA: future developments

The old view that sleep apnoea requires polysomnography to diagnose is rapidly being replaced with a more pragmatic and evidence-based approach using simpler equipment. Simpler ways to establish patients on CPAP are also evolving that will bring down costs further. Obesity surgery is improving and in appropriate cases may become the treatment of choice. Appetite suppressants are being developed that will greatly reduce the prevalence of obesity and hence OSA. Pharmacological agents are being tried that attempt to prevent the loss of tone in the pharyngeal dilators during sleep, mainly serotonergic agents, although progress in this area is slow (e.g. mirtazapine reduces OSA, but unfortunately causes sedation and weight gain!). New pharyngeal operations are being devised all the time, but none have been very effective when investigated properly: randomized controlled trials with objective outcome data are badly needed in this area.

Whether OSA is truly an independent risk factor for vascular disease (e.g. MI, strokes etc.) is hotly debated. Cross-sectional and non-randomized data suggest so. However, it is difficult to adequately control for confounding variables, such as visceral obesity, and non-randomized studies carry important bias. RCTs show small benefits to BP of treating OSA with CPAP.

Further information

Malhotra A, White DP. Obstructive sleep apnoea. *Lancet* 2002; **360**: 237–45.

Robinson GV *et al.* OSA/H syndrome and hypertension. *Thorax* 2004; **59**: 1089–94.

Sleep Apnoea Trust, Patients association, www.sleep-apnoea-trust.org.

SIGN/BTS guidelines (2003), http://www.sign.ac.uk/pdf/sign73.pdf.

NICE technology appraisal of CPAP for OSA, www.nice.org.uk/guidance/index.jsp?action=download&0=38198

Cochrane database on CPAP. Continuous positive airways pressure for obstructive sleep apnoea in adults. http://www.cochrane.org/reviews/en/ab001106.html.

Interventions to improve compliance with continuous positive airway pressure for obstructive sleep apnoea. http://www.cochrane.org/reviews/en/ab003531.html.

American commercial website showing all the CPAP equipment, www.cpapman.com

Main American Sleep Information website, www.sleephomepages.org.

American website with patient information on a variety of sleep disorders (simple), www.nlm.nih.gov/medlineplus/tutorials/sleepdisorders/nr249101.html.

Source of DIY dental device www.oscimedsa.com.

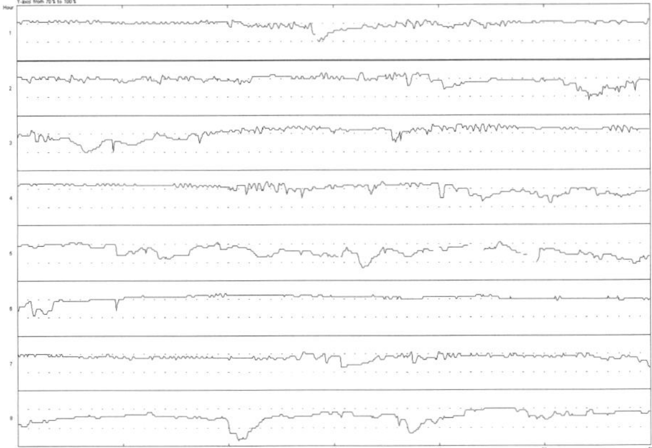

Fig. 47.7 Nocturnal hypoxia in COPD. Low baseline SaO_2, with more dramatic falls (often quite prolonged) during periods compatible with the occurrence of REM.

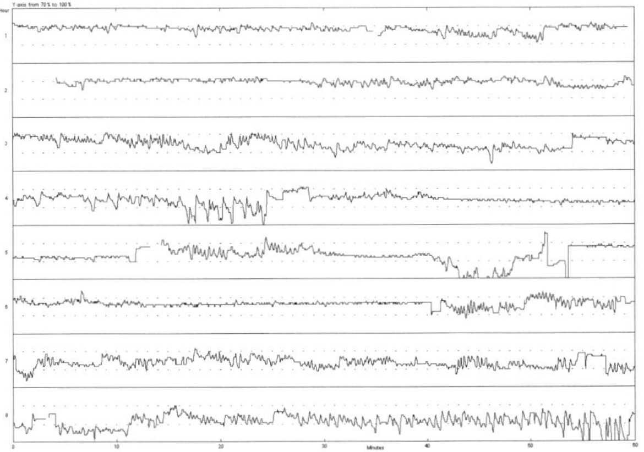

Fig. 47.8 Overlap syndrome—OSA and COPD. Low baseline SaO_2. Some periods with typical sawtooth dipping; other periods with prolonged falls in SaO_2.

Central sleep apnoea (CSA) and nocturnal hypoventilation

Definition and epidemiology 'Central sleep apnoea/hypopnoea', or 'hypoventilation', or 'periodic breathing' are said to occur when there is no evidence of upper airway obstruction as the cause for the reduced ventilation during sleep. Compared with OSA it is much less common.

- ***Central sleep apnoea*** tends to be used as a term when there are actual apnoeas, and referred to as Cheyne–Stokes breathing when there is regular symmetrical waxing and waning, usually in the context of left heart failure
- ***Periodic breathing*** is an alternative and can be used to describe regular fluctuations in breathing, with or without actual apnoeas
- The description ***nocturnal hypoventilation*** tends to be used when the hypoventilation and hypoxaemic dips are not particularly periodic in nature. However, these terms are imprecise and sometimes mixed indiscriminately.

Pathophysiology

Central sleep apnoea, or hypoventilation, or periodic breathing, can occur in a number of settings with different aetiologies (see also Chapter 15, p 92). At one end of a spectrum is pure loss of ventilatory drive, while at the other is pure loss of the ability to expand the chest adequately, with dependence on accessory muscles of respiration. Many clinical presentations are mixtures of these two.

Patients with ***reduced ventilatory drive*** (e.g. following brainstem damage) can often maintain adequate, or near adequate, ventilation whilst awake as there is a non-metabolic 'awake' ventilatory drive equivalent to about 4 or 5 L/min. During non-REM sleep, this awake drive is lost and ventilation becomes dependent on PaO_2 and $PaCO_2$. During REM sleep, an 'awake-like' drive sometimes returns partially and ventilation can improve again (seen in congenital forms of absent drive where REM sleep can temporarily restore SaO_2 levels).

In patients with ***impaired mechanical ability to ventilate***, accessory muscles of respiration become critically supportive (e.g. in many neuromuscular disorders and obstructive/restrictive respiratory conditions). However, during non-REM sleep, this reflex recruitment of accessory muscles is attenuated and hypoventilation follows. During REM sleep the physiological paralysis of all postural muscles (REM atonia) can remove all compensatory mechanisms, leaving only the diaphragm working, and produce profound hypoventilation or apnoea.

Chronic hypoventilation, often secondary to poor respiratory function (e.g. as evidenced by CO_2 retention in some patients with COPD or chest wall restrictive disorders) can eventually force resetting of ventilatory control mechanisms. This is an acquired blunting of ventilatory drive and leads to sleep-related changes in ventilation, similar to those described in the paragraphs above.

Unstable ventilatory control can lead to regular oscillations in ventilation, e.g. as occurs in heart failure and at altitude. During REM sleep it is normal to have fluctuations in ventilation, sometimes with complete apnoeas.

Sometimes sleep studies can be misinterpreted and apnoeas, really of obstructive origin, are mistakenly labelled as central. For example, if inspiratory muscles are very weak, their poor efforts during obstructive apnoeas may be missed.

Causes and clinical features of CSA/ hypoventilation 1

Although there are many different causes, only four relatively common clinical scenarios occur (but with overlap).

1. Absent or reduced ventilatory drive

Brainstem involvement from strokes, tumours, syringobulbia, surgical damage, post-polio syndrome, congenital (Ondine's curse—usually presents soon after birth, can be later, abnormalities of neural crest development due to increased number of 'alanine repeats' in one of the homeobox genes—PHOX2B). Presents clinically with unexplained ventilatory failure, much worse during sleep when the 'awake' drive is lost.

May be recognized early, cyanosis, morning confusion, ankle oedema.

May be recognized late, loss of consciousness and an emergency admission to ITU for ventilation.

Lung function is often normal, with no evidence of respiratory muscle weakness, indicating normal innervation from the voluntary motor system. Arnold–Chiari malformation with brainstem compression can present like this, but there is usually involvement of surrounding structures such as the lower cranial motor nuclei supplying the larynx and pharynx (with associated obstructive sleep apnoea, p 570).

These patients will have no apparent neuromuscular or respiratory cause for their hypoventilation, but may have a previous history of brainstem stroke (or other form of brain damage). The congenital form presents shortly after birth when the amount of REM sleep reduces and is replaced by non-REM.

Post-polio syndrome is:

- Ill defined syndrome—decline in function, decades after initial illness
- Return of weakness in previously affected areas (mechanism unclear)
- Late development of ventilatory failure is more likely if:
  - Inspiratory muscles were affected in the original illness
  - Additional scoliosis due to paravertebral muscle involvement (in which case vital capacity will be reduced)

This may be due to premature ageing of the upper and lower motor neurons due to their 'over-use'. This could follow the original destruction of some of the anterior horn cells to the inspiratory muscles, and the subsequent reinnervation by surviving neurons which then have to continuously supply more neurons than they were 'designed' for.

2. Weak or mechanically disadvantaged inspiratory muscles with/without secondary reduction of awake ventilatory drive

Neuromuscular inspiratory muscle weakness will produce diurnal ventilatory failure in its own right, particularly when the supine vital capacity falls below 20% predicted (approximately 1 L).

With increasing inspiratory muscle weakness, other accessory inspiratory muscles are recruited to maintain ventilation. When this is lost during non-REM sleep, and more so during REM sleep, ventilation will fall much more than in normal subjects. Whilst metabolic ventilatory drive is reasonably preserved, this will result in recurrent arousals to 'rescue' the ventilation and consequent marked sleep disturbance.

As ventilatory drive becomes progressively blunted, following the hypoventilation forced on the system by weak muscles, extra sleep hypoventilation (from loss of 'awake' drive) is tolerated and profound hypoxaemia is observed until there is finally an arousal that recovers the ventilation and SaO_2.

The above patients should have a history of a progressive neuromuscular disorder.

Chest wall restrictive diseases, such as scoliosis or post-thoracoplasty patients (p 579), can behave in a similar way with gradual onset of ventilatory failure, particularly when vital capacity <1 L. The muscles are not weak, but operating at severe mechanical disadvantage.

The same situation occurs in *COPD*, when muscles are overloaded and accessory muscles provide important support, but this too is reduced with non-REM sleep and lost during REM sleep. Again, any secondary reduction in ventilatory drive amplifies the sleep-related falls in SaO_2.

- Chest wall restrictive patients should have an obvious restrictive disorder with reduced VC to 1 L or below
- Increasing degrees of COPD will produce increasing degrees of sleep hypoventilation (p 581)
- If the awake SaO_2 is already low the sleep-related falls in ventilation will produce dramatic dips in SaO_2
- COPD and OSA together (overlap syndrome, p 570) provoke profound nocturnal hypoxic dipping (p 581), and probably a more rapid progression to diurnal hypoventilation with CO_2 retention, due to extra blunting of ventilatory drive (see p 570).

The diaphragm is the only respiratory muscle working during REM sleep, as all other postural muscles are profoundly hypotonic

- If the diaphragm is paralysed, then REM sleep is a particularly vulnerable time as there are no muscles of ventilation left working, producing particularly profound falls in SaO_2 during this period
- Patients with bilateral diaphragm weakness can present early with no obvious weakness elsewhere. Diaphragm weakness is best detected with the patient supine. Inspiration, particularly on sniffing, will provoke a paradoxical indrawing of the abdominal wall. The vital capacity will also fall on lying down, increasingly with greater degrees of paralysis (often a >30% fall in VC with complete paralysis).

In a progressive neuromuscular disorder, such as motor neuron disease, the above patterns will be variable between individuals, but will gradually worsen. Predominant diaphragm weakness, as occurs sometimes in motor neuron disease, spinal muscular atrophy, and particularly acid maltase deficiency, can lead to ventilatory failure at a time when the patient is still ambulant.

Causes and clinical features of CSA/ hypoventilation 2

3. Cheyne–Stokes breathing associated with LVF (p 575)

The raised left atrial pressure in left heart failure increases ventilatory drive through stimulation of J receptors. This is in addition to ventilatory stimulation due to any hypoxaemia from pulmonary oedema.

- This ventilatory stimulation lowers the awake $PaCO_2$ producing a respiratory alkalosis
- In addition the use of diuretics may produce a mild metabolic alkalosis,. especially if there is hypokalaemia
- This extra J receptor ventilatory stimulation appears to reduce at sleep onset. This, together with the loss of the awake ventilatory drive, allows central hypoventilation or apnoea to occur
- This hypoventilation or apnoea will continue until the $PaCO_2$ builds up to drive ventilation again, or until the attendant hypoxaemia causes arousal
- The return of ventilation itself may provoke arousal too. The arousal itself then injects increased ventilatory drive, reducing the $PaCO_2$ again
- Sleep returns, and once again the low $PaCO_2$ and alkalosis cause hypoventilation or apnoea

Thus a cycle is maintained that involves a fluctuating sleep state with arousals, and usually a fluctuating SaO_2. As with OSA, the patient may be completely unaware of these arousals. The delayed circulatory time of left heart failure may compound this instability by introducing a time delay between any change in $PaCO_2$ in the blood leaving the lungs and its arrival at the carotid body or central chemoreceptors.

4. Cheyne–Stokes breathing associated with altitude

The acute hypoxia following ascent to altitude provokes increased ventilation. The degree is variable between individuals and hence the degree of hypocapnia and respiratory alkalosis varies (see p 238). With sleep onset, with a lessening of the hypoxic drive, and removal of the awake drive, an uncompensated alkalosis will allow hypoventilation and even apnoea—similar to the situation described above for Cheyne–Stokes breathing. Again, ventilation will restart either when the $PaCO_2$ rises to a critical level, or the hypoxia provokes arousal. Sleep is fragmented with complaints of insomnia, but the cause of this is rarely recognized by the sufferer.

Skiing in Colorado, altitude 2400–3400 m (~10,000 f), is high enough to provoke significant periodic breathing in about a fifth of individuals. It seems that this fifth are the ones with the highest hypoxic ventilatory response. This gives them the largest respiratory alkalosis and hence the greatest tendency to sleep onset hypoventilation. In addition the tendency to arouse with the resultant extra hypoxaemia may be greater too, thus provoking large increases in ventilation on arousal and greater sleep disturbance. As the kidney excretes extra bicarbonate and produces a compensatory metabolic acidosis over a few days, the periodic breathing lessens.

Two pharmacological approaches have been taken to reduce this sleep-related periodic breathing.

- Pre-acclimatization with acetazolamide prior to ascent. This produces a mild metabolic acidosis and maintains the ventilatory drive at sleep onset, thus blocking the hypoventilation. Randomized controlled trials show the efficacy of this approach with doses between 250 and 500 mg/day, 1–3 days prior to ascent
- Hypnotics, such as temazepam, can reduce the degree of periodic breathing by reducing the tendency to arousal with each return of ventilation, and thus damping the system. Randomized trials suggest benefit for the early part of the night, with no impairment of nocturnal hypoxaemia or daytime functioning.

See also pp 238–39 (altitude sickness).

CSA/hypoventilation: investigations

Simple pulmonary function tests will characterize weakness of inspiratory muscles. Supine vital capacity is the best predictor of ventilatory failure as it incorporates diaphragm weakness that is masked during erect testing. Blood gases will reveal actual diurnal type II ventilatory failure and, if the base excess is raised with a normal $PaCO_2$ (therefore, a mild metabolic alkalosis), then this may indicate nocturnal hypoventilation and incipient ventilatory failure.

Sleep study

Examples on p 575, 579, 581.

Sleep studies in patients with suspected nocturnal hypoventilation or central sleep apnoea are required to confirm the diagnosis and to assess the degree of nocturnal hypoxaemia. Limited sleep studies will reveal falls in SaO_2 in association with hypoventilation, but no evidence of obstruction and, in particular, no snoring. Oximetry tracings alone will show a variety of patterns, often resembling OSA. The pattern in neuromuscular weakness will vary from oscillations all the time (due to recurrent arousal) to just REM sleep-related dips in SaO_2. The same will be true for chest wall restrictive disorders and COPD with only REM dips occurring initially, and more extensive hypoxaemia developing once there is an element of CO_2 retention and diurnal hypoxaemia.

- In OSA there is a slow fall in SaO_2 as oxygen is gradually removed from the lung stores, followed by a rapid rise engendered by the first deep inspiration as the apnoea breaks (so-called saw tooth pattern), p 571
- In Cheyne–Stokes of left heart failure the oscillations in SaO_2 are often more sinusoidal than in OSA as the pattern of breathing is usually more a symmetrical waxing and waning of ventilation, p 575. However, if each central apnoea is terminated by an arousal, rather than a smooth return of ventilation, then the pattern will look more like OSA.

In COPD, the degree of hypoxaemia on the sleep study will depend very much on the awake SaO_2. Because of the shape of the haemoglobin dissociation curve, a low awake SaO_2 makes it easier for the SaO_2 to fall further with a given reduction in ventilation. Thus during non-REM, with removal of awake drive, there will be a fairly stable reduction in SaO_2, but during REM sleep there will be further more dramatic dips. It is important not to diagnose OSA from just an oximetry tracing on the basis of SaO_2 oscillations in the presence of a low baseline SaO_2 and COPD. In this situation a fuller sleep study is required to provide evidence of additional upper airway obstruction. The combination of hypoxic COPD and OSA can produce particularly dramatic traces (p 581).

Management Intervention in central sleep apnoea or hypoventilation or periodic breathing, depends on symptoms. ***Better control of heart failure*** may improve Cheyne–Stokes breathing, but often does not. Further treatment will be required for two reasons: either to prevent the cyclical breathing and restore sleep quality, or to globally improve ventilation overnight and reset the respiratory control mechanisms such that the daytime respiratory failure reverses.

In situations where the hypoxia is playing a part in the pathogenesis (e.g. heart failure) then ***raising FiO2*** can help. There is limited literature on other forms of treatment for the Cheyne–Stokes of heart failure, although ***acetazolamide*** and ***benzodiazepines*** have been tried. The unstable breathing in heart failure has been treated with ***CPAP***, **however a large RCT has not confirmed long-term benefit.** More recently, treatment has been tried with specially designed ***servo ventilators,*** but whether these will provide better relief of symptoms than oxygen is not yet clear, but preliminary evidence suggests they might. There is some data to suggest that the recurrent arousal in Cheynes–Stokes may raise catecholamine levels and provoke deterioration of left ventricular function. Thus, measures to reduce the arousals may improve cardiac function as well as improve daytime vigilance.

Sedatives are contraindicated with a raised $PaCO_2$, and extra oxygen may increase the hypercapnia. In these situations, then ***overnight non-invasive ventilation***, via either nose or face mask, may be appropriate. In slowly progressive neuromuscular disorders, with either sleep fragmentation or diurnal type II respiratory failure (or both), the symptomatic and physiological response can be dramatic. The use of non-invasive ventilation in more rapidly progressive disorders is fraught with potential difficulties and is very much a specialist decision. Increasing dependence on equipment, not designed to be immediately life-sustaining, being a particular issue. In scoliosis there is rarely any question that treatment might not be appropriate, and again responses are dramatic.

Future developments

- Treatment of LVF (acute and chronic, no evidence yet for the latter) with overnight CPAP or non-invasive ventilation
- Introduction of overnight ventilation earlier in the course of a progressive neuromuscular disorder (such as motor neurone disease) to reduce symptoms and possibly prolong life
- Use of overnight ventilation on patients with stable COPD and hypercapnia. This may reduce exacerbations, hospital admissions, and prolong life. The evidence is inadequate yet to justify its wide use in this patient group.

Further information

Lanfranchi PA, Somers VK. Sleep-disordered breathing in heart failure: characteristics and implications. *Respir Physiol Neurobiol*. 2003; **136**: 153–65.

Wuyam B *et al.* Pathophysiology of central sleep apnea syndrome. *Sleep*. 2000; **23**(suppl. 4): S213–9.

Berry-Kravis EM *et al.* Congenital central hypoventilation syndrome. *Am J Respir Dis Crit Care Med* 2006; **174**: 1139–44.

Gray A etal. Noninvasive ventilation in acute cardiogenic pulmonary edema. NEJM 2008; 359:142–51.

BTS sleep training CD. Modular PowerPoint presentations on sleep and its disorders. Available from the BTS, +44 (0)2078318778

Obesity-related respiratory problems

Levels of obesity (BMI>30) are rising in all 'civilized' societies. In 1993, 13% of men and 17% of women in the UK (21% and 26% in the USA) had a BMI >30. In 2000 this was 21% and 22% in the UK (29% and 36% in the USA). This also has had many impacts on health care outside of respiratory medicine, particularly the components of the metabolic syndrome.

Obesity, particularly in conjunction with OSA and COPD, provokes ventilatory failure and cor pulmonale (see p 93). A common clinical scenario is the obese smoker, with a history of snoring and sleepiness, arriving in A&E with hypercapnia.

In addition to apportioning the relative contribution of obesity, COPD, and OSA to the hypercapnia, and treating accordingly, there are other obesity-related factors to consider:-

- **Intubation** The best predictor of a problematic intubation are neck circumference and a Mallampati score of 3 or more
- Tracheostomy tubes are often too short and too curved to cope with the increased distance between skin and trachea; tubes with adjustable flanges that allow customized intra tracheal lengths are useful here
- Percutaneous dilatational tracheostomy is more difficult and may have a higher complication rate
- Low FRCs mean that the oxygen stores are limited, leading to rapid falls in SaO_2 during apnoeas of any cause
- Abdominal loading of the diaphragm is increased, but the extra work of breathing can be reduced considerably by tilting the whole bed, head up, by as much as 20–30°.
- Abdominal loading of the diaphragm reduces basal lung expansion. Resultant basal atelectasis increases the A–a gradient. Raising the end-expiratory pressure during either invasive or non-invasive ventilation improves this
- Abdominal loading may increase perioperative risk of aspiration
- DVTs and pulmonary emboli are probably more common in the obese. It is not clear if DVT prophylaxis regimes need to be modified. Some recommend higher doses of low molecular weight heparin (LMWH), and this higher dose is more effective in patients undergoing bariatric surgery. Weight-based regimes of LMWH for the treatment of DVT and emboli appear satisfactory in the morbidly obese (BMI>40).
- Increased likelihood of failure to wean: non-invasive ventilation (inspiratory pressure 12, expiratory 4 cmH_2O) has been shown to aid weaning, post-open gastric-bypass surgery for obesity.
- Possible build-up of sedating anaesthetic agents in fat leading to prolonged half-life.

Further information

El-Solh AA. Clinical approach to the critically ill, morbidly obese patient. *Am J Respir Crit Care Med.* 2004; **169**: 557–61.

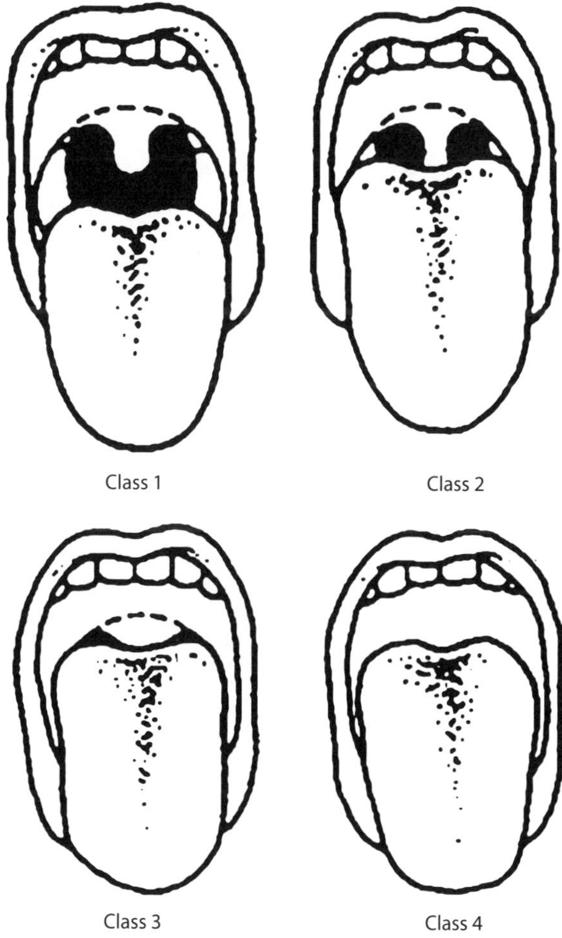

Fig. 47.9 Mallampati index. Simple scoring system for pharyngeal crowding. Affected by cranio-facial shape, tongue size, and obesity. Predicts difficulty of intubation and correlates with OSA severity. Reproduced with kind permission from Update in Anaesthesia; Issue 13, 2001.

Chapter 48

Toxic agents

Drug-induced lung disease: clinical presentations

Introduction A vast number of drugs can damage the respiratory system, from nose to alveoli. The most complete and useful list (plus references) is kept at **www.pneumotox.com** and can be queried by either drug (or drug type) or clinical/radiological presentation: all agents have equal prominence, but are coded with a star rating to indicate likely prevalence. This chapter describes the commoner drugs that produce respiratory problems.

Commoner presentations of drug-induced lung disease and examples of causative agents

- Interstitial lung disease, pneumonitis, fibrosis
  - Acute hypersensitivity pneumonitis (nitrofurantoin, methotrexate)
  - Interstitial pneumonitis ± eosinophilia (amiodarone, ACE inhibitors, sulfasalazine)
  - Chronic organizing pneumonia (amiodarone, bleomycin)
  - Pulmonary fibrosis (bleomycin, amiodarone, nitrofurantoin, β blockers)
- Airways disease
  - Bronchospasm (β blockers, contrast media)
  - Obliterative bronchiolitis (busulphan, penicillamine)
  - Cough (ACE inhibitors)
- Pleural changes
  - Pleural effusion/thickening (β blockers, nitrofurantoin, methotrexate, dopamine agonists)
  - Pneumothorax (bleomycin)
- Vascular changes
  - Thromboembolic disease (phenytoin)
  - Pulmonary hypertension (dexfenfluramine, other appetite suppressants)
  - Vasculitis (nitrofurantoin, L-tryptophan)
- Mediastinal changes
  - Node enlargement (bleomycin, phenytoin)
  - Sclerosing mediastinitis (ergot)
- Pulmonary oedema (methotrexate, contrast media)
- Pulmonary haemorrhage (methotrexate, nitrofurantoin, penicillamine, contrast media).

Drug-induced lung disease: examples 1

Amiodarone Iodinated benzofuran used to suppress supra- and ventricular tachycardias. Lung toxicity correlates loosely with total dose and therefore usually occurs after a variable number of months. Seen in 10% of subjects on >400 mg/day. Rare if <300 mg/day.

Risk factors

- Daily dose >400 mg
- Increasing age of patient
- Use for more than 2 months
- Pre-existing lung disease (although not a contraindication to its use)
- Recent surgical intervention or lung infection.

Diagnosis is usually one of exclusion, and response to cessation of drug (which can take months). Infiltrative lung disease varying from acute respiratory distress (rare) through to COP (cough, pleuritic pain, fever, dyspnoea, asymmetric patchy infiltrates, effusion), and the most indolent, chronic interstitial pneumonitis (cough, dyspnoea, weight loss, diffuse and/or focal opacities).

On ***CT*** the liver, thyroid, and lungs will usually show increased attenuation, indicating a significant amiodarone load. A baseline CXR is useful.

Lung biopsies exclude other diagnoses and provide compatible findings, but there is dissent as to how diagnostic they are (except for the finding of foamy macrophages in the airspaces, filled with amiodarone–phospholipid complexes, but may occur in absence of lung toxicity). Mechanisms of toxicity are unclear, and there are features to suggest hypersensitivity and direct toxic damage.

Treatment Steroids are effective and required in severe disease. The half-life of amiodarone in the tissues is in excess of a month and response to stopping the drug may be slow. Prognosis is good in the majority.

Anti-TNF agents (infliximab and etanercept) represent a large step forward in the treatment of rheumatoid arthritis and Crohn's disease. However, there is a small but important risk of reactivating TB, commonly extrapulmonary - see p 512. Pneumonia and development of antibodies are also more common; SLE develops only rarely.

Azathioprine Extensively used as an immunosuppressant but has remarkably little pulmonary toxicity other than via opportunistic lung infection. Case reports of pneumonitis only.

Bleomycin DNA-damaging glycopeptide used in the treatment of lymphomas, germ cell tumours, squamous carcinomas (cervix, head, neck, and oesophagus). Pulmonary fibrosis occurs in about 10%.

Risk factors

- Older age
- Those receiving total dose of >300,000 international units (1000 international units [or 1 old/USB unit] = 1.5-2.0 mgs)
- Increased FiO_2, probably via increased superoxide/free radical formation. Pneumonitis may be precipitated by supplementary oxygen for some time after drug administration—warn anaesthetist if surgery

planned in patients who have received bleomycin in previous 6-12 months
- Pulmonary irradiation, not just in the irradiated field
- Renal failure decreases drug elimination and thus toxicity
- Associated use of cyclophosphamide.

Symptoms (cough, dyspnoea, chest pain, fever) develop 1–6 months after bleomycin. There is hypoxia and a restrictive defect. Progressive basal subpleural shadowing, small lungs, and blunting of costophrenic angles.
Histology shows a dominant subpleural distribution of damage and repair with fibrosis; this appearance is non-diagnostic and common to many drugs/disorders. Toxicity is probably due to DNA damage or oxidative injury, with interindividual variation occurring due to differing activity of the enzyme bleomycin hydrolase; only low levels of this enzyme exist in the lung (and skin). A rare acute hypersensitivity form comes on within days of administration. Other unusual presentations include pulmonary nodules or organizing pneumonia.

Treatment
- Bleomycin must be stopped on suspicion of damage, and some units use lung function tests (kCO) to detect early damage
- Steroids are used, but there is little evidence they alter long-term prognosis (in the acute hypersensitivity subgroup there is a clear beneficial effect)
- Use the minimum FiO_2 to maintain an adequate SaO_2 (85-90%)
- Over 50% may experience a relentless decline in lung function.

Busulphan DNA alkylating, myelosuppressive, agent mainly used to treat chronic myeloid leukaemia, and prior to bone marrow transplantation, with a low rate of lung toxicity (4–10%) due to fibrosis.

Risk factors
- Cumulative doses over 500 mg (mostly over 120 days)
- Concurrent administration of other alkylating agents
- Pulmonary irradiation.

Presents with cough and progressive SOB, often years after exposure (usually about 4). CXR is typically unremarkable. Reduced kCO and restrictive defect. Diagnosis is usually by exclusion. The place of steroids is unproven.

Chlorambucil DNA alkylating agent mainly used to treat chronic lymphocytic leukaemia, lymphomas, and ovarian cancer. It has additional immunosuppressive actions, and is also used in conditions such as rheumatoid arthritis. Low risk (1%) of pulmonary toxicity and confined to those who have received >2 grams. Similarly to busulphan, presentation may be many years later. Presents with cough, dyspnoea, weight loss, and basal crackles. CXR shows diffuse basal reticular shadowing. Non-specific histology. On suspicion, chlorambucil should be stopped; use of steroids is unproven. Prognosis is poor (50% fatal).

Drug-induced lung disease: examples 2

Cyclophosphamide DNA alkylating agent mainly used to treat chronic lymphocytic leukaemia, small cell lung cancer, and other solid tumours. Particularly useful as an immunosuppressive agent in certain vasculitides and nephropathies. Lung toxicity is rare.

Risk factors

- Pulmonary irradiation
- Oxygen therapy
- Concurrent drugs causing pulmonary toxicity, e.g. bleomycin.

Clinical presentation is usually within 6 months, with a short duration of fever, cough, and fatigue. Reticular shadowing with ground-glass appearance on CT. Later onset progressive pulmonary fibrosis can also develop insidiously in those on therapy for many months with progressive SOB and dry cough. The histology of the more acute type can be similar to any of the acute interstitial pneumonias (e.g. COP, diffuse alveolar damage), whereas the more chronic form is indistinguishable from UIP. Cyclophosphamide is not itself toxic to the lung, but its metabolites are. There appears to be genetic variation to susceptibility, as there is no obvious dose–response relationship. Cessation of drug and steroid therapy is used successfully in the acute form, but the chronic form seems to progress inexorably, in a similar manner to UIP. Lung transplantation is an option. Note increased risk of PCP whilst taking cyclophosphamide.

Gold Used in rheumatoid arthritis, >500 mg cumulative dose can produce pneumonitis (possibly COP, obliterative bronchiolitis) with cough, dyspnoea, and basal crackles. Rare (1%), but associated with certain HLA types and distinctive histological feature of alveolar septal inflammation. Good prognosis following drug cessation; poor evidence for steroids.

Methotrexate Folic acid derivative, inhibiting cell division by blocking dihydrofolate reductase and nucleic acid production. Mainly used in leukaemia and as an immunosuppressive, e.g. rheumatoid arthritis and psoriasis. Commonly (4–10%) causes a variety of lung pathologies, not associated with folic acid deficiency.

Risk factors

- Hypoalbuminaemia
- Diabetes
- Previous use of drugs that modify disease progress in rheumatoid
- Rheumatoid or other lung/pleural disease
- Not particularly dose-related; can occur at doses of <20 mg per week
- Daily rather than intermittent (weekly) therapy
- >60 years.

Presents both acutely (interstitial pneumonitis, fever, and eosinophilia) and over very long time periods; however, the subacute form (within a year, dyspnoea, fever, cough, hypoxia, basal crackles, restrictive defect, and reduced kCO) is commoner. Bilateral diffuse pulmonary infiltrates or mixed pattern with alveolar shadowing on CXR, occasional effusions.

Histology more useful than in other drug toxicities, shows alveolitis, interstitial pneumonitis, epithelial cell hyperplasia, eosinophilic infiltration, and granuloma formation in the more acute, hypersensitivity, form, and more UIP-like changes in indolent form. Mechanism of damage unknown but likely to be multifactorial.

Treatment consists of drug withdrawal and unproven use of steroids. Anecdotal reports support use of steroids in the more acute, hypersensitivity form. Other methotrexate-related lung diseases include opportunistic lung infection (including PCP) and non-Hodgkin's B-cell lymphoma, which may regress with drug withdrawal, and may be associated with Epstein–Barr virus.

Nitrofurantoin is used commonly for long-term prophylaxis against urinary tract infections (UTIs). Acutely nitrofurantoin causes a hypersensitivity vasculitis, and, much less frequently, a chronic interstitial fibrosis. Most patients are women due to their much higher prevalence of chronic UTIs. The acute form presents abruptly with fever, dyspnoea, dry cough, rash, chest pain, hypoxia, crackles, and eosinophilia within a week or two of starting, and is dose-independent. Lower zone diffuse patchy infiltrates and sometimes unilateral effusions on CXR. Lung biopsy reveals vasculitis, eosinophilia, reactive type II pneumocytes, focal haemorrhage, and some interstitial inflammation. Treatment consists of discontinuation and improvement begins rapidly. Prognosis is good with or without steroids.

Oxygen Prolonged 80–100% oxygen therapy can provoke lung damage.

Penicillamine Used in the treatment of rheumatoid arthritis, penicillamine may increase the prevalence of obliterative bronchiolitis. This is dose-related but rare, with a subacute onset (after several months) of dyspnoea and cough. There is a progressive obstructive pattern without bronchodilator response. 50% mortality.

Sulphasalazine Used extensively in treatment of inflammatory bowel disease (mainly ulcerative colitis). Rarely causes side effects but can cause new onset dyspnoea and pulmonary infiltrates after any period of use. Cough, fever, lung crackles and blood eosinophilia is the usual presentation. Prior allergy history, rash and weight loss also seen with eosinophilic pneumonia the usual pathology. Withdrawal of drugs is usually successful within weeks, and recovery can be hastened by steroids. Rare deaths when the histology is more like usual interstitial pneumonitis and may be more related to the condition requiring sulphasalazine.

Talc is commonly used for pleurodesis (p 776). Talc particles may be small enough to enter the circulation after intrapleural instillation, being found throughout the body at post mortem. They appear to provoke a systemic reaction with fever, raised inflammatory markers, and hypoxia suggestive of an ARDS-like pathology. Occasional deaths after talc pleurodesis have been reported. Refined talc with fewer smaller particles seems less toxic.

Paraquat poisoning

Definitions

Paraquat (Weedol®, Pathclear®, Gramoxone®) and related bipyridyl compounds are used as contact herbicides. They kill plants by inhibiting NADP reduction during photosynthesis, which involves the production of superoxide radicals. The toxicity of paraquat in animals is also believed to be due to the production of damaging superoxides. Most cases of poisoning are deliberate, and the treatment should be commenced as soon as possible. Serious poisoning is usually by ingestion (although paraquat is absorbed through the skin and mucous membranes, including the conjunctiva and bronchial mucosa).

- More than 6 g is always fatal
- Less than 1.5 g is rarely fatal
- Between 1.5 and 6 g, the mortality is 60–70%
- A mouthful of 20% Gramoxone® liquid (10 g/50 mL) is almost certainly fatal
- Less than 1 sachet of Weedol® granules (1.4 g paraquat/57 g sachet) is unlikely to cause death
- Usually fatal if blood level >0.2 mg/mL at 24 h.

Clinical features

- Oral and oesophageal ulceration shortly after contact, with later formation of a pseudomembrane
- Renal failure (reversible) within a few days, but delayed excretion of paraquat prevents falls in blood levels
- Pulmonary oedema early on, evolving into 'acute respiratory distress syndrome'
- Death usually occurs within 1 to 2 weeks
- Pulmonary fibrosis if the patient survives, with varying degrees of recovery.

►► Management

- Gastric lavage with Fuller's earth/bentonite/activated charcoal/sodium resonium to reduce absorption
- Haemoperfusion (haemodialysis less effective) to reduce blood levels
- Lowest inspired oxygen tension possible (high concentrations probably increase superoxide formation)
- Supportive measures which may require intubation and ventilation
- Other treatments (e.g. immunosuppression, NO) are experimental.

Radiation-induced pulmonary disease

Manifestations of lung injury following radiotherapy include:

Radiation pneumonitis

- Often asymptomatic, although may cause dyspnoea and chronic ventilatory failure
- Radiographic abnormalities more common than clinical disease. Characteristically straight margins on CT infiltrate
- Pathological feature is of diffuse alveolar damage, with vascular intimal fibrosis
- Typically follows lung radiotherapy
- Treatment of symptomatic disease is with steroids (1mg/kg daily), although minimal evidence to support their use. Amifostine or pentoxifylline (used in the treatment of extrapulmonary manifestations of radiation-induced tissue damage) may be of benefit, although unproven.

Radiation-induced organizing pneumonia

- Often presents with cough (rather than breathlessness, which is more suggestive of radiation pneumonitis)
- Characterized by migratory patchy consolidation which always extends beyond radiation field on CT
- Typically follows breast radiotherapy
- Treatment is with steroids; often long courses are needed. Macrolides may have a role.

Radiation-induced chronic eosinophilic pneumonia

- Possible association; few cases reported.

Inhalational lung injury 1

Definition Agents damaging the lung and airways through direct toxicity. Much of the acute damage is common to many toxic agents including pneumonitis/pulmonary oedema, mucosal damage/sloughing/airway debris. Secondary infection is common due to breached defences.

►► Management of inhalational lung injury

- Following acute exposure, supportive therapy is critical
- Look for respiratory failure, stridor, or distress; may occur hours later
- CXR (poor sensitivity until pulmonary oedema develops)
- May need intubating/tracheostomy to bypass oedematous and sloughing upper airway mucosa
- Humidified oxygen:
  - Raise SaO_2 into low/mid 90s (higher levels may contribute to oxidative damage)
  - Raise PaO_2 as high as possible if CO poisoning suspected
- Treat cyanide poisoning if suspected (dicobalt edetate, little evidence)
- Bronchodilators
- Nebulized dilute heparin/acetylcysteine—variable opinions on value
- Steroids and prophylactic antibiotics—variable opinions on value
- Mechanical ventilation (low volume/pressure, permissive hypercapnia)
- Fluid replacement, but not excessive as encourages pulmonary oedema
- Enteral feeding.

Examples of toxic agents, listed alphabetically

Aldehydes (acetaldehyde, formaldehyde)
- Chemical and plastics industry, used for disinfection
- Highly irritant to mucosal membranes
- Acute damage
  - Pneumonitis and pulmonary oedema
- Chronic effects
  - Rhinitis/asthma

Ammonia
- Fertilizer and plastics production, used in many chemical industries
- Highly irritant to mucosal membranes
- Acute damage
  - Upper airway obstruction from secretions and mucosal oedema
  - Lung damage and secondary infection
- Chronic effects
  - Airways obstruction and bronchiectasis described

Chlorine
- Extensive use in the chemical industry, bleaching agent
- Acute damage
  - Overwhelming toxicity producing rapid hypoxia
  - Pneumonitis and pulmonary oedema
- Chronic effects (e.g. from repeated accidental exposure)
  - Airways obstruction; sometimes reversible

Cocaine (when smoked)
- Pneumothorax/pneumomediastinum
- Pulmonary haemorrhage
- Pulmonary oedema
- Allergic responses (asthma, pulmonary eosinophilia, hypersensitivity pneumonitis)

Metals and metal compounds (as fumes or nebulized solutions)
- Mainly used in the chemical industry
- Acute damage
  - Mucosal irritation
  - Pulmonary oedema
- Chronic effects
  - Pneumoconiosis
- Some specific effects such as:
  - Sarcoid-like reaction to beryllium
  - Asthma/from cobalt, chromium, nickel, vanadium
  - Fibrosing alveolitis from cobalt and zinc fumes

Methyl isocyanate (Bhopal disaster: 3800 dead, 170 000 injured)
- Chemical industry, carbamate pesticides
- Acute damage
  - Pneumonitis and pulmonary oedema
  - Secondary infection
- Chronic effects
  - Airways obstruction
  - Bronchiolitis obliterans
  - Pulmonary fibrosis

Hydrocarbons/mineral oils
- Used as lubricant and cooling agent
- Acute damage
  - Pneumonitis
- Chronic effects
  - Pneumonitis
  - Fibrosis
  - Asthma

Nitrogen dioxide
- Chemical industry (explosives)
- Agricultural silos
- Odourless and therefore high doses inhaled without knowing
- Acute damage (several hours after exposure)
  - Silo fillers lung (pneumonitis/pulmonary oedema)
- Later effects
  - Secondary pulmonary oedema 2–8 weeks after exposure
  - Steroid responsive, needs 2 months therapy after exposure.

Inhalational lung injury 2

More examples of toxic agents

Ozone

- Bleaching agent
- Product of welding
- Similar to NO_2
- Both immediate and late effects of pneumonitis/pulmonary oedema

Phosgene

- Chemical warfare, chemical industry, chlorination
- Released from heated methylene chloride (paint stripper)
- Acute damage
  - Pneumonitis and pulmonary oedema
  - Produces COHb; breath CO therefore reflects degree of exposure

Smoke

- Most smoke injury is due to heat damage to upper airway
- Hypoxia, vaporized toxins (e.g. formaldehyde, chlorine), systemic agents (e.g. CO and cyanide)
- Acute damage
  - Mucosal oedema and sloughing with airway blockage
- Look out for:
  - Peri-oral burns
  - Black sputum
  - Altered voice
  - Respiratory distress
  - Stridor (rapid inspiration to accentuate)
  - Additional CO and/or cyanide poisoning

Sulphur dioxide

- Used as a fumigant, and bleaching agent in the paper industry
- Very irritant as dissolves to form sulphuric acid
- Acute damage
  - Sloughing of airway mucosa
  - Pneumonitis and haemorrhagic pulmonary oedema
- Chronic effects
  - Airways obstruction

Welding fumes

- Many agents released
- Specific examples:
  - Cadmium—pneumonitis
  - Zinc—'metal fume fever'
  - Several agents may cause airways obstruction/COPD
- Siderosis (welders lung) non-fibrogenic pneumoconiosis
  - Iron deposits in lung producing small rounded opacities

Carbon monoxide poisoning

Definition and epidemiology

- Carbon monoxide is a colourless odourless gas formed when carbon compounds burn in limited oxygen
- It accounts for about 75 deaths per year in the UK, approximately 10% of which are accidental
- Accidental poisonings are commoner in the winter when faulty heating systems are in use
- Non-accidental deaths are mainly from car exhaust fumes
- Methylene chloride (industrial solvent, paint remover) is converted to CO in the liver and may present as CO poisoning
- Up to one-third die following acute high level exposure and another third may be left with permanent neurological sequelae
- Chronic low-grade CO exposure may present as non-specific ill health and may affect thousands of individuals.

Pathophysiology and related conditions

- Carbon monoxide competes avidly with O_2 (250 times greater) to bind with the iron in haemoglobin, making it less available for oxygen carriage
- The haemoglobin molecule is also distorted by combination with CO that makes it bind more tightly to O_2, shifting the O_2 dissociation curve to the left. The PaO_2 at which the haemoglobin is 50% saturated (P50) moves from about 3.5 to 2 kPa
- This further reduces oxygen delivery to the tissues: a 50% carboxyhaemoglobin level is far more dangerous than a 50% anaemia
- CO also binds to extravascular molecules such as myoglobin and some of the cytochrome chain proteins interfering with energy production, and in this respect is like cyanide
- Normal levels of carboxyhaemoglobin can be up to 3%, and up to 15% in heavy smokers
- Fetal haemoglobin combines even more avidly with CO; thus the fetus is especially vulnerable to CO poisoning of the mother.

Methaemoglobin

- Methaemoglobin is due to oxidation of Fe^{2+} to Fe^{3+} thus preventing O_2 carriage. This is due either to inherited deficiencies of enzymes (cytochrome b5 reductase) that reduce the Fe^{3+} back to Fe^{2+}, or toxic agents (e.g. nitrites (in 'poppers'), chloroquine) that overwhelm this reversal mechanism
- Methaemoglobin is slightly left shifted, but a 40% methaemoglobinaemia may be asymptomatic apart from the typical grey/blue colour of the patient, often mistaken for cyanosis.

Clinical features of CO poisoning

Immediate

- Nausea, headache, malaise, weakness, and unsteadiness
- Loss of consciousness, seizures, cardiac abnormalities (ischaemia, arrhythmias, pulmonary oedema)
- No cyanosis, healthy looking 'cherry red' colour
- Suspect if several members of household present with these features

Delayed (approximately 1 to 3 weeks, can be longer)

- Cognitive defects and personality changes
- Focal neurology and movement abnormalities

Investigations

- Pulse oximetry will appear ***normal*** due to COHb having similar absorption spectra to oxyhaemoglobin
- Arterial PaO_2 levels may be ***normal***
- COHb levels can be measured on a Co-oximeter
- Breath CO measured with devices used for smoking cessation work
- Routine tests to rule out other diagnoses.

►► Management of CO poisoning

- CO is only removed from the body through displacement by O_2; therefore use high concentrations of oxygen, e.g. via CPAP masks (p 732)
- Raise the PaO_2 as high as possible, intubate and 100% O_2 if necessary
- The half-life of COHb breathing air is about 6 h; breathing 100% O_2 it is about 1 h
- Hyperbaric O_2 more rapidly displaces CO and increases dissolved O_2. Reduces the frequency of delayed neurological symptoms from 46% to 25% following significant exposure in one randomized controlled trial, but needs to be instituted early. Still controversial, recent Cochrane report equivocal, and facilities poorly available.

Future developments Isocapnic hyperpnoea may further raise the PaO_2. Alkalosis must be avoided though, to prevent further left shift of the Hb dissociation curve. Can be done voluntarily with 5% CO_2 in O_2 or during intubation. Can double rate of CO elimination.

Further information

Blumenthal I. Carbon monoxide poisoning. *J R Soc Med* 2001; **94**: 270–2.

Cochrane review of hyperbaric oxygen, http://www.cochrane.org/reviews/en/ab002041.html

+44 (0)1752209999. Plymouth Diving Disease Research Centre, 24hr helpline and register of hyperbaric chambers.

Harper A, Croft-Baker J. Carbon monoxide poisoning: undetected by both patients and their doctors. *Age and Ageing* 2004; **33**: 105–9.

Kreck *et al.*, Isocapnic Hyperventilation Increases Carbon Monoxide Elimination and Oxygen Delivery. http://ajrccm.atsjournals.org/cgi/content/full/163/2/458

Chapter 49

Unusual conditions (BOLD)

British Orphan Lung Disease (BOLD) project

The British Orphan Lung Disease (BOLD) register was set up by the British Thoracic Society in 2001 to facilitate research into rare lung diseases and improve clinicians' knowledge of these conditions. It also aimed to help establish patient support groups.

In continental Europe there have been registers of rare lung diseases for many years. The term 'orphan' lung disease was coined because of the feeling that these diseases have, in the past, tended to be neglected because of their rarity, the limited knowledge of the conditions, and the limited available data on which to base practice.

The reporting system works via a web-based registration form, where consultants are encouraged to enter details of patients with any of the listed conditions. The data is anonymized, and the patient must sign a form (found on the BTS website at www.brit-thoracic.org.uk in the members only section) consenting for their details to be held on a central database. Interested parties are invited to submit research proposals, for which the collected data will be used.

The BOLD register collects data on:

- Alveolar proteinosis
- Churg–Strauss syndrome
- Ciliary dyskinesia
- Cryptogenic organizing pneumonia
- Langerhans' cell histiocytosis (histiocytosis X)
- Lymphangioleiomyomatosis
- Neurofibromatosis with lung disease
- Primary pulmonary hypertension
- Primary tracheal tumours
- Pulmonary arteriovenous malformations (including HHT)
- Tracheo/bronchial/pulmonary amyloidosis.

Rare lung disease patient support groups:

- Lymphangioleiomyomatosis Action—*www.lamaction.org*
- UK Histiocytosis Family Support Association—www.hrtrust.org
- Pulmonary Hypertension Association UK—www.pha-uk.com
- Churg–Strauss syndrome—*www.vasculitis-uk.org*
- Pulmonary Alveolar Proteinosis— www.papfoundation.org/ (USA)
- Primary Ciliary Dyskinesia Family Support Group—www.pcdsupport.org.uk/
- Alpha-1 antitrypsin deficiency—*www.alpha1.org.uk/*
- Amyloid—http://www.amyloidosis.org/whatisit.asp (USA)
- Hereditary Haemorrhagic Telangiectasia—www.telangiectasia.co.uk/

Alveolar microlithiasis

This is a rare interstitial lung disease of unknown aetiology, characterized by the accumulation of numerous and diffuse calcified microliths (calcium and phosphate hydroxyapatite bodies) in the alveolar space. There is no identifiable abnormality of calcium metabolism. Microliths are occasionally identified in the sputum. At post mortem the lungs are heavy and rock hard, often needing a saw to cut them. Fewer than 200 cases are reported.

Clinical features

- Typically presents in young adults, most commonly in the third and fourth decades of life
- May be an incidental CXR finding in asymptomatic patients
- Familial tendency—probable autosomal recessive inheritance
- Equal sex distribution in sporadic cases, 2:1 female preponderance in familial cases
- Usually slowly progressive, with progressive breathlessness, hypoxia, respiratory failure, and death
- CXR and chest CT show fine micronodular lung calcification, predominantly basally or around the hila. It may produce complete radiographic opacification. There is no associated lymph node enlargement. Progressive lung infiltration causes restriction of lung movement and impairs gas exchange, leading to progressive respiratory failure.

Treatment

- There is no effective medical treatment
- Lung transplantation has been successful.

Amyloidosis: pathophysiology and classification

Definition Amyloidosis is the extracellular deposition of low molecular weight protein molecules as insoluble fibrils. More than 20 such proteins have been described in different diseases and circumstances.

Pathophysiology The disease is one of abnormal protein folding, and is classified by the origin of the precursor proteins that form the amyloid. For example, AL amyloid forms from the light chains of immunoglobulins. In familial forms, genetic missense mutations produce abnormal folding of the protein. Little is known of the specific genetic and environmental factors that lead to the development of this abnormal folding. Despite their different origins, these protein molecules fold into alternative forms that are very similar to each other: in the classic 'β-pleated sheet' structure, fibrils form in an ordered fashion, with uniformity of fibril structure within the sheet. Substitutions of particular amino acids at specific positions in the light-chain variable region lead to destabilization of the light chains, increasing the chance of fibrillogenesis. In certain models, this abnormal folding can be initiated by the addition of 'amyloid enhancing factor', rather like the initiation of crystal formation in a supersaturated solution. Amyloid deposits accumulate in the extracellular space, disrupting normal tissue architecture and leading to organ dysfunction, both directly, and having space-occupying effects. The fibrils may be directly cytotoxic (possibly by promoting apoptosis). The subdivisions of amyloid are largely based on the origin of the amyloid protein and shown in the box opposite.

Epidemiology The epidemiology is difficult to define accurately as the disease is often un- or misdiagnosed. The age-adjusted incidence is estimated to be 5.1–12.8 per million person years.

Future developments Anti-amyloid drugs are under investigation, including drugs to stabilize the amyloid precursor proteins in their normal configuration and enhance fibril degradation.

Classification of amyloidosis

- Primary/light chain amyloid (AL), from immunoglobulin light chain fragments (λ or κ), usually monoclonal due to a plasma cell dyscrasia (a subtype of lymphoproliferative disorders)
  - 1 in 5000 deaths due to this type of amyloid
  - Median survival is 6–15 months
  - Frank myeloma is present in 20%, and a subtle monoclonal gammopathy in 70% (MGUS)
  - Systemic form due to circulating monoclonal light chains, widespread organ involvement, particularly heart, liver, and kidneys
  - Localized amyloid production by local clonal B cells; hence heterogeneous organ involvement is seen, commonly in the upper respiratory tract and orbit, with urogenital and gastrointestinal involvement—virtually any organ (except the brain) can be involved
- Secondary amyloid (AA)
  - A complication of chronic disease with ongoing/recurring inflammation, e.g. rheumatoid, chronic infections
  - The fibrils are fragments of acute phase reactant, serum amyloid A
  - Commonly renal, hepatic, and lower GI involvement, rarely neurological, lung, and cardiac involvement
  - Median survival 5 years
  - Only a small number of patients with chronic inflammation will develop AA amyloidosis, and the time period for the development of the disease is very variable
- Dialysis-related amyloid (DA), due to fibrils derived from β_2 microglobulin that accumulate in dialysis patients
- Inherited amyloidosis, e.g. due to abnormal pre-albumin (transthyretin, TTR), damaging neural and cardiac tissue
- Organ-specific amyloid, such as Alzheimer's disease; plaques of the β protein derived from the larger amyloid precursor protein (APP). Protein presumed to be generated locally.

Amyloidosis: lung involvement 1

Clinically significant respiratory tract disease is almost always AL in type, though the presence of a strong family history or chronic inflammatory disease may suggest other types.

Laryngeal amyloidosis Amyloid causes up to 1% of benign laryngeal disease. May present as discrete nodules or diffuse infiltration, and is usually localized, though can be a rare manifestation of systemic (AL) amyloid. Deposits are seen most commonly in the supraglottic larynx (presenting with hoarse voice or stridor). May present with choking and exertional dyspnoea that can be progressive or recurrent.

Tracheobronchial amyloid is rare (67 worldwide cases reported by the mid-1980s). Macroscopically is either diffusely infiltrative or 'tumour-like'. It is associated with tracheobronchopathia osteoplastica (a disorder characterized by the deposition of calcified submucosal airway nodules). It presents after the fifth decade with dyspnoea, cough, and rarely haemoptysis. Airway narrowing can lead to atelectasis or recurrent pneumonia; solitary nodules may lead to investigation for presumed lung cancer. Symptomatic disease is usually localized.

Parenchymal amyloid is the most frequently diagnosed amyloid respiratory disease. It is usually divided radiologically into solitary/multiple pulmonary nodules (usually localized AL amyloid) or a diffuse alveolar pattern (usually a manifestation of systemic AL amyloid). Parenchymal amyloid lung nodules are usually peripheral and subpleural, may be bilateral, and are more common in the lower lobes, ranging in diameter from 0.4 to 15 cm. They may cavitate or calcify. Clinical signs are non-diagnostic, PFTs may show a restrictive defect with reduced transfer factor. The differential diagnosis usually includes fibrosis. Cardiac amyloid may coexist, and distinguishing the contribution to the symptoms of the pulmonary and cardiac disease can be difficult. Median survival with clinically overt lung disease is about 16 months (similar to that of systemic amyloid).

Mediastinal and hilar amyloidosis are rarely associated with localized pulmonary amyloidosis and their diagnosis should lead to a search for a systemic cause of amyloid. Amyloid lymphadenopathy can also represent localized AL deposition in association with B-cell lymphoma.

Other Rare reports of:
- Ventilatory failure due to diaphragm or other respiratory muscle involvement
- Sleep apnoea from macroglossia due to amyloid
- Exudative pleural effusions.

Clinical features
- Dyspnoea and cough
- None—parenchymal disease may be an incidental finding on routine radiography
- Consider the diagnosis particularly in patients with odd upper airway symptoms and parenchymal involvement, or those with unexplained congestive cardiac failure or nephrotic syndrome.

Diagnosis Histological confirmation is usually required. Congo red stain producing 'apple green' birefringence in crossed polarized light is the gold standard. Positive histology must lead to immunohistochemistry to determine the fibril type.

- ***Histology*** Transbronchial biopsy or occasionally open or VATS biopsy (more likely if investigation for solitary pulmonary nodule).
- ***^{123}I labelled scintigraphy*** Radiolabelled serum amyloid P (SAP) localizes to amyloid deposits in proportion to the quantity of amyloid present, therefore allowing identification of the distribution and burden of disease. It is most sensitive for solid organ disease, though in lung disease is useful for determining the extent of disease in other organs. It is, however, expensive and carries an infection risk, as the serum amyloid P component is currently obtained from blood donors.
- ***HRCT*** may show nodules or parenchymal disease.
- ***Laryngoscopy and bronchoscopy*** may be needed to obtain samples for histology, depending on the clinical presentation.
- ***PFTs*** to assess the effect of disease on respiratory function. May show reduced transfer factor and a restrictive pattern. Tracheobronchial involvement may lead to abnormal flow–volume loops due to larger airway obstruction.
- Systemic disease
  - FBC, biochemistry, and urinalysis (?renal involvement)
  - Investigate for underlying blood cell dyscrasia, e.g. myeloma, Waldenstrom's macroglobulinaemia (bone marrow examination, and search for urine and serum monoclonal protein by immunofixation—the clonal proliferation underlying systemic AL amyloid is usually very subtle, and its identification may be difficult)
  - Echo for associated cardiac involvement (when congestive cardiac failure is present, survival is 4–6 months)
  - Thyroid/adrenal function are impaired in up to 10%.

Amyloidosis: lung involvement 2

Treatment There are limited clinical trials with which to guide management of respiratory tract amyloid. Management decisions are therefore often made empirically.

- No treatment may be needed
- Local measures may be warranted for endobronchial disease, e.g. symptomatic laryngeal disease—endoscopic excision, carbon dioxide laser evaporation (useful for small recurrent lesions), stenting. Steroids have no effect on laryngeal amyloid
- Tracheobronchial amyloid—management depends on symptoms and treatment may involve repeated endoscopic resection, YAG (yttrium–aluminium–garnet) laser therapy, and surgical resection. Repeated endoscopic procedures are thought to be safer than repeated open surgery
- Chemotherapy may be warranted for diffuse parenchymal amyloid if there is objectively measurable disease (prednisolone and melphalan, to suppress the underlying blood cell dyscrasia). More intensive chemotherapy has a better clinical response, but there are few trials.

Further Information

Falk RH, Raymond L *et al.* Systemic amyloidosis. *NEJM* 1997; **337**: 898–908

Gillmore JD, Hawkins PN. Amyloidosis and the respiratory tract. Rare diseases. *Thorax* 1999; **54**: 444–51

Hereditary haemorrhagic telangiectasia

(HHT; also referred to as Osler–Weber–Rendu syndrome)
Prevalence: 1 in 5000–8000.

Definition

An autosomal dominant disorder characterized by the development of abnormal dilated vessels in the systemic circulation, which may bleed leading to:

- Recurrent epistaxis
- Gastrointestinal bleeding
- Iron deficiency anaemia
- Other organ involvement, e.g. hepatic (in 30%, commonly asymptomatic), renal, pulmonary, and spinal arterio venous malformation (AVMs)

Screening Careful questioning of family members (Does anyone in the family have frequent nose bleeds?) and examination for telangiectasia should reveal those in whom screening should occur.

All those with HHT should be screened for pulmonary AVMs (PAVMs), and all of their offspring post-puberty and pre-pregnancy. There is increasing penetrance with increasing age (62% at age 16, 95% at age 40). Similarly, the detection of PAVMs in a patient should lead to screening for HHT in family members.

There is no consensus regarding the best screening method, but a combination of the following tests may be used:

- CXR
- Supine and erect oximetry
- CT chest
- Shunt quantification techniques, e.g. contrast echocardiogram, 100% oxygen rebreathing

Screening should continue throughout life (every 5–10 years) and during times of enlargement or development of AVMs—post-puberty and pre-pregnancy.

Management

- Usually involves liaison with ENT and gastroenterological colleagues for symptomatic treatment
- Iron replacement, transfusions
- Asymptomatic hepatic AVMs—no treatment usually required
- Cerebral AVMs (in 15% of HHT patients)—some specialists argue these should be treated prophylactically due to the risk of rupture and bleeding (2% per year, often fatal).

Further information

Shovlin CL, Letarte M. (Hereditary haemorrhagic telangectiasa and pulmonary AVMs: issues in clinical management and review of pathogenic mechanisms.) *Thorax* 1999; **54**: 714–39

Idiopathic pulmonary haemosiderosis

A rare disease of undetermined aetiology, characterized by recurrent episodes of alveolar haemorrhage and haemoptysis (in the absence of renal disease), usually leading to iron deficiency anaemia.

Pathophysiology The alveolar space and interstitium contain haemosiderin-laden macrophages, with variable degrees of interstitial fibrosis and degeneration of alveolar, interstitial, and vascular elastic fibres, depending on the chronicity of the condition. Electron microscopy shows damage to the endothelial and basement membranes, but no consistent or diagnostic features have been recognized.

No antibodies have been identified, though serum IgA levels are sometimes raised. With recurrent alveolar haemorrhage, the alveolar blood provokes a fibrotic reaction, with the development of diffuse pulmonary fibrosis.

Iron turnover studies show that the accompanying iron deficiency anaemia is due to loss of iron into the lung through haemorrhage.

Aetiology is uncertain, but likely to be multifactorial. Possible associations include toxic insecticides (epidemiological studies in rural Greece), premature birth, and fungal toxin exposure. The disease has an equal sex incidence in childhood, with twice as many men affected in adulthood.

Most patients present in childhood, with 85% of cases having onset of symptoms before 16 years. The actual prevalence is unknown, but a cohort study of Swedish children in the 1960s described an incidence of 0.24 per million children. Familial clustering is reported.

Pulmonary haemosiderosis is associated with rheumatoid arthritis, thyrotoxicosis, coeliac disease, and autoimmune haemolytic anaemia, suggesting a potential autoimmune mechanism.

Clinical features The clinical course is very variable and ranges from continuous low-level bleeding to massive pulmonary haemorrhage. The latter may be fatal, but is fortunately rare.

- Continuous mild pulmonary haemorrhage leads to a chronic non-productive cough with haemoptysis, malaise, lethargy, and failure to thrive in children
- Iron deficiency anaemia is common, as are positive faecal occult blood tests (due to swallowed blood)
- Generalized lymphadenopathy and hepatosplenomegaly are recognized.
- With an acute bleed, cough and haemoptysis may worsen, and dyspnoea, chest tightness, and pyrexia may develop
- Chronic bleeding leads to chronic disabling dyspnoea, chronic anaemia, and clubbing (in 25%). Cor pulmonale secondary to pulmonary fibrosis and hypoxaemia may develop.

Examination may be normal. Clubbing, basal crepitations, and cor pulmonale are all recognized, depending on the severity of the resulting lung disease.

Investigations The diagnosis is one of exclusion, with no evidence of other organ involvement. The main differential diagnosis is Goodpasture's syndrome, Wegener's granulomatosis, SLE, and microscopic polyarteritis.

- ***Blood tests*** Microcytic, hypochromic anaemia, with low iron levels. ANCA, dsDNA, and anti-GBM antibodies should be negative
- ***CXR*** May show transient patchy infiltrates, which worsen during an acute bleed. The apices are usually spared. Progressive disease leads to the development of reticulonodular infiltrates, and a ground-glass appearance that is typically perihilar or in the lower zones. Hilar lymphadenopathy may be seen
- ***PFTs*** kCO is transiently elevated during bleeding episodes (≥130% is abnormal), but this is only useful acutely. A restrictive defect with reduced kCO may develop with chronic disease
- ***CT chest*** The changes seen are fairly non-specific, showing a diffuse bilateral infiltrate, with patchy ground-glass change
- ***BAL*** (if done) contain haemosiderin-laden macrophages.

Management

There is no specific treatment.

- Steroids and immunosuppressive drugs may be of benefit during acute bleeding episodes, but do not appear to affect the long-term outcome. There are no published data to guide the optimal timing of treatment during the course of disease
- The iron deficiency anaemia responds to replacement therapy, and blood transfusion may be needed in severe bleeds.

At routine clinic appointments

- Check spirometry
- Measure haemoglobin and serum iron levels
- Ask about increases in SOB or haemoptysis.

Prognosis The prognosis is very variable, with some patients showing spontaneous remission. The duration of disease in the literature ranges from death within days following an acute severe illness, to survival with cor pulmonale associated with chronic disease after 20 years.

Langerhans' cell histiocytosis

Definition Pulmonary Langerhans' cell histiocytosis (LCH; previously termed pulmonary histiocytosis X or pulmonary eosinophilic granuloma) is a rare condition characterized by infiltration of the lung with histiocytes (Langerhans' cells). Pulmonary LCH overlaps with a number of other conditions with similar pathological findings but diverse clinical features. These range from localized infiltration of a single organ (e.g. eosinophilic granuloma of bone) to systemic diseases affecting multiple organs (Letterer–Siwe disease, a multi-organ disease affecting infants and elderly, associated with poor prognosis; also Hand–Schueller–Christian syndrome). Although the isolated pulmonary form most commonly presents to chest physicians, pulmonary manifestations also commonly occur in the systemic forms of the disease.

Epidemiology Rare, it tends to affect young adults aged 20–40 years. The vast majority of cases occur in current smokers, usually heavy smokers. May be more common in men, who tend to present at a younger age than women.

Pathogenesis Langerhans' cells are involved in antigen presentation, and are characterized by the presence of well-demarcated cytoplasmic organelles called Birbeck granules on electron microscopy. The Langerhans' cells seen in LCH appear to be monoclonal, although it is unclear if this represents a true neoplastic process. The antigen stimulus for activating Langerhans' cells in the lung is unknown, although cigarette smoke is a possible candidate. Langerhans' cells are typically organized into granulomata that are located in bronchiolar walls, and subsequently enlarge and invade adjacent structures. This results in the radiological appearance of nodules that at first cavitate and then become cystic.

Clinical features Typically exertional breathlessness and cough, sometimes with systemic symptoms (e.g. fever, weight loss). Pneumothorax occurs in at least 10% of patients and may be the presenting feature. Rib lesions may also give rise to chest pain. Around 25% of patients are asymptomatic. Examination is usually normal.

Investigations

- ***CXR*** Typically diffuse reticulonodular shadowing, sometimes with cystic change; upper and middle lobe predominance. May be normal
- ***HRCT*** Diffuse centrilobular nodules, sometimes with cavitation, and thin and thick-walled cystic lesions, reflecting lesions of varying age. These are interspersed with normal lung. Upper and middle lobe predominance; costophrenic angles are typically spared. Purely nodular or purely cystic appearances may occur. Unusual manifestations such as single nodules or large airways involvement are also described
- ***PFTs*** variable, ranging from normal to obstructive, restricted or mixed patterns. Reduced gas transfer and exertional hypoxia are common
- ***TBB*** may yield diagnostic material, although is often unhelpful; risk of pneumothorax is unknown although may be increased. Surgical lung biopsy is often preferable

- ***BAL*** Increased total cell counts and pigmented macrophages, reflecting simply the presence of cigarette smoking. Use of antibodies (e.g. OKT6) to detect Langerhans' cells in BAL fluid is limited by poor sensitivity
- ***Extrathoracic biopsy*** of involved sites (e.g. bone) may be diagnostic

Diagnosis Usually based on the combination of clinical and HRCT findings: typically a young adult smoker with cysts and nodules on HRCT. Confirmation by surgical lung biopsy may be considered in atypical presentations, such as the finding of solely nodular or cystic disease on HRCT. The appearance of purely cystic disease on HRCT may be confused with emphysema (where cysts lack walls) or lymphangioleiomyomatosis (where cysts are present uniformly in all regions of lung, including the costophrenic angles).

Associations

- Severe pulmonary hypertension—may be seen in the absence of significant parenchymal lung involvement; direct disease involvement of pulmonary vessels has been described
- Manifestations of systemic LCH—particularly diabetes insipidus from pituitary disease, skin involvement, lytic bony lesions, and rarely cardiac or gastrointestinal disease
- Lymphoma—may precede, complicate, or coexist with pulmonary LCH
- Lung cancer—more common, probably as a result of cigarette smoking.

Management Treatment other than smoking cessation is often not required. Oral corticosteroids may be tried in symptomatic disease, although there is little evidence to support their use; they are usually administered for at least 6 months. Lung transplantation should be considered in patients with severe respiratory failure or pulmonary hypertension. Pulmonary LCH may recur in transplanted lungs. Experimental treatments such as the use of IL-2 and anti-TNFα may be of benefit in the systemic forms of LCH seen in children.

Prognosis is variable. Spontaneous improvement is common, although later reactivation of disease may occur. A minority of patients deteriorate rapidly with respiratory failure and death within months. Overall life expectancy is reduced, with median survival 12–13 years from diagnosis. Death is most commonly due to respiratory failure. Poor prognostic factors include reduced FEV_1, increased residual volume, and reduced gas transfer.

Further Information

Sundar KM *et al.* Pulmonary Langerhans' cell histiocytosis. *Chest* 2003; **123**: 1673–83

Lymphangioleiomyomatosis (LAM): clinical features

Definition and aetiology A rare disorder characterized by abnormal proliferation of smooth muscle cells, affecting women of child-bearing age, usually in their 30s. The disease is hormone-dependent, so can occur in post-menopausal women on oestrogen replacement therapy.

- Incidence of 1 in 1.1 million population
- Unknown cause
- Not hereditary
- 40% of adult women with tuberous sclerosis (learning difficulties, sub-ungal fibromas, seizures, facial angiofibromas, autosomal dominant inheritance or spontaneous mutation) develop pulmonary changes identical to those of LAM.

Pathology Abnormal proliferation of atypical smooth muscle cells (LAM cells) throughout the lung, airways, blood vessels, and lymphatics. There is nodular infiltration, which is initially subtle. Progressive growth causes lymphatic and airway obstruction, leading to cyst formation throughout the lungs.

Clinical features

Common

- Secondary pneumothorax (in two-thirds of patients; occurs due to lung cystic change; recurrence is common)
- Dyspnoea (in 42%)
- Cough (in 20%)
- Haemoptysis (in 14%)
- Chylothorax (in 12%, thoracic duct leakage as a result of lymphatic obstruction by LAM cells, may be bilateral).

Less common

- Pleural effusion
- Chest pain
- Pulmonary haemorrhage (due to blocked blood vessels and increased intraluminal pressure).

Other organs affected

Kidney Angiomyolipoma, a benign tumour, occurs in 50% of LAM patients. Usually diagnosed on CT, these are mostly small and single, but can be multiple and larger in tuberous sclerosis. Smaller tumours are usually asymptomatic, but larger ones can cause flank pain and bleeding into the renal tract. Treatment options include tumour resection or embolization. Nephrectomy is not usually required. Screening for these lesions is important as it allows careful treatment planning in case they become symptomatic.

Abdomen Lymphadenopathy due to lymphatic obstruction. Occurs in one-third of patients and is usually asymptomatic.

Pelvis Lymphangioleiomyoma—a cystic mass that enlarges during the day and causes fullness and bloating.

Chylous ascites can occur in the absence of chylothorax.

Skin Cutaneous swellings, likely due to localized oedema.

Examination May be normal. There may be pulmonary crepitations or signs of pleural effusion. Palpable abdominal masses may be present.

Investigations

- ***PFTs*** may be normal, or show a predominantly obstructive pattern. Rarely restrictive. Decreased TLCO, with a normal or increased TLC
- ***CXR*** may be normal. Lungs may appear hyperinflated, with reticular shadowing and septal lines due to obstructed lymphatics. There may also be a diffuse interstitial infiltrate
- ***HRCT*** shows a characteristic appearance, with multiple cysts throughout the lung of varying size, which are usually small (<1 cm) and thin-walled. The adjoining lung parenchyma is normal. There may be pleural effusions.
- ***CT abdomen*** to examine for presence of angiomyolipomas and other lymphatic involvement.

LAM: diagnosis and management

Diagnosis Consider particularly in young or middle-aged women with:

- Recurrent pneumothoraces, especially those with pre-existing dyspnoea or haemoptysis
- Cystic lung disease, airflow obstruction, or chylous pleural effusions
- Angiomyolipomas or other retroperitoneal tumours
- Tuberous sclerosis and respiratory symptoms

The disease is easily missed in its early stages. The diagnosis can be made on the characteristic CT appearances, or with open lung biopsy. Transbronchial biopsies may not be diagnostic. Large retroperitoneal abdominal lymph nodes can also be biopsied.

Management

- There are no controlled trials of treatment
- The course of LAM is variable. Treatment should be aimed at those who are symptomatic and declining
- ***Diet*** Low-fat diet with medium chain triglyceride supplementation may prevent chylothorax recurrence, but there is not strong evidence for this. The diet is difficult to adhere to
- ***Bronchodilators*** may improve airflow obstruction
- ***Hormonal manipulation*** with progesterone has been tried. It may be beneficial in reducing the decline in FEV_1 and TLCO, particularly in patients with progressive disease, but there are no large studies. Tamoxifen and oophrectomy have also been tried
- ***Avoid oestrogens*** i.e. the oral contraceptive pill and hormone replacement therapy
- ***Contraception*** An increase in symptoms and accelerated disease decline are reported in pregnancy. Use the progesterone-only pill
- ***Pleural aspiration*** when required for pleural effusions. For recurrent effusions or chylothoraces, thoracic duct ligation or pleurectomy may be effective. Pleurodesis can be performed, but this is relatively contra-indicated if future lung transplant is an option
- ***Recurrent pneumothoraces*** Advise regarding flying and diving. Thoracic surgery may be necessary
- ***Avoid air travel*** if possible due to risk of pneumothorax
- ***Transplant*** Single (usually) or double lung, or heart–lung. LAM can recur in the transplanted lung
- ***Stop smoking*** as this accelerates the rate of decline
- Influenza vaccine
- Liaise with a specialist centre if required (this is Nottingham City Hospital in the UK).

Prognosis is very variable. The condition usually slowly progresses to respiratory failure. At 10 years 55% of patients have MRC grade 3 dyspnoea, 23% are on LTOT, and 10% are housebound. Survival: 70% of patients are alive at 10 years, 33% are alive at 15 years, and 25% are alive at 20 years.

Future developments Rapamycin may switch off the defect in LAM cells and prevent their proliferation. Studies are ongoing.

Further information

Johnson SR, Tattersfield AE. Clinical experience of LAM in the UK. *Thorax* 2000; **55**: 1052–7

Sullivan EJ. LAM: a review. *Chest* 1998; **114**: 1689–703

Ryu JH *et al*. Chylothorax in LAM. *Chest* 2003; **123**(2): 623–7

Primary ciliary dyskinesia (PCD)

A rare genetic cause of chronic respiratory disease, usually encountered in adult respiratory clinics as a cause of bronchiectasis. Cilia are found in:

- The whole length of the upper respiratory tract
- Brain ventricles
- Fallopian tube/ductus epididymis

They are made up of dynein arms, with outer and inner connecting rings, and beat at 14 beats/s. Many gene defects have been identified in PCD, causing a number of cilial abnormalities.

Abnormal cilia do not beat normally, leading to reduced mucociliary clearance, microbiological colonization (which further inhibits cilial action), chronic infection, and the development of bronchiectasis.

The main aim following diagnosis in childhood is the prevention of chronic respiratory disease and bronchiectasis.

Clinical features

- Autosomal recessive, >200 phenotypes
- May present with neonatal respiratory distress
- Situs inversus (in about 30%, as cilia determine the side of the organs. Random organ siting occurs with cilial dysfunction, hence the situs inversus of Kartagener's syndrome)
- Nasal blockage/rhinitis
- Persistent wet cough in childhood
- Hearing problems/history of glue ear/grommets in childhood
- Clubbing and signs of chest disease are rare in childhood
- Wheeze in 20%
- Infertility due to immotile sperm (sperm tails have same morphological defect as the cilia and do not beat correctly)
- In adults the disease usually presents with the clinical signs of bronchiectasis: cough productive of purulent sputum, recurrent chest infections, intermittent haemoptysis.

Diagnosis Saccharin test (see p 153). Nasal NO is very low in PCD (possibly because NO mediates ciliary function); this is the most sensitive and specific screening test. Cilial biopsy via the nasal route. Cilia are examined by high-speed digital video, where their beat frequency and pattern can be assessed, confirming the diagnosis. Most cases of PCD are diagnosed in childhood. There is an increased frequency in the children of consanguineous marriages.

Consider the diagnosis in:

- Bronchiectasis
- Situs inversus
- Persistent upper and lower respiratory infection from early childhood
- Infertility—males may present in infertility clinics.

Management

A national service for the diagnosis of PCD was set up in 2007, with three centres—London (Royal Brompton), Southampton, and Leicester.

In adults this involves the treatment of secondary bronchiectasis (see p 154), with:

- Antibiotics
- Physiotherapy
- Vaccinations
- Management of haemoptysis.

Pulmonary alveolar proteinosis (PAP): pathophysiology and clinical features

Pulmonary alveolar proteinosis (PAP), also referred to as alveolar lipoproteinosis, is a rare alveolar filling defect affecting around 3 per million people. There is a limited published literature: five reported case series of ≥10 cases, and only 410 total cases reported.

Pathophysiology PAP is due to failure of alveolar macrophages to clear spent surfactant, leading to the filling of alveoli with a phospholipid proteinaceous material. It is thought that the defect has an autoimmune basis, due to the presence of antibodies to granulocyte-macrophage colony-stimulating factor (GM-CSF), which cause inhibition of normal alveolar macrophage function, leading to abnormalities of surfactant homeostasis. Defects in GM-CSF signalling have been identified in animal models. Congenital disease is thought to be due to mutations in surfactant gene proteins. Other mechanisms for surfactant accumulation have also been identified:

- ***Heavy dust exposure*** leads to surfactant hypersecretion, which exceeds the lungs' normal clearance mechanism. Animal models have shown that this condition develops from endogenous lipoid pneumonia, with the accumulation of lipid-laden macrophages, which break down to release surfactant
- ***Amphiphilic drugs*** e.g. amiodarone, chlorphentermine
- ***Lymphoma, leukaemia, and immunosuppression*** The mechanism is uncertain, but it is thought that the lipoprotein may be generated from degenerating alveolar cells.

Appearances similar to alveolar lipoproteinosis may also be seen in endogenous lipoid pneumonia resulting from bronchial obstruction and are described in surfactant-secreting alveolar cell carcinoma.

Histology The alveoli are filled with a granular acellular eosinophilic PAS (periodic acid–Schiff) positive deposit. Cholesterol clefts and large foamy macrophages may also be seen. The alveolar architecture is usually well preserved. Surfactant protein can be identified using immunohistochemistry. Electron microscopy shows multiple osmiophilic bodies consistent with denatured surfactant.

Epidemiology

- Presents aged 30–50 (case reports in children and the elderly)
- Male to female ratio of 4:1
- Increased incidence in smokers
- Rare familial cases reported.

Clinical features

- Typically presents with breathlessness and a non-productive cough. Examination may be normal, or crackles may be heard on auscultation. Clubbing in one-third
- May present with superadded infection, causing an apparent acute onset of symptoms in association with fever
- Median duration of symptoms before diagnosis is 7 months
- Opportunistic infection is the major complication, most commonly *Nocardia* species, fungi, and mycobacteria. This occurs due to impaired macrophage function and impaired host defence due to surfactant accumulation.

PAP: diagnosis and treatment

Diagnosis is usually made on the basis of a characteristic CT appearance, although other tests may also be useful.

- Raised serum LDH
- ***ABGs*** Hypoxia and increased alveolar–arterial (A–a) gradient
- ***PFTs*** Restrictive defect, with reduced lung volumes and transfer factor
- ***CXR*** Bilateral consolidation with thickened interlobular septa. Usually bilateral. The pattern is very variable, and in up to 50% may be perihilar (bat-wing appearance)
- **CT** appearance is characteristic, with airspace shadowing in a geographical distribution, alternating with areas of normal lung, the so-called 'crazy paving' pattern. This CT appearance is not specific to alveolar proteinosis, but is also seen in lipoid pneumonia and bronchoalveolar cell carcinoma
- ***BAL*** reveals milky washings. Identification of antibodies to granulocyte-macrophage colony-stimulating factor in BAL washings is diagnostic. Cytological examination shows a granular extracellular deposit with foamy macrophages and cellular debris
- ***Transbronchial/open lung biopsies*** are occasionally needed if the CT is not characteristic.

Treatment of choice is repeated therapeutic whole lung lavage, which should be performed at a specialist centre. There are no randomized controlled trials of this treatment, but there is evidence of efficacy in terms of subsequent improvement of symptoms, physiology, and radiology.

- The indication for whole lung lavage is usually breathlessness limiting activities of daily living
- The procedure is done under general anaesthesia using 100% oxygen, and one-lung ventilation using a double-lumen tube. Repeated warm saline lavage using a closed circuit continues until the bronchial washing returns are clear—this may take up to 40 L lavage. One or both lungs may be treated at a time
- The response is variable—some patients need only one treatment, others may need multiple treatments, and about 10% fail to respond
- May be done on bypass if the patient is very hypoxic
- Characteristic milky lavage fluid is obtained.

Granulocyte colony-stimulating factor (subcutaneous injections) is a novel treatment option (only phase II studies, no RCT yet), which may prevent progression of disease.

There is no benefit from treatment with steroids, and they may exacerbate opportunistic infections.

Prognosis with whole lung lavage is generally good. Spontaneous remission occurs in one-third, one-third remain stable, and one-third progress to respiratory failure and death. There are reports of progression to pulmonary fibrosis (which may be a coincidental occurrence).

Further information

Shah P *et al.* Pulmonary alveolar proteinosis: clinical aspects and current concepts on pathogenesis. *Thorax* 2000; **55**: 67–77

Trapnell MD *et al.* Pulmonary alveolar proteinosis: mechanisms of disease. *NEJM* 2003; **349**: 2527–39

Pulmonary arteriovenous malformations (PAVMs): aetiology and diagnosis

Aetiology

- Pulmonary arteriovenous malformations (PAVMs) are abnormal blood vessels replacing normal capillaries, making a direct low-resistance connection between the pulmonary arterial and systemic venous circulations. They vary in size from tiny clusters of vessels (telangiectasia) to larger, more complex aneurysmal-type sacs
- The disorder is rare, affecting 1 in 15, 000–24 000
- Several genetic susceptibility loci have been identified on chromosomes 9 and 12. One identified mutation is in the endoglin gene. This modulates signalling via the transforming growth factor-β family of growth factors. This gene is also implicated in the development of primary pulmonary hypertension
- Subjects with significant PAVMs have low pulmonary vascular resistance, a low mean pulmonary artery pressure, and a high cardiac output—due to longstanding adaptive mechanisms to the effects of the shunt, in addition to vascular remodelling effects
- Most patients present post-puberty, as AVMs probably develop at this time. They probably grow throughout life, especially during puberty and in pregnancy. They may rarely regress spontaneously.

Diagnosis

- Most patients present with an abnormal ***CXR***, classically showing a smooth rounded intrapulmonary mass, with draining or feeding vessels
- Mild ***hypoxaemia*** An AVM is a direct communication between the pulmonary artery and pulmonary vein. Blood therefore bypasses the pulmonary capillary bed, with reduced oxygenation, which poorly corrects with supplementary oxygen
- ***Orthodeoxia*** is desaturation on standing, due to an increase in blood flow in the dependent lung areas. 70% of PAVMs are basal; hence the desaturation seen
- ***CT*** identifies all AVMs, and can determine those suitable for embolization. Contrast is not required
- Patients may present with the complications of a PAVM, particularly bleeding or peripheral abscess formation. The absence of a normal filtering capillary bed means small particles can reach the systemic circulation, leading to sequelae, particularly in the cerebral circulation—strokes and cerebral abscesses. These abnormal vessels are also at risk of rupture.

Shunt quantification

- ***100% oxygen rebreathing study***, a non-invasive method of shunt quantification
- ***^{99m}TC perfusion scan***, a tracer study; the size of the shunt can be assessed from the proportion of radiolabelled macro-aggregates reaching the systemic circulation compared with the total number injected. In a normal study, aggregates accumulate in the kidneys
- ***Contrast echocardiogram*** to measure the circulatory transit time of injected echocontrast
- ***Angiography*** at specialist centre only
- In normal individuals the anatomical shunt is <2–3.5% of the cardiac output (due to post-pulmonary drainage of bronchial veins into pulmonary vein, and drainage into the left atrium).

Clinical features

- Asymptomatic (50%)
- Dyspnoea
- Haemoptysis (10%), probably due to additional bronchial telangiectasia, which can also cause haemorrhage into bronchi or the pleural cavity
- Chest pain (12%); aetiology is uncertain
- Clubbing
- Cyanosis
- Orthodeoxia
- Vascular bruits
- Telangiectasia; 80% of PAVM patients have hereditary haemorrhagic telangiectasia (HHT), and their families should be screened because of the risk of stroke (see p 618)
- May present with acute stroke, with focal neurological signs

PAVMs: management and complications

Management

Embolization is usually done with coils, which generate local thrombin, leading to cessation of blood flow in AVM feeding vessels. This results in a reduction in the right–left shunt and improvement in hypoxaemia, and should be done by an expert in a specialist centre only. The small risk of neurological sequelae and angina/arrthymias is reduced with operator experience.

60–70% of patients are left with a small persisting shunt following treatment, and retain a small risk of abscess formation. Patients are therefore given prophylactic antibiotics for dental and surgical procedures (ensure the patient has a MedicAlert card).

Surgical resection may be more appropriate than embolization in some cases.

Anti-platelet therapy (rarely) in individual cases, if ongoing transient ischaemic attacks.

Transplantation is not advised as there is no increased survival benefit over medical treatment.

Screening The majority of patients with PAVMs have HHT and so screening of family members is important.

Follow-up All patients need regular follow-up with shunt assessment post-surgical resection or embolization, as removal of one shunt may unmask or provoke the development of others.

Female patients should be advised to defer pregnancy until completion of formal assessment, because of the risks of growth and rupture of PAVMs in pregnancy (see below).

Complications

- PAVM patients never die of respiratory failure in the absence of additional respiratory disease
- All patients are at risk of stroke and cerebral abscesses
- Transient ischaemic attack/stroke (in 25%) due to rupture of abnormal capillaries in aneurysms
- Abscess (in 10%) due to paradoxical emboli through the right to left shunt, and the absence of a filtering capillary bed

Pregnancy is associated with an increase in size of AVMs, and new ones may develop, with potentially catastrophic consequences. Careful shunt assessment is therefore needed prior to pregnancy, with contraceptive advice prior to specialist assessment. Close liaison between the specialist centre and obstetric team is paramount. AVMs may need embolization in the third trimester to allow safe delivery.

Recurrent respiratory papillomatosis

These are essentially warts of the upper respiratory tract, caused by the human papilloma virus (HPV 6 or 11). The virus infects epithelial cells and mucous membranes, similar to that seen in cutaneous and anogenital infection. The infection is most commonly acquired during ororespiratory exposure from the mother during vaginal delivery, and typically presents in childhood from 6 months onwards, with signs and symptoms of upper respiratory tract infection. It may also present for the first time in adulthood. It is associated with HLA DR3, and with sexual transmission in adults. Recurrent respiratory papillomatosis is rare (2 per 100 000), but oral HPV infection is common.

Clinical course

This is variable.

- May remit spontaneously
- Progressive voice loss and airway obstruction
- Most cases are confined to the larynx, although up to 25% of patients subsequently develop extralaryngeal spread to the bronchial tree
- 1% have malignant change to squamous cell carcinomas

Management

- Surgical excision to maintain airway patency
- Laser therapy—but potential problems of thermal injury, stricture formation, and spread of papillomas
- Photodynamic therapy reduces recurrence rate, using oral or intravenous photosensitizing agent, then a laser to destroy photosensitive tissue
- Microdebrider is now used more commonly
- Medical treatment—interferon, aciclovir, ribavirin, isoretinoin, and methotrexate have all been tried
    - ***Interferon-*α** as a daily subcutaneous injection leads to complete remission in 30–50%, and partial resolution in 30%. One-third recur when treatment is stopped. Adverse reactions are common: flu-like symptoms, deranged LFTs, leucopenia, and alopecia
    - ***Cidofovir*** is a nucleoside monophosphate analogue and inhibits viral polymerase. It is given as an intralesional injection. Potential side-effects include nephrotoxicity and neutropenia.

Chapter 50

Upper airway diseases

Acute upper airway obstruction

Presentation Sudden respiratory distress with cyanosis and aphonia. Airway obstruction can occur at any level within the airway. Partial airway obstruction leads to noisy breathing, with stridor, gurgling, or snoring. Complete airway obstruction is associated with distress and marked respiratory effort, with paradoxical chest and abdominal movement ('seesaw breathing'), and use of accessory muscles of respiration. This may be followed by collapse with loss of consciousness, and progress to cardiorespiratory arrest. Look for chest and abdominal movements, and listen and feel for airflow at the nose and mouth.

Causes

- Pharyngeal occlusion by tongue and other muscles, secondary to loss of muscle tone. This may be secondary to drugs, alcohol, a neurological event, or cardiorespiratory arrest
- Vomit or blood
- Inhaled foreign body, which may also cause laryngeal spasm
- Laryngeal obstruction due to oedema from burns, inflammation, or anaphylaxis
- Excessive bronchial secretions, mucosal oedema, bronchospasm: may cause airway obstruction below the larynx
- Infection, such as epiglottitis
- Any cause of chronic airway obstruction, such as an airway tumour or extrinsic compression due to tumour or lymphadenopathy, may deteriorate precipitously.

▶▶ Management of upper airway obstruction

Call for senior anaesthetic help early

- Open the airway with backwards head tilt, chin lift, and forward jaw thrust. In cases of trauma, do not tilt the head, but perform a jaw thrust only
- If unsuccessful at restoring normal respiration, visually inspect the mouth for obvious occlusion and remove it with a finger sweep. Leave well-fitting dentures in place
- If there is a witnessed history of choking, consider performing the Heimlich manoeuvre to dislodge the particle (firm and rapid pressure applied beneath the diaphragm in an upwards movement), or directly visualize the airway with a laryngoscope and use McGill's forceps to remove the particle, or with bronchoscope and the use of biopsy forceps
- If the patient is breathing, consider inserting an airway to maintain patency: oropharyngeal (Guedel) or nasopharyngeal. Maintain oxygenation, using mask with reservoir bag, delivering 10–15 L/min. If there is no spontaneous respiratory effort, insert a laryngeal mask or endotracheal tube and deliver oxygen via self-inflating bag with supplemental oxygen 10 L/min and reservoir bag. If they are not breathing and cannot be ventilated, a cricothyroidotomy may be necessary (p 763)
- Suction out secretions
- Maintain circulation with cardiac compression if necessary
- Seek definitive treatment for the cause of airway obstruction, as appropriate.

Heliox Helium–oxygen mixtures can be used for patients with airway obstruction, often due to tumour compression or invasion. Helium has a lower density than nitrogen and can improve ventilation rapidly when used with oxygen. It can be used as an interim measure until more definitive management is available, such as radiotherapy, or to allow time for radiotherapy to take effect. The evidence relating to its use is mainly case studies, with no randomized control trials.

Nebulized adrenaline may also be helpful in upper airway obstruction, especially laryngeal oedema. This is only a stabilizing measure to buy time until definitive treatment is available.

Anaphylaxis

This is a potentially life-threatening medical emergency. Call for help

Causes IgE-mediated type 1 hypersensitivity reaction to allergen. Histamine release causes the clinical syndrome. Typical allergens include bee or wasp sting, peanuts, fish, drugs, foods, latex, contrast media, muscle relaxants, anaesthetic agents.

Presentation Varying severity of:

- Angio-oedema
- Urticaria
- Dyspnoea
- Wheeze
- Stridor
- Hypotension
- Arrhythmias
- Also rhinitis, abdominal pain, vomiting, diarrhoea, sense of impending doom
- May have had previous episodes of severe allergic-type reactions.

►► Management of anaphylaxis

- Remove likely allergen
- Cardiopulmonary resuscitation if necessary
- ***Airway and breathing*** Administer high-flow oxygen through non-rebreathe mask. If airway obstruction present, consider tracheal intubation. Airway swelling may make this difficult and cricothyroidotomy may need to be performed (see p 763)
- ***Circulation*** Give adrenaline (epinephrine) IM 1:1000 solution 0.5 mL (500 μg). Repeat after 5 min if no improvement or deterioration
- In those with profound shock and immediately life-threatening anaphylaxis, such as during anaesthesia, or those with no pulse. IV adrenaline can be given slowly, 100 μg per min or 1 mL of 1:10 000 solution/min. Stop as soon as there is a response. This can be hazardous and needs cardiac monitoring
- IV fluids if hypotension persists: 1–2 L rapidly infused
- Antihistamines, such as chlorphenamine 10–20 mg IV
- Consider steroids: 100–500 mg hydrocortisone IV
- Consider nebulized salbutamol or adrenaline if bronchospasm
- On discharge, provide epipen (IM self-administered adrenaline) and advise on future episodes, MedicAlert bracelet, and card
- Consider immunology referral if allergen unknown.
- Consider C1 esterase inhibitor deficiency, especially if repeated episodes.

Future developments Allergen immunotherapy aiming to desensitize to the allergen. Useful in those who cannot avoid allergen exposure. Small amounts of the allergen are injected usually weekly, with slowly increasing dose strengths until the maximum dose of the allergen is administered, which can take up to 12 months. Mechanism unknown, but probably related to increased IgG binding to the allergen, falling allergen-specific IgE levels, and decreased amount of circulating inflammatory cytokines. Can protect against anaphylaxis for 3–5 years, but 'top-up' doses necessary. Effective for dust, grass, tree, and weed pollen, mould spores, latex, and insect venom, as well as some animal allergens. Side-effects of administration: anaphylaxis, bronchoconstriction, local reaction. Some centres may not perform in people with chronic asthma because of the risk of death.

Further information

Abramson M, Puy R *et al.* Allergen immunotherapy for asthma. *Cochrane Database Syst Rev* 2003; **4**: CD001186

Advanced Life Support Provider Manual, 5th edn, 2006. Resuscitation Council UK

Upper respiratory tract infections 1

Acute upper respiratory tract infections (URTIs) include rhinitis, pharyngitis, tonsillitis, and sinusitis.

Upper respiratory tract infections are the commonest cause of people taking time off work in the United Kingdom. The majority are managed by general practitioners and will not reach a respiratory specialist. They are usually self-limiting and often do not require specific treatment.

Acute rhinitis Nasal congestion with rhinorrhea, mild malaise, and sneezing. Most commonly due to viral infection (the common cold).

Topical decongestants may be useful. There is no evidence for the use of antibiotics or antihistamines.

Candidiasis Oral candida infection is common in those who have received antibiotics, are immunosuppressed, or on oral or inhaled steroids. Seen as white plaque-like lesions on the tongue and pharyngeal mucosa. Treat with oral nystatin or amphotericin lozenges, and with oral hygiene. Severe infection can be debilitating, leading to difficulties with eating, especially in the elderly. Exclude underlying immunocompromise (e.g. HIV, leukaemia) in those with persisting infection despite treatment.

Acute epiglottitis (supraglottitis) is infection mainly localized to the epiglottis and surrounding supraglottic structures. It is commoner in children than adults, but a mortality of up to 7% is reported in adults. This is due to upper airways obstruction from grossly oedematous upper airway tissue.

- *Haemophilus influenza*, *Streptococci*, and *Staphylococci* are causative organisms
- Acute epiglottitis typically presents with a sore throat and dysphagia. Inspiratory stridor is less common, but it can also present with acute upper airway obstruction and CXR infiltrates consistent with pulmonary oedema (due to high negative intrathoracic pressure)
- May need airway protection with an endotracheal tube or tracheostomy: liaise with ENT/anaesthetic colleagues early
- In severe infection, epiglottic swabs may be of diagnostic use, but beware of precipitating airway obstruction. Treat with third-generation cephalosporin for 2 weeks (to cover β-lactam producing *H. influenzae*). Change to amoxicillin if sensitive

Sinusitis The sinuses are normally sterile. The paranasal sinuses communicate with the nose, and are therefore susceptible to infection from this route. All the sinuses drain by means of the mucociliary escalator. Blockage of free sinus drainage is a predisposing factor for bacterial infection. Sinusitis is a common cause of persistent cough (see p 18). Dental sepsis may lead to maxillary sinusitis, by direct spread.

Acute sinusitis complicates 1 in 200 upper respiratory tract infections and usually presents with fever, nasal congestion/discharge, and sinus pain which is worse on leaning forward. It may be associated with systemic upset. Respiratory viral infection interrupts normal defences of the mucosal lining, producing mucous exudates, with secondary bacterial infection. *S. pneumoniae* and *H. influenzae* are the commonest pathogens. *S. aureus* and *S. pyogenes* are also causes, with *Pseudomonas* in cystic fibrosis.

Mixed infections with anaerobes are seen in 10%. Specific diagnostic tests are not usually needed. If symptoms persist, antibiotic treatment may be indicated.

Chronic sinusitis by definition, if present for >3 months. The ciliated epithelial sinus lining is replaced by thickened stratified squamous lining, with absent cilia, due to repeated infection. Anaerobic infection is more common. Fungal infection is more common in atopic people with nasal polyps. Sinus mycetoma is a rare complication in neutropenic patients, diabetics, and the immunocompromised.

Presents with frontal headache (frontal sinusitis), maxillary pain, pain over bridge of nose (ethmoidal sinusitis), retro-orbital headache (sphenoidal sinusitis), with purulent nasal discharge and blockage. Wegener's granulomatosis may mimic the symptoms of sinusitis.

Investigations are not usually warranted, but a sinus radiograph may show an air-fluid level, with thickened mucosal lining, or sinus opacification. CT is more sensitive, but not usually warranted unless surgical intervention planned or malignant disease suspected.

Treatment Analgesia, topical decongestants, antibiotics if severe infection (amoxicillin first line, trimethoprim if penicillin allergic).

Surgery may be warranted if prolonged infection, anatomical abnormality, or other complications, e.g. if infection has spread to the cranial cavity or orbit. Spreading infection is uncommon if there has been prior antibiotic treatment.

Upper respiratory tract infections 2

Acute pharyngitis and tonsillitis 80–90% are caused by viruses, most commonly adenoviruses, coronaviruses, rhinoviruses, and influenza viruses. Group B streptococci, *Streptococcus pneumoniae*, and *Haemophilus influenzae* may cause secondary infection. Mycoplasma and chlamydia are seen less commonly.

- Pharyngitis and tonsillitis present with a sore throat, which is usually self-limiting. May be associated with fever, malaise, lymphadenopathy, conjunctivitis, headache, nausea, and vomiting
- Infectious mononucleosis (Epstein Barr Virus) is associated with pharyngitis in 80% of cases. Diagnose with Paul Bunnell test for heterophil antibodies, and atypical mononuclear cells in peripheral blood
- Coxsackie A and herpes simplex cause 'herpangina syndrome'—ulcerating vesicles on the tonsils and palate
- CMV can also cause pharyngitis associated with lymphadenopathy and splenomegaly
- Lemierre's syndrome (jugular vein suppurative thrombophlebitis) is a rare anaerobic pharyngeal infection (see p 446).

Other causative agents

- *Corynebacterium diptheriae* in unvaccinated populations. A pharyngeal membrane may form, with systemic symptoms, and 'bull neck' due to cervical lymphadenopathy. Low-grade fever, with a relatively high pulse rate. Treat urgently with diphtheria antitoxin
- Vincent's angina is anaerobic infection in those with poor mouth hygiene. Caused by Gram-negative *Borrelia vincenti* and other anaerobic infections. Treat with penicillin
- Group A streptococcus may cause a more unpleasant illness, with systemic upset and dysphagia due to pharyngotonsillar oedema.

Treatment is usually supportive, but anti-streptococcal antibiotics may be warranted if there is severe infection. There is no evidence that antibiotics reduce the duration of symptoms, but they may reduce complications (e.g. sinusitis, quinsy, and rheumatic fever, which is rare in the Western world). Oral penicillin is the first-line treatment (or a macrolide if penicillin allergic). Amoxycillin can cause a rash in infectious mononucleosis and so should be avoided. Throat swabs for group A streptococcus may be helpful in directing treatment.

Complications of untreated infection include peritonsillar abscess (quinsy), retropharyngeal abscess, and cervical abscess. Treat with appropriate antibiotics. Surgical drainage is occasionally required.

Laryngitis This is usually part of a generalized upper respiratory tract infection. *Moraxella catarrhalis* is the causative agent in up to 50%. It may cause a hoarse voice or aphonia.

Other causes include inhaled steroids, occupational exposure to inhaled chemicals, and gastro-oesophageal reflux disease. If a hoarse voice persists in a smoker, a laryngeal or lung cancer (with recurrent laryngeal nerve involvement) must be excluded. Other causes include tuberculous infection, HSV, CMV, diphtheria, fungal infections, and actinomycoses.

Treatment Usually no specific treatment is required, as the illness is typically self-limiting.

Acute bronchitis, tracheitis, and tracheobronchitis Inflammation due to infection can occur in any part of the tracheobronchial tree, and is termed tracheitis, tracheobronchitis, or bronchitis depending on the anatomical site. It usually follows viral infection, especially of the common cold type, and is commoner during influenza epidemics. Secondary bacterial infection is common, with *H. influenza* and *S. pneumoniae* commonest. There is increased prevalence in the winter months.

Presents with a productive cough, small volume streaky haemoptysis, and fever. Breathlessness and hypoxia are uncommon unless there is coexistent cardiorespiratory disease, or a concomitant pneumonia. Retrosternal chest pain is common in tracheitis. Examination is often normal.

Diagnosis is usually on the basis of the history. A persisting cough, especially in a smoker, may warrant further investigation.

Treatment is usually symptomatic, particularly in the previously well. Use antibiotics for persistent cough productive of mucopurulent sputum, or if there is coexistent cardiopulmonary disease.

Chapter 51

Vasculitis and the lung

Classification

These are rare conditions, but are often seen in the specialist chest clinic (see p 25 for an approach to diffuse alveolar haemorrhage). Clinical features can be non-specific and similar to those seen in other diseases and diagnosis can therefore be difficult. Vasculitides are great 'mimickers' of other diseases, such as lung cancer or ARDS, and have a high untreated mortality. There is considerable overlap between the different vasculitides, which can make definitive diagnosis difficult. Suspect a diagnosis of vasculitis if:

- Weight loss
- Low-grade fever
- Raised inflammatory markers
- Chest disease is not improving or responding to treatment as expected:
  - Unexplained dyspnoea
  - Hypoxia
  - Unexplained desaturation on exercise
  - Haemoptysis
  - Sinus or nasal disease
  - Wheeze
  - CXR abnormalities/infiltrates
  - Abnormal KCO
- Associated renal impairment or positive urine dip for blood or protein
- Raised autoantibodies
- No other clear diagnosis

The primary pathology in vasculitis is inflammation and necrosis of differing sized blood vessels. The pulmonary vessels are involved as part of a multi-systemic vasculitis process.

Small vessel vasculitides are the most common to involve the lung. Arterioles, capillaries, and venules located within the lung interstitium are affected. Neutrophil infiltration and subsequent fibrinoid necrosis causes vessel wall destruction. Necrotizing pulmonary capillaritis can also occur: characterized by a marked neutrophilic infiltration of the interstitium. Interstitial capillaries become damaged, allowing red blood cells to enter the alveolus; thus alveolar haemorrhage is a feature of many of the small vessel vasculitides.

Further information

Schwarz M, Brown K. Small vessel vasculitis of the lung. Rare diseases 10, *Thorax* 2000; **55**: 502–10

Table 51.1 Classification of vasculitis, based on the Chapel Hill International Consensus, 1992

Primary vasculitis	Lung involvement	ANCA
Small vessel		
Wegener's granulomatosis	Frequent	c-ANCA in 75%, p-ANCA in 15%
Churg–Strauss	Frequent	p-ANCA in 70%
Microscopic polyangiitis	Frequent	c/p-ANCA
Goodpasture's disease	Frequent	p-ANCA in 10–20%
Medium size vessel		
Polyarteritis nodosa	Rare	Negative
Large vessel		
Giant cell arteritis	Rare	Negative
Takayasu arteritis	Frequent	Negative

ANCA

Anti-neutrophil cytoplasmic antibodies react with cytoplasmic granule enzymes in neutrophils and stain them in one of two ways:

- Diffusely cytoplasmic pattern or **c-ANCA**
- Perinuclear pattern or **p-ANCA**

These autoantibodies may have a direct role in pathogenesis as well as being disease markers.
ANCA have 2 major specificities:

- Antiproteinase 3 antibodies (anti-PR3)—associated with c-ANCA pattern
- Antimyeloperoxidase antibodies (anti-MPO)—associated with p-ANCA pattern.

c-ANCA (anti-PR3) targets proteinase 3 and may suggest Wegener's granulomatosis (75% of cases are c-ANCA positive). Levels correlate with disease activity and extent. Also found in patients with microscopic polyangiitis (45% of those with clinical disease will be c-ANCA positive).
p-ANCA (anti-MPO) targets myeloperoxidase and has a wider range of disease associations, including other vasculitides and autoimmune diseases, HIV, lung cancer, pulmonary fibrosis, and pulmonary emboli.

Further information

Bosch X *et al.* ANCA. *Lancet* 2006; **368**: 404–18

Wegener's granulomatosis: presentation and diagnosis

Definition and epidemiology Necrotizing vasculitis affecting small and medium size vessels, especially in the upper and lower respiratory tract and also the kidneys. Associated granulomata.
- Unknown cause
- Male = female
- 3/100 000, 80–97% Caucasian
- Any age, but most common between 40 and 55 years

Clinical features
- **ENT** In 90%, upper airways involvement will be the first presenting sign. Nasal congestion and epistaxis, with inflamed crusty ulcerated nasal mucosa. Nasal septum perforation. Late sign is a saddle nose deformity. Sinusitis is common and may be painful. Otitis media. Subglottic stenosis, causing upper airway obstruction, dyspnoea, voice change, and cough. Abnormal flow–volume loops
- **Lung** Affected in 85–90% of patients. Haemoptysis, cough, dyspnoea. Pleuritic chest pain
- **Kidney** Affected in 77% of patients. Haematuria, proteinuria, and red cell casts. Only 10% have renal impairment initially, but 80% will have involvement during their disease course. Characteristic progressive deterioration of renal function
- **Systemic** Fever and weight loss
- **Other organ systems (skin, eyes, joints, CNS)** Vasculitic skin rash with granulomatous involvement in 46%. Muscle and joint pains. Conjunctivitis, scleritis, proptosis, eye pain, visual loss. Mononeuritis multiplex and CNS disease.

Investigations
Consider:
- ***CXR*** Flitting cavitating pulmonary nodules, consolidation, or pulmonary infiltrates, alveolar haemorrhage, parenchymal distortion, large and small airway disease, pleural effusion, bronchiectasis. Can look like neoplasms, infection, or fluid overload
- ***HRCT*** of chest
- ***Oxygen saturations***
- ***FBC, U&E, CRP, ESR***
- ***Serum ANCA***, especially c-ANCA, is sensitive and fairly specific. Present in 90% of patients with extensive Wegener's and 75% with limited. p-ANCA positive in 5–10% of patients with Wegener's. Combining indirect immunofluorescence with specific immunoassays for antibodies to PR3 and MPO increases sensitivity and specificity for Wegner's and microscopic polyangiitis to over 90%. **Remember ANCA can be negative, especially in disease confined to the respiratory tract.** ANCA titres rise prior to a relapse and are higher when disease is active, and this can act as a guide to starting treatment. However, high ANCA levels in the absence of clinical symptoms or signs may not represent active disease,

and therefore ANCA levels should not be used in isolation to determine treatment. Consider CRP ± ESR also

- ***Urine dipstick and microscopy*** Red cell casts
- ***Pulmonary function tests, including kCO***
- ***Image sinuses*** Bony destruction makes Wegener's likely
- ***Bronchoscopy*** May show inflammation and ulceration of larynx, trachea, and bronchi. Scarring and stenosis may be seen. BAL is neutrophilic, also with eosinophils and lymphocytes. Transbronchial biopsy is unlikely to be diagnostic
- ***Biopsy***
    - *Respiratory tract and nose*—granulomata in association with medium and small vessel necrotizing vasculitis and surrounding inflammation. Nasal biopsies are often non-specific and may not be diagnostic
    - *Renal biopsy*—focal segmental or diffuse necrotizing glomerulonephritis. Pauci-immune and granulomata rare. Not specific for Wegener's
    - *Skin biopsy*—leucocytoclastic vasculitis ± granulomata

Diagnosis Biopsy and ANCA are key to diagnosis. Biopsy whichever site is affected. May be nasal, lung (open or thoracoscopic), skin, or renal. If there is evidence on urine dip of renal vasculitis, this may be the best and easiest biopsy site. Disease may be patchy in nature, requiring repeat biopsies if the first is negative. High c-ANCA and anti-proteinase 3 (PR3) is highly suggestive of Wegener's.

Differential diagnosis of Wegener's granulomatosis

Malignancy, TB, sarcoidosis, allergic bronchopulmonary aspergillosis, Goodpasture's disease (anti-glomerular basement membrane disease with pulmonary haemorrhage and nephritis), SLE, microscopic polyangiitis, connective tissue disease.

Wegener's granulomatosis: management

Involve the renal team and share care of the patient. See p 675 for immunosuppressive drug details.

- Standard regimen for **generalized or organ-threatening disease** (e.g. active/progressive pulmonary or renal disease or CNS disease):
  - Induce remission with oral prednisolone (1 mg/kg/day, tapering weekly to a dose of 15 mg or less daily by 3 months) and cyclophosphamide orally (2 mg/kg/day, up to 200 mg/day) or IV (pulses at 2- or 3-week intervals, 15 mg/kg) for 3–6 months. Reduce cyclophosphamide dose in elderly (e.g. reduce oral dose by 25% if >60 years, and by 50% if over 75 years) and in setting of renal impairment. Taper cyclophosphamide dose to maintain WCC>4 × 10^9/L and neutrophils >2 × 10^9, to reduce infection risk (see p 679 for more detail)
  - The aim is to prevent irreversible tissue necrosis. There is evidence that this regime induces remission in 80% of patients at 3 months and 90% at 6 months
  - After induction of remission (at 3–6 months), consider switch from cyclophosphamide and prednisolone to maintenance therapy with prednisolone and either azathioprine (2 mg/kg/day for 12 months, then reduce to 1.5 mg/kg/day; check TPMT levels, p 678) or methotrexate (15 mg once/week, increase to maximum of 20–25 mg once/week by week 12; p 680). This avoids the morbidity associated with long-term cyclophosphamide use. Both azathioprine and methotrexate have been demonstrated to maintain remission, although the evidence favours use of azathioprine
  - Restart the regime if the patient relapses—this may occur in 50%
- For **severe life-threatening disease** (e.g. rapidly progressive renal failure or massive pulmonary haemorrhage):
  - Plasma exchange/plasmapheresis (7 x 4 L exchanges over 2 weeks) has been shown to be more effective than methylprednisolone in the treatment of Wegener's granulomatosis. In patients with severe pulmonary haemorrhage it is also effective and can be given along with fresh frozen plasma
  - In addition, treat with pulsed methylprednisolone (500–1000 mg/day depending on body weight for 3 days) and intravenous cyclophosphamide (15 mg/kg, reduce if elderly or renal impairment)
  - Dialysis for renal failure
  - After induction of remission (over 3–6 months), switch from cyclophosphamide to azathioprine or methotrexate with prednisolone as maintenance therapy
- For **localized disease or early systemic disease** (without threatened organ involvement):
  - Prednisolone with either methotrexate or oral/pulsed cyclophosphamide. Use of methotrexate avoids cyclophosphamide-related toxicity, but may be associated with a higher relapse rate. Localized disease may still be serious (e.g. retro-orbital involvement), and in these situations cyclophosphamide should be considered.

- **Duration of treatment** Maintenance therapy is recommended to continue for at least 24 months after initial disease remission, as relapses are common. Some recommend continuing treatment for up to 5 years, particularly if the ANCA remains positive
- PCP prophylaxis with co-trimoxazole is recommended (960 mg 3×/week) in patients receiving cyclophosphamide and prednisolone. There is some evidence that co-trimoxazole alone may be effective in the treatment of especially limited Wegener's, although the reasons for this are not clear—it may be due to suppression of nasal *Staphylococcus aureus* carriage, the presence of which is associated with an increased risk of relapse
- Osteoporosis prophylaxis should be considered
- **Follow-up** monthly for 3 months, then 3–6 monthly. Monitor FBC, U&E, CRP, LFT, ANCA, CXR, and kCO. Rising ANCA titres are a poor predictor of relapse; in the absence of other features of a relapse, follow up more closely, but do not increase immunosuppression solely on this basis. Withdrawal of immunosuppression in the setting of a persistently positive ANCA is associated with relapse, however
- **Relapses** Treat minor relapses with an increase in the prednisolone dose. Treat major relapses with cyclophosphamide and increasing prednisolone; consider IV methyprednisolone, plasma exchange
- **Refractory disease** Liaise with specialist; consider alternative therapies such as infliximab, high-dose IV immunoglobulin, rituximab, anti-thymocyte globulin, or CAMPATH 1H (alemtuzumab, anti-CD52). Mycophenolate or leflunomide are alternatives to azathioprine or methotrexate. Exclude underlying infection, malignancy, and non-compliance

Prognosis *Limited disease* with pulmonary but no renal involvement and an often negative c-ANCA test has a better prognosis. However, this can progress over time to *extensive disease*, with classical destructive sinusitis, nephritis, and vasculitis and strong c-ANCA positivity, and is associated with higher mortality. Untreated, 80% of people with extensive Wegener's will die in 1 year. Overall, 75–90% of patients can be brought into remission with treatment, although 50% relapse in 5 years and long-term follow-up is required.

Microscopic polyangiitis

At least as common as Wegener's and may be hard to distinguish. Managed in the same way.

- **Incidence** Male = female, mean age 50, mainly Caucasians
- **Kidneys** Main organ affected by a small vessel necrotizing vasculitis, causing proteinuria, and haematuria. Renal biopsy shows focal segmental glomerulonephritis with fibrinoid necrosis and sparse immune deposits
- **Pulmonary involvement** occurs in 30–50% of patients, with pleurisy, asthma, haemoptysis, and pulmonary haemorrhage. CXR may be suggestive of pulmonary haemorrhage
- **p-ANCA** positive, often c-ANCA also.

Treatment with immunosuppression: steroids and cyclophosphamide (see previous page).

Future developments

It had been thought that anti TNFα agents were likely to have a role in acute vasculitis and seemed to work best in granulomatous disease. A randomized controlled trial of etanercept plus standard therapy for Wegener's granulomatosis showed no significant effect on remission rates (*NEJM* 2005; **352**: 351–61). Further studies are ongoing of other anti-TNFα agents.

B-cell depletion with the monoclonal anti-CD20 antibody rituximab. This is used for non-Hodgkin's lymphoma, SLE, rheumatoid arthritis. Encouraging results in small studies of ANCA positive vasculitis, but no RCT as yet.

Mycophenolate for immunosupression in vasculitis to induce remission. Used post-transplant. A large study vs. azathioprine is underway.

Further information

Lapraik C *et al.* British Society of Rheumatology and British Heath Professionals in Rheumatology guidelines for the management of adults with ANCA associated vasculitis. *Rheumatology* 2007; **46**: 1615–16

Langford C, Hoffman G. Wegener's granulomatosis. Rare diseases 3, *Thorax* 1999; **54**: 629–63

Frankel SK *et al.* Update in the diagnosis and management of pulmonary vasculitis. *Chest* 2006; **129**: 452–65

Goodpasture's disease

Definition and epidemiology Linear deposition of IgG on the basement membranes of alveoli and glomeruli, which damages collagen and in the lungs allows leakage of blood.

- Anti-glomerular basement membrane antibodies are detectable in blood
- Alveolar haemorrhage and glomerulonephritis
- Important differential diagnosis of pulmonary–renal syndrome
- Annual incidence of 1 case per million
- Male:female = 4:1
- Commonest age 20–30 years
- Second peak when women in their late 60s are affected by glomerulonephritis alone
- Cause unknown. Often a preceding viral infection. Smokers at greater risk of pulmonary haemorrhage, but not of Goodpasture's disease
- HLA DR2 association in 60–70%.

Clinical features

- Haemoptysis in 80–90%—more common in smokers
- Cough, dyspnoea, fatigue, and weakness
- Examination: inspiratory crackles common.

Investigations

- ***Serum electrolytes*** show impaired renal function and often renal failure
- ***FBC*** Iron deficiency anaemia
- ***Urine dip and microscopy*** Haematuria, proteinuria, granular and typically red blood cell casts. Occasionally macroscopic haematuria
- ***Anti-GBM*** and autoantibody screen
- ***CXR ± CT*** Diffuse bilateral patchy air space shadowing in mid and lower zones. May see air bronchograms
- ***PFTs*** Restrictive defect with raised kCO if alveolar haemorrhage present.

Diagnosis Renal biopsy usually shows diffuse crescentic glomerulonephritis. Linear IgG deposition detected by immunofluorescence or immunoperoxidase. Lung biopsy shows active intra-alveolar haemorrhage with collections of haemosiderin laden macrophages. These are not specific changes, but may also show linear immunofluorescence staining of IgG.

Differential diagnosis Wegener's granulomatosis, other pulmonary renal syndromes.

Management

- Involve the renal team and share care of the patient
- Plasma exchange improves the speed of response to immunosuppression
- High-dose steroids and cyclophosphamide
- May need dialysis. Renal function may not improve and renal transplant is only an option later if anti-GBM antibody levels become low
- Recurrence is uncommon once disease is controlled. It usually responds to further immunosuppression. Residual defects in PFTs frequent.

Prognosis Rapidly progressive pulmonary haemorrhage and renal failure. Usually fatal if not treated.

Churg–Strauss syndrome

Definition and epidemiology Asthma, blood eosinophilia, and an eosinophilic granulomatous inflammation of the respiratory tract, with necrotizing vasculitis affecting small and medium sized vessels.

- Rare, 2.4 per million population, but 64 per million of an asthmatic population (who may have been misdiagnosed with asthma)
- Middle-aged adults
- 2 male:1 female
- Unknown cause. Montelukast was postulated as a possible cause, but this is now thought unlikely. Development of Churg–Strauss syndrome in people on montelukast probably related to their decreased steroid dose 'unmasking' Churg–Strauss syndrome, or as part of an increasing treatment regime in those with uncontrolled asthma, later diagnosed as Churg Strauss syndrome.

Clinical features A diagnosis of Churg–Strauss syndrome can be made if 4 of the following 6 criteria are present:

- Asthma—may have had for years, often maturity onset, difficult to control, associated with rhinitis and nasal polyps
- Blood eosinophilia >10%
- Vasculitic neuropathy, such as mononeuritis multiplex (occurs in 75%)
- Pulmonary infiltrates
- Sinus disease
- Extravascular eosinophils on biopsy findings.

(American College of Rheumatology criteria, 1990)

- Also may have:
  - Myositis and cardiac failure, cardiomyopathy, coronary artery inflammation, pericardial effusion
  - Eosinophilic infiltration of mesenteric vessels causing GI disturbance
  - Alveolar haemorrhage
  - Rarely, proteinuria caused by renal disease with focal segmental glomerulonephritis. Renal failure is rare
  - Skin nodules and purpura
  - Myalgia and arthralgia
  - Fever and weight loss.

Typical pattern of disease has three phases: beginning with asthma, then developing blood and tissue eosinophilia, then going on to systemic vasculitis. The asthma precedes the vasculitis, often by years (mean 8 years).

Investigations

- ***CXR*** Fleeting peripheral pulmonary infiltrates and bilateral multifocal consolidation
- ***HRCT*** Ground-glass inflammation, pulmonary nodules, bronchial wall thickening, or alveolar haemorrhage
- ***Bronchoscopy*** BAL: marked eosinophilia
- ***Pathology*** Extravascular tissue eosinophilia, necrotizing angiitis, granulomata
- ***Serum markers*** Peripheral blood eosinophilia. p-ANCA and anti-MPO positive in two-thirds. ANCA levels may not correlate with disease activity, but blood eosinophilia is a good guide.

Diagnosis Predominantly a clinical diagnosis. Pathological confirmation of eosinophilic tissue infiltration or vasculitis desirable. Biopsy easiest site affected, such as skin, kidney, or open or thoracoscopic lung biopsy.

Differential diagnosis Allergic bronchopulmonary aspergillosis, sarcoidosis, drug and parasitic causes of eosinophilic pneumonias, hypersensitivity pneumonitis, hypereosinophilic syndrome.

Management Depends on severity of disease at presentation.

- ***If isolated pulmonary disease***, oral prednisolone 1 mg/kg (max 60 mg/day) for 1 month or until no evidence of disease, then slowly decrease over 1 year, with increases if symptoms recur
- ***If unwell, or with alveolar haemorrhage***, pulsed methylprednisolone IV for 3 days, followed by high-dose oral steroids, with or without cyclophosphamide (see p 678 and 680)
- ***In cardiac or GI disease, relapse, or life-threatening situations***, such as requiring organ support, cyclophosphamide should be added (see p 680)
- Plasma exchange is of no benefit
- Treatment is aimed at reversing organ damage and reducing relapse rate
- ***To maintain remission***, prednisolone and one other immunosuppressant drug are usually required. Cyclophosphamide is often changed to azathioprine after 4–6 months
- Prophylactic co-trimoxazole should be given (960 mg 3×/week) and consider bone protection for steroids
- ***Follow-up***: regularly, with checks on FBC and eosinophil count, CXR.

Prognosis Good prognosis if isolated pulmonary disease. Good response to steroids. May continue to have asthma despite control of vasculitis, which can be severe and difficult to control. Poor prognosis associated with cardiac disease and severe gastrointestinal disease, causing bleeding, perforation, or necrosis. Untreated, 5-year survival rate is 25%. Also associated with worse prognosis: proteinuria >1 g/24 h, renal insufficiency, CNS involvement. Cardiac disease is the main cause of death.

Further information

Noth I *et al.* Churg–Strauss syndrome. *Lancet* 2003; **361**: 587–94

www.vasculitis.org

Rare pulmonary vasculitides

Polyarteritis nodosa

- Similar to microscopic polyangiitis, but affects medium-sized vessels
- May exist as an 'overlap' disorder with Wegener's or Churg–Strauss
- Lung involvement is rare
- Sometimes associated with previous hepatitis B or rarely hepatitis C infection.

Takayasu's arteritis

- Predominantly young women, often Asian
- Vasculitis affecting the aorta and its major branches. Large and medium-sized pulmonary vessels affected, but involvement is usually silent. Pulmonary artery stenosis and occlusion common, occasionally with mild pulmonary hypertension
- **Presents** with fevers and weight loss. Absent or weak upper limb peripheral pulses, particularly on left (as left axillary artery comes off aortic arch) and arterial bruits
- **Diagnosis** made by angiography
- **Treatment** Steroids may reduce symptoms, but do not affect mortality. Angioplasty and surgical procedures may reduce the complications. Spontaneous remissions may occur.

Giant cell arteritis

- Commonest form of systemic vasculitis affecting large- and medium-sized vessels
- 24 cases per 100 000. Predominantly elderly females
- **Presents with** non-specific symptoms of fever and weight loss, also headache, scalp tenderness, and jaw pain. Amaurosis fugax and visual loss due to optic neuritis
- **Pulmonary complications** occur in 9–25% of cases. They are relatively minor, with cough, sore throat, and hoarseness. Pulmonary function tests and CXR normal
- **Diagnosis** High ESR, temporal artery biopsy showing pan-arteritis and giant cell formation
- **Treatment** Good response to oral steroids. Continue for 1–2 years.

Part 3

Supportive care

Chapter 52
Ethical issues

Background

Most ethical issues faced by doctors arise at the end of a patient's life. This particularly applies to respiratory physicians, where difficult decisions about the appropriateness of treatment and the prolongation of life in patients with chronic underlying lung disease may need to be made. In some situations artificial ventilation may prolong the dying process; life has a natural end and the potential to prolong life in the intensive care unit can sometimes cause dilemmas.

The General Medical Council (GMC) states that doctors have an obligation to respect human life, protect the health of their patients, and put their patients' best interests first. This means offering treatments where the benefits outweigh any risks, and avoiding treatments that carry no net gain to the patient. If a patient wishes to have a treatment that in the doctor's considered view is not indicated, the doctor and medical team are under no ethical or legal obligation to provide it, but the patient's right to a second opinion must be respected.

The discussion about resuscitation and formal ventilation is never an easy one, but should ideally be taken with nursing staff, the patient, and their next of kin, in advance of an emergency situation. In practical terms, clearly this is not always possible. Ideally all decisions regarding resuscitation and the ceiling of treatment (particularly relating to ventilation) should be documented in advance, and handed over to the on-call team. Most possible outcomes can be anticipated.

Where it has been decided that a treatment is not in the best interests of the patient, there is no ethical distinction between stopping the treatment, or not starting it in the first place (though the former may be more difficult to do), and this should not be used as an argument for failing to initiate the treatment in the first place.

Some clinical scenarios are more commonly encountered by the respiratory physician. These are discussed on the next pages.

COPD

COPD is the 4th commonest cause of death in America, and most patients die of respiratory failure during an exacerbation. A commonly encountered clinical situation is where a patient with COPD is admitted with an exacerbation, and is in type II respiratory failure. Standard treatment does not improve the respiratory acidosis, so non-invasive ventilation is commenced. Before starting NIV, a decision must be clearly documented as to whether or not NIV is the ceiling of treatment. It may be, especially if the patient has severe or end-stage COPD.

Formal ventilation in the intensive care unit may be appropriate in certain specific situations; for example:

- In a relatively young patient (i.e. <65 years)
- A patient with a relatively new diagnosis of COPD, in whom the episode is the first or second admission
- In the patient in whom there is a very obviously potentially reversible cause for the exacerbation, e.g. pneumonia

Sometimes in this situation, a defined time period for intensive care input may be decided, e.g. ventilation for 48 h (to allow treatments to work and to allow time to assess for any improvement), with extubation after that time period if no improvement has been made.

Decisions about formal ventilation and intensive care admission can only be made with knowledge of the patient's usual level of functioning and previous quality of life. The difficulty in this situation is that quality of life is a very subjective measure. Objective measures of usual functioning, such as measures of daily activity, usual exercise tolerance, and whether home care or assistance with activities of daily living is required are more useful in guiding the appropriateness of escalating therapy. With particular reference to the patient with COPD, the number of hospital admissions and exacerbations, and the need for home oxygen or nebulizers will also be useful. Helpful information may be obtained from the GP, especially if the previous hospital notes are unavailable.

Neither the next of kin nor those with Enduring Power of Attorney (EPA) have the legal right to determine any treatment; the responsibility remains with the doctor and multidisciplinary team, occasionally involving the courts of law. Lasting Power of Attorney (LPA) replaced EPA from October 07. This allows an appointed attorney to make decisions about personal welfare, including giving or refusing consent to treatment, if the patient loses their capacity.

Where limited information is available about the patient and therefore uncertainty exists about the appropriateness of ventilation, it should be started until a clearer assessment can be made. This may be relevant for a patient attending the accident and emergency department, in whom little information is available. The above point concerning the withdrawal of therapy, should it subsequently be found to be inappropriate, also holds.

There are downsides to invasive ventilation: the risk of pneumothorax is increased in those with end-stage emphysema, and the risk of ventilator-acquired pneumonia increases with time ventilated. Knowledge of the risk of these adverse events helps the medical team to balance the argument and make a decision about whether the risks of ventilation are likely to outweigh its benefits. The issue of limited resources should not influence a decision about formal ventilation or ITU admission.

The average length of intubation of patients with COPD admitted to ITU is 3.2 days. These patients have a 20–25% in-hospital mortality, with 50% of patients surviving 1 year post-ITU discharge. About 50% will be living independently 1 year post-hospital discharge. Clearly, only a very selected subgroup of patients are admitted to ITU, but concerns about prolonged periods of ventilation in this group of patients seem to be unfounded. Patients in whom a clear cause for the exacerbation can be identified (e.g. pneumonia) tend to do better, as there is a treatable cause for the exacerbation and not just progression of the underlying disease.

Lung cancer and neurological disease

Lung cancer The use of antibiotic treatment for pneumonia in a patient with advanced lung malignancy may be inappropriate in some circumstances. The stage and extent of disease, response to other treatments (e.g. chemotherapy), and the patient's wishes and quality of life are all paramount. This is another situation in which it might be appropriate to define at the outset the treatments that are appropriate, e.g. 10 days total of intravenous and oral antibiotics. Note that treatments such as antibiotics can lead to improvement in symptoms (e.g. by reducing fever), without necessarily prolonging life, and it may be kinder to continue antibiotics in this situation.

Progressive neurological disease The decision about non-invasive ventilation in a patient with a progressive neuromuscular disease can be difficult. In this setting the clinical deterioration can usually be anticipated, and in most situations, discussion should have taken place early on (unless the patient presents in respiratory failure, for example, due to pneumonia, and subsequent ventilator weaning is difficult). Different centres, patients, and their relatives will have differing views as to whether life-prolonging non-invasive ventilation in the face of progressive neuromuscular disability is warranted. Some centres take the view that if the quality of life and higher mental functioning are good, and the respiratory muscles are affected early on (and other functions and mobility remain good), then NIV is warranted. Further decisions about withdrawal of treatment with progression of the underlying neurological disease of course will still be needed. In, for example, motor neurone disease with bulbar palsy, aspiration is a relative contraindication to non-invasive/mask ventilation. Aspiration in these patients is a poor prognostic sign, and often a sign of imminent death.

Advance directive documents the patient's wishes in the event of serious illness. It will usually include a decision about resuscitation and other potential life-prolonging treatments. The patient must understand the implications of his/her decision.

Further information

Withholding and withdrawing life-prolonging treatments: good practice in decision-making. General Medical Council 2002

Chapter 53

Financial entitlements

Patient financial entitlements

Patients with chronic lung disease and their carers may be eligible for financial support. There are a large number of potential benefits that can be claimed, and the process is often time-consuming and complicated. The best sources of information are:

- Benefits Enquiry Line 0800 882200 (0800 220674 in Northern Ireland)
- Website www.dwp.gov.uk. Forms can be completed on-line
- The Citizens Advice Bureau www.nacab.org.uk
- The ward social worker is usually a good source of information

Patients who are unable to work may be eligible for:

Statutory sick pay (SSP) A doctor's certificate is usually required for more than 1 week's sick pay. New rules now make the doctor's certificate the responsibility of the hospital consultant under whom the patient was admitted, and it should be completed on discharge, to cover the advised period off work. This also applies to patients needing time off work, but not admitted to hospital. Nursing staff usually complete the forms for the period during which the patient was in hospital.

Incapacity benefit is more complicated and is paid to people not eligible for SSP. It runs for up to a year. After 196 days (the first period is usually covered by a medical certificate) the patient may have to pass a personal capability assessment to show they are incapable of work.

Severe disablement allowance

Income-related benefit

Benefit for the extra cost of disability

Disabled persons tax credit (DPTC) This is not a benefit as such, but a tax credit from the Inland Revenue (paid in addition to benefits).

Severe disablement allowance if a test of 80% disablement is passed.

Disability living allowance or attendance allowance are benefits for the extra costs of disability and depend on age (>or <65 years)

Costs for care needs and mobility needs

Industrial diseases disablement benefit. See pneumoconiosis p 363 and asbestosis p 118.

Reduced earning allowance

Form DS1500, the 'special rules form', is for more urgent benefits for patients with terminal disease, in whom life expectancy is not likely to exceed 6 months. Patients with a terminal illness can also usually claim attendance allowance, incapacity benefit, and disabled living allowance under 'special rules'. This means that the claim is processed as a priority, with no qualifying period, allowing higher rates of payment, and without the individual having to prove how much care is needed. The application can be made on behalf of the patient, who does not have to sign the form. This may be appropriate if the patient has not been told the exact details of their life expectancy.

Further information

There are a number of charities who give grants/aid towards the cost of buying equipment.
www.charitiesdirect.com
www.charity-commission.gov.uk

Chapter 54

Immunosuppressive drugs

Patient advice and monitoring

Immunosuppressive drugs are used mainly in the management of pulmonary vasculitis, but also in asthma, sarcoidosis, and interstitial lung diseases. Centres differ in their use of these drugs and local guidelines are often available.

General advice for patients on immunosuppressive drugs

- Increased risk of infections and increased likelihood of severe infections. Check FBC if develop febrile illness
- May have atypical presentation of infections
- Avoid live vaccines, such as measles, mumps, rubella, BCG, yellow fever, oral typhoid, oral polio
- If never had varicella zoster:
  - Avoid contacts with chickenpox or shingles
  - Consider passive immunization
  - Immunoglobulin therapy if exposed
  - Hospital treatment with close monitoring if develop chickenpox
- Avoid measles exposure. Prophylaxis with immunoglobulins if exposed.

Table 54.1 Summary of tests to perform before and during immunosuppressive drug treatment

Drug	Check before starting	Follow-up
Corticosteroids	BP, glucose. Consider bones/osteoporosis	BP, glucose if symptoms of diabetes
Azathioprine	FBC, LFT, TMPT test (see text)	FBC every 2 weeks for 3 months, then monthly LFT monthly
Methotrexate	FBC, U&E, LFT CXR Folic acid	Bloods every 2 weeks for 3 months, then monthly
Cyclophosphamide	FBC, U&E, LFT Urine dip Semen store	Check all every week for 1 month, then every 2 months

Corticosteroids and azathioprine

Corticosteroids

- First-line treatment for suppressing inflammation. At high doses, also cause immunosuppression. Ineffective as sole therapy for induction of remission in systemic vasculitis
- IV methylprednisolone (500–1000 mg/day) for 3–5 days can be used for aggressive induction of remission, e.g. Wegener's granulomatosis, followed by maintenance oral steroids (prednisolone 30–40 mg/day)
- Usually taken in the morning as they may disturb sleep
- Dose should be slowly reduced when control of the disease is achieved. Gastric and bone protection may be necessary as the patient will be on high doses for some months. Also ensure BP and glucose are controlled
- Ensure patients have steroid treatment card.

Side-effects include skin and hair thinning, obesity, cataracts, diabetes, and aseptic bone necrosis. Inform patient of these and document. PCP infection can occur secondary to steroid treatment, particularly with high doses for prolonged periods. Some centres use PCP prophylaxis.

Steroids and osteoporosis

Current guidelines suggest patients being started on long-term steroids, with one other osteoporosis risk factor (such as being over 65 or having had a previous osteoporotic fracture), should also start on a bisphosphonate.

In other patients who will be on 7.5mg/day or more for more than 3 months, consider checking bone mineral density via DEXA scan of hip and spine, and offer lifestyle advice and bisphosphonates if this is reduced (T score –1.5 or lower).

(see Royal College of Physicians guidelines, www.rcplondon.ac.uk and National Osteoporosis Society, www.nos.org.uk)

Azathioprine

- Mainly used as a steroid-sparing agent, or when vasculitis is under control to enable cyclophosphamide to be stopped. Takes approx. 4 weeks to work
- Cytotoxic drug, less effective than cyclophosphamide. May be reasonable alternative if side-effects of cyclophosphamide are unacceptable
- Maximal effect on disease may not be evident for 6–9 months, but can be used long term
- TPMT (thiopurine methyltransferase) testing should be performed prior to commencement. TPMT breaks down azathioprine to an inactive product. 90% of the population have normal TPMT levels, 10% have intermediate activity, so azathioprine should be given with caution; 0.3% have no TPMT activity and azathioprine should be avoided

- For vasculitis, start with 2 mg per kg/day after cyclophosphamide. Maximum dose usually around 150–200 mg/day
- As steroid sparing regime: could start 50 mg od for 2 weeks, increasing to 100 mg od for 2 weeks, if FBC satisfactory and increasing to 150mg od (or 75mg bd) after further 2 weeks FBC satisfactory. Reduce prednisolone by 5 mg every 4 weeks
- **Check FBC** every 2 weeks for 6 weeks, then at 2 and 4 weeks after each dose increase and thereafter monthly. **Check LFTs** monthly. Stop treatment if WCC <3, platelets <100, or ALP and transaminases 3× normal. Restart when they recover.

Side-effects include sore mouth, ulcers, nausea and vomiting, diarrhoea, skin rash, alopecia (rare). Most respond to stopping the drug and restarting at a lower dose. Interacts with allopurinol and leads to increased toxicity.

Methotrexate and cyclophosphamide

Methotrexate

- Can be used as a second-line treatment
- Dose: 7.5–25 mg once/week. Usual starting dose is 10 mg. Can increase after 6 weeks to 15 mg, in increments of 2.5 mg weekly
- Baseline CXR. Monitor FBC, U&E, and LFTs every 2 weeks for 3 months then monthly. Give folic acid 5 mg 3–4 days after dose, to reduce toxicity.

Side-effects include mouth ulcers, skin rashes, nausea, macrocytosis, myelosuppression, pneumonitis (dyspnoea and dry cough). Avoid if significant renal or hepatic impairment, or if pleural effusions or ascites, as it can accumulate in these fluids. Stop if WCC <3, platelets <100, transaminases 3× normal, pneumonitis.

Cyclophosphamide

- The primary cytotoxic drug used for treating systemic vasculitis
- Causes immunosuppression without anti-inflammatory effects
- Used particularly if there are life- or organ-threatening features, e.g. ventilation for lung vasculitis, systemic features, renal involvement
- Takes 12–14 days to work; hence is combined with high-dose steroids at the beginning of treatment. When combined with steroids, it induces remission of vasculitis in 90% of patients
- Perform a baseline urine dip for blood prior to treatment (although note microscopic haematuria is common with active vasculitis). Check routinely for macroscopic haematuria in patients receiving IV cyclophosphamide and, if it is present, stop drug and arrange cystoscopy (rare if mesna is used, and rare with oral cyclophosphamide regimes)
- PCP prophylaxis with co-trimoxazole is recommended (960 mg 3×/week) in patients receiving cyclophosphamide and prednisolone
- Semen storage for men prior to starting treatment.

Usual treatment duration of cyclophosphamide is 3–6 months. Courses longer than 6 months should generally be avoided; they are no more effective and carry the risk of side-effects from the cumulative dose. Induce remission with cyclophosphamide and prednisolone and maintain remission with prednisolone and another immunosuppressant (azathioprine, or methotrexate) for at least 2 years.

Side-effects Haemorrhagic cystitis is a potentially serious side-effect of cyclophosphamide therapy. Risk of bladder cancer is increased (and is greater with increasing cumulative dose), and indefinite monitoring of urinalysis 3–6-monthly after treatment with cyclophosphamide is recommended. Other side-effects include nausea, vomiting, infection (including PCP), hair thinning or alopecia, bone marrow suppression (2%), leucopenia, infertility, lymphoma (0.7%) and leukaemia, pulmonary and bladder fibrosis. Risk of cervical cancer may be higher—recommend annual cervical smear for 3 years, and thereafter as per population screening programme.

Cyclophosphamide regimes

Oral cyclophosphamide is used if possible in active vasculitis, at a dose of 2 mg/kg (up to 200 mg/day). Reduce dose in elderly (by 25% if >60 years, and by 50% if over 75 years) and in setting of renal impairment

Monitoring Check FBC and renal function weekly for the first month, 2-weekly for the 2nd and 3rd month, and monthly thereafter.

- If WCC $<4 \times 10^9$/L, neutrophils $<2 \times 10^9$/L, stop oral cyclophosphamide and restart with dose reduced by at least 25 mg when WCC recovered, and then monitor weekly for 4 weeks
- If prolonged (WCC $<4 \times 10^9$/L, neutrophils $<2 \times 10^9$/L for >2 weeks) or severe (WCC $<1 \times 10^9$/L, neutrophils $<0.5 \times 10^9$/L) leucopenia/neutropenia, stop cyclophosphamide and restart at 50 mg daily when WCC recovered; then increase to target dose weekly, WCC permitting
- If WCC is falling ($<6 \times 10^9$/L and fall of $>2 \times 10^9$/L since previous count), reduce dose by 25%.

Pulsed intravenous cyclophosphamide is given if patients cannot take oral preparations, using doses of 15 mg/kg (reduced for age and renal function, maximum dose 1500 mg) every 2 weeks for the first 3 pulses and then at 3-weekly intervals. The lowest white cell count occurs 10 days after a pulse. A randomized study has shown that pulsed doses give a lower cumulative dose than oral regimes, but there is no difference in remission rates between the two. The infection rate is higher with oral regimes (European Vasculitis Study Group).

If giving IV cyclophosphamide, patients should be well hydrated before (1 L normal saline) and after (3 L/day oral fluids for 3 days), and given mesna, which chelates with the urotoxic cyclophosphamide metabolite, acrolein. Dose varies according to the cyclophosphamide dose and is available on product literature. Give during cyclophosphamide infusion, and also 4 and 8 h after. Prescribe anti-emetics.

Monitoring Check FBC and renal function on day of pulse or previous day.

- If WCC $<4 \times 10^9$/L, neutrophils $<2 \times 10^9$/L, postpone pulse until WCC $>4 \times 10^9$/L, neutrophils $>2 \times 10^9$/L, whilst checking FBC weekly, and reduce dose by 25%
- After first pulse, check FBC between days 10 and day of next pulse: reduce dose of next pulse by 40% of previous dose if WCC nadir $1–2 \times 10^9$/L or neutrophil nadir $0.5–1.0 \times 10^9$/L
- Reduce dose of next pulse by 20% of previous dose if WCC nadir $2–3 \times 10^9$/L or neutrophil nadir $1–1.5 \times 10^9$/L
- Thereafter check FBC on day of pulse or previous day, unless dose adjustment when checked additionally at day 10.

Further information

Lapraik C *et al.* British Society of Rheumatology and British Heath Professionals in Rheumatology guidelines for the management of adults with ANCA associated vasculitis. *Rheumatology* 2007; **46**: 1615–16

Chapter 55

Inhalers and nebulizers

Background

Inhalers

- There are many different inhaler devices that deliver drugs directly to the airways
- Ideally patients should try a range of devices to choose the most appropriate for them
- Patients should receive advice on techniques for inhaler use. Technique should be checked regularly, and if patients cannot manage a particular device, they should be switched to another
- The percentage of a drug delivered to the airway varies for each device (from 15% to 60% according to the manufacturers) and depends on good technique
- Spacer devices improve this delivery and are particularly useful for the elderly, children, and those who find it difficult to coordinate inhaler administration with breathing
- Try to use the same inhaler device for all the drug classes used by a patient
- Advise the patient how to recognize when a device is empty: some have dose counters; others are shaken to hear if they still have contents
- Titrate inhaler doses with clinical response.

Nebulizers are used by patients who gain greater relief from nebulized therapy than from inhaled therapy. This may be during acute respiratory illnesses, because of disease severity, or because they are unable to use inhalers. Patients who are being considered for nebulizer therapy should be referred to a respiratory physician. If antibiotics are being nebulized, a more powerful nebulizer is required.

How to use Open the ampoule containing the drug solution and squirt the solution into the nebulizer chamber. Salbutamol and ipratropium bromide can be taken together, but nebulized budesonide or antibiotics should be used separately. If ipratropium bromide only is being used, this should be delivered via a mouthpiece, as it can lead to glaucoma if used via a mask. Reattach the chamber to the nebulizer mask or mouthpiece. Put the mask over nose and mouth, or position mouthpiece between the lips in the mouth. Switch the nebulizer machine on. Breathe slowly in and out. Continue until all the solution is gone. Switch off the machine. Rinse the nebulizer chamber with hot soapy water after each use. If nebulization takes more than 10 min, change the neb-set (mask, chamber, tubing—lasts 1–3 months). If no improvement, consider servicing the machine. If the patient is using oxygen, this can still be used during nebulization, either via nasal prongs under the nebulizer mask or by using oxygen tubing attached directly to the nebulizer chamber to drive the nebulization; at home most cylinders do not provide sufficient flow rates to allow this. Nebulizer machines should be serviced annually.

Different inhaler types and instructions for their use

Table 55.1 Different inhaler types

Generic name of drug (with product names)	Mechanism of action	Inhaler colour
Salbutamol (Ventolin®, Asmasal®, Pulvinal®, Salbutamol, Salamol®, Salbutamol Cyclocaps®, Airomir®, Asmasal Clickhaler®, Salamol Easi-Breathe®) **Terbutaline** (Bricanyl®)	Short-acting β_2 agonist Duration 3–5 h	Blue
Salmeterol (Serevent®) **Formoterol** (Foradil®, Oxis®, Atimos Modulite®)	Long-acting β_2 agonist Duration 12 h	Green Green/turquoise
Ipratropium bromide (Atrovent®) **Ipratropium and salbutamol** (Combivent®)	Short-acting anticholinergic	White/grey
Tiotropium (Spiriva®)	Long-acting anticholinergic	Grey Handihaler®, Respimat®
Beclometasone dipropionate (Becotide®, Becloforte®, Pulvinal®, Beclometasone, Beclomethasone Cyclocaps®, AeroBec®, AerobecForte®, Asmabec Clickhaler®, Beclazone Easi-Breathe®, Qvar®) **Budesonide** (Pulmicort®, Budesonide Cyclocaps®, Novolizer®) **Fluticasone propionate** (Flixotide®) **Mometasone furoate** (Asmanex®) **Ciclesonide** (Alvesco®)	Corticosteroid	Brown Brown Red Red Red
Salmeterol and fluticasone (Seretide®) **Eformoterol and budesonide** (Symbicort®)	Combination steroid and bronchodilator	Purple Red and white
Sodium cromoglicate (Intal®, Cromogen Easi-Breathe®) **Neocromil sodium** (Tilade®)	Unknown, stabilize mast cells	Yellow and white

Table 55.2 Instructions for use of different inhaler types

Type of device	Instructions for use
Pressurized aerosol metered dose inhaler (MDI) Aerosol Evohaler®	Remove the mouthpiece and shake the inhaler well. Hold the inhaler upright with the thumb on the base below the mouthpiece and the first finger on the metal canister. Breathe out as far as is comfortable then place the mouth piece between the teeth and close lips around it. Do not bite it. As you start to breathe in through the mouth, press on the top of the inhaler to release the medication whilst still breathing in steadily and deeply. Hold your breath, take the inhaler from your mouth, and continue holding your breath for up to 10 s if possible. Wait 30 s prior to taking second puff. Use with spacer device to improve drug delivery. CFC-free inhalers need washing every 2–3 weeks, as they can block.
Spacer Nebuhaler® Nebuchamber® Volumatic® Aero Chamber® Able Spacer® PARI Vortex Spacer®, Pocket Chamber® OptiChamber® OptiHaler®	Ensure spacer is compatible with patient's inhaler. Remove cap of inhaler and shake it. Insert it into end of spacer device. Place the other end of the spacer in the mouth. Press the inhaler canister once to release one dose of the drug. Take one deep breath in and hold, or take 3–4 steady breaths in and out. Repeat as indicated. Valve should rattle. Clean the spacer once a month with mild detergent, rinse, and air-dry. Replace after 6–12 months.
Breath-actuated devices Autohaler® Easi-breathe®	If an autohaler, remove the cap and lift the red lever. Insert device into mouth. Inhale slowly and deeply. Continue inhaling when the device 'clicks'. Hold breath for up to 10 s if possible. Slowly breathe out. To take a second inhaled dose, lower the red lever and lift again. If an Easi-breathe, open the hinged cap. Insert device into mouth. Inhale slowly and deeply. Continue inhaling when the device 'clicks'. Hold breath for up to 10 s if possible. Slowly breathe out. Close the cap and reopen for further doses. If Easi-breathe spacer used, it will need to be removed between each inhalation so that cap can be opened and closed.
Dry powder devices Accuhaler® Turbohaler® Clickhaler® Twisthaler Easyhaler® Cyclohaler® Aerocaps® Spincaps® Novolizer®	Prime the device. ***Turbohaler***: hold upright, remove the cap, twist the base as far as possible until the click is heard and then twist back again. ***Clickhaler***: shake the device, remove the cap, click the top down and release. ***Twisthaler***: remove the cap by twisting and the dose is then ready. ***Accuhaler***: Open inhaler cover, mouthpiece facing you and push lever down to pierce the blister containing dose. ***Diskhaler***: insert disc into device by opening and pulling out mouthpiece section. To prepare dose, lift up back of lid to 90° until the blister is pierced, then lower the lid. To use all the devices, hold them level, exhale fully, place the mouthpiece into mouth between teeth, and inhale steadily. Hold your breath and remove the inhaler. For a second dose, repeat the above actions.

Table 55.2 Instructions for use of different inhaler types—(contd.)

Type of device	Instructions for use
Handihaler®	Flip lid and white mouthpiece open and insert capsule. Close the mouthpiece back down until it clicks. Pierce the capsule by pressing the green button at the side. Exhale as far as is comfortable. Place mouthpiece into mouth and breathe in slowly and deeply. Remove inhaler from your mouth and hold your breath for 10 s if possible. Slowly breathe out. Repeat if necessary to ensure all the powder from capsule is gone.
Respimat®	Hold inhaler upright with cap closed. Turn the transparent base until it clicks. Open the cap. Breathe out slowly and insert the mouthpiece and seal with lips. Point towards the back of the throat. While taking a deep breath, press the button and continue to breathe. Hold your breath for 10 s if possible and breathe out slowly.

Chapter 56

Intensive therapy unit (ITU): when to involve

Ideally communicate with ITU early, as it is much better that they know about a potentially sick patient who may need ITU input, than to find your patient (and you!) in difficulty later on, with no ITU bed.

Scoring systems for the early recognition of sick patients are in use in many hospitals, enabling doctors and nursing staff to readily identify and assess a deteriorating patient. An example is shown on the opposite page.

The common situations in which ITU input may be required in relation to respiratory disease are principally those relating to decisions about formal ventilation. Most commonly these will be:

- Respiratory failure (either type I or type II)
  - Exacerbation of COPD (usually type II failure). Patients with COPD admitted to ITU have a hospital mortality of 20–25%. Poor prognostic factors include low baseline FEV_1, long-term oxygen use, low sodium and albumin, low BMI, poor functional status, and comorbid disease. Age does not add prognostic information
  - Pneumonia (to maintain an adequate pO_2—usually type I failure). In this situation, ITU input may not necessarily lead to intubation, as adequate oxygenation may be achieved by the proper use of a non-rebreathable mask or CPAP, with the additional benefits of one-to-one nursing. Altered mental state and difficulty clearing secretions may make invasive ventilation necessary
- Upper airway emergencies
- ≥1 organ failure (not necessarily with respiratory failure)
- Sepsis requiring organ support
- Inotropic support.

PAR (patient at risk) scoring system

This is an example of a ward-based patient illness severity scoring system. It is used to assist medical and nursing staff in the early identification of sick patients, to enable prompt and appropriate HDU/ITU liaison.

Table 56.1 Scoring systems for the early recognition of sick patients

Score	**3**	**2**	**1**	**0**	**1**	**2**	**3**
Heart rate/min		≤40	41–50	51–100	101–110	111–130	≥131
SBP	≤70	71–80	80–100	101–199		≥200	
Resp rate/min		≤8		9–14	15–20	21–29	≥ 30
Temp/°C		≤35				≥39.5	
Conscious level				Alert	Drowsy/ confused	Painful stimuli	Unres- ponsive
Urine output					<60 mL/2 h	<40 mL/2 h	0 mL

Calculate the PAR score by the addition of the scores in each column.
Total score 1–3: increase observations to 4-hourly.
Total score 3 in one category: contact doctor for immediate review.
Total score total ≥3: contact doctor for review within 30 min. SHO should consider senior review.
Total score >6: patient needs immediate review, contact ITU outreach team if appropriate.
Respiratory rate is the most sensitive marker of illness severity

Chapter 57

Non-invasive ventilation

Terminology

Ventilatory support may be invasive (via endotracheal tube or tracheostomy) or non-invasive (via nose mask or face mask). Non-invasive ventilation may be subdivided into positive or negative pressure ventilation.

Positive pressure ventilators (also NIV, bi-level, BiPAP (trade name)) deliver volume or pressure support; many different types are available. Bi-level pressure support devices are used extensively, and provide pressure support between inspiratory and expiratory positive airway pressures (IPAP and EPAP) that are selected by the prescriber. They function in several modes, including patient-triggered inspiratory support with provision of an underlying back-up rate that will cut in if the patient fails to breathe. Non-invasive positive pressure support may be provided by specialized portable ventilators, or by standard critical care ventilators.

Negative pressure ventilators assist inspiration by 'sucking out' the chest wall; expiration occurs through elastic recoil of the lungs. Includes devices such as tank ventilators and chest 'shell' ventilators. Other devices such as the rocking bed and 'pneumobelt' displace abdominal contents to aid diaphragmatic contraction. Used extensively in the polio epidemics of the 1950s; now only rarely used to manage chronic respiratory failure.

Continuous positive airway pressure (CPAP) supplies constant positive pressure during inspiration and expiration, and is therefore not a form of ventilation. It provides a 'splint' to open the upper airway and collapsed alveoli (thus improving V/Q matching). CPAP is used extensively in the community to treat obstructive sleep apnoea, but also has a role in improving oxygenation in selected patients with acute respiratory failure, e.g. patients with cardiogenic pulmonary oedema, pneumocystis pneumonia (p 476).

Abbreviations

NIV-non-invasive ventilation, also referred to as non-invasive mechanical ventilation (NIMV).
NIPPV-non-invasive positive pressure ventilation; confusingly it is also sometimes interpreted as nasal intermittent positive pressure ventilation, and sometimes referred to as 'NIPPY', after the name of a particular type of ventilator.
IPAP-inspiratory positive airways pressure.
EPAP-expiratory positive airways pressure, also referred to as positive end-expiratory pressure (PEEP).
BiPAP-bi-level positive airway pressure (IPAP greater than EPAP), refers to a commercial product, but now used to refer to similar machines.
CPAP-continuous positive airway pressure (IPAP equal to EPAP).

Further information

Mehta S, Hill NS. Noninvasive ventilation. *Am J Respir Crit Care Med* 2001; **163**: 540–77

Indications

NIV may be used in an attempt to avoid invasive ventilation and its complications (e.g. upper airway trauma, ventilator-acquired pneumonia); alternatively, NIV may represent the 'ceiling' of treatment in patients deemed unsuitable for intubation. NIV is not an alternative to invasive ventilation in patients who require this definitive treatment.

Acute exacerbation of COPD

- Consider NIV in patients with an acute exacerbation of COPD who have a respiratory acidosis (pH <7.30) despite initial medical treatment and controlled oxygen therapy
- Benefits include reduced mortality and need for intubation, more rapid improvement in physiological outcomes (respiratory rate, pH), and symptomatic relief from breathlessness, when compared with standard medical treatment
- NIV only assists ventilation; the pressures used are not enough to take over ventilation due to the high airways resistance
- Invasive ventilation, if deemed appropriate, should be considered particularly in patients with a severe respiratory acidosis (pH <7.25), as this is associated with treatment failure and increased mortality with NIV
- High expiratory pressures (e.g. 6–8 cmH_2O, PEEP) may help reduce the work of breathing by offsetting intrinsic PEEP, but will lessen the IPAP–EPAP difference, thus reducing the ventilation component.

Acute cardiogenic pulmonary oedema

- Use of CPAP via face mask is effective and should be considered in patients who fail to improve with medical management alone
- Bi-level NIV has not been shown to be superior to CPAP and there is a suggestion of increased myocardial infarction rates following its use. It may, however, have a role in patients who do not respond to CPAP.

Decompensated obstructive sleep apnoea

NIV is effective in the treatment of obstructive sleep apnoea and the overlap syndrome (i.e. raised $PaCO_2$, typically with associated obesity hypoventilation or COPD, p 582) when CPAP alone fails to reverse the CO_2 retention. NIV is generally recommended as the first choice over CPAP when an acute respiratory acidosis is present, but conversion to CPAP later may be possible.

Respiratory failure from neuromuscular weakness

- NIV is the treatment of choice for ventilatory failure resulting from neuromuscular weakness or chest wall deformity
- The pressures used may be adequate to fully take over ventilation, because the chest and lung compliance are often little impaired

Immunocompromised patients

- Immunocompromised patients who develop acute respiratory failure have an extremely high mortality following endotracheal intubation and ventilation
- In immunocompromised patients with pulmonary infiltrates, fever, and hypoxaemic acute respiratory failure, intermittent NIV results in lower intubation rates and hospital mortality when compared with standard treatment
- CPAP is effective in the treatment of pneumocystis pneumonia.

Community-acquired pneumonia

- Use of NIV may result in a reduction in need for intubation compared with standard medical treatment, although no significant differences in hospital mortality or length of hospitalization have been shown
- CPAP may have a role in improving oxygenation in severe pneumonia
- In patients who would potentially be candidates for intubation, use of NIV or CPAP should not inappropriately delay invasive ventilation, and so should only be attempted in an ITU setting.

Other conditions

- There is no evidence to support the use of NIV in acute severe asthma
- There is no strong evidence to support the use of NIV in exacerbations of bronchiectasis and cystic fibrosis, although NIV may be useful as a 'ceiling' of treatment in patients with severe underlying disease who would not be considered suitable candidates for invasive ventilation
- Bi-level NIV or CPAP may have a role in improving gas exchange following trauma or surgery.

Contraindications

Relative contraindications to the use of NIV are listed below. They should be considered in the context of individual patients; for example, severe hypoxaemia may not be considered a contraindication for NIV in a patient who is unsuitable for invasive ventilation.

Contraindications to NIV

- Cardiac or respiratory arrest
- Impaired consciousness or confusion
- Severe hypoxaemia
- Copious respiratory secretions
- Haemodynamic instability
- Facial surgery, trauma, burns, or deformity
- Upper airway obstruction
- Tracheal injury
- Undrained pneumothorax
- Inability to cooperate or to protect the airway
- Vomiting, bowel obstruction, recent upper gastrointestinal tract surgery, oesophageal injury.

Further information

BTS guidelines on non-invasive ventilation in acute respiratory failure. *Thorax* 2002; **57**: 192–211

Plant *et al.* Early use of non-invasive ventilation for acute exacerbations of chronic obstructive pulmonary disease on general respiratory wards: a multicentre randomised controlled trial. *Lancet* 2000; **355**: 1931–5

NIV in acute respiratory failure: practical use

The decision to start NIV should follow a period of initial standard medical treatment including appropriate supplementary and controlled oxygen therapy; a proportion of patients will improve and will no longer require ventilation. Prior to commencing NIV a senior doctor should make a decision with the patient and their family regarding suitability for invasive ventilation should NIV fail and document this clearly in the medical notes. ***If the patient is a candidate for invasive ventilation, care must be taken to avoid inappropriate delays in intubation through the use of NIV or CPAP. Liaise with ITU staff early.***

Setting up NIV

1. Select an appropriate mask type and size for the patient. Masks may be nasal or oronasal (full face). Nasal masks require clear nasal passages and may allow mouth leaks, particularly in the acutely breathless patient, but they are more comfortable. Full-face masks avoid mouth leakage and are generally favoured for initial use in acute respiratory failure.
2. Allow the patient to hold the mask to their face prior to attaching the head straps—this may increase confidence and compliance. Mask adjustments are often necessary to minimize air leaks, although some leakage may have to be accepted. Avoid excessive strap tension; 1 or 2 fingers should be able to fit under the strap.
3. Set up the ventilator. Typical initial pressures for ventilating a patient with hypercapnic respiratory failure due to an exacerbation of chronic obstructive pulmonary disease (COPD) would be EPAP 4 cmH_2O and IPAP 12 cmH_2O, with a back-up rate of 15/min and inspiratory: expiratory ratio of 1:3 in spontaneous/timed mode. Increase the IPAP in increments of 2 cmH_2O to a maximum of 20, as tolerated by the patient. Similar settings can be used for patients with hypercapnic respiratory failure resulting from neuromuscular weakness. Consider increasing the EPAP (e.g. to 8 or 10 cm) in obese patients with an 'overlap' syndrome of COPD and obstructive sleep apnoea.

   Pressure support ventilators can also be set to provide CPAP by equalizing the IPAP and EPAP; typical pressures range from 5 to 12.5 cmH_2O. CPAP may improve oxygenation in selected patients with cardiogenic pulmonary oedema or pneumonia.
4. Supplementary oxygen concentration (FiO_2) should be guided by the underlying disease process and by oximetry monitoring. For many hypercapnic patients with COPD, maintenance of oxygen saturations between 88% and 92% effectively balances the risks of hypoxia and hypercapnic respiratory acidosis.
5. Patient monitoring should involve assessment of comfort, respiratory rate, synchrony with the ventilator, mask leaks, pulse rate, blood pressure, and oxygen saturations.
6. Arterial or capillary blood gas analysis should be performed after 1 h and again after 4 h if there has been no improvement. Improvement in acidosis, and decline in respiratory rate after 1 and 4 h of treatment are

associated with a better outcome. Repeat the blood gas analysis if the clinical condition changes.

7. Lack of response may be indicated by a worsening acidosis or persistently abnormal arterial blood gases, or by a reduced conscious level and clinical deterioration. Consider invasive ventilation, if appropriate. The decision to halt NIV depends on the circumstances of the individual patient, and should be made by a senior doctor.
8. Subsequent management depends on the patient's response. Optimal duration of NIV is unclear, but it is typically administered for up to 3 days in acute respiratory failure. NIV does not need to be continuous, and the patient may have breaks for meals and nebulizers.

Table 57.1 Troubleshooting

Problem	Possible solution
Clinical deterioration or worsening respiratory failure	Ensure optimal medical therapy Consider complications, e.g. pneumothorax, aspiration, sputum retention Does the patient require intubation, if appropriate?
pCO_2 remains high (persistent respiratory acidosis)	Exclude inappropriately high FiO_2 Check mask and circuit for leaks Check for patient–ventilator asynchrony Check expiration valve is patent. Consider increasing IPAP
pO_2 remains low (<7 kPa)	Consider increasing FiO_2 Consider increasing EPAP
Irritation or ulceration of nasal bridge	Adjust strap tension Try cushion dressing Change mask type
Dry nose or mouth	Consider humidifier Check for leaks
Dry sore eyes	Check mask fit
Nasal congestion	Decongestants
Hypotension	Reduce IPAP (or EPAP if high)

NIV in chronic respiratory failure

Chest wall deformity and neuromuscular weakness (p 582)

- NIV has a well-established role in the management of chronic respiratory failure due to chest wall deformity or neuromuscular weakness, and has been shown to improve symptoms, gas exchange, and mortality
- Common underlying diagnoses include chest wall deformity and kyphoscoliosis, post-polio syndrome, motor neurone disease, spinal cord injury, neuropathies, myopathies, and muscular dystrophies. The nature of the underlying disease must influence the appropriateness of initiating ventilation: progressive conditions such as motor neurone disease often result in increasing dependence on the ventilator, and the patient and their care-givers should be made aware of this
- NIV is administered at home overnight and this improves daytime gas exchange. The mechanism for this is unclear: it probably resets the central respiratory drive, although respiratory muscle rest and improved chest wall and lung compliance may also play a part
- Small portable positive pressure ventilators with either face or nasal masks are used in the majority of cases; negative pressure or abdominal ventilators may rarely have a role in patients who are intolerant of masks, although their use may be limited by upper airways obstruction
- The decision to introduce overnight NIV is difficult, and is based on both symptoms (morning headaches, hypersomnolence, fatigue, poor sleep quality) and evidence of ventilatory failure (daytime hypercapnia (pCO_2 >6.0 kPa) and/or nocturnal hypoventilation with O_2 saturations <88% on overnight oximetry). Daytime ventilatory failure, however, is often a late feature, and is typically preceded by hypercapnic hypoventilation during sleep.
- A recent study in patients with myopathies demonstrated supine inspiratory vital capacity to be an accurate predictor of respiratory reserve: supine IVC <40% of predicted was significantly associated with hypercapnic hypoventilation and such patients should be considered for treatment with NIV. Supine IVC <20% was typically associated with daytime respiratory failure, whereas supine IVC >60% indicated a minimal risk of respiratory complications. Other factors include signs of cor pulmonale or hospital admission with respiratory failure
- Patients with excessive secretions may not be suitable for non-invasive ventilation, although face mask ventilation is possible even in the setting of bulbar weakness
- Regular follow-up of patients on overnight ventilation is important. Ask about symptoms and compliance, and repeat arterial or capillary blood gas analysis. Lack of improvement in gas exchange may reflect non-compliance, excessive air leakage, inadequate pressure support, or progression of underlying disease; consider repeating nocturnal oximetry monitoring. Patients with persisting severe hypoxia may benefit from long-term supplementary oxygen, although this may worsen CO_2 retention.

Sleep apnoea (p 574)

Overnight NIV may have a role in patients with central hypoventilation, Cheyne–Stokes respiration, obesity hypoventilation, overlap syndromes of obstructive sleep apnoea with coexisting COPD or obesity.

Cystic fibrosis (p 218)

Overnight NIV may have a useful role as a 'bridge' to transplantation in patients with cystic fibrosis and chronic respiratory failure.

COPD (p 179)

Use of NIV in the management of chronic stable COPD is controversial. Trials have shown conflicting results, although some possible benefit in a subgroup of patients with severe hypercapnia, extra nocturnal hypoventilation, and recurrent admissions for worsening ventilatory failure.

Further information

Clinical indications for noninvasive positive pressure ventilation in chronic respiratory failure due to restrictive lung disease, COPD, and nocturnal hypoventilation—a consensus conference report. *Chest* 1999; **116**: 5 21–34

Ragette R *et al.* Patterns and predictors of sleep disordered breathing in primary myopathies. *Thorax* 2002; **57**: 724–8

Chapter 58

Oxygen therapy

Acute oxygen therapy

Acute oxygen therapy is either 'controlled' or 'uncontrolled'.

- *Uncontrolled* Use when extra O_2 is required to raise the SaO_2 above 92%, to ensure adequate O_2 delivery to the tissues *and* where there are no concerns that high PaO_2 values will depress ventilatory drive to the point that $PaCO_2$ will rise, and pH fall, dangerously, e.g. pneumonia, pneumothorax, pulmonary emboli, asthma, LVF, etc.
- *Controlled* Use when extra O_2 is required, but ventilation critically depends on hypoxic drive, e.g. exacerbations of COPD (particularly when there has been a chronically raised $PaCO_2$, as evidenced by a significant base excess), chronic ventilatory failure due to scoliosis, neuromuscular disease, and any other cause of 'pump' failure.
- With stable type II ventilatory failure, ventilation still seems to be dominantly driven by $PaCO_2$/pH, but in exacerbations (when PaO_2 usually falls), peripheral chemoreceptor drive from low PaO_2 becomes dominant. Thus, O_2 therapy must not raise PaO_2 above 8 kPa (~92% SaO_2) as this will 'turn off' ventilatory drive, allowing hypoventilation, hypercapnia, acidosis, and potentially death. There is some evidence that high alveolar PO_2 also 'turns off' pulmonary hypoxic vasoconstriction. This allows an increase in pulmonary blood flow to poorly ventilated areas and reducing CO_2 excretion (accounts for ≈ 20% of the $PaCO_2$ rise following excessive FiO_2 in COPD exacerbations).

Delivering uncontrolled oxygen This can be done in many ways, essentially by blowing O_2 over the face, whilst limiting inhalation of surrounding air or exhaled CO_2.

- Standard O_2 masks (sometimes called high-flow masks). Set the O_2 regulator to at least 4 L/min, much more if very breathless, to prevent dilution by air drawn into mask by high inspiratory flows via exit holes. Can deliver about 50–60% O_2.
- Nasal cannulae/prongs/catheters are uncontrolled and deliver unpredictable levels of O_2 (depending on flow rate, minute ventilation, and oral vs. nasal breathing route). Titrate using an oxygen saturation monitor.
- Non-rebreathe reservoir masks can deliver FiO_2 values over 60% by means of a soft plastic bag between the end of the tubing and mask, plus one-way valves between the bag and mask and on the mask exit ports. This mechanism ensures that most of the inspired air is pure O_2. The ability of the reservoir to empty on inspiration briefly allows higher inspiratory flows than the actual O_2 regulator setting, and the bag valve prevents inhalation of very much exhaled CO_2; the mask exit valves close, preventing air inhalation. The usual problem is kinking of the junction between the mask and bag when the head tilts forward, reducing the effectiveness of the reservoir.
- Very high FiO_2 requires a tight seal, and is generally delivered with CPAP masks (using pressures of about 5–7 cmH_2O). This ensures no air is entrained through blow off vents or leaks, as well as improving V/Q matching by recruiting collapsed alveoli.

Delivering controlled oxygen therapy This requires the ability to reliably control the FiO_2 in order to keep the patient's SaO_2 less than 92% (some suggest 90%), but high enough to prevent anaerobic metabolism. This lower acceptable level is debatable: 88% is generous, 85% is likely to be adequate, and 80% may be acceptable if cardiac output is adequate.

- FiO_2 is controlled through Venturi masks—O_2 is directed through a narrow nozzle and exits at speed, lowering the air pressure at this point. This draws in surrounding air, diluting the O_2
- A proper Venturi mask mixes O_2 and air in the same proportion, regardless of the oxygen flow
- The minimum flow setting of the regulator, written on the nozzle, ensures adequate overall flow to prevent air being drawn through the exit holes during inhalation, e.g. a 28% Ventimask has a 1:10 entrainment ratio, 1 L/min O_2 entrains 10 L/min air (total flow 11 L/min), 2 L/min O_2 entrains 20 L/min (total flow 22 L/min)
- Nasal cannulae are definitely not controlled O_2 therapy and are in fact the opposite. If nasal cannulae do deliver too high an FiO_2, and ventilation decreases as a consequence, the proportion of the minute ventilation containing the fixed flow nasal oxygen will rise, increasing the FiO_2 and hence PaO_2 still further—a vicious cycle
- Controlled and very low flow oxygen is also needed sometimes with NIV when the patient is still required to trigger inspiration. Added O_2 should be avoided if possible and rarely requires more than 1 L/min to be entrained; again it should be titrated using the SaO_2. When adding too much oxygen, it is easy to be lulled into a false sense of security by an SaO_2 over 92%, while the $PaCO_2$ gradually rises undetected.

Oxygen alert card should be given to all patients with a previous episode of hypercapnic respiratory failure. This alerts ambulance crews and medical staff to the potential risk of hypercapnia with high-flow oxygen and documents usual resting baseline SaO_2. However, the ambulance staff protocols are sufficiently rigid that they are not allowed to override them. In some areas, letters from the patient's consultant and head of the ambulance service must be with the patient.

Patient details

Sticky label

Introduction

If you have a sudden worsening of your lung disease (usually due to a chest infection) it is essential that you do not receive too much or too little oxygen, either can be dangerous. Too much oxygen can cause a rise in the level of carbon dioxide in your blood and this can make you drowsy and slow your breathing. Too little oxygen can also be dangerous.

Purpose of this card

The purpose of this oxygen alert card is to make sure that the doctors or ambulance staff involved in your care are made aware of your special needs regarding oxygen therapy. The card recommends the appropriate amount of oxygen therapy for you based on your previous blood gas tests.

Carry the card with you at all times

If you need to call the ambulance service or attend the hospital accident and emergency department, show this card to the GP, paramedics, doctor or emergency department staff looking after you, as it provides them with essential information regarding your personal oxygen needs.

Latest blood gas recordings:

Date: ___/___/______

On: Air, or % oxygen ____%

pH:___ pCO_2____ pO_2____

Oxygen saturation: ______ %

You should receive enough Oxygen to achieve a $\%O_2$ saturation of no higher than 92%, but higher than 86%, if possible. This is usually done with either a 24% or 28% venturi mask.

Signed .... Name....................

Designation....................

Fig. 58.1 Oxygen alert card.

Home oxygen therapy

Home oxygen is delivered with essentially three different aims. First, to reduce the long-term complications of chronic hypoxia such as cor pulmonale, usually called long-term oxygen therapy or LTOT. This requires ≥15 h a day to be successful. Home oxygen can also be supplied for the relief of breathlessness, usually called 'short' burst oxygen therapy or SBOT. If SBOT is used for many hours a day, it is sometimes incorrectly called LTOT, particularly by the oxygen supply companies. Oxygen can also be supplied to ambulant patients so that they can leave the house and travel (ambulatory oxygen).

Long-term oxygen therapy (LTOT)

Background and indications

Two landmark trials of LTOT in the 1980s: the British MRC Working Party trial and the American Nocturnal Oxygen Therapy Trial (NOTT).

The *MRC trial* compared COPD patients receiving oxygen for 15 h/day with controls receiving no oxygen. The *NOTT trial* compared continuous daily oxygen (average 17.7 h/day) with overnight oxygen (average 12 h). The patients in the MRC trial were on average hypercapnic (mean $PaCO_2$ 7.3 kPa), whereas those in the NOTT trial were on average normocapnic (mean $PaCO_2$ 5.7 kPa). The main outcome in both trials was improved survival in those patients receiving oxygen for at least 15 h/day, though this improved survival was not seen in the MRC trial until after a year of oxygen therapy.

The *NOTT trial* showed a reduced exercise pulmonary artery pressure (PAP) after 6 months of continuous or nocturnal oxygen therapy. The 8-year survival was related to the fall in mean PAP during the first 6 months of continuous oxygen use.

The *MRC trial* failed to show a fall in mean PAP with LTOT, but the mean annual increase in PAP (3 mmHg) in patients in the control arm was not seen in the oxygen treated group.

The reason for the improved survival with LTOT is not clear, and is unlikely to relate to the small changes in pulmonary haemodynamics seen.

COPD is the disease for which LTOT is most commonly prescribed, and the disease in which the original studies were completed. Subsequent oxygen studies have shown improved exercise endurance in COPD patients breathing supplemental oxygen, with improved walking distance and ability to perform daily activities. FEV_1 is the strongest predictor of survival in COPD; LTOT does not influence the decline in FEV_1.

Additional benefits of LTOT include:

- Reduction of secondary polycythaemia
- Improved sleep quality, by reducing hypoxia-associated brain arousals
- Reduced cardiac arrthymias, and potentially reducing the risk of nocturnal sudden death
- Reduced sympathetic outflow leading to improved renal function, with increased salt and water excretion, and reduced peripheral oedema

Indications for LTOT in COPD patients

Criteria for prescription of LTOT in the UK are based on the clinical parameters of patients showing improved survival in the two LTOT trials.

- PaO_2 <7.3 kPa (55 mmHg) breathing air (i.e. a saturation on air ≤88%), in a stable clinical state. Borderline results may need reassessment after 3 months, particularly if oximetry SaO_2 <92%
- PaO_2 7.3–8 kPa (56–59 mmHg, SaO_2 89–90%) if pulmonary hypertension (i.e. symptoms and signs of cor pulmonale), polycythaemia, or additional nocturnal hypoxaemia (SaO_2 ≤90% for at least 30% of the night). There is no evidence that treating solely nocturnal hypoxaemia leads to improved survival
- Clinical stability is the absence of an exacerbation for the previous 4 weeks. This is usually assessed twice, several weeks apart, to ensure stability and ideally at least 6 weeks following an exacerbation
- LTOT is usually prescribed for those with FEV_1 <1.5 L or <40% predicted. If the FEV_1 is higher in the presence of hypoxia/hypercapnia, it suggests an additional cause for the ventilatory failure, such as additional obstructive sleep apnoea; further investigations may be indicated
- Medical management of the disease must be optimized prior to the prescription of LTOT
- $PaCO_2$ does not influence the prescription of LTOT for COPD. There is a small risk of precipitating worsening hypercapnia with LTOT in those who are already hypercapnic, particularly if the patient has OSA or is experiencing an exacerbation
- Blood gases should be checked on LTOT to ensure the absence of worsening hypercapnia, if symptoms such as headache and confusion suggest that this has occurred, and to ensure a satisfactory increase in PaO_2. Aim for PaO_2 values of 8–9 kPa (60–65 mmHg, SaO_2 90–92%)
- Patients should have stopped smoking: the benefit of LTOT in continued smokers is limited, and there is an increased risk of fire. However, most studies suggest that around 18% of patients on LTOT continue to smoke; they should be warned of the risks.

Indications for LTOT in non-COPD patients

There is very limited evidence to support the use of true LTOT in these patient groups and no data showing improved survival; the prescription thresholds are therefore not evidence-based. Ensure optimal medical management first. LTOT is a term best reserved when one is trying to ward off complications of hypoxia, but is often confused with prolonged use of oxygen for palliative purposes; even guidelines confuse the two. Consider in:

- Interstitial lung disease if PaO_2 <8 kPa (SaO_2 90%)
- Cystic fibrosis if PaO_2 <8 kPa (SaO_2 90%)
- Pulmonary hypertension with PaO_2 <8 kPa, in the absence of parenchymal lung disease
- Neuromuscular or skeletal disorders causing ventilatory failure. Consider either oxygen alone (very rarely appropriate), or in combination with NIV (usually via a specialist centre)
- Chronic heart failure if PaO_2 <7.5 kPa.

Guidelines also include the following, but this is not really LTOT, but prolonged SBOT.

- Palliative care—for the dyspnoea of lung malignancy, or other causes of disabling dyspnoea due to terminal disease.

Indications for SBOT

- Short-burst oxygen therapy usually refers to intermittent supplemental oxygen to relieve dyspnoea, for periods of 10–20 min, but the periods may become much longer. Often the resting PaO_2/SaO_2 may be normal. Some would argue there is a large placebo effect due to the cooling effect of the oxygen on the face; a similar effect may be achieved by using a fan. Traditionally used in the following situations, although very little data exist to support its use in COPD, interstitial lung disease, heart failure, etc.:
- Pre-oxygenation before exercise
- Recovery from exercise
- SOB at rest
- Palliative care
- Overnight to reduce sleep disruption of Cheyne–Stokes breathing in heart failure.

Should only be prescribed if clear proven benefit, preferably with objective improvement in hypoxia and symptoms. It is expensive to prescribe, based on a daily rate and hours prescribed, irrespective of actual usage. It is best provided by using one or more oxygen cylinders placed strategically round the house. Use of an O_2 concentrator becomes more economical above a certain h/day usage. To supply a cylinder to stay in the wardrobe 'just in case' is now a very expensive placebo.

Indications for ambulatory oxygen

Ambulatory oxygen is oxygen delivered by portable equipment, and may be suitable for:

- Patients on LTOT who are mobile
- Those with exercise desaturation, and who show an improvement in exercise capacity or dyspnoea with oxygen; titrate oxygen to limit the exercise desaturation, aiming for SaO_2 >90%.

This indication is poorly researched and defined. Ideally clear benefit should be demonstrated, and guidelines recommend laborious assessment, but facilities to do this often do not exist. It is up to the specialist prescriber to decide whether to order through the oxygen supply company, and then up to the supply company to decide on the best way to deliver. A 2-month assessment is usually required, to determine the likely number of hours of use. A reasonable initial prescription might be for 1–2 h/day. Ideally usage should be regularly reviewed and withdrawn if of no benefit, or not being used. It is usually provided via portable cylinders, although liquid oxygen is a more convenient option, providing 6 h use per recharge.

Practical issues

- Home O_2 should not be supplied to patients who still smoke, due to added fire risk, and probable reduced efficacy by the increased HbCO
- LTOT is best provided by an oxygen concentrator, set at 1–4 L/min depending on PaO_2 or SaO_2. Some concentrators can deliver 8 L/min. Concentrators contain a molecular sieve containing zeolite, which traps gas molecules depending on size and polarity. Can produce up to 96% oxygen, depending on flow (the argon is also concentrated, to 4%)
- Patients can use nasal prongs or a fixed concentration mask (uncontrolled or controlled oxygen, e.g. 24% and 28%) depending on physiological requirements and their preference. A back-up cylinder should be prescribed in case of power cuts
- Oxygen humidification is possible, but difficult to arrange and rarely necessary. Only works well above 4 L/min, and tube lengths <1.5 m
- LTOT should be used for ≥15 h/day in patients with COPD, although survival improves when used for longer; therefore use should not be restricted to 15 h/day
- Patient education in the use of LTOT and machine maintenance are important. Specialist respiratory nurses may be involved with this
- If using SBOT at >3 oxygen cylinders/week, an oxygen concentrator is more economical (the oxygen supply company decides on this).

How to organize home oxygen

- The UK-wide integrated oxygen service (2005) ensured that provision of all modalities of domiciliary O_2 is from one contractor in each area. Prescription should, in theory, come from respiratory specialists only (doctors, specialist nurses). Local arrangements are defined by primary case trusts (PCTs); in some areas almost anyone is defined as a 'respiratory specialist', able to prescribe O_2, with consequential escalation of O_2 costs
- The prescriber completes *and signs* a Home Oxygen Order Form (HOOF), providing the oxygen supplier with the patient's details and an exact prescription of the oxygen required
- The HOOF is used for the prescription of LTOT, short burst, and ambulatory oxygen; includes details of the oxygen flow rate, % oxygen, and delivery device/mask required
- The oxygen supplier will invoice the PCT (Local Health Board in Wales); it is vital that this information is completed otherwise the HOOF will be returned
- A Home Oxygen Consent Form (HOCF) form must be signed by the patient, consenting for the disclosure of relevant medical information, address, telephone number to the oxygen supplier and fire brigade
- The HOOF and HOCF are faxed to the oxygen supplier, with copies to the PCT, GP, and clinical lead for home oxygen services
- An LTOT prescription does not automatically include provision for oxygen outside the home; a separate form must be completed
- The response time for the delivery of LTOT, short-burst oxygen, and standard ambulatory supply is 3 days.

Follow-up is needed to ensure:

- Compliance; withdraw if not using despite support and explanation. Home visit within 4 weeks by specialist nurse recommended

- Confirm the ongoing requirement for LTOT. Some patients improve and no longer need LTOT. Arterial blood gas tensions at 3 months, and then yearly monitoring (may be performed by specialist nurses)
- Cancellation with the O_2 company as soon as a patients dies
- Inform O_2 company of any changes in flow rates/%O_2
- Inform O_2 company of any changes in patient address etc.
- Inform O_2 company of admission to hospital for more than a week (reduces cost).

Emergency supply is a separate category and should only be prescribed when the patient has no O_2 at home. The supplier is required to deliver this within 4 h of receipt of the order. It should not be ordered for more than 3 days.

Portable oxygen options

- DD—460 L. Lightweight and easily portable. Lasts 3 h 50 min at 2 L/min
- F size—1360 L. Lasts approximately 11.5 h at 2 L/min
- PD—300 L. Much smaller, but heavier than DD. Lasts 2.5 h at 2 L/min
- E size—600 L. Lightweight and portable. Lasts 5 h at 2 L/min. (Not available on the NHS.)
- Liquid oxygen
- Use O_2 conserver devices (reduce O_2 wastage during expiration).

Table 58.1 Oxygen supplier 24 h contact details

Supplier	Region	Telephone	Fax
Air products plc	North West, Yorkshire and Humberside, East Midlands, West Midlands, London North Wales	0800 373580	0800 214709
Air Liquide	North East SW London, Thames Valley, Hants & Isle of Wight SE London, Kent, Surrey & Sussex South West	0808 2020999 0500 823773	0191 4974340 0800 7814610
BOC Medical	Eastem England	0800 136603	0800 1699989

Further information

http://www.primarycarecontracting.nhs.uk/uploads/HOS/june_2007/appendix_10.pdf

http://www.lunguk.org/oxygen-suppliers.asp

NICE COPD Guidelines. http://guidance.nice.org.uk/CG12/niceguidance/pdf/English/download.dspx

Guidelines for emergency oxygen use in adult patients. BTS website—in preparation

Venturi principle. http://www.flexicare.com/content/education/education_oxygen_fixedmask.htm

Oxygen alert cards and controlled oxygen: preventing emergency admissions at risk.. Gooptu *et al.* Emerg Med J.2006; 23: 636-638

http://www.dh.gov.uk/en/Policyandguidance/Medicinespharmacyandindustry/Prescriptions/Homeoxygenservice/index.htm. DOH website

http://www.homeoxygen.nhs.uk/lookup.php

Chapter 59
Palliative care

Palliative care is defined by the World Health Organization as an approach that improves the quality of life of patients and their families facing the problems associated with life-threatening illness, through the prevention and relief of suffering by means of early identification, impeccable assessment, and treatment of pain and other problems, physical, psychosocial and spiritual. Palliative care is moving away from being involved just at the end of life, especially in developing countries when curative possibilities are less readily available and palliative treatments may be the only option. In the UK, patients may be under palliative care teams intermittently for symptom control, respite care, etc., and may not see the service again for months or years.

Within chest medicine, palliative care is most commonly considered for patients with lung cancer and mesothelioma; many other patients with progressive end-stage respiratory disease (such as COPD, CF, and fibrotic lung disease) also benefit from specific palliative interventions. These two areas are discussed separately below, although there is much overlap in the management.

Lung cancer and mesothelioma

- Involve the specialist palliative care team early
- Treat symptoms promptly
- Recognize problems are often mixed, complex and multiple
- Recognize that delirium, dyspnoea, and decreased mobility often herald the terminal phase of cancer.

Pain

- Aim to determine cause, type, and site
- Start with simple analgesia and increase according to the WHO analgesic ladder, moving from non-opioid analgesia through weak opioids to strong opioids. Reassess repeatedly and regularly
- If moving to morphine from weak opioid, 5–10 mg should be adequate. 10–20 mg or more required to replace a strong opioid (60 mg codeine qds is equivalent to 5 mg morphine 4-hourly. If pain was not previously controlled, start at 10 mg morphine 4-hourly). If first dose of morphine no more effective than previous analgesia, increase next dose by 50%
- Prescribe analgesia as required for breakthrough pain (see box)
- Give drugs a chance to work at appropriate doses, particularly if they have not had strong opioids before. Allows assessment of analgesic effect and side-effects. Usually increase every 3rd day if required
- Once pain is reasonably controlled, morphine dose can be converted to slow release morphine by dividing total amount by two and giving that dose as modified release morphine 12-hourly. The breakthrough dose is one-sixth of the total 24-h dose (e.g. 15 mg slow release morphine bd, then 5 mg (immediate release morphine sulphate) for breakthrough pain)

- Treat drug side-effects, e.g. constipation, nausea. Prescribe prophylactic laxatives with morphine. Warn people they may feel more drowsy if starting morphine or having dose increase, but this usually settles within a few days
- Patients with renal failure are more likely to develop opioid toxicity (drowsiness, confusion, myoclonus) as they have difficulty excreting morphine metabolites. They may need alternatives to morphine (e.g. methadone, alfentanil, fentanyl) if their pain is not controlled on low-dose morphine
- The addition of an anti-inflammatory drug can be effective for bone pain and for liver capsule pain if there are hepatic metastases
- Consider radiotherapy for localized pain in the chest related to cancer
- *Pleuritic pain* Consider PE, treat any infection. Consider non-steroidal anti-inflammatory drug ± intercostal nerve block
- *Bone metastases causing local tenderness* Start a strong opioid. If there is no improvement after 3 dose increases, add a non-steroidal anti-inflammatory drug for a 1-week trial. If single site, consider radiotherapy or intercostal nerve block. If multiple sites, consider bisphosphonates (so long as not hypocalcaemic), e.g. 90 mg of pamidronate IV every 4 weeks.
- *Neuropathic pain* can be treated with specific antidepressants (e.g. amitriptyline 10–50 mg) or anticonvulsants (e.g. carbamazepine or sodium valproate 200 mg/day, gabapentin)
- Consider referral to pain clinic or specialist centre for further intervention, such as a intercostal nerve block, transcutaneous electrical nerve stimulation (TENS), cervical cordotomy, or complementary therapies.

Treatment of breakthrough pain

- *If already on non-opioid analgesic*: give one extra dose of the regular analgesic
- *If already on a regular oral opioid*: give 4-hourly oral dose (= one sixth of total 24 hour dose), e.g. 60 mg/day = 10 mg dose
- *If on transdermal opioid patch*: Fentanyl—give 1-hourly dose e.g. 25 μg/h patch, give 25 μg SC or sublingually. Buprenorphine—give 6-hourly dose, e.g. 35 μg/h patch = 200 μg SC or sublingually
- *If already on continuous SC infusion of opioid*: Diamorphine—give 4-hourly dose, e.g. 30 mg/24 h = 5 mg dose SC. Fentanyl—give 1-hourly dose, e.g. 500 μg/24 h = 20 μg dose SC

Consider increasing regular analgesic dose if the breakthrough pain occurs before the next regular dose. If there is no response to the additional breakthrough pain treatment, repeat after 4 h if non-opioid or 1 h if opioid, with same dose. If still no response, consider changing from non-opioid to weak opioid, or weak opioid to strong opioid.

Conversions between opiates

More potent opioids or routes do not provide greater analgesic efficacy, but may provide an alternative route to ensure adequate absorption, or if patient experiencing side-effects (usually toxicity and confusion)

- *Oral morphine to subcutaneous morphine* Conversion factor is ÷ 2, e.g. 60 mg/24 h oral morphine = 30 mg SC morphine
- *Oral morphine to diamorphine infusion* Conversion factor is ÷ 3, e.g. 60 mg/24 h oral morphine = 20 mg/24 h SC diamorphine
- *Oral morphine to transdermal fentanyl (patch)* Oral morphine in mg/24 h÷ 3 = transdermal fentanyl in μg/h, e.g. 75 mg oral morphine in 24 h = 25 μg/h transdermal fentanyl. Use transdermal fentanyl for patients with stable pain.

Dyspnoea

- Consider possible causes (see box opposite). Dyspnoea may be due to the underlying lung disease, or due to an additional pathology
- Dyspnoea is frightening and made worse by anxiety and panic
- Lung cancer and pulmonary metastases are associated with the sensation of shortness of breath, often due to stimulation of receptors by malignant infiltration or lymphangitis carcinomatosis
- Optimize treatment of any underlying lung disease with bronchodilators and steroids if appropriate
- Treat concurrent chest infection
- Opioids (e.g. 2.5–5 mg morphine sulphate solution 4-hourly) relieve the sensation of dyspnoea without affecting respiratory function
- Oxygen cylinders for intermittent short burst/prn use may help symptoms
- Fan blowing cool air onto the face can be helpful
- Consider the need for tumour debulking by bronchoscopy or an airway stent in a patient with lung cancer experiencing dyspnoea due to bronchial obstruction or compression with tumour
- If PE diagnosed, consider treatment with low molecular weight heparin as warfarin can cause INR to be variable and difficult to optimize
- Subcutaneous opiate infusion may relieve symptoms as death approaches; use with haloperidol, midazolam or levomepromazine.

Causes of breathlessness in patients with lung cancer

- Pneumonia
- Underlying chronic lung disease (e.g. COPD, UIP) or concomitant cardiac disease
- Lobar collapse
- Pleural effusion
- Pneumothorax
- SVCO
- Upper airway obstruction
- Pulmonary emboli
- Lymphangitis carcinomatosis
- Chest wall infiltration
- Phrenic nerve paralysis
- Pericardial effusion
- Respiratory muscle weakness, due to cachexia, paraneoplastic syndromes, steroid myopathy
- Anaemia
- Depression
- Anxiety and panic.

Other symptoms

Anxiety

- Leads to dyspnoea, which in turn worsens anxiety
- Explain they will not suffocate, symptoms will pass
- Benzodiazepines (such as short-acting lorazepam 0.5–1 mg sublingually 8–12-hourly) are effective for respiratory panic.
- Acute panic may be helped by midazolam 2.5 mg IV, increased in increments of 1 mg, given in a controlled environment with oxygen
- Amitryptiline or citalopram may be effective longer-term treatments - probably best used as first line, as tolerance can develop to benzodiazepines
- Relaxation exercises, diaphragmatic breathing training, and complementary therapies may help some patients.

Cough

- Treat the underlying cause
- Try simple or codeine linctus
- Nebulized saline may help expectoration
- Methadone linctus 1–2 mg nocte or bd may be of benefit
- Nebulized local anaesthetic may help (specialised setting only), e.g. 5ml 2% lidocaine 6-hourly or bupivacaine 5 mL 0.25% 6-hourly (avoid in asthmatics, as it causes bronchospasm). Pharyngeal numbness is likely to occur, so avoid fluids for 1–2 h afterwards.
- Consider radiotherapy if haemoptysis due to lung cancer. Consider discontinuing antiplatelet drugs or anticoagulants
- If massive haemoptysis, consider tranexamic acid, plus emergency supply of opioids and benzodiazepines to ensure pain control and reduction of fear by decreasing awareness.

Pleural effusion

- Drain if symptomatic and pleurodese early if recurrent, although not if prognosis is poor (less than 3 months)
- Consider in-dwelling tunnelled catheter to drain fluid if effusion is symptomatic and pleurodesis has failed due to trapped lung.

Poor appetite

- Common symptom; may be primary due to cachexia–anorexia syndrome, or secondary due to mouth problems such as candidiasis, nausea, hypercalcaemia, drugs, or depression
- May be improved in the short term (about 6 weeks) by a course of oral steroids, such as prednisolone 20 mg daily
- Cachexia leads to decreased respiratory muscle strength and increased shortness of breath
- Consider nutritional supplements.

Brain metastases

- Steroids relieve the cerebral oedema associated with brain metastases, e.g. dexamethasone 4 mg bd–qds initially and then decrease
- Avoid steroid dosing in the evening, as sleep is affected
- Cranial radiotherapy may be considered if there is a good response to steroids.

Non-malignant respiratory disease (COPD, CF, fibrotic lung disease)

The main problems associated with severe non-malignant respiratory disease are dyspnoea, hypoxia, immobility, and psychosocial problems, including depression. End-stage COPD patients may have very frequent exacerbations for some years before a final terminal event. One study has shown those with end-stage COPD are more likely to have depression ± anxiety than those with terminal cancer, but they are less likely to receive specific treatment for their emotional problems or any targeted palliative care. It may be appropriate therefore to shift the focus in patients with severe end-stage respiratory disease away from management of acute exacerbations towards a more palliative approach to care.

Dyspnoea

- Dyspnoea is frightening and made worse by anxiety and panic
- Patients may decrease their mobility to avoid dyspnoea, and subsequently become more deconditioned.
- Dyspnoea may be due to the underlying lung disease or an additional pathology (PE, infection, pneumothorax, cardiac failure)
- Sitting upright reduces airway obstruction and optimizes ventilation. Relaxing and dropping the shoulders can improve ventilation, when anxiety has caused patient to 'hunch up'
- Calm gentle reassurance can decrease anxiety and reduce dyspnoea
- Fan blowing cool air onto the face can be helpful
- Optimize treatment of any underlying lung disease with bronchodilators and inhaled steroids
- Treat concurrent exacerbations with antibiotics and oral steroids
- Stop smoking
- Consider pulmonary rehabilitation, if appropriate
- Opioids (e.g. 2.5–5 mg morphine sulphate solution 4-hourly) relieve the sensation of dyspnoea without affecting respiratory function
- Oxygen cylinders for intermittent short burst use may help symptoms. Consider concentrator if multiple cylinders being used

Hypoxia

- SaO_2 <92%
- LTOT may be appropriate (see p 706)
- Oxygen cylinders for intermittent or ambulatory use may help symptoms, but little data to support their use.

Anxiety and depression

- May be due to fear and uncertainty over prognosis
- Lead to dyspnoea, which in turn worsens anxiety
- Explain they will not suffocate; symptoms will pass
- Benzodiazepines (such as short-acting lorazepam 0.5–1 mg sublingually 8–12-hourly) are effective for respiratory panic
- Acute panic may be helped by midazolam 2.5 mg IV, increased in steps of 1 mg, given in a controlled environment with oxygen

- Depression rates are high in patients with COPD. Consider antidepressant treatment and counselling. Amitriptyline or citalopram may be effective at helping anxiety also
- Relaxation exercises, diaphragmatic breathing training, and complementary therapies may help some patients

Cough

- Treat the underlying cause
- Refer to physiotherapy to improve cough efficacy, particularly if large volume secretions
- Consider mucolytics, steroids, antibiotics
- Try simple or codeine linctus
- Nebulized saline may help expectoration
- Methadone linctus 1–2 mg nocte or bd may be of benefit
- Oral local anaesthetics, such as benzocaine and lignocaine lozenges may be useful for laryngeal, pharyngeal or tracheal irritation, but associated risk of aspiration
- Nebulized local anaesthetic may helps, e.g. 5 mL 2% lidocaine 6-hourly or bupivacaine 5 mL 0.25% 6-hourly (avoid in asthmatics, as it causes bronchospasm). Pharyngeal numbness is likely to occur, so avoid fluids for 1–2 h afterwards.

Other problems

- Malnutrition, thirst
- Nausea, vomiting, constipation
- Sleep disturbance
- Chest pain
- Fatigue
- Oral candidiasis
- Impact on carers and family of patient with chronic respiratory disease

Further information

British National Formulary—useful information on prescribing in palliative care in its first section

Palliative care formulary www.palliativedrugs.org (free to register)

Liverpool Care Pathway—care pathway designed by palliative care team to enable generic care workers to deliver optimum hospice type care to a dying patient, whatever their location or diagnosis. Sample care pathway available online: www.mcphil.org.uk/liverpool_care_pathway

Chapter 60

Pulmonary rehabilitation

Aims and patient selection

Pulmonary rehabilitation is a well-established multidisciplinary programme of care for patients with chronic respiratory impairment. The programme is individually tailored for each patient. Pulmonary rehabilitation is not available yet in every centre, although it is probably the most cost-effective intervention in COPD.

Aims of rehabilitation

- To reduce disability and handicap in people with chronic lung disease
- To improve quality of life and restore independence
- To diminish the health care burden of disease.

Early studies measured pulmonary function tests and found there was no improvement after pulmonary rehabilitation. The first positive study of pulmonary rehabilitation measured functional status.

Meta-analysis of 14 RCTs using a variety of different style programmes has confirmed the benefit of rehabilitation, with improvements in functional exercise.

- Further UK RCT of patients with severe airflow obstruction showed improvements in exercise, health status, and health economic advantages
- Patients who had completed rehabilitation courses had no fewer hospital admissions for exacerbations than those who had not had rehabilitation, but hospital stays were shorter (10 days vs. 21 days)
- Patients with COPD who have completed rehabilitation courses perform better than controls on walking tests and have less subjective dyspnoea
- Rehabilitation programmes containing lower-extremity training are better, when compared with controls, than those using just respiratory muscle training
- Short-term programmes achieve overall similar outcome benefits across the spectrum of patient disability. A minimum programme length of 6 weeks is recommended
- Decline in exercise tolerance and health status tends to occur between 6 and 12 months after completion of a course. Sustained improvement with ongoing rehabilitation sessions has yet to be evaluated.

Candidates

- Anyone with chronic lung disease causing functional impairment
- The majority of candidates will have COPD, but also asthma, pulmonary fibrosis, and bronchiectasis
- Any stage of a lung disease, when symptoms are affecting a patient's activity. Ideally receiving optimum medical treatment
- Well-motivated patients seem to benefit most
- Patients with poor lower limb mobility may benefit from upper limb exercise
- Oxygen therapy is not a contraindication to rehabilitation
- Stable ischaemic heart disease is not a contraindication to rehabilitation.

Candidates in whom rehabilitation may not be indicated

- Unstable ischaemic heart disease, severe valvular heart disease, cognitive impairment, locomotor difficulties
- Poorly motivated people with geographical or transport problems making attendance difficult tend to do less well.

Programme

Programmes are usually run on an out-patient basis, but can be done in the community, in the home, or as an in-patient. They are run by a multi-professional team—physician, physiotherapist, occupational therapist, dietician, nurse, pharmacist, social worker, and psychologist. A minimum programme length of 6 weeks is recommended. Programmes should be regularly audited by the department.

- **Physical training** The main component of the programme, with aerobic exercise such as walking and cycling 2–3 times per week, with 2 supervised/class sessions. May include upper limb strength exercise with weights. Individually prescribed exercise programmes, designed for each patient to work to high intensity. Benefit increases with training intensity. Oxygen supplementation may be required if significant desaturation occurs during exercise to below 80%
- **Disease education**
- **Psychological and social intervention** with advice on anxiety and depression, smoking cessation, plus physiotherapy and occupational therapy input
- **Nutritional education** to optimize body weight and muscle mass.

Pre-rehabilitation assessment

- Optimize medical treatment
- Oxygen saturation on exercise
- ECG may be warranted, especially if history of cardiac disease.

Outcome assessment measures

- **Physical** Often with shuttle walk tests (SWT) or 6-min walk test (6MWT) to assess ability and progress (see box opposite)
- **Health status** Disease-specific questionnaires:
  - Chronic Respiratory Questionnaire (CRQ)
  - St George's Respiratory Questionnaire
  - Generic questionnaires
  - Short Form-36 (SF-36)
  - Hospital Anxiety and Depression scores (HADS) are measured, but are insensitive to change during pulmonary rehabilitation
- **Practical** Pulmonary Function Status–Dyspnoea Questionnaire (PFS-DQ) may be used to measure performance and satisfaction relating to activities of daily living.

Shuttle walk test (SWT)

10-m course between two points. Walking speed determined by external audio-tape signals ('beeps'), and the patient should pace their walk to reach each point at a beep. The patient is required to incrementally increase their speed as the beeps occur more frequently. Test finishes when the patient needs to stop and distance achieved calculated.

6-min walk test (6MWT)

30-m course between two points on a hard flat surface. Patients do as many 60-m laps as they can around the 2 points in 6 min. They determine their pace and intensity of exercise. They are allowed to rest in the time if they need to. Total distance walked in 6 min is counted. Results vary according to mood and encouragement.

Future developments

- Determining which components of rehabilitation are the most valuable to improvements in exercise: intensity of exercise programme, type of exercise
- How to optimally maintain the improvements following a rehabilitation programme
- Performance enhancement using oxygen, steroids, nutrition, creatine, heliox, non-invasive ventilation.

Further information

Nici L *et al.* ATS/ERS statement on pulmonary rehabilitation. *Am J Respir Crit Care Med* 2006; **173**: 1390–413

Troosters T *et al.* Pulmonary rehabilitation in COPD. *Am J Respir Crit Care Med* 2005; **172**: 19–38

Lacasse Y, *et al.* Pulmonary rehabilitation for COPD (Cochrane Review). CD003793

Salman *et al.* Rehabilitation for patients with COPD: meta-analysis of RCTs. *J Gen Int Med* 2003; **18**(3): 213–21

BTS Statement on Pulmonary Rehabilitation. *Thorax* 2001; **56**: 827–34

Griffiths TL *et al.* Results at one year of outpatient multidisciplinary pulmonary rehabilitation: a randomised controlled trial. *Lancet* 2000; **355**: 362–68

Lacasse Y *et al.* Meta-analysis of pulmonary rehabilitation in COPD. *Lancet* 1996; **348**: 1115–19

Chapter 61

Smoking cessation

Aims and nicotine replacement therapy

Smoking is the main cause of chronic obstructive pulmonary disease and lung cancer. The NHS spends £1.7 billion per year caring for people with smoking-related conditions. Government targets have been set to reduce the number of smokers in the UK and health authorities have been allocated funding for smoking cessation services.

- Approximately 31% of men and 29% of women in the UK smoke and 82% of smokers start as teenagers
- The incidence of smoking is increasing in developing countries
- Smoking is also associated with bladder, oesophageal, cervical, and renal cancers, as well as cardiovascular and cerebrovascular disease
- Nicotine exerts its effects on the CNS and is very addictive
- Peak nicotine withdrawal time is 2–3 days
- 0.4% of smokers manage to stop each year
- Stopping smoking is associated with an average weight gain of 2 kg
- Government legislation in the UK banned smoking in the workplace and public places from 1st July 2007 and increased the age for sale of tobacco from 16 to 18 on 1st October 2007.

Aims of smoking cessation interventions In order to achieve the goal of sustained abstinence, the aim is to reduce short-term cravings for nicotine (nicotine and non-nicotine replacement therapy) and in the long term to modify behaviour (counselling, telephone or group support (buddy systems)). It is vital that the smoker is motivated to stop or attempts will fail. It is important as a health professional to address smoking cessation at all opportunities. Health professionals can trigger quit attempts by giving brief advice to all smokers. This can lead to 1–3 out of 100 people stopping smoking for 6 months. Doctor advice often has the strongest impact. People may be more receptive to smoking cessation advice during times of concern for their own or their families health. A guide to approaching the topic is:

- Ask how much a person smokes and document pack-years
- Advise on risks of continued smoking. Assess commitment to quitting
- Assist by offering behavioural therapy ± pharmacotherapy
- Provide self-help material and refer to stop smoking services
- Arrange follow-up.

Some hospitals or primary care trusts have smoking cessation counsellors. The best results in terms of quit rates are achieved by combining counselling with nicotine replacement therapy (NRT), bupropion, or varenicline, with regular support and follow-up. These can improve quit rates to around 25%. The National Institute of Health and Clinical Excellence has issued guidance on the use of nicotine replacement therapy, bupropion, and varenicline for smoking cessation. This advises pharmacotherapy should only be for a smoker committed to a target stop date. Choice of therapy is based on a patient's likely compliance, availability of counselling, previous experience of therapies, contraindications, and patient preference. Prescribe 2 weeks of NRT or 3–4 weeks of bupropion/varenicline and only give further prescription if individuals show a continuing attempt to quit. If they fail to quit, a second attempt within 6 months should not be funded.

Nicotine replacement therapy (NRT) allows short- and medium-term nicotine withdrawal symptoms to be minimized, by replacing nicotine. Should not be used whilst still smoking, as it is possible to overdose on nicotine (symptoms: agitation, confusion, restlessness, palpitations, hypertension, dilated pupils, SOB, abdominal cramps, vomiting). Can be bought over the counter or be prescribed by general practitioner, and is cheaper than cigarettes. Most NRT products are contraindicated in pregnancy, breast-feeding mothers, and children under 18, but are used under supervision.

- ***Patches*** Give small amounts of nicotine via transdermal patch to decrease cravings before they occur. Different strength patches (15, 10, 5 mg) according to how much is smoked. Use higher dose patch if 10+ cigarettes per day smoked. Convenient. Worn continuously throughout day, but removed at night due to vivid nature of dreams. Can get localized irritation at patch site. Patches should be used for 6–8 weeks at the higher dose, then weaned to a lower dose for 2–4 weeks. Available to buy over the counter
- ***Chewing gum*** Different strengths of gum that release nicotine as they are chewed. (Smoke <20/day - chew one 2-mg piece slowly for 30 min when urge to smoke occurs. Smoke >20/day or needing >15 pieces of 2-mg gum daily—use 4-mg strength gum. Max 15 4-mg pieces/day). Relieves cravings as they occur. When mouth tingles and has peppery taste, should stop chewing and 'park' the gum inside the cheek. Nicotine is then absorbed through the lining of the mouth. Should not chew continuously or may become nauseated. Nicotine needs to be absorbed through mouth and not swallowed in saliva. Therefore don't drink with gum. Physical act of chewing can relieve craving. Can taste unpleasant and may need to use several packs of gum a day. Use for 3 months, then reduce the strength and the amount of gum used. Available to buy over the counter
- ***Sublingual tablets*** used on demand to help with cravings. Useful for smokers wanting a discreet form of treatment. 1–2 tablets should be placed under the tongue every hour when needed. Dissolve over 30 min. Licensed for use in pregnancy (1 tablet only). Use for 3 months and then gradually reduce the number of tablets used a day. Available on prescription
- ***Lozenges*** Available to buy over the counter
- ***Inhalator*** Cigarette style appliance giving small amounts of nicotine when used. Useful for people who are habitual or ritualistic in when they have a cigarette and want the 'hand to mouth' routine. Nicotine is absorbed through the lining of the mouth, not via the lungs. Use for 2 months, and then gradually reduce. Available on prescription
- ***Nasal spray*** provides rapid relief of craving. Faster absorption than other forms of NRT. May cause local irritation. Use for 2 months; then reduce. Available on prescription.

Non-nicotine replacement therapy

Drugs

Bupropion (Zyban®) is promoted as an aid to smoking cessation in combination with motivational support. It is an antidepressant that was found to reduce the desire to smoke, regardless of whether people were depressed or not. It weakly inhibits dopamine, serotonin, and noradrenaline reuptake in the CNS. It counteracts nicotine withdrawal symptoms by increasing these levels in the brain. It is suitable if people smoke 10 or more cigarettes a day. Liver metabolism and 20 h half-life. Smokers start taking bupropion 1–2 weeks before their intended 'quit day'. Continue taking it for 7–9 weeks after. Leads to improved abstinence rates compared with placebo or nicotine patch if associated with counselling (30% 12-month abstinence rate with bupropion, 16% with nicotine patch, 15% with placebo, 35% with patch and bupropion). (*NEJM* 1999; 340: 685–91) Also thought to lessen weight gain associated with stopping smoking. Contraindicated in patients with epilepsy or at risk of fits, those with a CNS tumour, those acutely withdrawing from alcohol or benzodiazepines, pregnancy, those with eating disorders and those on monoamine oxidase inhibitors. Reduce dose if elderly or hepatic or renal impairment. Recognized adverse effects include dry mouth, hypersensitivity, insomnia, seizures (1 in 1000 users) and death. Prescription only.

Varenicline (Champix®/Chantix®) is a new drug, also promoted as an aid to smoking cessation in combination with motivational support. It binds to the $\alpha_4\beta_2$-nicotinic acetylcholine receptor and acts as a partial agonist. Its binding alleviates symptoms of craving and withdrawal, and reduces the rewarding and reinforcing effects of smoking by preventing nicotine binding to the $\alpha_4\beta_2$ receptors. Smokers start taking varenicline 1–2 weeks before their intended 'quit day' and continue for 12–24 weeks. Starting dose is 500 μg od for 3 days, 500 μg bd for 4 days, then 1 mg bd for 11 weeks, if tolerated. If smokers are abstinent after 12 weeks, they should continue for another 12 weeks to avoid relapse. Avoid abrupt withdrawal. Side-effects include nausea, vomiting, appetite change, change in taste, headache, difficulty sleeping, abnormal dreams, dry mouth, tiredness. Use with caution if breast feeding, history of psychiatric disease, renal impairment. RCTs have shown significantly higher quit rates with varenicline than with bupropion or placebo. Quit rates are higher with higher doses (e.g. continuous quit rate for any 4 weeks: 48% with 1 mg bd ($p = 0.01$ vs. placebo), 37% with 1 mg od ($p = 0.01$), 33% with bupropion ($p = 0.02$, 17% with placebo), Drug-side effects leading to stopping treatment were lower than with bupropion (*Arch Int Med* 2006; **166**: 1561–8). Prescription only.

Hypnosis aims to improve will power in the subconscious state with therapeutic suggestion. Anecdotal success, but Cochrane review of trials showed no greater abstinence rate with hypnosis than with any other treatment or placebo treatment.

Acupuncture/acupressure No evidence in favour of it over placebo acupuncture.

Future developments

- Increasing and improving hospital-based smoking cessation services with links to community-based services
- Nicotine immunotherapy. Laboratory-based models to create a 'nicotine vaccine' to try and prevent abstinent smokers from re-starting are in progress. Induce specific nicotine antibodies to prevent inhaled nicotine from binding to nicotine receptors and causing neurological stimulation.

Further information

BTS powerpoint 'toolkit' for smoking cessation www.brit-thoracic.org.uk/cessationcompetencies

Brief interventions and referral for smoking cessation in primary care and other settings. March 2006. www.nice.org.uk

ABC of smoking cessation series. *BMJ* Feb-April 2004

Riemsma RP *et al.* Systematic review of the effectiveness of stage based interventions to promote smoking cessation. *BMJ* 2003; **326**: 1175

West R *et al.* Smoking cessation guidelines for health professionals. *Thorax* 2000; **55**: 987–99

www.doh.gov.uk/tobacco

www.nosmokingday.org.uk

Quitline 0800 002200

Chapter 62

Tracheostomy

Temporary tracheostomy is most often performed as an adjunct to assisted ventilation. Such patients are now often returned to respiratory wards for 'decannulation'.

Indications for tracheostomy on the ICU (no uniform agreement)

- Usually performed after a period of time following intubation with an endotracheal tube
- Improved patient communication (with appropriate cuff deflation and/or tube fenestration)
- Possible reduction in laryngeal damage. The evidence for this is very limited
- Nursing care potentially easier
- Facilitation of weaning.

(There is no evidence for a reduced incidence of aspiration or pneumonia with tracheostomy versus endotracheal tube.)

The usual practice is to convert from endotracheal tube to tracheostomy at 7 days if ventilation is likely to be needed beyond 14 days. Conversion beyond 14 days is considered best practice and certainly by 21 days.

Percutaneous versus surgical tracheostomy Percutaneous tracheostomy (PT) can be performed on the ICU immediately once the decision is made and is quicker than conventional tracheostomy. There are a variety of PT techniques: Griggs' guidewire with dilating forceps, and the Ciaglia multiple or single (Blue Rhino) dilator approach, preferably with endoscopic verification of placement. In the Blue Rhino system a curved, cone-shaped dilator is slid over a guidewire and introduced into the tracheal lumen between the 2nd and 3rd tracheal rings until the hole is large enough to accept the required tracheostomy tube. This technique requires controlled force and there is significant potential for traumatic damage. The fit of the tracheostomy tube is tighter, with less stomal infection, less post-operative haemorrhage, but the long-term complications of the two techniques are similar. However, units with prompt access to surgical tracheostomy tend to use this whenever possible, due to the potential traumatic damage from the PT approach. Humidification of the inspired gas is always required to prevent the build-up of thick viscid mucus. Humidification can only be withdrawn in long-term tracheostomy patients after several weeks or months.

Decannulation Tracheostomy may still be required to administer intermittent ventilation, reduce ventilatory deadspace, aid respiratory secretion clearance, limit aspiration (when cuffed), and bypass any upper airway obstruction. This is weighed against the consequences of a tracheostomy: increased tendency to aspirate (because of a reduced ability to swallow), reduced ability to talk, and the increased infection brought about from a foreign body in the trachea and bypassing the upper airway. Thus, decannulation should be carried out as soon as:

- Adequate clearance of secretions, i.e. good cough and thin secretions
- No upper airway obstruction

- No significant aspiration (can be checked by drinking methylene blue and then suctioning), although a small amount is not an absolute contraindication
- No need to continue ventilation for maintenance of gas exchange
- Conversion to non-invasive ventilation is possible, and has been demonstrated to work adequately.

The ability to cope adequately without the tracheostomy can be repeatedly determined (and for increasing periods) by capping the tube with the cuff fully deflated and preferably with a fenestrated tube.

Once a tube has been removed, the stoma can close over very quickly and make reinsertion difficult. Introducing a 'guidewire', over which the old tube is removed and the new can be inserted, is often useful (a suction tube, with the connector cut off, will suffice).

The final decision to decannulate is often delayed unnecessarily. Sooner rather than later is usually better.

Available tube options Tracheostomy tubes can be cuffed or uncuffed. If ventilation is not necessary, and aspiration is not a problem, cuffs are not required. Some patients can be adequately ventilated even with the cuff down (or no cuff at all): this is usually in patients with normal lungs where the compliance is good and inflation pressures therefore low.

Tracheostomy tubes can be either single or double (i.e. with an inner and outer tube). Double tubes allow better cleaning and therefore reduce the chance of the lumen obstructing, but the diameter of the lumen is of course less for a similar sized external diameter.

Tracheostomy tubes can be fenestrated to allow exhalation via the larynx to aid talking. The fenestration can be closed off with a non-fenestrated inner tube, should intermittent ventilation still be required.

Speaking valves are available that fit on the tracheostomy, allowing inspiration via the tracheostomy, but close and allow expiration via the larynx (if cuff down and/or fenestration open). They effectively maintain a reduced deadspace, maintain access for suctioning, but allow talking.

Further information

Commercial video of Blue Rhino insertion, http://www.cookmedical.com/cc/educationMedia.do?mediaId=1558

Part 4

Practical procedures

Chapter 63

Airway management

Simple airway

▶▶ Call for anaesthetic help early

Patients may require support of their airway and ventilation/oxygenation in situations when they are unable to adequately maintain these. Such situations may be related to a Glasgow Coma Score of <8, which can cause difficulties with airway maintenance, or related to respiratory compromise or arrest in the critically ill patient.

Simple airway adjuncts are used to overcome backward tongue displacement in an unconscious patient.

Oropharyngeal airway (Guedel) A curved plastic tube with a flanged end that is inserted into the mouth. Size is estimated by holding it at the side of the patient's face and estimating required length from angle of the mouth to angle of the jaw. Ensure the mouth is clear, then insert the airway 'upside down', with the curved side towards the tongue. When it is in as far as the soft palate, turn it around by 180° and push it in further, so the flange is at the patient's mouth. If the patient has a gag reflex, remove the airway. Suction can be performed through the airway and oxygen administered via a mask.

Nasopharyngeal airway A soft plastic tube with a bevelled end and a flange at the other end. Better tolerated in the semi-conscious, and should not be used in those with base of skull fractures. Sizes 6–7mm are suitable for adults. If necessary, insert a safety pin through the flange. Lubricate it with water-soluble jelly and insert the bevelled end into a nostril and gently push back with a twisting action. Do not force if obstruction is encountered, but remove and try in the other nostril. Nasal bleeding can be caused if the mucosa is damaged. The safety pin ensures the airway is not dislodged into lung. Oxygen can be administered through a mask.

Intubation

Endotracheal tube The optimal method of managing a patient's airway and providing airway protection from aspiration of gastric contents. Requires training in tube insertion. The tube is bevelled at one end with an inflatable cuff and has a connector at the other end. The connector can be removed if the tube needs to be cut, but can be replaced.

- Patient lies flat, with neck flexed and head extended (the 'sniffing the morning air' position). A pillow is placed under the head, not the neck, to aid this
- Pre-oxygenate with bag and mask ventilation
- Using the laryngoscope in left hand and standing behind the head, the mouth is opened, and the laryngoscope placed over the right side of the tongue and advanced
- It may be necessary to apply suction to clear the mouth of secretions
- When the epiglottis is seen, the laryngoscope is advanced into the vallecula, between the root of the epiglottis and the base of the tongue Upward pressure in the direction of the laryngoscope handle is applied to lift the jaw slightly and the cords should come into view, taking care not to damage the teeth
- Slide the tube through the cords and then withdraw the laryngoscope
- Inflate the cuff

- Confirm adequate tube position by auscultating for breath sounds over the chest bilaterally
- End tidal CO_2 measurement should be used if available; 5 breaths showing CO_2 confirm an adequate tube position
- If the tube is not in position, usually because it has been passed into the oesophagus or the right main bronchus, deflate the cuff, remove the tube, and re-oxygenate with the bag and mask, before trying again. Pull the tube back slightly if the breath sounds are only on the right as this suggests the tube is in the right main bronchus
- Secure the tube
- Administer oxygen with a self-inflating bag with oxygen and reservoir bag
- CXR to confirm correct tube position 2–3 cm above the carina
- Suction can be performed through the tube

Laryngeal mask airway

An alternative to formal intubation. A wide-bore tube with an inflated cuff at one end, which is positioned over the larynx and inflated, hence forming a seal; thus aspiration of gastric contents and gastric inflation are minimized. It is easy to insert, and is used in anaesthetic practice and also used in emergencies. Requires minimal head tilt, so is ideal for use in patients with possible cervical spine injuries. Not suitable for patients with high airway resistance, such as pulmonary oedema, bronchospasm, or COPD. Select a size 4 or 5 tube and, after ensuring the cuff works, deflate it. Put water-soluble lubricating jelly over the cuff. The patient should be lying flat, with head extension if possible. Hold the tube like a pen and insert from behind the patient's head, with the point of the cuff positioned to the back of the mouth. Advance along the roof of the mouth and then press it downwards and backwards until resistance is felt. Inflate the cuff, which will cause the tube to lift out of the mouth a little. Confirm adequate airway position by auscultating for breath sounds over the chest bilaterally. Secure the tube.

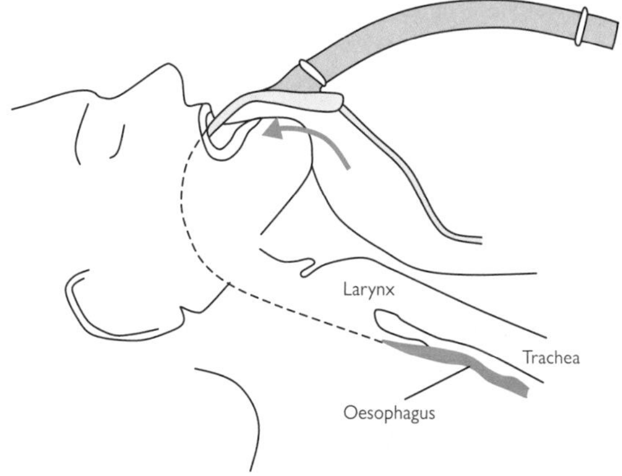

Fig. 63.1 Diagram of laryngeal mask insertion.

Chapter 64

Bronchoscopy

Indications and risks

Bronchoscopy is the procedure of passing a telescope or camera into the trachea to inspect the large and medium-sized airways. It may be performed with a flexible scope using local anaesthetic ± sedation, favoured by physicians, or under a general anaesthetic with a rigid scope, used mostly by surgeons. Airways can be visually inspected, samples taken, and therapeutic procedures can be performed. This chapter focuses on flexible bronchoscopy.

Indications for bronchoscopy

- ***Suspected lung cancer*** Patients who have a central mass <4 cm from the origin of the nearest lobar bronchus, which is likely to be accessible for biopsy at bronchoscopy
- ***Suspected pulmonary infection*** such as TB in a patient who is unable to produce sputum, or in immunocompromised patients, with fever, cough, hypoxia, or CXR changes (induced sputum with hypertonic saline may be an alternative; see p 769)
- ***Suspected interstitial lung disease*** if a transbronchial biopsy will provide an adequate sample for diagnostic purposes, such as in sarcoid. Only indicated in a limited number of interstitial lung diseases, as more adequate biopsies are often obtained through open lung biopsy, which may be preferable
- ***Foreign body removal*** if this is located proximally
- ***Therapeutic indications*** include central airway obstruction, sputum plugging, and possibly emphysema (endobronchial lung volume reduction, see p 180) and asthma (bronchial thermoplasty, see p 137).

Relative contraindications/take care

- If a patient has saturations below 90% on air at rest, or PaO_2 less than 8 kPa, the risk of significant hypoxia during bronchoscopy is increased
- FEV_1 <40% predicted
- Blood clotting abnormalities, particularly platelet level <50 000/mm^3
- Uraemia, pulmonary hypertension, SVCO, liver disease, and immunosuppression predispose to haemorrhage
- Recent myocardial infarction may be associated with cardiac ischaemia during bronchoscopy. Wait until 4–6 weeks after.

Risks associated with bronchoscopy Flexible bronchoscopy is a safe procedure, with reported mortality rates in large series being 0.01–0.04% and major complications of 0.08–0.12%. Complications include respiratory depression, pneumonia, pneumothorax, airway obstruction, laryngospasm, cardiorespiratory arrest, arrhythmias, pulmonary oedema, vasovagal episodes, fever (especially following BAL), septicaemia, haemorrhage, nausea, and vomiting.

Bleeding and bronchoscopy

- Bleeding occurs in approximately 0.7% of patients due to mechanical trauma from the scope, suctioning, brushing, or biopsy, but is more common with transbronchial biopsy (1.6–4.4%). Patients with malignancy, immunocompromise, or uraemia have an increased bleeding tendency
- If bleeding does not stop spontaneously, the bronchoscope should be wedged to tamponade the bleeding in the segmental bronchus. Use minimal suction, to allow clot formation. 1 mL aliquots of 1:10 000 adrenaline solution are administered via the bronchoscope as near to the bleeding point as possible, until it stops. Iced saline may be useful
- If massive haemorrhage occurs, the patient should be turned on to the side of the bleeding to protect the other lung. Balloon tipped vascular catheter may be used to tamponade the bleeding point. If bleeding continues, emergency or thoracic surgery may be indicated.

Further information

Lee P *et al.* Therapeutic bronchoscopy in lung cancer. *Clin Chest Med* 2002; **23**: 241–56

BTS Bronchoscopy guidelines. *Thorax* 2001; **56**(suppl. 1)

Bungay HK *et al.* An evaluation of CT as an aid to diagnosing patients undergoing bronchoscopy for suspected bronchial carcinoma. *Clin Radiol* 2000; **55**(7): 554–60

Laroche C *et al.* Role of CT scanning of the thorax prior to bronchoscopy in the investigation of suspected lung cancer. *Thorax* 2000; **55**(5): 359–63

Ernst A et al. Effect of routine clopidogrel use on bleeding complications after TBB in humans. Chest 2006; **129**: 734–7.

Patient preparation and procedure

Patient preparation

- ***Information*** Patients should be given written information about the procedure ideally more than 24 h prior to the procedure. Provide an information sheet for the patient to take home following the bronchoscopy, with advice about the effects of any sedation and possible complications, as well as telephone numbers in case help is needed
- ***Consent*** The physician performing the bronchoscopy should obtain written consent, with a description of the procedure and its associated risks
- ***Nil by mouth*** Patients should have no food for 4 h beforehand and clear fluids only until 2 h beforehand
- ***Blood tests*** Patients do not need routine pre-procedure blood tests, unless there are specific concerns (uraemia, deranged LFTs, low platelets). Many physicians check platelet counts and clotting times prior to transbronchial biopsy (platelets >75 000/mm^3, PT, and APTT within 1–2 s of control) and warfarin/heparin/low molecular weight heparin may be temporarily stopped
- ***Bedside tests*** Consider performing an ECG in patients with a history of cardiac disease. Check blood sugar in patients with diabetes
- ***Prophylactic antibiotics*** recommended in those at risk of endocarditis, i.e. asplenic, heart valve prosthesis, previous infective endocarditis: amoxicillin 3 g PO 1 h pre-bronchoscopy, or if penicillin allergic, clindamycin 600 mg PO or azithromycin 200 mg PO. Recent guidelines, however, from British Society of Antimicrobial Chemotherapy suggest this is not necessary (Gould FK *et al. J Antimicrob Chemother* 2006; **57:** 1035–42)
- ***In those with asthma***, a nebulized bronchodilator should be given before the bronchoscopy
- ***Those at high risk of infection (TB)*** should be last on the list.

Procedure

- Practices vary between centres. Some perform bronchoscopy with the patient sitting up facing the operator; some from behind with the patient lying flat
- ***IV access*** should be present in all patients
- ***Nasal oxygen*** should be administered and oximetry measured throughout
- ***Premedication*** may be given in addition for mild sedation, anxiolysis, and anterograde amnesia. A benzodiazepine such as midazolam 2 mg, with 1 mg increments as necessary, may be used with fentanyl. Some patients and operators prefer not to use sedation, due to concerns particularly in elderly patients, those with COPD, or those with cardiac disease. Midazolam can make some patients more agitated. Premedication with anticholinergics is not beneficial during bronchoscopy

- ***Lidocaine*** Local anaesthetic spray or gel is applied to the nostrils and the vocal cords are anaesthetized by spraying local anaesthetic (lidocaine 10 mg/spray) to the back of the throat and allowing time to work. Peak plasma levels occur after 15 min.
    - Transcricoid injection may be used to administer 4% lidocaine into the trachea, or this may be anaesthetized under direct vision through the bronchoscope, when the vocal cords are open
    - Aliquots of 1–2% lidocaine may be administered to right and left main bronchi via the bronchoscope when it is passed through the vocal cords into the trachea. Use the minimal dose required for cough suppression. Peak plasma levels occur after 5 min via the scope. Airway inflammation increases lidocaine absorption
    - Maximum dose of lidocaine is 8 mg/kg (= 29 mL of 2% solution in 70 kg patient); 5 mg/kg if hepatic or cardiac insufficiency. Toxic effects include seizures and arrhythmias
    - The half-life of lidocaine is 1.5–2 h
- Most access the trachea via the nasal route, as this gives increased stability when taking biopsies and allows the patient to cough and spit out secretions more easily. If this is not possible, a mouth guard is used and access obtained through the mouth
- All sections of the bronchial tree should be visually inspected, including the cords and trachea. CXR or CT may help localize the area of concern so specimen site can then be targeted. This increases the diagnostic yield of bronchoscopy in cases of suspected lung cancer
- Avoid unnecessary suction, as this can increase hypoxia.

Sampling techniques

Bronchial washings are taken by instilling about 10 mL of saline and then collecting it in a pot/trap to obtain superficial airway cells.

Bronchial brushings are taken by inserting a covered brush into a bronchial segment, uncovering it, rubbing the bronchial wall, covering it, removing it, and wiping it on a slide. The slide is then sprayed with a cell fixing solution.

Bronchial biopsies are taken with biopsy forceps. 5–7 should be taken to optimize yield. These may be taken blindly or from a visibly abnormal area, which gives a higher diagnostic yield than blind biopsies. They can be placed in formalin or saline solution depending on whether they are for histology or microbiology.

Bronchoalveolar lavage (BAL) is performed by inserting 50–100 mL of saline through the bronchoscope when it is wedged well in a small airway. Ideally instil fluid during inspiration and, after allowing the fluid to dwell for 10–30 s, aspirate back into the syringe during expiration or collect in a trap. Best performed in the area of abnormality on CXR or CT, or non-dependent lobes such as the right middle lobe or lingula. Poor return if the patient is coughing excessively or if they have emphysema. Can cause hypoxia proportional to amount of lavage fluid used.

Transbronchial biopsy (TBB) Technique of passing transbronchial biopsy forceps down a terminal bronchus until resistance is first felt and taking a sample of parenchymal tissue. Safe to perform if patient is taking aspirin or on subcutaneous heparin, but omit clopidogrel for 5 days before (as well as aspirin if taking both) and, if on warfarin, wait until INR <1.3. Some perform with radiological screening.

Associated with a significant risk of bleeding in 9% and pneumothorax in 3.5%, but up to 14% if patient is mechanically ventilated. Half of all pneumothoraces require chest drains. Therefore perform on one side only and minimize risk by performing TBB in the lower lobes, in dependent segments. Perform CXR 1 h after the bronchoscopy. Pneumothorax should be managed according to standard guidelines (p 376). Small pneumothoraces often resolve spontaneously, but the patient may need admission if there are concerns.

Transbronchial needle aspiration (TBNA) (see p 286) is used to sample mediastinal and hilar lymph nodes in suspected malignancy, TB, or sarcoidosis. It is also useful in sampling extrabronchial masses or necrotic endobronchial tumour. When added to other sampling techniques in lung cancer, it increases the diagnostic yield by 18%.

When performing bronchoscopy

- Wear gloves, face mask and eye shields
- Use particulate (duck) masks if there are concerns about TB or HIV

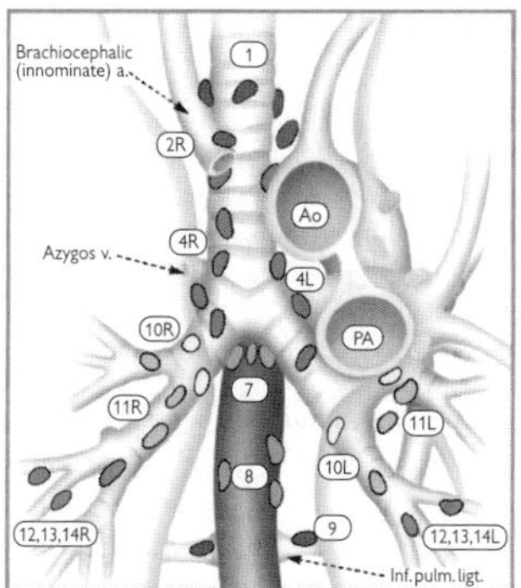

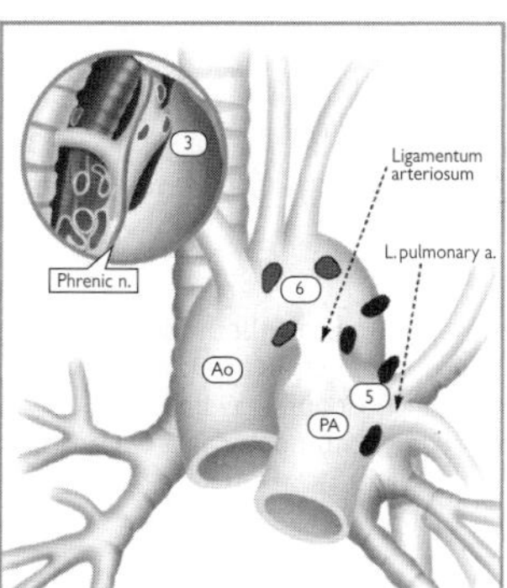

Superior Mediastinal Nodes

- **1** Highest Mediastinal
- **2** Upper Paratracheal
- **3** Pre-vascular and Retrotracheal
- **4** Lower Paratracheal (including Azygos Nodes)

N_2=single digit, ipsilateral
N_3=single digit, contralateral or supraclavicular

Aortic Nodes

- **5** Subaortic (A-P window)
- **6** Para-aortic (ascending aorta or phrenic

Inferior Mediastinal Nodes

- **7** Subcarinal
- **8** Paraesophageal (below carina)
- **9** Pulmonary Ligament

N_1 Nodes

- **10** Hilar
- **11** Interlobar
- **12** Lobar
- **13** Segmental
- **14** Subsegmental

Fig. 64.1 Mediastinal lymph node stations. Reproduced with the kind permission of the American College of Chest Physicians.

Central airway obstruction

(see also upper airway obstruction, p 640)

Central airway = trachea and mainstem bronchi

Obstruction can be:

- Extrinsic, such as tumour pressing on airway causing obstruction
- Intrinsic, such as tumour occluding airway lumen
- Mixed, a combination of extrinsic and intrinsic

Symptoms and signs

- May be asymptomatic if obstruction is mild
- Productive cough, due to mucosal swelling and mucous production
- Wheeze, unilateral wheeze, positional wheeze
- Stridor
- Secondary atelectasis and pneumonia
- Dyspnoea

Investigations

- Flow–volume loops, FEV_1
- CXR—may be normal
- CT chest + 3D airway reconstruction if possible
- Bronchoscopy to make tissue diagnosis of underlying disease

Treatment

- Secure airway
- Consider bronchoscopy – senior physician ± anaesthetist should perform. Bronchoscopy itself can cause obstruction in a compromised airway. Adrenaline administered via bronchoscope may be helpful
- Consider endobronchial treatment: core out tumour, dilate a stenosis, or place a stent (see p 755)
- Consider heliox (see p 641)

Causes of central airway obstruction

- Malignant
  - Primary endoluminal cancer, especially lung cancer or carcinoid
  - Metastatic cancer
  - Laryngeal cancer
  - Oesphageal cancer
  - Mediastinal tumour
  - Lymphadenopathy, lymphoma

- Non-malignant
  - Lymphadenopathy
  - Relapsing polychondritis
  - Tracheomalacia
  - Papilloma
  - Hamartoma
  - Amyloid
  - Web
  - Goitre
  - Foreign body
  - Granulation tissue

Further information

Ernst A *et al.* Central airway obstruction. *Am J Respir Crit Care Med* 2004; **169**: 1278–97

Janssen JP *et al.* Series: Interventional pulmonology. *Eur Respir J* 2006; **27**: 1258–71; **28**: 200–18

Wood DE *et al.* Airway stenting for malignant and benign tracheobronchial stenosis. *Ann Thorac Surg* 2003; **76**: 167–74

ERS/ATS Statement on Interventional Pulmonology. *Europ Respir J* 2002; **19**: 356–73

Interventional bronchoscopy

Used particularly in the diagnosis and palliative treatment of patients with lung cancer and central airway obstruction due to local tumour growth, where the relief of the obstruction will have symptomatic benefits.

Diagnostic procedures

Transbronchial needle aspiration and endobronchial ultrasound allow mediastinal node sampling without the surgical procedure of mediastinoscopy. Some lymph nodes are accessible for sampling in this way, which cannot be accessed via mediastinoscopy.

Transbronchial needle aspirate (TBNA) Technique of inserting a biopsy needle blindly through the bronchial wall into an enlarged lymph node or extrabronchial mass, and aspirating cells. Used to give additional staging information in lung cancer. Appropriate lymph nodes should be identified on CT first. Should be performed initially, so the bronchoscope is not contaminated with malignant cells from the airway, and start with the highest-stage lymph nodes first. Push sheath out through end of bronchoscope until the hub is just visible. Extend the needle and then position over nodal position and insert through bronchial wall. Subcarinal and right hilar nodes are the easiest to sample. Aim for 5–7 needle passes.

Endobronchial ultrasound (EBUS) Technique of visualizing the bronchial wall and the immediate surrounding structures via an ultrasound probe either incorporated into the tip of the bronchoscope or passed down the scope. A balloon surrounding the probe is inflated with water, in order to achieve close circular contact and view surrounding structures. Useful to assess lymph node involvement in malignancy and to guide TBNA: left and right paratracheal, carinal, subcarinal and some hilar nodes can be assessed. Mediastinal structures or masses next to the airways can be identified, the depth of bronchial wall tumour invasion assessed, or masses within the lung localized for biopsy. RCT shows improved yield compared with 'blind' TBNA. Oesophageal endoscopic ultrasound (EUS) is an alternative strategy, which allows examination of the posterior and inferior mediastinum, the liver, the coeliac axis, and the left adrenal gland. It is more accurate at diagnosing mediastinal metastases than CT and PET.

Autofluorescent bronchoscopy (AFB) Technique to differentiate central malignant areas from normal tissue, including dysplasia and pre-invasive tumours *in situ*. However, the progression of these abnormalities is not known, so the role of AFB is unclear. Used in conjunction with usual white light bronchoscopy. Uses blue light to induce tissue autofluorescence, which means normal and abnormal tissues appear different colours when viewed through a specialized bronchoscope. Airway trauma, however, can also cause a different mucosal appearance and the test has low specificity. It is being used in some centres as a surveillance tool following surgical resection of lung cancer, or in patients with head and neck cancer suspected of having a lung primary, or following positive sputum cytology. Its role is not, however, clear and advances in standard white light bronchoscopes (such as using narrow band imaging) may be found to be as good at identifying abnormal mucosa.

Rigid bronchoscopy Visualize bronchial tree to level of segmental bronchi. Can remove or core out endobronchial tumours, insert a stent, dilate tracheal or bronchial stenosis, and manage massive haemoptysis. Useful to provide information regarding resectability in lung cancer by measuring airway length. Incidence of serious complications <5%: hypoxia, laryngospasm, pneumothorax, bleeding.

Therapeutic procedures

Bronchial laser resection, electrocautery, argon–plasma coagulation, photodynamic therapy (PDT) and cryotherapy These are all procedures that can be used to debulk obstructing endobronchial lesions or coagulate a bleeding point. Electrocautery is the use of an electrical current via a probe to heat tissue, causing coagulational vaporization, which enables cutting. Laser achieves the same effect. These are used predominantly for obstructing malignant lesions, but may be used to remove benign lesions, e.g. papilloma, or to treat benign stenoses, e.g. due to intubation, sarcoidosis, Wegener's, trauma, etc. Avoid using FiO_2 >40% with both laser and electrocautery, to minimize the fire risk. Shave skin on thigh if necessary before placing electrode for electrocautery and avoid placing it over metal prosthetic joints. Argon–plasma coagulation is a non-contact method using argon gas. These are all effective immediately. Cryotherapy is the technique of freezing and then thawing an area with a probe in order to destroy tissue, such as an endobronchial obstructing lesion. It takes hours–days to have its effects. It can also be used to remove a foreign body, as freezing attaches foreign body to the end of the probe.
Photodynamic therapy Intravenous administration of a photosensitizer drug to the patient, followed by bronchoscopic exposure of the pre-sensitized tumour to a light of specific matching wavelength in order to cause tumour necrosis. Airways cleared of debris immediately after and again a few days later.
Bronchial stent insertion via the bronchoscope to re-establish airway patency if there is extrinsic compression. Self-expanding metal stents used in cases of external compression, such as lung cancer, for palliation of breathlessness. These are inserted over a guidewire with flexible bronchoscopic visualization. Repositioning can be tricky after placement. Retained secretions can cause stent blockage. Silicone stents are used in mainly benign disease and are inserted via rigid bronchoscopy. They are easily removed and manoeuvred, but can migrate and lead to problems with retained secretions.
Brachytherapy Procedure of endobronchial irradiation using iridium-192 via bronchoscope for endobronchial and intramural tumours. The radioactive source can be implanted into the tumour. Delayed effect, requires several sessions. Complementary to other bronchoscopic therapies. Can cause fistulas and haemorrhage.

Chapter 65

Chest drains

Indications, drain types, complications

Chest drain insertion is associated with significant morbidity and mortality, and careful consideration should be given to the precise indication for drainage. Ultrasound guidance may be required for small or loculated effusions (e.g. empyema).

Indications

- Tension pneumothorax (following needle decompression)
- Symptomatic pneumothorax with failed aspiration or underlying lung disease
- Complicated parapneumonic effusion and empyema
- Malignant pleural effusion for symptomatic relief and/or pleurodesis
- Haemothorax
- Traumatic haemopneumothorax
- Rarely, for symptomatic effusions of other aetiology.

Contraindications

- Inexperienced operator
- Lung adherent to chest wall
- Bleeding tendency (a relative contraindication; routine measurement of platelet count and clotting in the absence of risk factors is not required)
- Post-pneumonectomy (not a contraindication, but discuss with cardiothoracic surgical team; imaging may be required for drain placement).

Types of chest drain Traditional ***trocar*** drains consist of a flexible plastic tube surrounding a metal rod with a blunt tip and are available in a variety of sizes. When inserted incorrectly or with excess force by an inexperienced operator, they can cause significant harm and even death. Blue ***portex*** drains are inserted over a flexible plastic introducer in a similar manner to trocar drains; they are available in a range of sizes, up to 28F. Newer **Seldinger**-style drains involve sliding the drain into the pleural cavity over a guidewire. They are safer than trocar drains, but still require experience and care to be inserted safely and comfortably. Small (10–14F) drains are more comfortable and are adequate for the majority of situations. Large bore chest drains (28–32F) are only rarely required, e.g. secondary pneumothorax with large air leak and/or surgical emphysema, acute haemothorax.

Complications

- Pain—very common. Opiate analgesia frequently required
- Inadequate drain position—may require withdrawal or insertion of new drain
- Surgical emphysema (in pneumothorax)—air leaks into subcutaneous tissues. May occur if tube blocked or positioned with holes subcutaneously, or with very large air leaks. See p 383 for management
- Infection—empyema rate around 1%, perhaps higher in trauma patients
- Organ damage (e.g. lung, liver, spleen, heart, great vessels, stomach)—particularly if sharp trocar used. Intrapulmonary placement results in significant continuous bubbling and bleeding; this may occur in up to

6% of all drain insertions. Drainage of gastrointestinal contents suggests bowel perforation (or oesophageal rupture as the cause of the effusion)

- Haemorrhage into drain—bloody pleural fluid is a common finding (e.g. in malignant effusions), but unexpected large volume drainage of frank blood suggests damage to organs or intercostal vessels. Clamp the drain and leave it in place. Urgent imaging and surgical referral
- Re-expansion pulmonary oedema (p 383)
- Vasovagal reaction
- Sudden death due to vagus nerve irritation reported.

Insertion technique

An assistant is required.

1. Discuss procedure with patient and obtain written consent (unless emergency situation)
2. Insert IV cannula
3. Consider sedation (e.g. midazolam 2–5 mg IV or diamorphine 2.5–5 mg IV) with oxygen saturation monitoring; be cautious in patients with severe underlying lung disease or respiratory failure
4. Position patient lying with bed head at 30°, with insertion side of trunk rotated about 45° upwards, and arm on insertion side behind their head; stand behind the patient. Alternative position is with patient sitting forward, leaning over a table
5. Double-check correct side from chest examination and CXR
6. Choose insertion site: ideally within 'triangle of safety', which avoids major vessels and muscles (boundaries: anteriorly, anterior axillary line, and border of pectoralis major; posteriorly, posterior axillary line inferiorly, horizontal to level of nipple in man or fifth intercostal space in woman). More posterolateral approaches are safe, but less comfortable for the patient when lying; avoid posteromedial approaches close to spine, as intercostal artery drops medially to lie in mid-intercostal space
7. Sterile skin preparation. Wear sterile gloves and gown
8. Infiltrate skin, intercostal muscle, and parietal pleura with 10 mL of 1% lidocaine. Aim just above the upper border of the appropriate rib, avoiding the neurovascular bundle that runs below each rib. The subcutaneous fat lacks pain receptors and does not require anaesthetic. The parietal pleura, however, is extremely sensitive; use the full 10 mL of lidocaine
9. Verify that the site is correct by aspirating pleural fluid or air. Occasionally, a green (21G) needle may be too short in obese patients, and a longer needle is required. If unable to aspirate fluid or air, do not proceed with drain insertion; consider image-guided drainage
10. Whilst waiting for anaesthetic to work, prepare drain and connections. Assistant should prepare underwater seal
11. Insert drain:
    - **Trocar drains** Small (1-cm) skin incision parallel to rib. Consider horizontal mattress stitch across incision to facilitate later closure. Dissect intercostal muscles with blunt forceps (e.g. Spencer–Wells)—the fibres can be teased apart by opening and then removing the forceps; do not close forceps within the chest, this may damage underlying structures. This blunt dissection may take some time. Insert trocar and drain smoothly and gently—there should not be any significant resistance. ***Never apply force when inserting a chest drain.*** Once the chest wall has been entered, withdraw the trocar a few centimetres and insert the drain into the pleural cavity. Never insert the trocar blindly into pleural cavity. An alternative approach is to remove the trocar and grip the end of the chest tube with blunt forceps, and use these to guide the tube into the chest. Aim towards the apex for a pneumothorax, and the lung base for a pleural effusion

(Note—in emergencies, or in patients with extreme obesity or subcutaneous emphysema, it may be appropriate to make a larger initial incision and insert an index finger to assist the drain track)

- **Seldinger drains** Gently insert the introducer needle and check that air or fluid can be easily aspirated through it with a syringe. Remove syringe. Smoothly insert the guidewire through the introducer needle. Remove introducer needle. Slide plastic dilator around guidewire to enlarge the entry-track. Remove the dilator and slide the drain into the pleural cavity over the guidewire. Do not let go of the guidewire at any time. Remove the wire when the drain is within the chest

12. Connect the drain to underwater seal bottle via a three-way tap and tubing. If the drain is correctly positioned in the pleural space it should swing in time with respiration, and drain air or fluid
13. Stitch and tape the drain in place on the chest wall
14. Ensure adequate analgesia
15. Warn the patient not to disconnect the tubing or lift the underwater bottle above the level of the insertion site on the chest; supply a 'chest drain information leaflet'
16. Obtain CXR to check position. The 'ideal' tube position (apex for pneumothorax, base for effusion) is not necessary for effective drainage, so do not reposition functioning drains on this basis. CT may be useful in confirming drain position in certain circumstances. Drains are often positioned in fissures, but in most cases this does not affect their functioning
17. Small drains may need regular flush to ensure potency; prescribe 10 mL normal saline flush to drain tds

Further information

Laws D, *et al.* BTS guidelines for the insertion of a chest drain. *Thorax* 2003; **58**(suppl. II): ii53–9

Drain management

General points

- Patients should ideally be managed on a specialist ward by experienced nursing staff. 'Chest drain observations' should be charted regularly, including swinging, bubbling, and volume of fluid output
- If drain water level does not swing with respiration, the drain is kinked (check underneath dressing, as tube enters skin), blocked, clamped, or incorrectly positioned (drainage holes not in pleural space; check CXR). Occluded drains may sometimes be unblocked by a 30 mL saline flush. Non-functioning drains should be removed (risk of introducing infection)
- Suction is sometimes used to encourage drainage, although there is a lack of evidence regarding its use. Consider in cases of pneumothorax with persistent air leak, or following chemical pleurodesis. Suction should be high volume/low pressure, typically starting at a level of 5 cm H_2O and increasing to 10–20 cm H_2O. It is often painful and may not be tolerated by the patient.

To clamp or not to clamp?

Never clamp a bubbling chest drain (risk of tension pneumothorax). Clamping may be considered in two situations:

- To control the rate of drainage of a large pleural effusion. Rapid drainage of large volumes may result in re-expansion pulmonary oedema; clamping, e.g. for 1 h after draining 1 L, may prevent this
- To avoid inappropriate drain removal in cases of pneumothorax with a slow air leak, when bubbling appears to have ceased. Clamping of a drain for several hours followed by repeat CXR in such situations may detect very slow or intermittent air leaks. This is controversial, however, and should only ever be considered on a specialist ward with experienced nursing staff. If the patient becomes breathless, the drain should be immediately unclamped.
- **Drain removal** Quickly and smoothly remove the drain, whilst patient is breath-holding in expiration (although opinions on this differ—some recommend removal in maximal inspiration). Tie previously placed mattress suture, if applicable. Apply dressing. CXR to document lung position.

Chapter 66

Cricothyroidotomy

Indication

In some situations of upper airway obstruction or facial trauma, ventilation and tracheal intubation of a patient is impossible. It may therefore be necessary to create an immediate surgical airway below the level of obstruction.

Cricothyroidotomy

►► ***Call for anaesthetic and ENT help***

- Extend the head, with the patient lying flat. Place a pillow under the patient's shoulders, not their head
- Identify cricothyroid membrane: soft triangular area above cricoid ring and below the thyroid cartilage. (Put your fingers on the larynx and move them down to the soft area below, where you are aiming for). Clean with antiseptic swab
- Puncture the membrane in the midline with a large bore cannula (18G or larger). Remove the needle, attach a syringe, and aspirate air to confirm correct position. Specific cricothyroidotomy kits are available
- Angle the cannula downwards at 45° and advance. Ensure air can still be aspirated and then connect to high-pressure oxygen supply, with a Y connector if possible
- Occlude one limb of Y connector with a finger until chest rises and then release to allow exhalation, ideally via larynx. Inflate for 1 s and deflate for 4 s. Must allow air to be exhaled. If there is no Y connector, a hole is cut in the oxygen tubing, which can be intermittently occluded
- Secure the cannula
- Perform a formal surgical cricothyroidotomy with ENT help, as needle method does not allow adequate ventilation as the tube is too small and the larynx is blocked. Vertical skin incision; press lateral edges outwards to minimize bleeding. Transverse cricothyroid membrane incision, take care not to damage cricoid cartilage. Dilate tract with tracheal spreader or scalpel handle, and insert a cuffed tube.

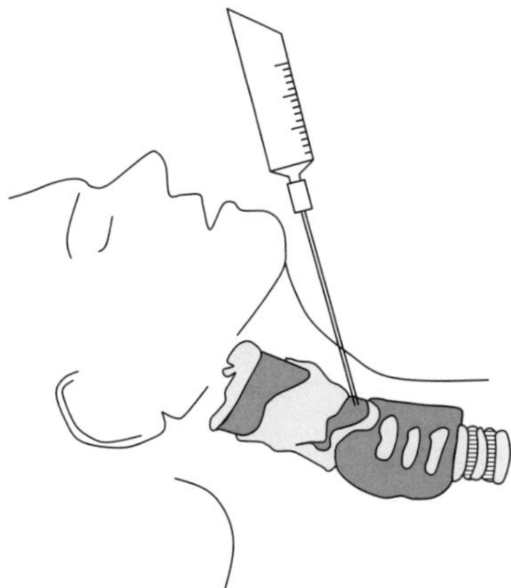

Fig. 66.1 Diagram of needle cricothyroidotomy. Reproduced from Wyatt *et al.* Oxford Handbook of Emergency Medicine 3e, 2006, with permission from Oxford University Press.

Further information

Advanced Life Support Provider Manual, 5th edn 2006. Resuscitation Council UK

Chapter 67

Miscellaneous diagnostic tests

Skin prick tests

These may be useful in identifying specific allergens causing immediate hypersensitivity reactions. They may influence management and guide allergen avoidance. They are also used to help define atopy. Triggers in contact urticaria, atopic eczema, and suspected food allergy may also be identified. The results are available almost immediately (compared with a RAST test for specific IgE) and correlate well with RAST test results. They should be carried out by staff trained to read the tests and manage adverse reactions.

The allergens tested should be identified from the history, and usually include common aeroallergens, e.g. grass, house dust mite (*Dermatophagoides pteronyssinus*), and cat dander.

Practical points

- Testing should be performed off steroids and anti-histamines
- There is a very small risk of anaphylaxis; adrenaline and resuscitation equipment should be available. Particular care is needed with food and latex testing
- Put a drop of allergen on the skin (usually the inside forearm). A range of allergens are available commercially. Fresh produce should be used for suspected fruit and vegetable hypersensitivity
- Lance the skin through the allergen drop using a needle (do not draw blood). This should be with a calibrated lancet (1 mm), held vertically, or a hypodermic needle held at 45° to the skin
- The positive control is usually histamine, and the negative control the dilutent (usually saline)
- Read the test after 15 min
- A positive result is an itchy weal, which should be compared with the controls, as some subjects react to the skin prick alone (dermatographism)
- Test solutions are standardized to give a mean weal diameter of 6 mm
- A weal of 3 mm or more is considered positive (indicating allergen sensitization)
- A positive result does not prove that the clinical symptoms are due to bronchial hyperresponsiveness to the tested allergen, but do raise clinical suspicion. Positive results can occur in those without symptoms, and false negatives do occur.

RAST or radio-allergosorbent blood tests are more specific, but less sensitive and more expensive than skin prick tests, but give similar information. There is no risk of anaphylaxis and the patient does not need to stop steroids or antihistamines for the test to be performed.

Unconventional tests Electrodermal allergy testing (using a Vegatest machine) was developed as an aid to homeopathic prescribing, and is widely used in complementary medicine to assess allergic status to food and environmental allergens. It is based on small changes in skin electrical impedance at acupuncture points, in response to allergens placed in an electrical circuit. There are no RCT data to show that this method can identify atopic from non-atopic individuals, as identified from skin prick tests.

Technique of induced sputum

- Used to investigate for infection (e.g. TB, PCP) or airway inflammation
- Patients rinse their mouth and clean their teeth to minimize oral contamination. Give inhaled salbutamol, to minimize bronchoconstriction
- Nebulized hypertonic (2.7–5%) saline is administered via a face mask. Afterwards the patient expectorates sputum into a sterile pot
- If transmission of infection (e.g. TB) is likely, perform the test in a negative pressure room, with appropriate protection of staff and other patients. Do not perform on the open ward or out-patient department
- Send sputum promptly to microbiology for staining and culture, and direct immunofluorescent testing for PCP (if indicated). Sputum for cell counts is mixed with 0.1% dithiothreitol, diluted with saline, and then filtered and centrifuged.

Methacholine challenge testing

- Methacholine induces bronchospasm in people with hyperreactive airways. Helpful if there is diagnostic doubt regarding the diagnosis of asthma
- Should be performed by experienced personnel, with facilities to deal with acute bronchospasm
- Increasing nebulized doses of methacholine are given systematically, with the FEV_1 measured after each dose
- If there is a 20% fall in FEV_1, or if the highest dose of methacholine has been given, the test is stopped
- The concentration of drug causing the 20% fall is known as the PC_{20}
- Asthma is indicated by a $PC_{20} < 8$ mg/mL. Normal subjects have a PC_{20} >16 mg/mL.

Chapter 68

Pleural biopsy

Indications for Abrams' pleural biopsy

- Diagnosis of tuberculous pleural effusion
- Abrams' biopsy is used for the diagnosis of malignant pleural disease in many centres, although a recent randomized controlled trial has shown that CT-guided cutting-needle biopsy has a greater sensitivity (sensitivity 87% in CT-guided biopsy group vs. 47% in Abrams' group).

Technique

An assistant is required.

1. Discuss procedure with patient and obtain written consent
2. Insert IV cannula
3. Consider sedation (e.g. midazolam 2–5 mg IV, with oxygen saturations monitoring)
4. Position patient sitting forward, leaning on a pillow over a table with their arms folded in front of them
5. Double-check correct side from chest examination and CXR
6. Choose biopsy site: 1–2 intercostal spaces below upper level of effusion on percussion. Use posterior or lateral approach (although avoid very posterior approaches close to spine, as intercostal artery drops medially to lie in mid-intercostal space)
7. Sterile skin preparation. Wear sterile gloves and gown
8. Infiltrate skin, intercostal muscle, and parietal pleura with 10 mL of 1% lidocaine. Aim just above the upper border of the appropriate rib, avoiding the neurovascular bundle that runs below each rib. Anaesthetize area behind rib below the insertion point
9. Whilst waiting for anaesthetic to work, assemble Abrams' reverse bevel biopsy needle. The needle consists of an outer sheath with a triangular opening (biopsy port) that can be opened or closed by rotating an inner sheath
10. Verify that the insertion site is correct by aspirating pleural fluid with a green (21G) needle. If unable to aspirate fluid, do not proceed
11. Make small (5 mm) skin incision; dissect intercostal muscles with blunt forceps (e.g. Spencer–Wells)
12. Insert biopsy needle gently with biopsy port closed. Do not apply force; the needle should slip into the pleural space without resistance. When in the pleural cavity, fluid can be withdrawn by attaching a syringe to the needle and opening the biopsy port
13. To take a biopsy, attach a syringe to the needle. Open the biopsy port and angle it downwards, and then pull the biopsy port firmly against the parietal pleura on the rib beneath the entry point (6 o'clock position relative to entry point). Close the biopsy port, thereby pulling a sample of parietal pleura into the needle
14. Remove the biopsy needle, open the biopsy port, and remove biopsy sample
15. Repeat procedure 4–6 times in positions 4–8 o'clock, always sampling below the insertion point (to avoid the neurovascular bundle beneath the rib above)
16. Send biopsy samples in saline for analysis for tuberculosis and in formalin if malignancy is suspected

17. Apply dressing to biopsy site. May require a single stitch
18. CXR to exclude pneumothorax.

Complications include pain, pneumothorax, haemothorax, and empyema. Haemorrhage from trauma to an intercostal artery may necessitate emergency thoracotomy. Fatalities are well documented, but rare.

Further information

Maskell NA *et al.* Standard pleural biopsy versus CT-guided cutting-needle biopsy for diagnosis of malignant disease in pleural effusions: a randomised controlled trial. *Lancet* 2003; **361**: 1326–31.

Chapter 69

Pleurodesis

The aim of pleurodesis is to seal the visceral pleura to the parietal pleura with adhesions to prevent pleural fluid or air accumulating. Successful pleurodesis is dependent upon two factors.

- Lung re-expansion following removal of pleural fluid or air, which allows the apposition of visceral and parietal pleura. This may be encouraged by applying suction to an intercostal drain
- Inflammation of the pleural surfaces, which is required to produce pleural fibrosis and adhesions. This may be induced by a chemical sclerosing agent or by pleural abrasion at thoracoscopy.

Indications

- Recurrent and symptomatic pleural effusion (most commonly as a result of malignancy, although pleurodesis is also rarely used in benign recurrent effusions)
- Recurrent pneumothorax (due to concerns regarding the long-term safety of intrapleural talc, surgical abrasion pleurodesis is usually the procedure of choice in younger patients; chemical pleurodesis may be used as a last resort in older patients who are unfit for surgery).

Chemical pleurodesis

Types of sclerosant Choice of sclerosing agents varies. The most commonly used agents are sterile talc, tetracycline, and bleomycin.

- Talc is the most effective (success rate about 90%), and can be administered either as a slurry via a chest drain or as a poudrage at thoracoscopy, but it carries a risk of inducing ARDS (see later)
- Tetracycline is successful in about 65% cases
- Bleomycin has success rates of only 60%, and is expensive.

Other rarely used agents include doxycycline, minocycline, interferon, interleukins, cisplatin, or the patient's own blood.

Corticosteroids may increase the failure rate of pleurodesis by inhibiting the pleural inflammatory response and development of adhesions, and should be discontinued beforehand. The effect of NSAIDs on the success of pleurodesis is unclear.

Technique Most centres will have a written pleurodesis protocol, usually involving premedication and intrapleural local anaesthesia. A typical protocol is set out below.

1. Discuss procedure with patient and obtain written consent
2. Insert chest drain (p 760): small bore (10–14F) chest tubes are sufficient for fluid drainage and pleurodesis, and are more comfortable than larger drains. Flush drain with 20 mL normal saline 6-hourly
3. Commence heparin 5000 IU bd as prophylaxis against thromboembolism (increased risk following pleurodesis, especially in patients with malignancy)
4. Drain fluid in a controlled manner. There is a small risk of re-expansion pulmonary oedema if large effusions are drained too quickly; control output by clamping drain; aim to drain a maximum of 1 L/h

5. CXR when drain output slows (<150 mL/day):
   - Consider pleurodesis if fluid removed and lung fully or partially expanded on CXR (although success rates are much lower in the setting of an incompletely expanded lung)
   - Consider trial of suction if lung only partially re-expanded. Aim to gradually increase pressure to –20 cmH_2O. Use of suction may be limited by pain.

For pleurodesis

6. Insert IV cannula and attach pulse oximeter
7. Pleurodesis is often extremely painful. Consider premedication with opioid (diamorphine 2.5 mg IV), anti-emetic (metoclopramide 10 mg), and benzodiazepine (midazolam 1–2 mg IV, titrate to conscious level; care in elderly and in patients with respiratory failure). The patient should be comfortable, but cooperative
8. Administer intrapleural local anaesthetic (e.g. lidocaine 3 mg/kg, maximum 250 mg) via the chest drain, as intrapleural administration of sclerosants is frequently painful. Clamp drain and wait several minutes
9. Administer sterile talc slurry (4 g talc in 30 mL normal saline)
10. Flush drain with 20 mL saline
11. Further analgesia if required
12. Clamp drain for 1 h after administration of sclerosant. Then unclamp drain and consider applying suction, –20 cmH_2O. Restart drain flushes
13. Monitor pulse, blood pressure, temperature, respiratory rate, and oxygen saturations half-hourly for 2 h and then 6-hourly
14. Analgesia and antipyretics as required
15. Optimal duration of drainage following pleurodesis is unknown; consider drain removal within 12–72 h if there is adequate drainage of fluid and lung expansion on CXR. Can usually remove tube at 48 h
16. In cases of mesothelioma arrange prophylactic radiotherapy for the drain site (total of 21 Gy in 3 fractions over 1 week). Malignant seeding at drain sites in non-mesothelioma malignant effusions is uncommon and prophylactic radiotherapy is not required.

Complications All sclerosants may cause chest pain and fever as side-effects. Use of sterile talc may rarely (<1%) result in respiratory failure due to adult respiratory distress syndrome, manifest as hypoxia and diffuse pulmonary infiltrates within 48 h of pleurodesis. The risk appears to be reduced with lower talc doses (<5 g). 'Mixed' talc (containing small particles) appears to be associated with greater systemic inflammation and greater deterioration in gas exchange than 'graded' talc (which has small particles removed), so routine use of graded talc is now recommended.

Future developments are likely to focus on more effective and safer sclerosing agents for pleurodesis, for example, transforming growth factor-β, which has been demonstrated to produce an effective pleurodesis in rabbits.

Chapter 70

Pneumothorax aspiration

Indications

- ***Primary pneumothorax*** Consider aspiration if patient breathless and/or pneumothorax large (rim of air >2 cm on CXR)
- ***Secondary pneumothorax*** Consider aspiration if patient aged <50 years, with small pneumothorax (rim of air <2 cm on CXR) and minimal breathlessness.

Technique Refer to pp 380–1 for treatment algorithms.

1. Discuss procedure with patient and obtain written consent (unless emergency situation)
2. Insert IV cannula
3. Position patient sitting upright, supported on pillows
4. Double-check correct side from chest examination and CXR
5. Choose aspiration site: second intercostal space in mid-clavicular line on side of pneumothorax
6. Infiltrate skin, intercostal muscle, and parietal pleura with 10 mL of 1% lidocaine. Aim just above the upper border of the appropriate rib, avoiding the neurovascular bundle that runs below each rib. Parietal pleura is extremely sensitive; use the full 10 mL of lidocaine
7. Sterile skin preparation. Wear sterile gloves and gown
8. Whilst waiting for anaesthetic to work, connect 50 mL syringe to 3-way tap, with tap turned 'off' to patient
9. Confirm presence of pneumothorax by aspirating air with green (21G) needle
10. Insert large bore (e.g. 16G) cannula over upper border of rib. Remove inner needle, quickly connect cannula to three-way tap and 50 mL syringe
11. Aspirate 50 mL air with syringe, turn tap and expel air into atmosphere. Repeat until resistance felt, or 2.5 L of air aspirated (aspiration of >2.5 L suggests a large air leak, and aspiration is likely to fail). Halt procedure if painful or patient coughing excessively.
12. Remove cannula; cover insertion site with dressing
13. Repeat CXR. Ideal timing of CXR following aspiration is unknown; it may be advisable to wait several hours before performing the CXR in order to detect slow air leaks
14. Aspiration is successful if lung is fully re-expanded on CXR
15. If initial aspiration of a primary pneumothorax fails, repeat aspiration should be considered (unless ≥2.5 L has already been aspirated). At least one-third of patients will respond to a second aspiration.

Chapter 71

Thoracentesis

Thoracentesis ('pleural tap', or pleural fluid aspiration) may be diagnostic or therapeutic.

Diagnostic thoracentesis

Indication Undiagnosed pleural effusion.
There are no absolute ***contraindications*** to pleural aspiration, although care should be taken if the patient is anticoagulated.

Technique

1. Explain procedure to patient
2. Position patient sitting forward, leaning on a pillow over a table with their arms folded in front of them
3. Double-check correct side from chest examination and CXR
4. Choose aspiration site 1–2 intercostal spaces below upper level of effusion on percussion. Use posterior or lateral approach (although avoid very posterior approaches close to spine, as intercostal artery drops medially to lie in the mid-intercostal space)
5. Sterile skin preparation and aseptic technique
6. Infiltrate skin, intercostal muscle, and parietal pleura with 10 mL of 1% lidocaine. Aim just above the upper border of the appropriate rib, avoiding the neurovascular bundle that runs below each rib. The parietal pleura is extremely sensitive; use the full 10 mL of lidocaine
7. Aspirate pleural fluid with a green (21G) needle and 50 mL syringe
8. Following diagnostic tap:
   - Note pleural fluid appearance
   - Send sample in sterile pot to biochemistry for measurement of protein and LDH
   - Send a fresh 20 mL sample in sterile pot to cytology for examination for malignant cells and differential cell count. Use of a 3.8% sodium citrate tube may help preserve cells in cytology samples
   - Send samples in sterile pot and blood culture bottles to microbiology for Gram stain and microscopy, culture, and AFB stain and culture
   - Process non-purulent heparinized samples in arterial blood gas analyser for pH (consult biochemistry laboratory for local policy of pH analysis beforehand; never put purulent samples in the arterial blood analyser)
   - Consider measurement of cholesterol and triglycerides, haematocrit, glucose (with paired blood sample), and amylase, depending on the clinical circumstances
9. There is no need for a routine CXR following aspiration

If unable to aspirate fluid, further attempts should be made with ultrasound guidance. Ultrasound guidance may also be required for small or loculated effusions, or to distinguish fluid from pleural thickening.

If ***mesothelioma*** is likely, 'tattoo' the aspiration site with India ink (to guide prophylactic radiotherapy; pierce skin through ink) and perform aspiration in mid-axillary line 6th–7th intercostal space (corresponding to the site of thoracoscopy port, to minimize area of radiotherapy required).
Complications of thoracentesis include pneumothorax, cough, bleeding, empyema, spleen or liver puncture, and malignant seeding down aspiration site (particularly in mesothelioma).

Therapeutic thoracentesis

Indication Symptomatic relief of breathlessness due to a pleural effusion, most commonly due to malignancy.

Technique In many cases, can be performed as a day-case procedure.

1. The initial procedure is identical to that of diagnostic thoracentesis (steps 1–7 opposite). It is important to verify that the insertion site is correct by first aspirating pleural fluid with a green (21G) needle. If unable to aspirate fluid, abort the procedure and ultrasound the chest to check the presence and location of fluid
2. Carefully advance a large bore intravenous cannula along the anaesthetized track
3. Remove the inner needle and attach the cannula to a 3-way tap
4. Aspirate fluid from the chest with a 50 mL syringe via the 3-way tap, and flush the fluid into a pot through extension tubing. Drain a maximum of 1.5 L of fluid in one sitting (risk of re-expansion pulmonary oedema following sudden removal of very large volumes). Stop the procedure if resistance is felt, or the patient experiences discomfort or severe coughing
5. Apply dressing to aspiration site
6. Repeat CXR to document extent of improvement in effusion size and to exclude pneumothorax or trapped lung

Chapter 72

Thoracoscopy (medical)

Thoracoscopy is the procedure of examining the chest wall, parietal pleura, visceral pleura, and diaphragm with a thoracoscope and taking biopsies. Chemical pleurodesis can also be performed. Performed by chest physicians using sedation and local anaesthetic.

There needs to be an adequate space into which the thoracoscope is inserted without damaging the underlying lung. Patients suitable for thoracoscopy are therefore those who have an underlying pleural effusion or a pneumothorax, where the lung is away from the instrument insertion site.

Indications for thoracoscopy

- Undiagnosed pleural effusion—usually an exudate (diagnostic sensitivity of medical thoracoscopy is 95%)
- Suspected mesothelioma
- Staging of pleural effusion in lung cancer
- Treatment of recurrent pleural effusions with pleurodesis
- Pneumothorax requiring chemical pleurodesis, as an alternative to surgery, e.g. the patient unfit for surgical thoracoscopy.

Contraindications/proceed with caution

- Obliterated pleural space
- Pleural adhesions, as these may tear when pneumothorax is induced
- Bleeding disorder
- Hypoxia <92% on air
- Unstable cardiovascular disease
- Persistent uncontrollable cough.

Risks associated with thoracoscopy

Mortality rates are low (<0.01% of cases)

- Haemorrhage—may need diathermy in the pleural space. Rare
- Pulmonary perforations. Rare
- Air or gas embolism during pneumothorax induction. Rare <0.1%
- Local wound infection
- Empyema
- Fever, ARDS with talc poudrage (see p 777).

Preparation of patient and consent

- Patient should have written information >24 h before the procedure. Written consent taken by doctor performing procedure
- Check recent CXR and any CT scans available
- Check FBC, coagulation, U&E
- Send blood for group and save
- Nil by mouth for 4 h pre-procedure
- IV cannula in arm on the same side as the thoracoscopy to make repeated sedative administration during the procedure easy
- Premedication with analgesia, such as a single dose of oral ibuprofen 800 mg, 1–2 h before. Also antibiotics, such as cefuroxime 1.5 g IV, for infection prophylaxis
- Baseline oxygen saturations, pulse, BP, temperature. Measure oximetry throughout.

Procedure The patient is placed in the lateral decubitus position, with the side of the pleural effusion uppermost. Sedation is administered and allowed time to work. Oxygen (2–4 L/min) is administered via nasal cannulae. The skin is cleaned and local anaesthetic inserted, in the same way as for a chest drain. The aspiration of fluid or air from the pleural space confirms it is safe to proceed to thoracoscopy. An incision is made and blunt dissection performed through the parietal pleura. The thoracoscope port is then inserted. The pleural effusion is drained via a suction tube through the thoracoscope port. Air is allowed to enter the pleural space through this port so the lung does not re-inflate, and effectively a pneumothorax is created. The thoracoscope, with its light source, can then be inserted through the port and the chest cavity inspected. A second smaller incision allows forceps or other instruments to be inserted and biopsies taken.

Thoracoscopic biopsies are usually large and yield good diagnostic results. If the pleural surfaces have appearances consistent with malignancy, pleurodesis can be performed at the end of the procedure, using talc inserted via an insufflator. There is no evidence that pleurodesis performed at thoracoscopy is more efficacious than pleurodesis performed via chest tube, but it may save the patient having a further procedure.

Post thoracoscopy care

- Monitor oxygen saturations, pulse, blood pressure, and temperature
- The patient will have a chest drain *in situ*. This should be on free drainage initially, but continuous suction is required when the drain stops bubbling
- Analgesia as required, such as IV diamorphine 2.5 mg, dihydrocodeine 30–60 mg PO, paracetamol 1 g
- DVT prophylaxis with subcutaneous heparin (increased coagulopathy with talc pleurodesis)
- Mobile CXR on the morning after thoracoscopy
- Remove chest drain when the lung is re-inflated on CXR with minimal fluid or air drainage. Trapped lung occurs if the visceral pleura is too thick to allow lung re-inflation (see p 350)
- If mesothelioma is diagnosed, refer for radiotherapy to thoracoscopy and chest drain tract sites.

Further information

Daniel T. Diagnostic thoracoscopy for pleural disease. *Ann Thorac Surg* 1993; **56**: 639–40

Loddenkemper R, Boutin C. Thoracoscopy: present diagnostic and therapeutic indications. *Eur Respir J* 1993; **6**: 1544–55

Appendices

Appendices

Appendix 1

Blood gases and acid–base balance

Interpretation of arterial blood gases: 1

Normal ranges

Breathing air: PaO_2 > 12 kPa (>10 in normal elderly), $PaCO_2$ 4.6–5.9.

How to take

- **Arterial blood gases** Best taken from radial, rather than brachial, artery due to dual radial/ulnar supply to hand. Use a heparinized syringe, analyse immediately, or within 30 min if kept on ice.

Always record date, time and the % inspired O_2

- ***Arterialized capillary sample*** An under-used technique. Uses small glass pre-heparinized tube to draw up blood from a puncture on the ***end*** of the ear lobe. Blood gas machine must take microsamples (most do). $PaCO_2$ levels are accurate enough for clinical practice, but good arterialization, with rubefacients (Algipan/Deep Heat) or heat and vigorous rubbing, required for accurate PaO_2: the latter is less important as oxygenation can be assessed by oximetry. Can easily be performed by nursing staff, to monitor response to NIV and O_2 therapy.

The three main things blood gases tell you about gas exchange

- How much is the patient ventilating their alveoli? This is derived from the $PaCO_2$. $PaCO_2 \geq 6$ kPa = underventilating, $PaCO_2 \leq 4.5$ kPa = over-ventilating
- Is the PaO_2 high enough to adequately oxygenate tissues and prevent anaerobic metabolism? $PaO_2 > 6$ kPa ($SaO_2 \approx 80\%$) is probably adequate; $PaO_2 > 7$ kPa ($SaO_2 > 87\%$) is definitely adequate
- Is there evidence of V/Q mismatch? Evidence of low V/Q units is derived from the calculated alveolar to arterial (A–a) O_2 gradient

The two main things blood gases tell you about acid/base balance

(see later section on acid–base balance)

- What is the respiratory component to an abnormal pH? This is derived from the $PaCO_2$
- What is the metabolic component to an abnormal pH? This is derived from the standard base excess/deficit.

The A–a gradient calculator graph sets out the graphical representation of gas exchange

- Point ❶ = pO_2 and pCO_2 (virtually zero) of *inspired air* (atmospheric pressure ≈ 100 kPa, air is 21% O_2, and air is slightly 'diluted' by water vapour pressure (7 kPa) following humidification by upper airways). 21% of 100–7 = 20 kPa. (Point ❷ = pO_2 and pCO_2 when breathing 24% O_2 via a Ventimask and point ❸ = pO_2 and pCO_2 when breathing 28% O_2 via a Ventimask)
- Point❹ = theoretical pO_2/pCO_2 of *inspired gas* when breathing air, if all the O_2 removed and replaced by CO_2 (equivalent to extreme hypoventilation and impossible!), when the respiratory quotient (RQ = CO_2 produced/O_2 consumed) is 0.8 (usual value)
- The line between ❶ and ❹with a gradient of 0.8 describes all possible combinations of alveolar gas, moving towards ❶ if breathing more, and towards ❹if breathing less, called the *alveolar air line*.

- Point ❺ = area in which PaO_2 and $PaCO_2$ of *arterial blood* sit normally. If lungs are perfect gas exchangers, then blood leaving the lungs and entering systemic arterial circulation (❺) should be perfectly equilibrated with the alveolar gas (A).

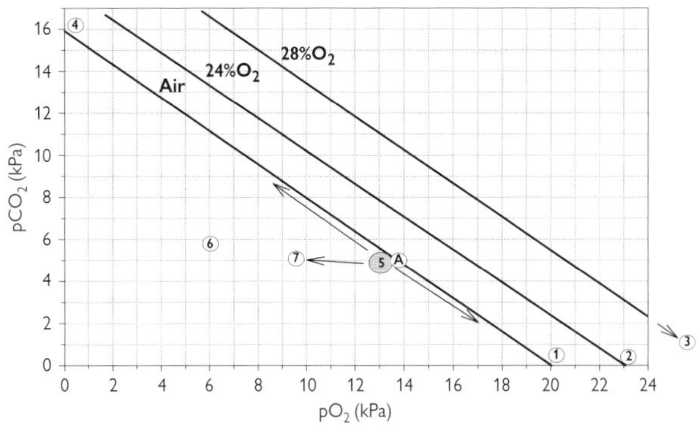

Fig. A1.1 pCO_2 vs pO_2: alveolar air lines and A–a gradient calculator.

- Point ❻ = However, the *mixed venous point* (or the *pulmonary arterial* blood) is well to the left of the alveolar air line. This is because capillary PO_2 falls more kPa than the PCO_2 rises during gas exchange in the tissues (CO_2 solubility curve is steeper than PaO_2–SaO_2 dissociation curve).
- Thus, if the lungs fail to oxygenate mixed venous blood properly (e.g. area of consolidation, or low V/Q due to asthma/COPD) then it is as if mixed venous blood has bypassed the lung and leaked into the arterial blood, which therefore moves the eventual arterial PaO_2/$PaCO_2$ point to the left of the alveolar air line, point ❼

Interpretation of arterial blood gases: 2

- The horizontal distance between the actual arterial point and the 'ideal' alveolar air line is called the ***alveolar to arterial (A–a) gradient*** and is a measure of how efficiently mixed venous blood is equilibrated with alveolar gas, i.e. it is a measure of V/Q mismatch, right-to-left shunts, and very severe lung fibrosis through reduced diffusion across the alveolar-capillary membrane. As well as being read off the graph it can be mathematically calculated as shown in Fig. A1.2.

Arterial PO_2 Arterial PCO_2

$$\text{A–a gradient} = PIO_2 - \left(PaO_2 + \frac{PaCO_2}{0.8}\right)$$

*Inspired PO_2 Respiratory quotient

*Calculation of inspired PO_2 breathing air or 24/28% O_2:
Air, 21% of (100–7) ≈ 20 kPa (where 100 kPa is atmospheric pressure and 7 kPa is water vapour pressure due to the inspired air being humidified); 24%, 24% of (100–7) ≈23 kPa; 28%, 28% of (100–7) ≈26 kPa

In Fig. A1.1 the alveolar air line depends on the % inspired O_2, and the two extra lines, for 24% and 28% O_2, are shown. In the calculation the PIO_2 has to be adjusted accordingly, (see Figure A1.2).

In normal lungs matching of V/Q is not totally perfect due to relative under-perfusion of the apices and over-perfusion of the bases (gravity effects on pulmonary arterial blood flow, not fully compensated for by hypoxic vasoconstriction of pulmonary arterioles). These imperfections in V/Q, and direct drainage of some of the cardiac muscle venous blood into the left ventricular cavity and thus systemic arterial circulation, lead to a small A–a gradient, 1–2 kPa in the young and middle aged, and 2–3 kPa in the elderly. Figures in excess of these values are abnormal and indicate areas of low V/Q or increased shunt.

Use of A–a gradient diagram: examples

Case 1 Consider point W in the pO_2–pCO_2 graph (Fig. A1.3), the blood gases on air of a young non-smoker complaining of chest pain 7 days post-operatively. The PaO_2 of 13 is normal. Does this reassure you or does it provide supporting evidence for a pulmonary embolus? Ask the following questions

- How much is the patient ventilating? $PaCO_2 = 2$; therefore ≤4.5 kPa and indicates hyperventilation
- Is the patient adequately oxygenated? PaO_2 >7 kPa; therefore, OK
- Is there an abnormal A–a gradient? Read off graph, horizontal line between W and alveolar line, or calculate:

  $20 - [13 + (2/0.8)] = 4.5$ kPa

  >2 kPa, hence yes; therefore the V/Q matching is not normal.

This provides supporting evidence for a pulmonary embolus, but could just as well be due to consolidation from pneumonia, for example

- Remember, PaO_2 cannot be used to assess V/Q matching in the lung without an associated $PaCO_2$ to tell you 'what the PaO_2 ought to be'.

Case 2 Consider point X on the pO_2–pCO_2 graph. These are the gases on air from a young man following an overdose of methadone tablets.

- How much is the patient ventilating? $PaCO_2 = 11$; therefore ≥6 kPa and indicates hypoventilation
- Is the patient adequately oxygenated? PaO_2 only 6 kPa; therefore not enough and needs extra O_2
- Has the patient got an A–a gradient?

  $20 - [6 + (11/0.8)] = 0.8$ kPa

<2 kPa, hence no; therefore there is nothing wrong with the lungs, despite the abnormal gases, this represents pure hypoventilation.

After a messy stomach wash-out he is sent to the ward and 24 h later is febrile. Gases on 24% O_2 are point Y on the graph; thus both $PaCO_2$ and PaO_2 are better.

- How much is the patient ventilating? $PaCO_2$ just ≥6 kPa; therefore is still hypoventilating a bit
- Is the patient adequately oxygenated? PaO_2 >7 kPa; therefore adequately oxygenated
- Has the patient got an A–a gradient?

  $23 - [11 + (6.5/0.8)] = 4.2$ kPa

(remember, the PIO_2 is 23 because he is on 24% O_2)

>2 kPa hence, yes; therefore may have developed an aspiration pneumonia.

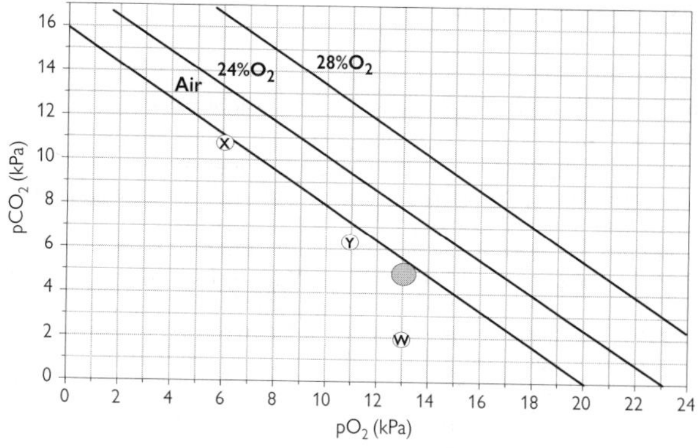

Fig. A1.3 Examples of using A–a gradient.

Three things blood gases tell you about gas exchange

- How much is the patient ventilating their alveoli?—$PaCO_2$
- Is the PaO_2 high enough to adequately oxygenate tissues and thus prevent anaerobic metabolism?
- Is there any evidence of a V/Q mismatch, assessed from the alveolar–arterial (A–a) gradient for oxygen?

Acid–base balance

Normal ranges

pH 7.37–7.43 (H^+ 37–43 nmol/L), $PaCO_2$ 4.7–5.9, base excess ±3 mmol/L.

Interpretation Acid–base relationships are best plotted as a $PaCO_2$ vs. pH graph, because these are the two primary measurements made by a blood gas machine (everything else to do with acid–base balance is calculated). This is shown opposite.

Normal acid–base is the area labelled N, the pH between 7.37 and 7.43, the $PaCO_2$ around 5 kPa. As ventilation is decreased or increased ($PaCO_2$ going up or down, respectively), the pH will change, the amount depending on the buffering capacity of the blood (CO_2 is an acid gas, combining with water to give [H^+] and [HCO_3^-] ions). Without buffering, the pH would fall disastrously following small rises in $PaCO_2$. This buffering capacity depends mainly on haemoglobin and other proteins, producing the normal buffer line running through N on the graph.

Therefore, ***acute hypoventilation and hyperventilation*** will move the patient up and down this line, in the direction *b* or *c*, respectively. If the ***hypoventilation*** at point *b* comes ***chronic*** (e.g. as it may in COPD), then the kidney retains bicarbonate (by excreting hydrogen ions) to try and correct the pH towards normal, and the patient moves onto a new iso [HCO_3^-] buffer line displaced to the right, e.g. the one labelled + 10 meq/L (35 meq/L). The degree of displacement represents the ***metabolic component to the acid–base status***, and in this case, because the [HCO_3^-] has risen, will be higher than the normal figure of about 25 meq/L. When the raised figure is quoted relative to the normal 25 meq/L (by subtracting 25), this is called the *base excess*. Thus, buffer lines to the right of the normal buffer line represent a metabolic alkalosis or base excess.

These figures are calculated assuming a normal or 'standard' $PaCO_2$, called the 'standard bicarbonate' (SBC on the blood gas machine printout), or 'standard base excess' (usually BE). The other similar figures on some printouts (usually HCO^-_3 and TCO_2) are calculated at the patient's actual $PaCO_2$ and are not much use.

Chronic hyperventilation (e.g. at altitude due to the hypoxia) produces the opposite, a resorption of [H^+] by the kidney, and the buffer line shifts to the left giving a negative value for the 'base excess', a *base deficit*. Thus, a metabolic acidosis compensates for a respiratory alkalosis. Note that these corrections rarely bring the pH back to normal as there needs to be an error signal to keep the correction process going.

A *metabolic acidosis* (such as in ketoacidosis) will also move the line to the left (*a*), producing a base deficit (or negative base excess), followed by hyperventilation to try and correct it (i.e. a respiratory alkalosis to correct a metabolic acidosis). This pure ventilatory stimulation in the absence of abnormal lungs often produces deep breathing with little increase in rate and is called ***Kussmaul's breathing***. Thus, lines to the left of the normal buffer line represent a metabolic acidosis or base deficit. A metabolic acidosis due to anaerobic metabolism (and hence lactic acid production) can reverse the compensatory metabolic alkalosis secondary to chronic hypercapnia during a severely hypoxic COPD exacerbation, removing the evidence for chronic CO_2 retention.

Finally, a *metabolic alkalosis*, e.g. during hypokalaemia (when the kidney is forced to use hydrogen ions instead of potassium ions to swap for the sodium that needs resorbing from the tubular fluid) moves the buffer line to the right (*d*), but with only limited hypoventilation available to compensate, due to the inevitable ventilatory stimulation the attendant hypoxaemia produces.

Thus, the mixture of respiratory and metabolic contributions to a patient's acid–base disturbance can be established by plotting the $PaCO_2$ and pH on the graph.

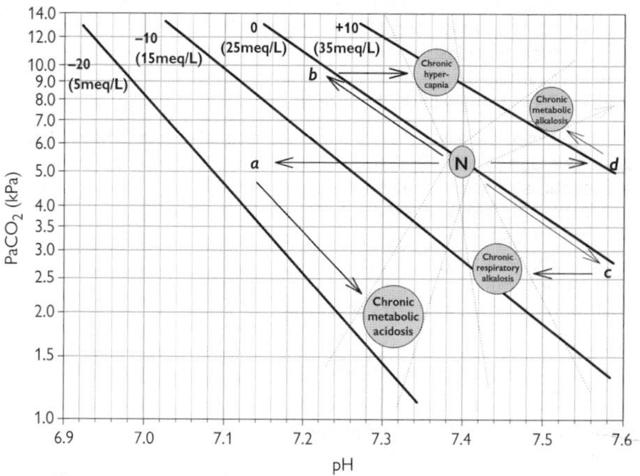

Fig. A1.4 Acid–base balance: $PaCO_2$–pH.

Anion gap

The anion gap $[(Na^+ + K^+)-(Cl^- + HCO_3^-)]$ shows the amount of other anions, apart from $Cl^- + HCO_3^-$, that exist, and helps differentiate the cause of any metabolic acidosis. Depending on methods of measurement, the normal value is between 8 and 16 mmol/L (or meq/L) and mainly due to albumin. High anion gap indicates loss of HCO_3^- without a subsequent increase in Cl^-. Electroneutrality is maintained by increase in anions such as ketones, lactate, PO_4^-, and SO_4^-. Because these anions are not part of the anion-gap calculation, a high anion gap results.

An acidosis with a normal anion gap will be a simple HCO_3^-/Cl^- exchange such as might occur, for example, in:

- Renal tubular acidosis
- Acetazolamide therapy
- HCO_3^- loss from profuse diarrhoea.

An anion gap is likely to be present, for example, when the metabolic acidosis is due to:

- Diabetic, starvation, or alcohol induced ketoacidosis (ketones are acids)
- Renal failure (although can be in the normal range too)
- Lactic acidosis
- Salicylate poisoning
- Methanol poisoning
- Ethylene glycol (anti-freeze) poisoning.

Three things arterial samples tell you about acid–base balance

- Is there a ventilatory/respiratory contribution from an abnormally high or low $PaCO_2$?
- Is there a metabolic component evidenced by a shift of the buffer line to the left or right, numerically the base excess (or deficit)?
- If there is an acidosis, is there an increased anion gap?

Further information

Williams AJ. ABC of oxygen. http://www.bmj.com/cgi/content/full/317/7167/1213

Conversion between arterial oxygen saturation and oxygen tension (haemoglobin dissociation curve)

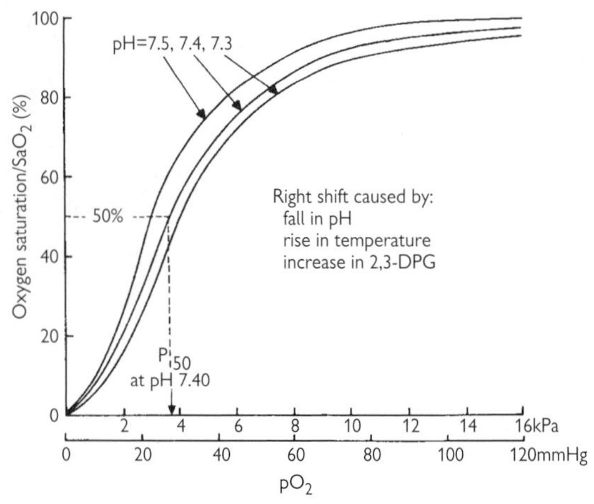

Fig. A1.5 Haemoglobin dissociation curve.

A ***fall in pH*** (more acidotic), or a rise in ***body temperature***, will move the dissociation curve to the ***right***. This has the effect of making the ***PaO_2 higher for any given SaO_2***, e.g. at pH 7.20 a measured saturation (e.g. by oximetry) of 90% is equivalent to a higher PaO_2 of 9.7 kPa (73 mmHg) than the usual 7.7 kPa (58 mmHg): a rise in body temperature to 41°C will do the same, and the effects of pH and temperature are additive.

Conversely, for a given PaO_2, pyrexia and acidosis will ***lower the SaO_2*** and thus oxygen carriage to the tissues. A PaO_2 of 7.7 kPa (58 mmHg) will normally give a SaO_2 of 90%, but if the temperature rises to 41°C, and pH falls to 7.20, then the SaO_2 falls to 70%. Increasing 2,3-DPG levels shift the curve to the right, but levels fluctuate unpredictably and any changes are small.

Changes in body temperature are often the reason why measured pulse oximetry saturations apparently 'do not agree' with the measured blood gases (pH is taken into account in the *theoretical* calculation of SaO_2 by blood gas analysers, but the patient's correct body temperature is rarely entered and thus not taken into account). This is particularly important in hypothermia when the curve is left shifted leading to impaired oxygen unloading anyway. Furthermore, an apparently adequate oximetry reading can mask a low PaO_2, which will further lessen oxygen availability to the tissues (although somewhat mitigated by the reduced metabolic rate of hypothermic tissues).

Table A1.1 Conversion chart*

% Saturation	kPa	mmHg
98	15.0	112
97	12.2	92
96	10.8	81
95	9.9	74
94	9.3	70
93	8.8	66
92	8.4	63
91	8.1	60
90	7.7	58
88	7.3	55
86	6.8	51
84	6.5	49
82	6.2	47
80	5.9	45
75	5.4	40
70	4.9	37
65	4.5	34
60	4.2	31
55	3.8	29
50	3.5	27

*Assumes a normal position of the haemoglobin dissociation curve.

kPa and mmHg: conversion factor, 7.5 x kPa = mmHg.

Appendix 2

BMI calculator; height and weight converter

BMI = weight in kilograms, divided by height in metres squared
e.g. 70 kg man, 1.8 m tall. BMI = 70/(1.8 × 1.8) = 21.6

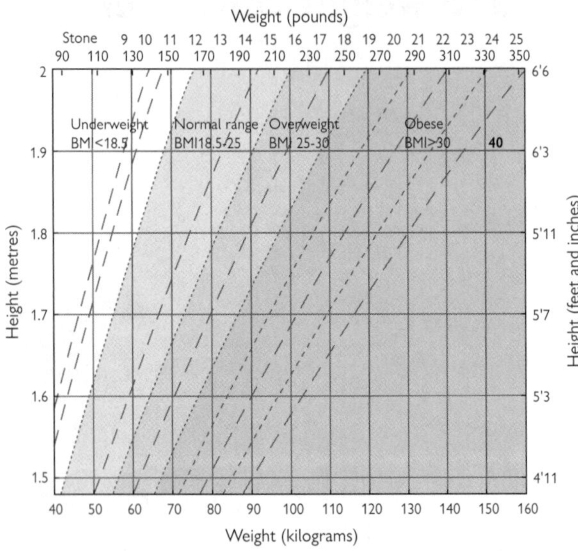

Fig. A2.1 BMI calculator.

Appendix 3

CT anatomy of the thorax

These are not standard images set for mediastinal or lung viewing, but have been adjusted to aid anatomical labelling. Contrast was used to highlight the vessels.

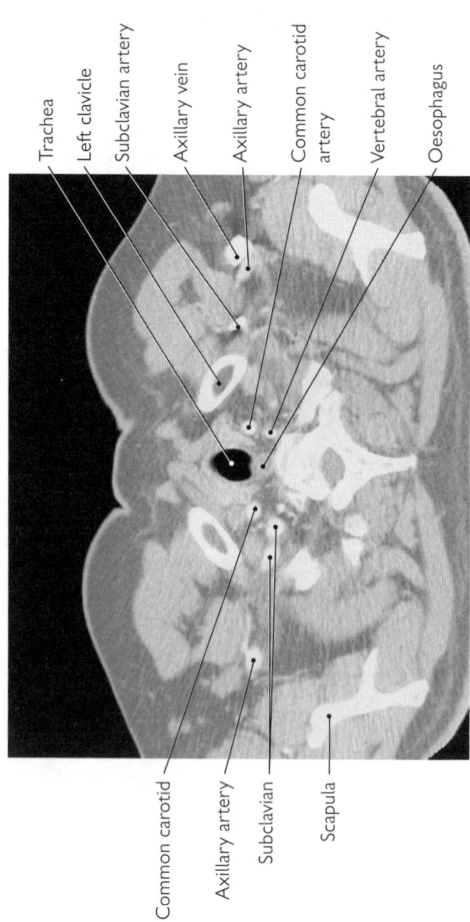

Fig. A3.1 CT anatomy of the thorax: level of C7.

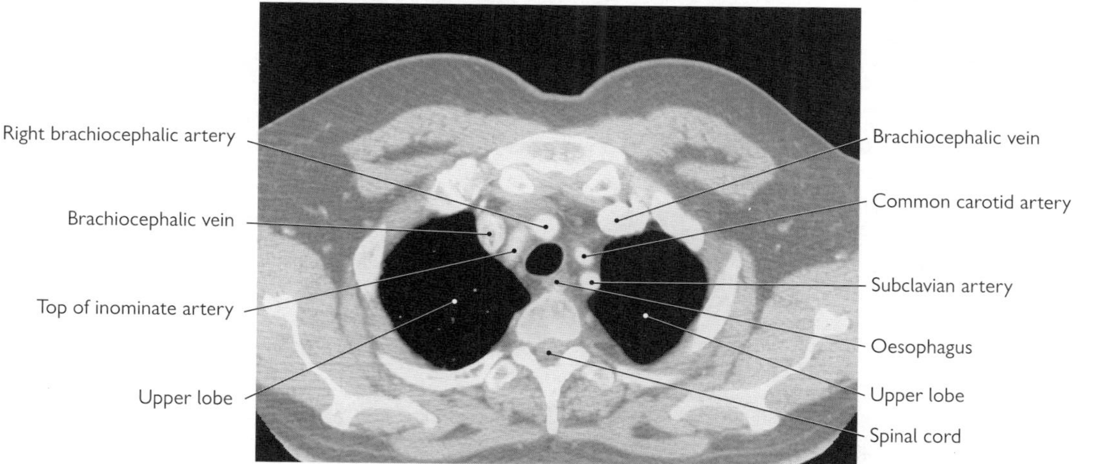

Fig. A3.2 CT anatomy of the thorax: level of T2.

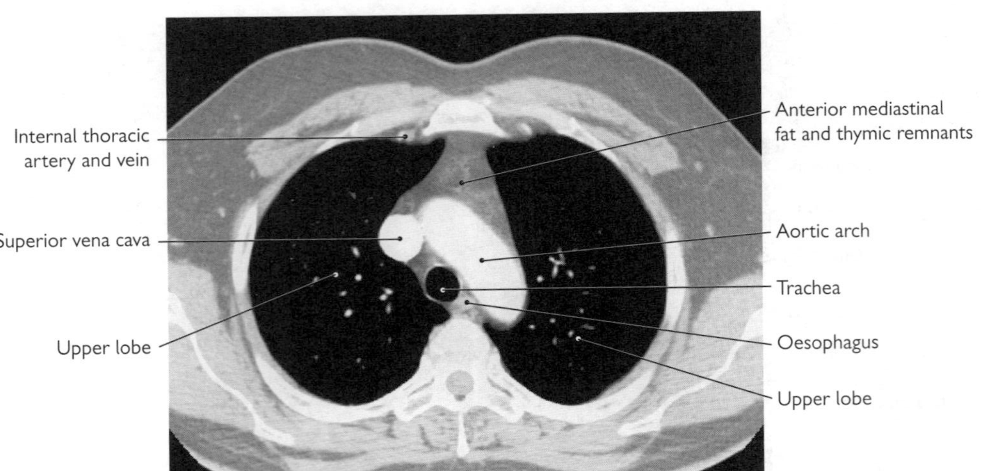

Fig. A3.3 CT anatomy of the thorax: level of T4.

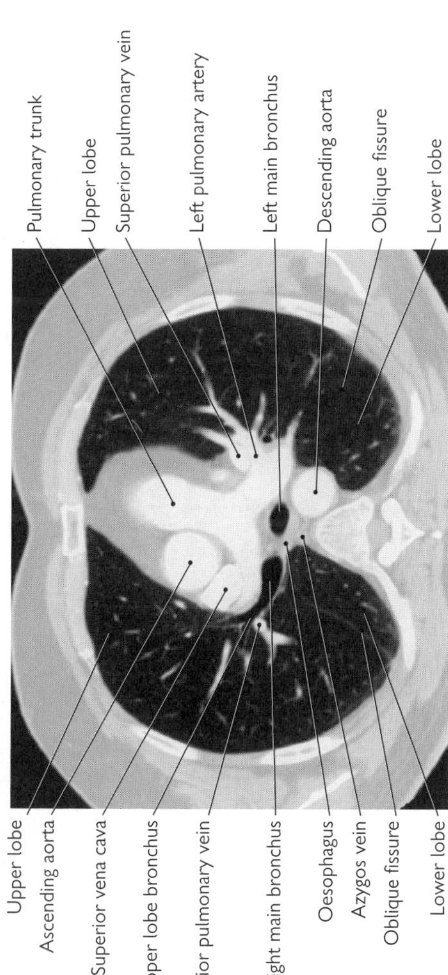

Fig. A3.4 CT anatomy of the thorax: level of T6.

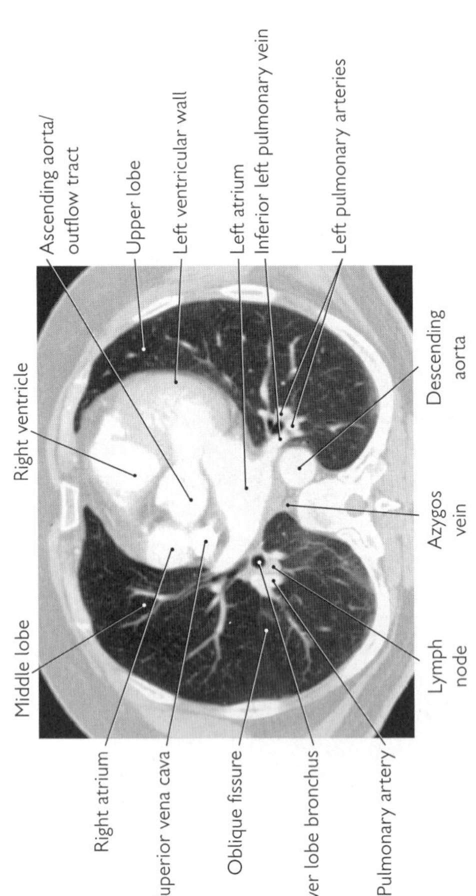

Fig. A3.5 CT anatomy of the thorax: level of T7.

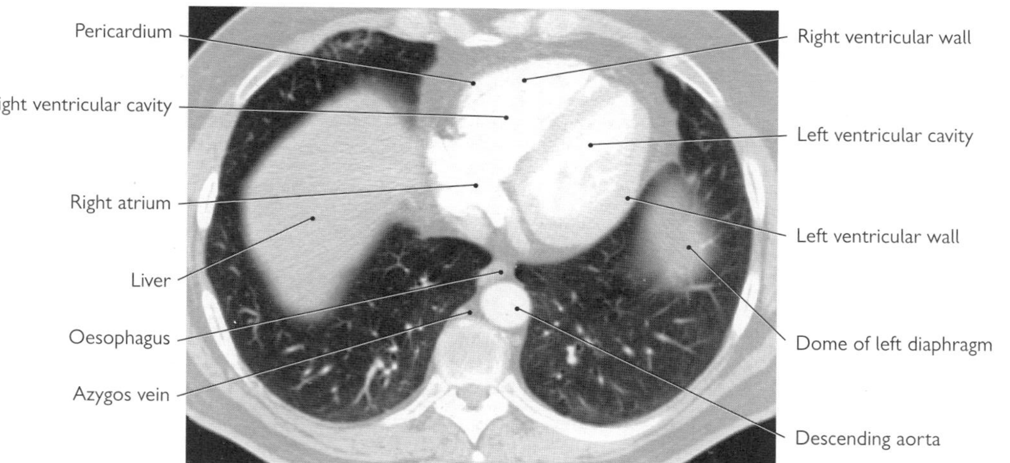

Fig. A3.6 CT anatomy of the thorax: level of T9.

Appendix 4

CT patterns of lung disease

Term	Process	Causes
Air space consolidation	Fluid/secretion accumulation in alveoli	Pneumonia, pulmonary oedema or haemorrhage, ARDS, COP, lymphoma, drugs, bronchoalveolar cell carcinoma, eosinophilic pneumonia

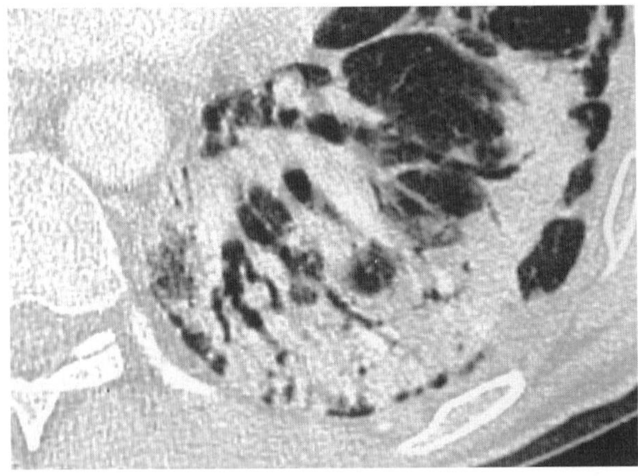

Fig. A4.1 Chronic organizing pneumonia (COP). Air bronchograms clearly present.

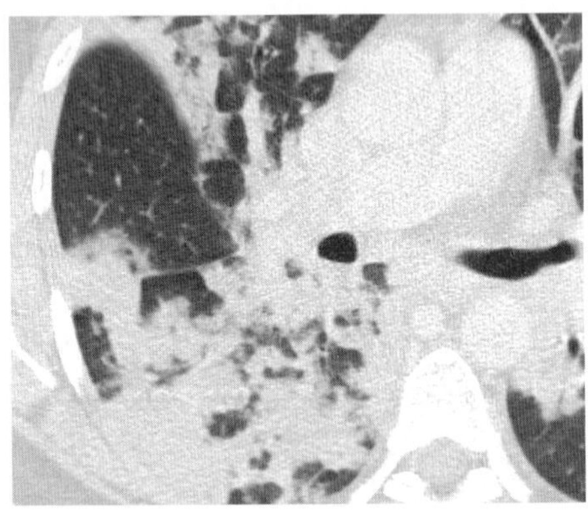

Fig. A4.2 Extensive airspace consolidation due to eosinophilic pneumonia.

Term	Process	Causes
Air trapping	Partial small airway obstruction	Asthma, obliterative bronchiolitis, COPD

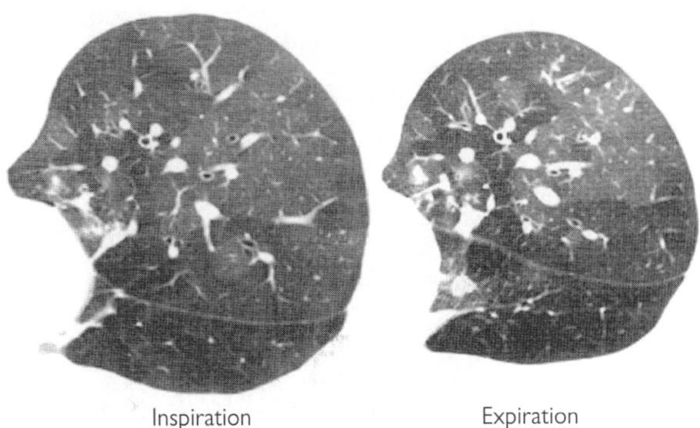

Fig. A4.3 Subject prone. On expiration the denser area becomes more dense indicating the lung has deflated: other parts of the lung remain lucent, indicating that air is trapped behind narrowed airways.

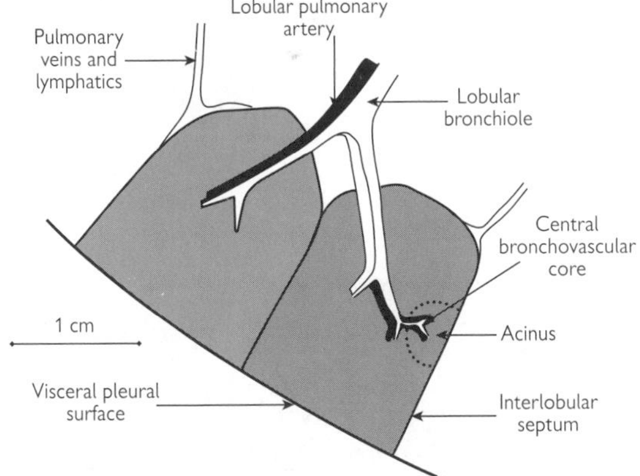

Fig. A4.4 Structure of two secondary pulmonary lobules abutting the pleural surface. The secondary pulmonary lobule is the smallest anatomical area visible on CT. Tree in bud appearance will be in the acinus around the central bronchovascular core. Reticular patterns will be centred on the interlobular septae and/or draining lymphatics. Mosaic patterns and air trapping will tend to follow outlines of the lobule or sets of lobules.

Term	Process	Causes
Cystic air spaces	Clearly defined air-containing space with definable wall	LAM, LCH, end-stage UIP, PCP, LIP, septic emboli

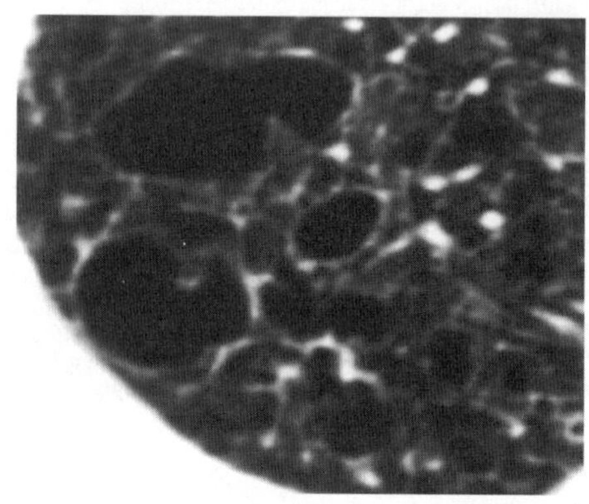

Fig. A4.5 Langerhans' cell histiocytosis (LCH). Walls are thin, but more pronounced, irregular, and widely spread than emphysematous holes.

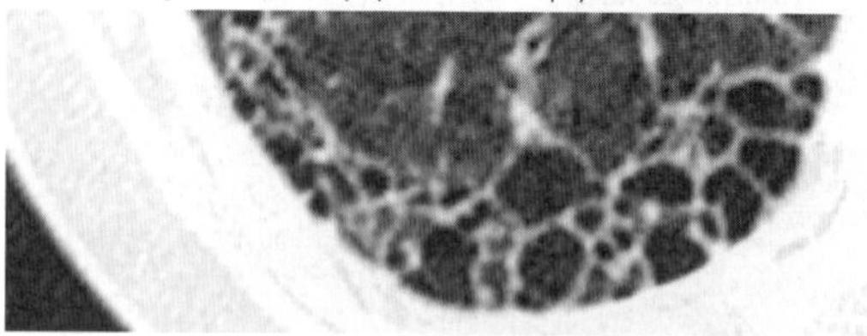

Fig. A4.6 Peripheral cysts (honeycombing) of usual interstitial pneumonitis (UIP), characteristic subpleural distribution.

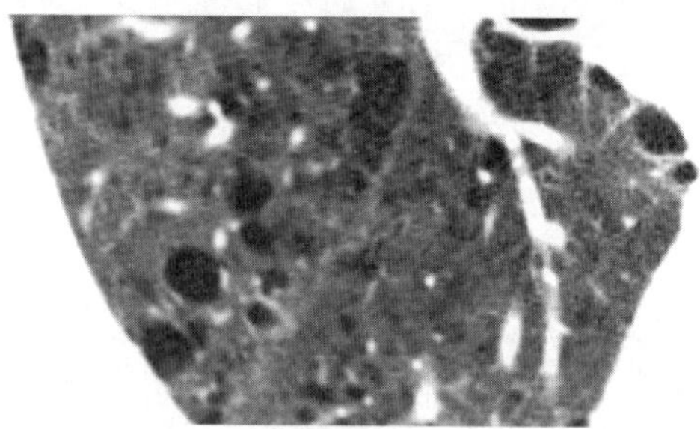

Fig. A4.7 Holes in the lungs due to emphysema. No real 'walls'.

Term	Process	Causes
Fissural, bronchovascular, and sub-pleural nodularity	Nodules seen along the pulmonary fissures, along the bronchovascular bundles, and sub-pleurally	Sarcoidosis. Also described in Kaposi's sarcoma

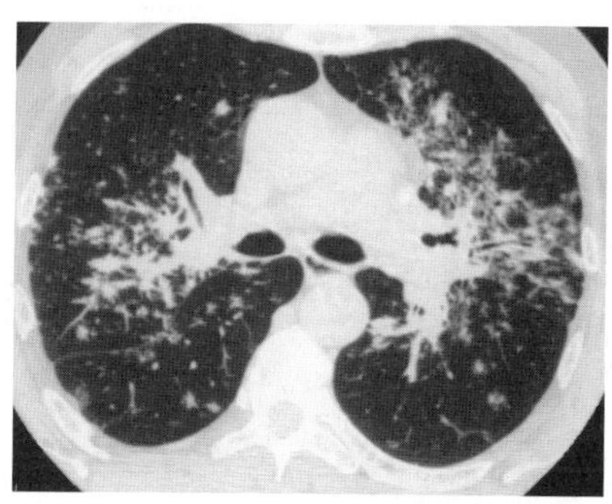

Fig. A4.8 Sarcoidosis, perihilar, and bronchovascular distribution of nodularity.

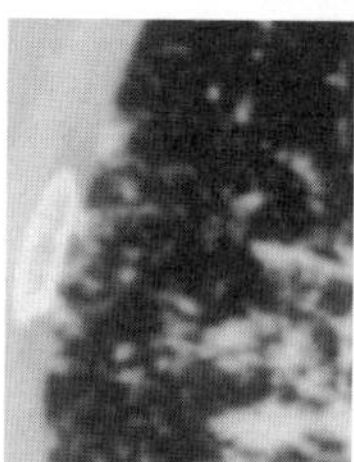

Fig. A4.9 Sarcoidosis, subpleural nodules.

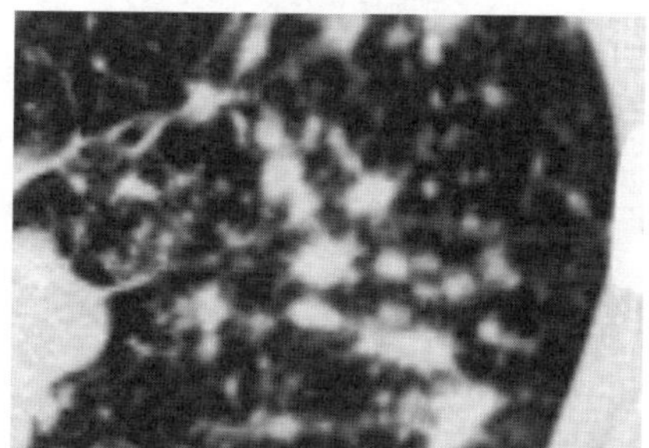

Fig. A4.10 Irregular/nodular thickening of fissures and bronchovascular bundles.

Term	Process	Causes
Ground-glass shadowing	Grey appearance to lung interstitium; air in bronchus looks blacker	Parenchymal inflammatory conditions, such as sarcoidosis, alveolitis, early UIP and other IIPs, hyper-sensitivity pneumonitis, pulmonary oedema or haemorrhage, PCP, alveolar proteinosis, drug/radiation injury

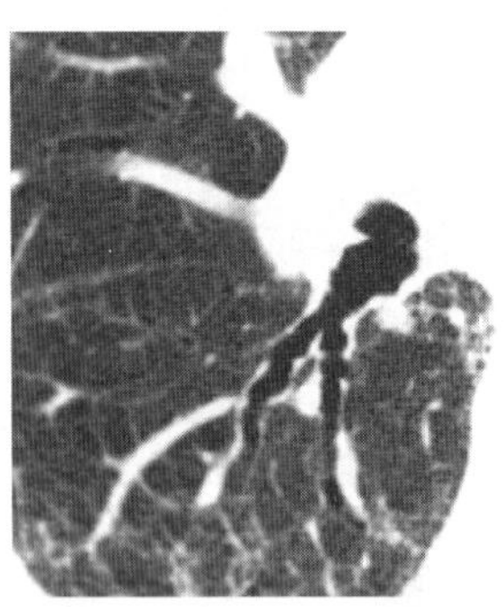
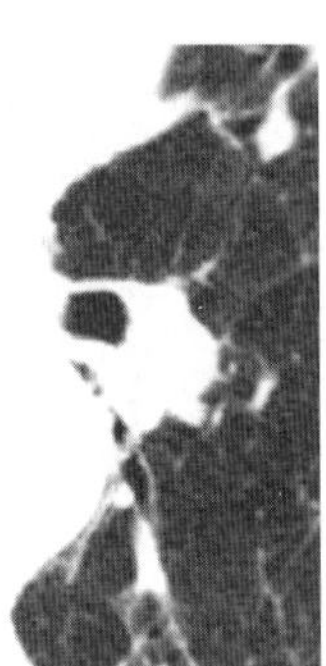

Fig. A4.11 Subtle ground-glass shadowing in early usual interstitial pneumonitis. Airways appear blacker, but lung is diffusely more dense. Early reticular pattern at right base also.

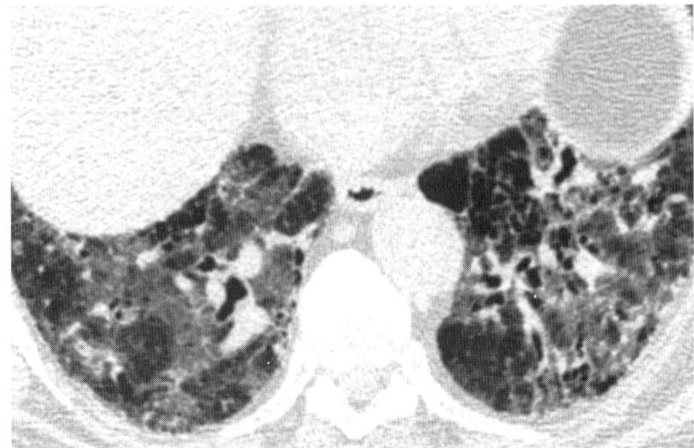

Fig. A4.12 More marked ground-glass shadowing in UIP. Very early honeycombing and traction bronchial dilatation (bronchiectasis) as well.

Term	Process	Causes
Honeycomb lung	End-stage fibrotic lung	UIP, asbestosis

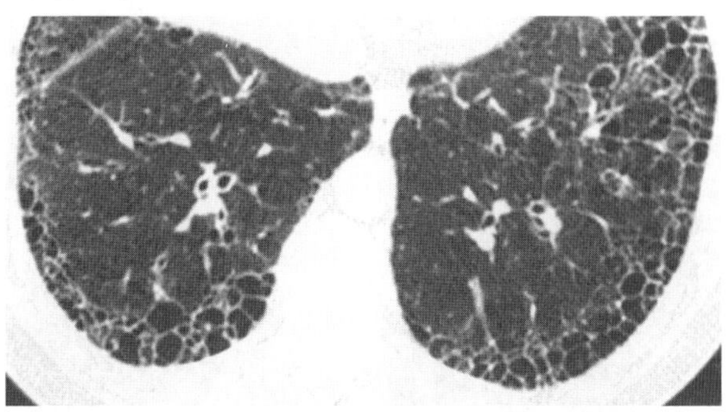

Fig. A4.13 Honeycombing in usual interstitial pneumonitis (UIP). Usually mainly peripheral.

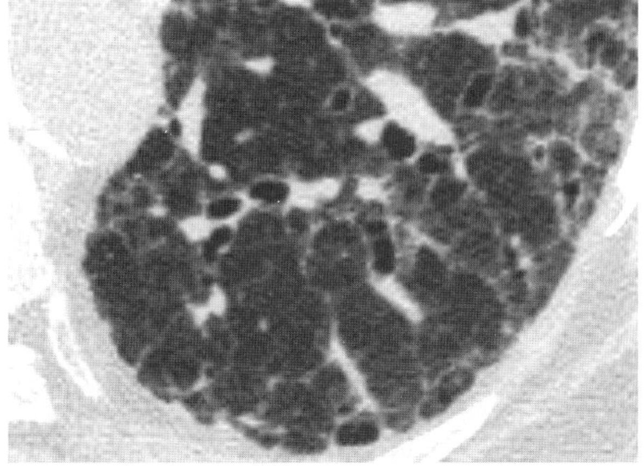

Fig. A4.14 More subtle honeycombing at the lung periphery with other features of UIP. Traction bronchial dilatation due to surrounding lung fibrosis and a reticular pattern beginning to outline the secondary pulmonary lobule.

Term	Process	Causes
Mosaic attenuation pattern	Well-defined areas of normal lung abutting abnormal lung, giving a mosaic pattern. Seen particularly in expiration	Indicates small airways disease such as asthma, vascular disease such as PE, or infiltrative disease such as obliterative bronchiolitis, hypersensitivity pneumonitis

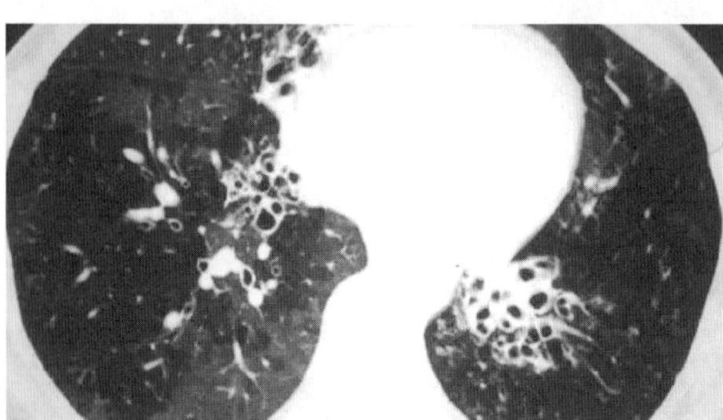

Fig. A4.15 Bronchiectasis with small airways disease that is causing the mosaic pattern. In addition, there are markedly bronchiectatic airways in the left lower lobe with considerable airway crowding due to distal lung collapse.

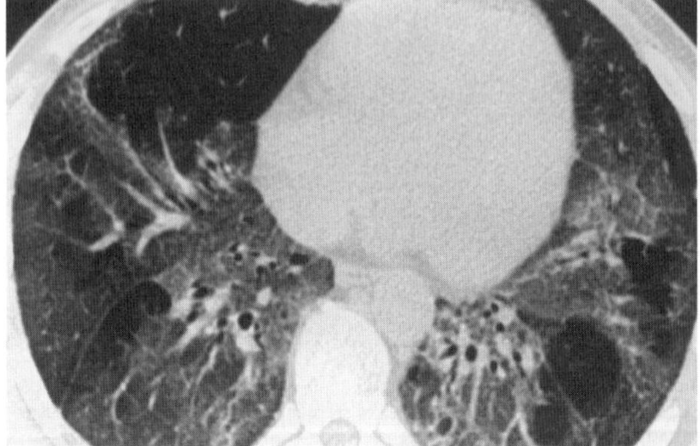

Fig. A4.16 Non-specific interstitial pneumonitis (NSIP) showing patchy and mosaic-like pattern of increased attenuation.

Term	Process	Causes
Nodularity	Small discrete dots 1–10 mm, may be in air spaces or interstitium	Metastases, sarcoidosis, pneumoconiosis, hypersensitivity pneumonitis, miliary TB, fungal infection, idiopathic pulmonary haemorrhage, alveolar microlithiasis, varicella pneumonitis

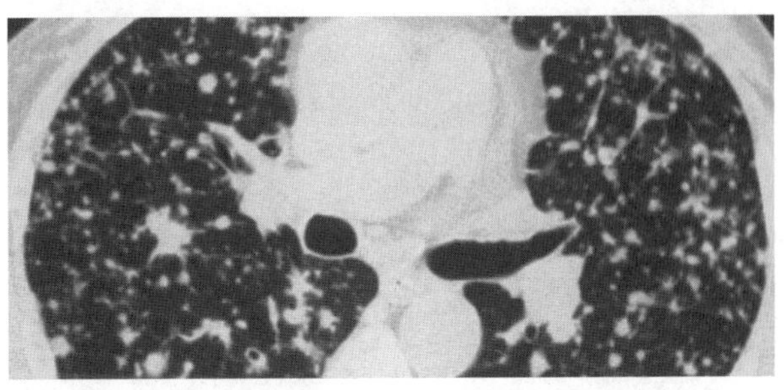

Fig. A4.17 Multiple dense nodules of varying size due to metastases.

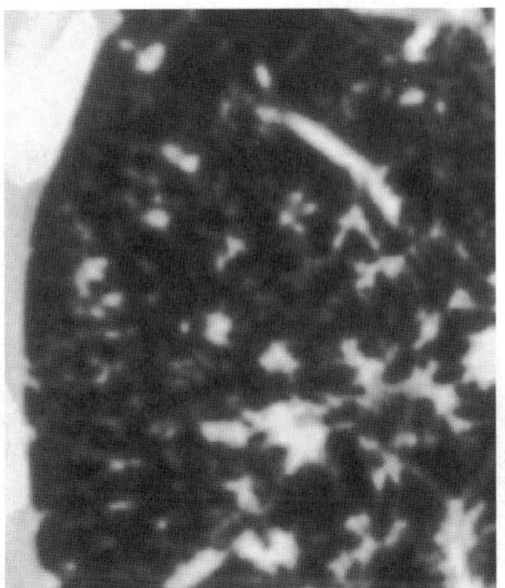

Fig. A4.18 Sarcoid. Multiple small nodules throughout lung, but usually associated with other features of sarcoid, such as fissural nodularity and bilateral hilar node enlargement.

Term	Process	Causes
Poorly defined centrilobular nodules	Peribronchiolar inflammation in the absence of intraluminal secretion	Hypersensitivity pneumonitis, RB-ILD

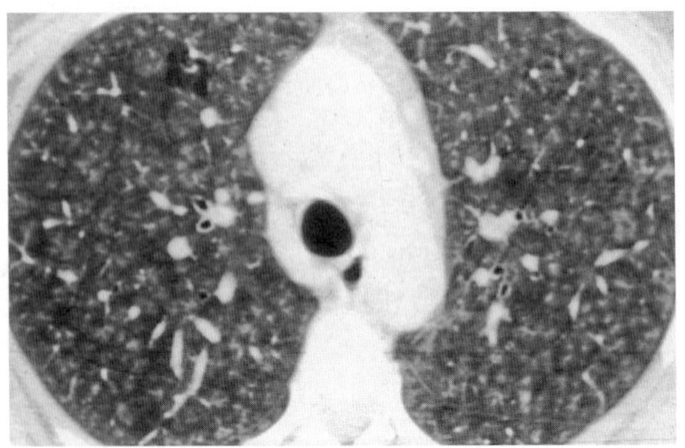

Fig. A4.19 Soft centrilobular nodularity due to hypersensitivity pneumonitis (also called extrinsic allergic alveolitis, EAA).

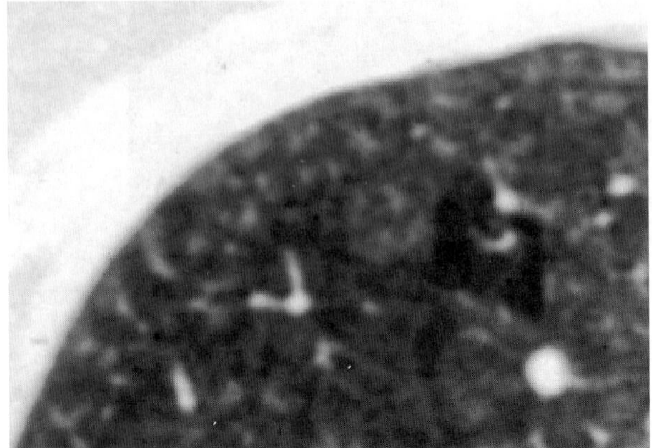

Fig. A4.20 Another example of hypersensitivity pneumonitis enlarged to show position of soft nodules in the centre of the secondary pulmonary lobules.

Term	Process	Causes
Reticular (or linear) pattern	Linear fine lines, indicating thickened interlobular septa. Sub-pleural reticulation	ILD (e.g. UIP, asbestosis), pulmonary oedema, drug-induced fibrosis, pulmonary haemorrhage, lymphangitis

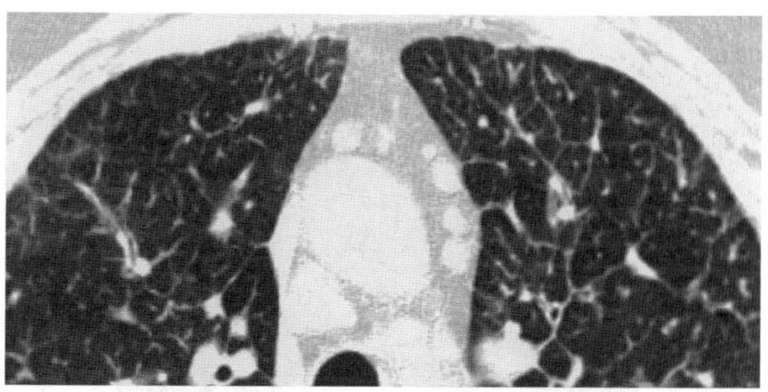

Fig. A4.21 Lymphangitis carcinomatosis. Infiltrated lymphatics widen and thicken the interlobular septa.

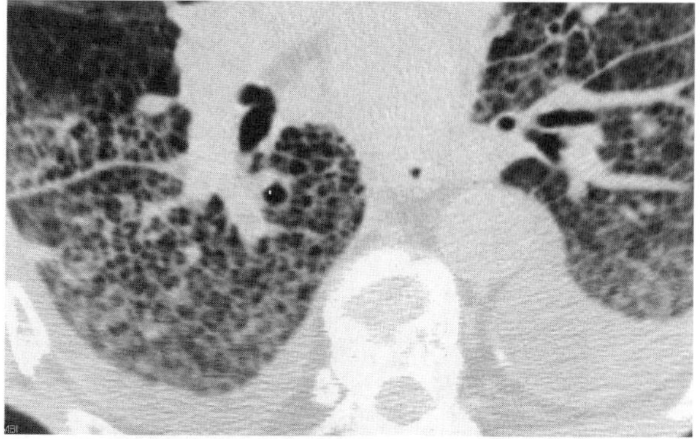

Fig. A4.22 Pulmonary oedema due to left heart failure. Fluid-distended lymphatics outlining the secondary pulmonary lobules. Worse in dependent areas. Fluid in the fissures, bilateral pleural effusions, and some air-space filling with pulmonary oedema.

Term	Process	Causes
Tree in bud	Mucus/pus/secretions filling bronchioles and causing dilatation	Small airways disease, particularly infection including mycobacteria, *Haemophilus influenzae*, diffuse panbronchiolitis, CF, yellow nail syndrome, primary pulmonary lymphoma

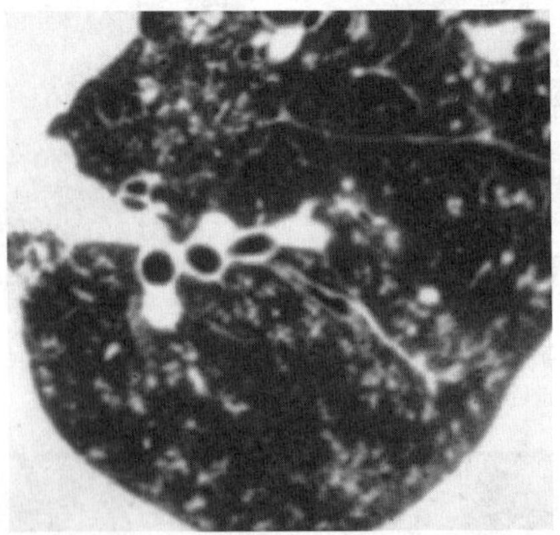

Fig. A4.23 Extensive tree in bud appearance in the left lower lobe from opportunistic mycobacterial disease.

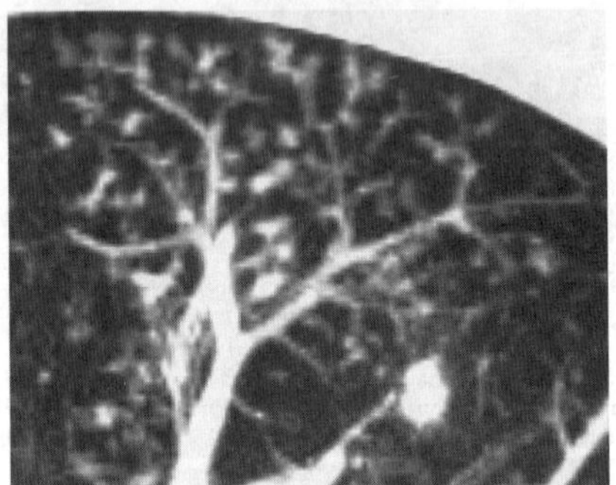

Fig. A4.24 Tree in bud appearance enhanced by a post-processing technique called 'maximum intensity projection'. Effectively this squashes denser structures from several thin cuts into one allowing branching structures to be viewed in their entirety.

Appendix 5
Lung function testing

Flow–volume loop 1

A good starting point to the understanding of lung function tests is the flow–volume loop. This plots inspiratory and expiratory flow against lung volume during a maximal expiratory and maximal inspiratory manoeuvre.

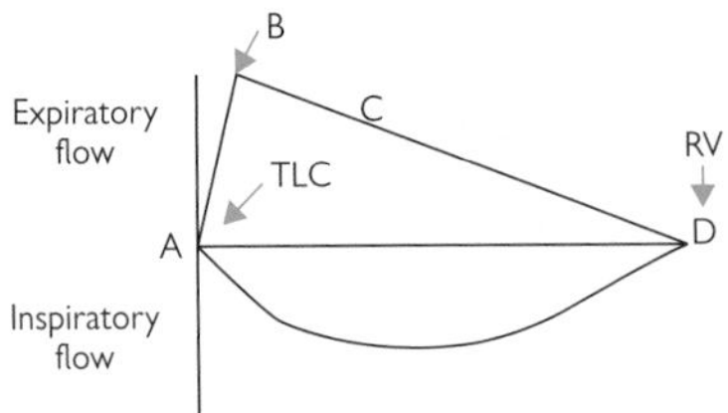

Fig. A5.1 Flow–volume loop.

At the beginning of ***expiration*** from a full breath in, the expiratory muscles are at their strongest, the lungs at their largest, and hence the airways are at their most open (A). Because the lungs are at their largest, the radial attachments to the airways, effectively the alveolar/capillary membranes and their connective tissue, are pulling the hardest and supporting the airways against ***dynamic compression*** during the exhalation manoeuvre.

This means that the highest flow rates are possible at the beginning of the blow; hence, the sudden rise to a ***peak expiratory flow rate*** in the first 100 ms or so of the forced breath out (B). This is the ***peak flow*** and is essentially what a peak flow meter measures.

As the lung empties and the lung volume drops, the dilatory pull on the airways from the radial attachments of the surrounding lung tissue reduces (C). Hence the airways narrow and become less supported, and are less able to resist dynamic compression. This means that the maximal airflow obtainable, regardless of effort, falls too.

Eventually, the expiratory muscles come to the end of their 'travel' and cannot squeeze the chest anymore. Also, increasingly with age, the small airways may actually close off, preventing anymore emptying (D). The volume at which this begins to happen is called the ***closing volume***.

As maximal ***inspiration*** starts, although the inspiratory muscles are at their strongest, the airways are at their smallest. Thus, flow rates start low and increase as the airways open up. However, as the lung expands the inspiratory muscles are approaching the end of their 'travel' and are weakening; this means the flow rates fall again, hence the different, rounded appearance of the inspiratory limb of the flow–volume curve.

Thus, normally the inspiratory and expiratory flow rates depend on lung volume and are termed 'volume-dependent'. If there is a ***fixed upper airway narrowing***, such as from a solid hard tumour partially blocking the trachea, then the size of the airway at this point may become so narrow that it now limits maximal flows. However, its diameter will vary very little with lung volumes and hence flow will become 'volume-independent'. Figure A5.2 shows this.

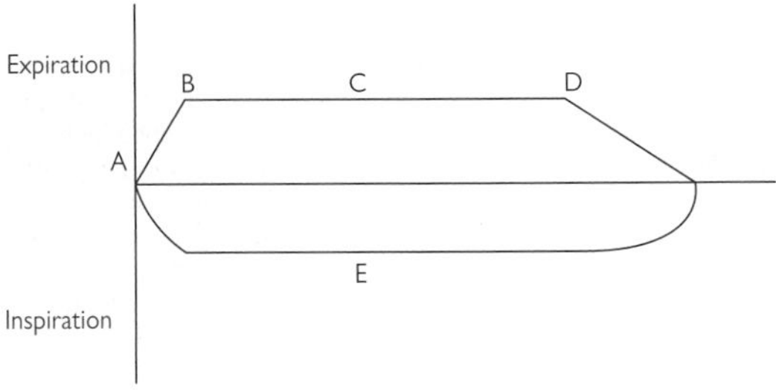

Fig. A5.2 Volume-independent flow.

At A, the rise in flow will initially be normal, but at some point the maximum flow imposed by the upper airway narrowing will cut in (B). From that point onwards the flow rate will be fixed at this maximum (C) until at much lower lung volumes the lower recoil and narrowing small airways again determine the maximum flow (D). The flow–volume curve has been severely 'clipped' with a squarish appearance. The same clipped appearance will be present on the inspiratory limb (E), giving rise to the so-called 'square box' appearance.

Sometimes, such upper airways restriction may be *variable*, rather than fixed, and only obstruct during inspiration (e.g. paralysed and collapsing vocal cords) due to the obstructing elements being sucked in, and then blown open again on expiration.

- Thus, a square inspiratory limb, but normal expiratory limb, provides evidence of a mobile ***extrathoracic* upper airways obstruction.**

Conversely, a mobile intrathoracic upper airway obstruction (e.g. soft fleshy tumour at the carina, or retrosternal thyroid) may obstruct more during expiration (when the expiratory effort is compressing the lung), compared with inspiration when the chest is being expanded.

- Thus, a square expiratory limb, but normal inspiratory limb, is evidence of a ***variable intrathoracic upper airways obstruction.***

Sometimes ratios of maximal inspiratory to maximal expiratory flows are used to characterize intra- or extrathoracic airway obstruction.

Flow–volume loop 2

The other, more common, causes of airway obstruction are due to narrowing of the lower airways (asthma, COPD). In these conditions the airway calibre (and thus flow rates) still remains dependent on lung volume. Hence, the flow rates decrease as the lung volume decreases, but particularly so at low lung volumes. This is because resistance to flow is proportional to the airway radius raised to the power of 4 (r^4) and therefore most significant when airways are already small. Hence, increasing airflow obstruction produces expiratory flow–volume curves like those in Figure A5.3. This greater effect of small airways narrowing at low lung volumes has led some units to report flow rates at, for example, 25% expired lung volume, or averaged between 25% and 75% of the total expired lung volume.

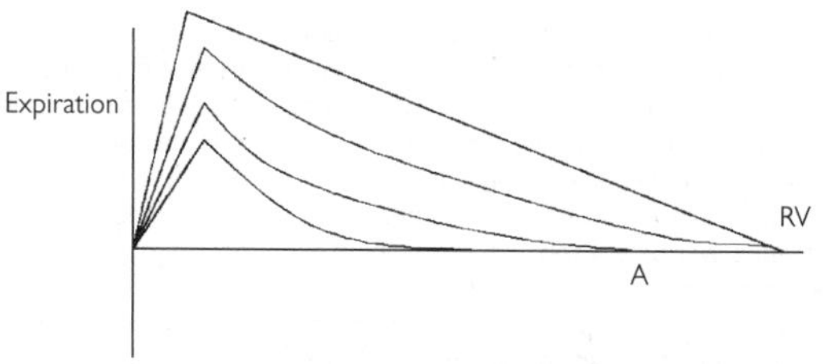

Fig. A5.3 Expiratory flow volume curves–lower airways obstruction.

Airways can be so small so that during expiration they begin closing off earlier than normal (the ***closing volume***); hence a full breath out is not possible, producing air trapping and a raised residual volume (RV) (A). Sensitive tests of small airways narrowing have to concentrate on flows at low lung volumes, and peak flow measurements are relatively insensitive.

- Note, however, that peak flow measurements are the most sensitive to ***upper airway narrowing*** and a good way to follow changes in upper airway narrowing during, for example, radiotherapy for a central airway obstructing lung cancer.

Spirometry, peak flow measurements, and CO transfer

- The ordinary spirometer (mechanical or electronic) records ***volumes against time***, rather than ***flows against volume***
- The two essential measures are ***FEV_1*** and ***VC***.

The vital capacity (VC) is the maximum amount of air that can be blown out completely. This will be ***reduced*** if the lungs are ***stiff*** (preventing a full breath in), the ***inspiratory muscles are weak*** (preventing a full breath in), or the ***airways are narrowed*** such that the small airways collapse during expiration (preventing a full breath out).

The FEV_1 is the amount (forced expiratory volume) that can be blown out in 1 s. Because the value is taken over a second, much more flow is being captured during the breath out than the PEFR, but it is still occurring when the airways are larger. It is less dependent on effort and generally more robust. The ratio of the two figures (FEV_1/VC) tells us about the degree of airflow obstruction.

- A ratio of FEV_1/VC of less than about 70–75% indicates airflow ***obstruction***.

This ratio is very useful because it is hardly affected by age, sex, height, ethnic origin, etc.—it is self-normalizing. The individual measures of FEV_1 and VC ***do*** need corrections for the above factors and are usually quoted as % predicted. The range of normality is considerable, and it may not be clear if results are simply at the bottom end of normal, or considerably reduced from the patient's normally much higher figures. Serial measurements indicating continuing deterioration may be the first clue. If the FEV_1/VC ratio is *normal*, then the VC *can* be interpreted as to whether there is a reduced total lung volume, such as from interstitial lung disease. This is called a ***restrictive*** pattern, and a low FEV_1/VC ratio is called an ***obstructive*** pattern. The FEV_1/VC ratio may actually be raised in interstitial lung disease as the airways are better supported by the fibrosed radial attachments, which reduces dynamic compression, improving expiratory flow.

The ***slope*** of the volume–time plot from a spirometer is effectively the *flow rate* at any particular point: because flow is dropping during expiration the slope progressively flattens off. However, if there is any fixed upper airways obstruction (as discussed above) the expiratory flow rate will be constant for a while, and hence the spirometer line will be straighter than usual. An interesting index to detect possible upper airway obstruction, the ***Empey index***, has been described:

Empey Index = [FEV_1 (mL)/PEFR (L/min)]

Because PEFR is clipped first by the presence of upper airflow obstruction, relative to the FEV_1, the above index gets larger with such a problem. A figure over 10 is suggestive of upper airflow obstruction, but it is only a pointer, and there will be false positives and negatives.

Although one-off measures of lung function can be made, more interesting information comes from serial measurements, e.g. in asthma, PEFR will fluctuate with characteristic morning 'dips'.

Spirometry – how to do it

Everyone has their own way to do spirometry, but this is a way that works for the authors. Say to the patient:- 'This is a test of how big your lungs are, and how fast you can empty them. What I would like you to do is take an enormous breath in, the biggest you can manage, then seal your lips around the tube, and blow as hard and as fast and as long as you possibly can'. Then demonstrate the manoeuvre yourself with a spare tube (not connected to the spirometer) so that they can then mimic it. Whilst they are blowing, say 'Excellent, well done, keep blowing, come on, come on, come on, keep blowing'. There are various recommendations as to numbers of blow etc. These are the arguments.

Standing or sitting?	High intrathoracic pressure generated may cause the patient to pass out. Therefore, sitting down is safer, but better and more consistent figures are obtained standing. Have a chair behind patient to sit on if dizzy.
Nose clip?	Prevents escape through the nose which would give falsely low figures, but is uncomfortable. Vast majority of patients do not need it, but if the line appears to fall off towards the end of the blow, or inconsistent volumes, try a nose clip.
Best of 3 blows?	Need to demonstrate that maximal blow has been achieved, usually by seeing two identical tracings. A device showing the actual spirometer tracing is extremely helpful. If two tracings are identical, this is probably enough, but may need more if blowing is erratic, until satisfied it is maximal.
Keep going to end of page (6 s) or not?	Need to establish correct VC. Therefore if line still rising, then VC not reached, but have to stop somewhere. In restrictive disease, or normals, usually maximal by 3 s; in obstructive disease may need to do slow VC to establish real value.
Repeat with a sub-maximal effort?	Sometimes useful to ask patient to repeat with slightly less effort, when emphysema suspected. Will often give better expiratory volume in 1 s, and VC, suggesting major dynamic airways compression.

Carbon monoxide (CO) transfer

Usually done in the lung function laboratory and essentially measures the amount of ***gas exchanging surface area*** available. A gas mixture containing CO is inhaled, the breath held for 10 s, then exhaled. The amount of CO that has disappeared (by crossing the alveolar capillary membrane and being taken up by red cells) is calculated. A correction for the haemoglobin concentration is required, as the amount of CO transferred will fall as the available haemoglobin is reduced. The ***total amount of CO transferred is the TLCO*** (total lung, TL). When divided by the total lung volume during the breath hold, it is called the ***kCO, gas transfer per unit lung volume***. The total lung volume 'reached' by the CO is the amount breathed in *plus* the amount of air already in the lung at the start of the breath in. This is measured by including helium in the inhaled gas mixture that is diluted by the air already in the lung; by comparing inspired helium concentration with expired, this total lung volume can be calculated.

- The kCO is *reduced* most in emphysema when alveoli have been destroyed
- The kCO is also *reduced* in interstitial lung diseases where the alveolar capillary membrane may be thick enough to reduce CO passage
- The kCO may also be *raised* when lungs are poorly expanded by, say, weak respiratory muscles, because the lung is 'more concentrated' and transfers CO *better* when quoted per unit volume
- The kCO may also be *raised* for a few days when there has been profuse lung haemorrhage, as can occur in, SLE, Wegener's, and Goodpasture's. This is because the free red cells lining the alveoli take up CO directly and 'falsely' elevate the figure. As the haemoglobin is broken down, the kCO returns to normal, unless there is another bleed. This helps to distinguish re-bleeding from other causes of lung infiltrates such as infection

This test requires more cooperation than simple spirometry, as well as a minimum inspired volume, and therefore cannot always be obtained.

Respiratory muscle function, body plethysmography, and lung volumes

Respiratory muscle function

Respiratory failure and small VCs may be due to weak respiratory muscles. It is therefore useful to be able to assess inspiratory and expiratory muscle power. There may be global weakness, or specific inspiratory weakness, usually due to diaphragm paralysis. In the clinic the simplest test is a ***lying and standing VC***. If the diaphragm is paralysed then on lying down the abdominal contents will push up the diaphragm and limit inspiration. On standing the abdominal contents drop and aid inspiration.

- A fall in VC of less than 10% on lying down is probably normal
- A fall of 10–20% is suspicious of diaphragm paralysis
- A fall of more than 20% is abnormal and suggests significant, usually bilateral, diaphragm paralysis.

In the laboratory there are various ways to test respiratory muscle function. The patient can blow against a *pressure meter* after a maximum inspiration, and inspires against the meter after a full expiration. This is, of course, highly effort dependent. A manoeuvre such as a ***sniff*** is very stereotypic and patients can reproduce this. Measuring the inspiratory pressure produced at the nose during this manoeuvre is a reasonably reliable way of screening for inspiratory muscle weakness. More accurate assessments of inspiratory muscle function, particularly the diaphragm, can be obtained using two oesophageal balloons placed above and below the diaphragm and connected to pressure transducers. The *transdiaphragmatic pressures* during maximal inspiratory efforts, sniffing, and breathing to TLC all provide reproducible measures of diaphragm function, but depend on good co-operation and effort by the patient. Activating the phrenic nerve directly with a superficial electrical stimulator, or by using high-intensity magnetic stimulation over the nerve roots of C3–C5, provides non-effort-dependent ways to test diaphragm function.

Body plethysmography requires the patient to climb into an airtight cabinet and breathe through a shuttered mouthpiece connected to the outside world. It has two particular advantages over simpler lung function tests. It is able to measure the ***total lung volume or capacity*** (TLC) in the thorax, and it provides a measure of airways obstruction involving little or no effort by the patient.

The other main method of measuring TLC involves helium dilution as described during the TLCO measurement above. However, in the presence of lower airways obstruction, the helium may not 'reach' all parts of the lung during the 10 s breath hold, and the volume of dilution will therefore be lower than the real TLC. The body plethysmograph relies on the pressure changes that occur when all the air in the chest is alternately compressed and expanded by the patient making breathing efforts against an airway closed by a shutter at the mouth. The pressure changes produced in the oral cavity versus in the box are then proportional to the volume of air being compressed and rarefied, thus allowing calculation of the volume in the chest at the time. Note that this volume will include any bullae and the *difference* between the *plethysmographic lung volume* and the *helium dilution volume* will reflect the *bullae volume*, as well as areas not reached by the helium due to increased airways resistance.

Measurement of ***airways resistance*** with the body box relies on a similar principle. If there were no airways resistance, then breathing in and out would not compress or rarefy the air in the chest. With increasing resistance, the air in the chest will be compressed during expiration and rarefied on inspiration. It is this phenomenon that allows calculation of the airways resistance during quiet breathing or panting (the latter ensures the vocal chords are fully open and not contributing to the measured resistance).

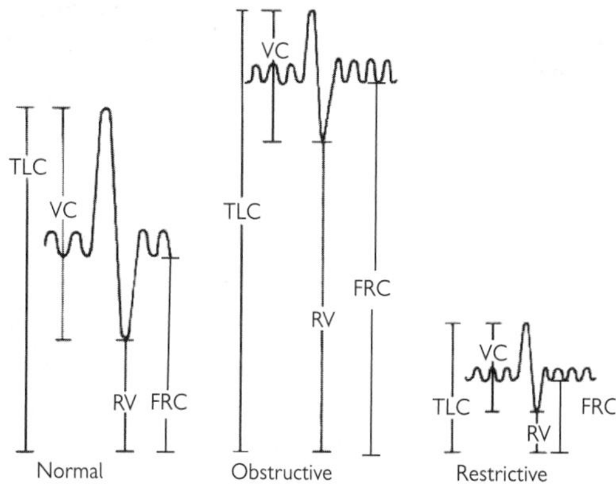

Fig. A5.4 Lung volumes in normal, obstructive, and restrictive lung conditions. TLC = total lung capacity; VC = vital capacity; RV = residual volume; FRC = functional residual capacity; FEV_1 = forced expiratory volume in 1 s.

Derivative	Obstructive	Restrictive
FEV_1 (% predicted)	↓↓	↓
VC (% predicted)	↓ or →	↓
FEV_1/VC ratio	↓	→ or ↑ (increased recoil)
TLC (% predicted)	↑ or →	↓
RV (% predicted)	↑	↓
FRC (% predicted)	↑	↓
RV/TLC ratio	↑ (gas trapping)	→ or ↓

Further reading

Gibson GJ. *Clinical Tests of Respiratory Function*, 2nd edn. Hodder Arnold, 1995.

Peak flow reference ranges

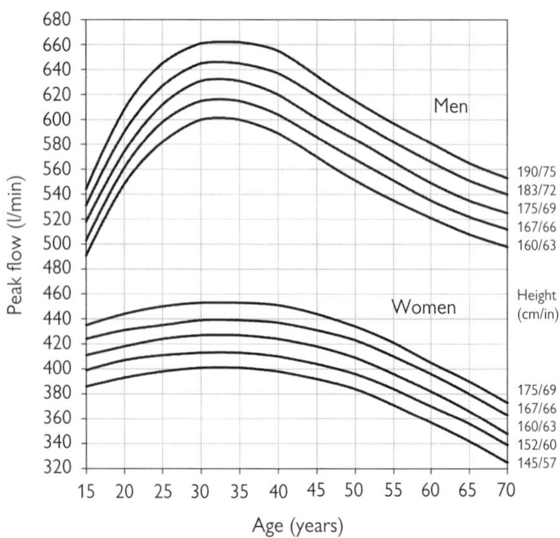

Fig. A5.5 Normal values for peak flow based on original Gregg and Nunn values (*BMJ* 1973), but corrected for new EU scale peak flow meters. Normal range is about ±15% or roughly 100 l/min in men and 50 l/min in women. Old Wright peak flow meters over-read in the middle of the scale (e.g. reading about 400 when actual value was 350 l/min), and were replaced from October 2004 by a corrected scale.

Conversion calculator available at: http://www.mortonmedical.co.uk/clement_clarke_mini_wright_EU.htm

Appendix 6

Plain radiograph and lobar collapses

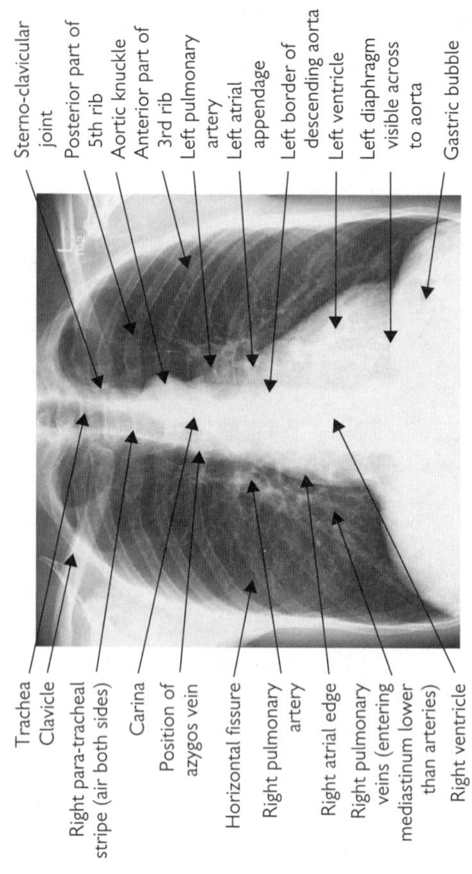

Fig. A6.1 Normal PA chest radiograph.

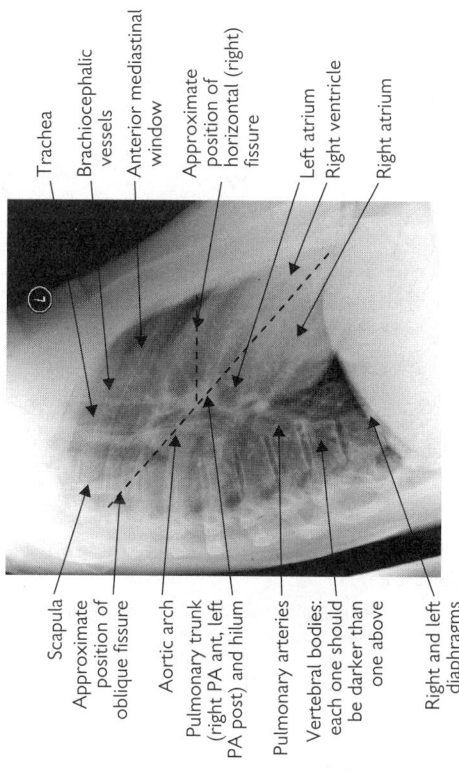

Fig. A6.2 Normal left lateral chest radiograph.

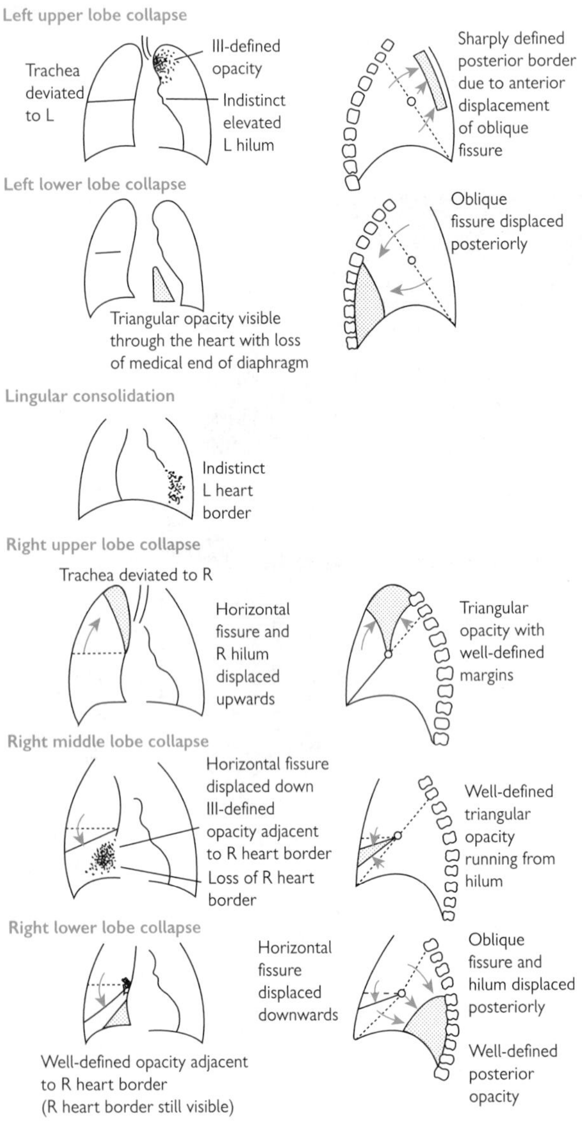

Left upper lobe collapse

Trachea deviated to L

Ill-defined opacity

Indistinct elevated L hilum

Sharply defined posterior border due to anterior displacement of oblique fissure

Left lower lobe collapse

Triangular opacity visible through the heart with loss of medical end of diaphragm

Oblique fissure displaced posteriorly

Lingular consolidation

Indistinct L heart border

Right upper lobe collapse

Trachea deviated to R

Horizontal fissure and R hilum displaced upwards

Triangular opacity with well-defined margins

Right middle lobe collapse

Horizontal fissure displaced down

Ill-defined opacity adjacent to R heart border

Loss of R heart border

Well-defined triangular opacity running from hilum

Right lower lobe collapse

Horizontal fissure displaced downwards

Well-defined opacity adjacent to R heart border (R heart border still visible)

Oblique fissure and hilum displaced posteriorly

Well-defined posterior opacity

Fig. A6.3 Lobar collapse.

Appendix 7

Radiological investigations and radiation exposure

Table A7.1 Common radiological investigations used in respiratory practice

	Plain CXR (AMBER) one view	Staging chest and abdo CT	HRCT	CT pulmonary angiogram	Low dose CT	V/Q scan ^{99m}TcMAA and ^{133}Xe	PET scan	MRI	Head CT
Indication	Best technique for plain chest radiography	e.g. for staging lung cancer, usually with IV contrast to identify vascularity of structures	For diffuse lung disease, giving good resolution at level of secondary pulmonary lobule	For pulmonary emboli and visualization of pulmonary vasculature	Used in lung cancer screening	For identifying perfusion defects without accompanying ventilation defects, as in pulmonary emboli	For detection of malignant deposits, and increasingly for areas of inflammation	Better detection of malignant tissue invasion	e.g. for brain metastases
Technique	Multiple beam equalization improves contrast by varying beam intensity depending on tissue density	Commonly, 5 mm slices at 5 mm intervals with thinner slices reconstructed from same data. Whole lung scanned. 200–400 mA beam intensity	1.25 mm at 10 mm intervals i.e. only abut 10% of the lung scanned	Approx 2 mm slices at 2 mm intervals	0.6 mm slices at 0.6 mm intervals i.e. whole lung scanned at approx ¼ standard beam intensity (50 mA)	IV radio labelled albumin macro-aggregates that lodge in the pulmonary arterioles to image vasculature, and inhaled xenon gas to image ventilated areas	Radio-labelled glucose (^{18} F-FDG) – uptake proportional to metabolic activity		5 or 10 mm slices at 5 or 10 mm intervals i.e. whole brain scanned

Radiation dose mSy or mGy (x 100 for mrad)	0.04	Variable, approximately 4 to 8 (higher in US where 400 mA more common). Larger doses of contrast medium scatter more radiation into nearby tissues	1	4 Probable higher effective dose due to contrast medium scattering of radiation	Variable, approximately 1	1.5–2	7	0	2
Radiation dose (equivalent to background radiation in UK)	5 days	2 years	4 months	1.3 years	4 months	7 months	2.3 years	0	8 months
Radiation dose (equivalent to numbers of CXRs)	1	150	25	100	23	44	175	0	50
Limitations		Poorer resolution so secondary pulmonary lobule not visualized	8.5 mm gaps, so early cancers may be missed	Same as ordinary CT	Lower beam intensity produces lower resolution	No structural information or the ability to make alternative diagnoses	Usually combined with CT so add on up to another 6 mSy	Lower resolution	

Different departments/countries will use different protocols, e.g. some will always do a standard CT as well as an HRCT in case a malignant nodule is missed.

Radiation dose estimates are fraught with many assumptions and estimates, there is significant uncertainty in some areas.

1 mSy in the dose of absorbed radiation produced by exposure to 1 mGy of radiation
1 mSy=100 mrad absorbed dose (mSy includes quality factor (type of radiation and nature of tissue), but for Xrays and most tissues, mSy and mGy are numerically identical (for alpha emitters 1 mGy causes 20mSy)).

Background radiation approximately 3 mSy/year (mainly from radiation in the home, and varies across the country); transatlantic flight = extra 0.03 mSy.

Useful websites

Thoracic societies

American College of Chest Physicians www.chestnet.org
American Thoracic Society www.thoracic.org
British Society for Allergy and Clinical Immunology www.bsaci.org
British Thoracic Society www.brit-thoracic.org.uk
Canadian Thoracic Society www.lung.ca
European Respiratory Society dev.ersnet.org
Society of Thoracic Surgeons www.sts.org
Thoracic Society of Australia and New Zealand www.thoracic.org.au

Thoracic journals

American Journal of Respiratory and Critical Care Medicine ('Blue journal') ajrccm.atsjournals.org
American Journal of Respiratory Cell and Molecular Biology www.ajrcmb.atsjournals.org
Chest www.chestjournal.org
European Respiratory Journal access via www.ersnet.org
Thorax thorax.bmj.com

General journals

British Medical Journal bmj.bmjjournals.com
Free medical journals site www.freemedicaljournals.com
Journal of the American Medical Association jama.ama-assn.org
The Lancet www.thelancet.com
National Library of Medicine (Pub Med) www.ncbi.nlm.nih.gov/entrez/query.fcgi
New England Journal of Medicine content.nejm.org

Teaching resources

Drugs that cause lung disease www.pneumotox.com
Evidence-based medicine site www.bestbets.org
Simple thoracic and other anatomy site www.anatomy.uams.edu
Cardiothoracic imaging www.info.med.yale.edu/intmed/cardio/imaging/
Supercourse lectures on public health www.pitt.edu/~super1
University of New South Wales teaching/pathology site web.med.unsw.edu.au/pathmus

Fitness to drive

www.dvla.gov.uk

Charities

British Lung Foundation www.lunguk.org
www.charitiesdirect.com
www.charity-commission.gov.uk

Index

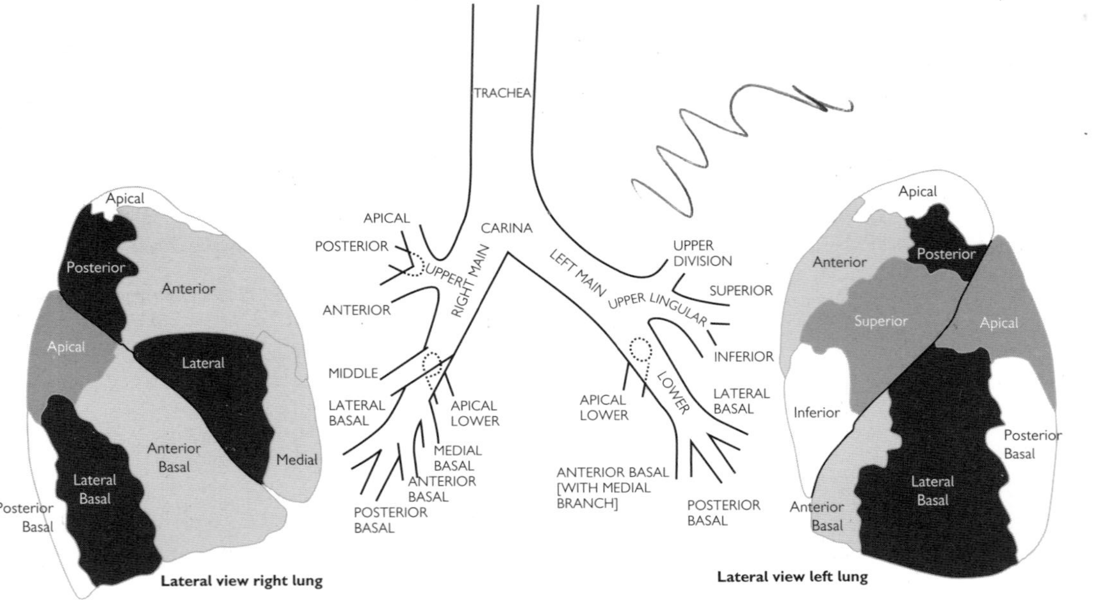

Lateral view right lung

Lateral view left lung